Memorizing Medicine
A Revision Guide

Paul Bentley

Specialist Registrar Neurology

Imperial College

London, UK

The ROYAL
SOCIETY of
MEDICINE
PRESS Limited

© 2007 Royal Society of Medicine Press Ltd

Reprinted 2008

Published by the Royal Society of Medicine Press Ltd
1 Wimpole Street, London W1G 0AE, UK
Tel: +44 (0)20 7290 2921
Fax: +44 (0)20 7290 2929
E-mail: publishing@rsm.ac.uk
Website: www.rsmpress.co.uk

British Library Cataloguing in Publication Data
A catalogue record for this book is available from the British Library
ISBN 978-1-85315-420-1

Distribution in Europe and Rest of World:

Marston Book Services Ltd
PO Box 269
Abingdon
Oxon OX14 4YN, UK
Tel: +44 (0)1235 465500
Fax: +44 (0)1235 465555
Email: direct.order@marston.co.uk

Distribution in the USA and Canada:

Royal Society of Medicine Press Ltd
c/o BookMasters, Inc.
30 Amberwood Parkway
Ashland, Ohio 44805, USA
Tel: +1 800 247 6553/ +1 800 266 5564
Fax: +1 419 281 6883
Email: order@bookmasters.com

Distribution in Australia and New Zealand:

Elsevier Australia
30-52 Smidmore Street
Marrickville NSW 2204, Australia
Tel: +61 2 9349 5811
Fax: +61 2 9349 5911
Email: service@elsevier.com.au

Typeset by IMH(Cartrif), Loanhead, Scotland
Printed in Great Britain by The Alden Group, Oxfordshire

Contents

Introduction   vi

Examples of Effective Memorizing   vii

Book Guide   viii

Memorizing Medicine – 6 Tips   x

Acknowledgements and Dedication   xii

Cardiology   1

Chest Pain **2**; Cardiology Examination **4**; Murmurs **6**; Aortic Stenosis **8**; Aortic Regurgitation **9**; Mitral Stenosis **10**; Mitral Regurgitation **11**; ECG Interpretation **12**; Tachycardia **16**; Atrial Fibrillation **18**; Ventricular Tachycardia **20**; Bradycardia **22**; Acute Coronary Syndromes **24**; Myocardial Infarction **26**; Management of NSTEMI, UA, and STEMI **28**; Shock **30**; Hypertension **32**; Heart Failure **34**; Cardiology Treatments **36**; Rheumatic Fever **38**; Infective Endocarditis **40**; Pericardial Disease **42**; Myocarditis **44**; Myxoma **45**; Cardiomyopathy **46**; Congenital Heart Disease **48**

Respiratory Medicine   53

Respiratory Examination **54**; Clubbing **56**; Cyanosis **57**; Respiratory Failure **58**; Respiratory Function Tests **60**; Chest X-ray Patterns **62**; Pneumonia **64**; Asthma **66**; Acute Severe Asthma **72**; COAD **74**; Fibrosing Alveolitis **76**; Occupational Lung Diseases **78**; Sarcoidosis **80**; Bronchiectasis **82**; Lung Abscess **83**; Cystic Fibrosis **84**; Pheumothorax **86**; Pleural Effusion **88**; Pulmonary Oedema **90**; Lung Carcinoma **92**; Obstructive Sleep Apnoea **94**; Pulmonary Embolism **96**; Pulmonary Hypertension **98**

Gastroenterology   101

Abdominal Pain **102**; Diarrhoea **104**; Constipation **105**; Nausea and Vomiting **106**; Sore Throat **108**; Oral Ulceration **109**; Dysphagia **110**; Haematemesis **112**; Rectal Bleeding **113**; Abdominal Examination **114**; Abdominal Masses **115**; Oesophagitis **116**; Oesophageal Carcinoma **118**; Peptic Ulcers **120**; Gastric Neoplasia **124**; Inflammatory Bowel Disease **126**; Colorectal Carcinoma **130**; Malabsorption **132**; Coeliac Disease **134**; Acute Pancreatitis **136**; Chronic Pancreatitis **138**; Jaundice **140**; Liver Failure **142**; Liver Transplant **145**; Portal Hypertension **146**; Oesophageal Varices **148**; Ascites **150**; Acute Liver Failure **152**; Chronic Liver Disease **154**; Infective Hepatitis **156**; Primary Biliary Cirrhosis **158**; Chronic Autoimmune Hepatitis **159**; Haemochromatosis **160**; Wilson's Disease **161**; Liver Tumours **162**; Pancreatic Tumours **163**; Gallstones **164**

Infectious Diseases 167

Infectious Organisms **168**; Bacteria **172**; Antibiotics **174**; Viruses **176**; Pneumonia **178**; Food Poisoning **180**; Gastroenteritis **181**; Genital Discharge **188**; Genital Ulceration **190**; Viral Exanthema and Related **192**; Herpes Simplex Virus **194**; Epstein-Barr Virus **195**; HIV **196**; Tuberculosis **200**; Mycobacteria **204**; Leprosy **205**; Syphilis **206**; Non-Venereal Treponemes **207**; Borreliosis **208**; Leptospirosis **209**; Rickettsia **210**; Malaria **212**; Nematodes (Roundworms) **214**; Cestodes (Tapeworms) **216**; Trematodes (Flukes) **217**

Rheumatology 219

Osteoarthritis **220**; Rheumatoid Arthritis **224**; Seronegative Arthropathies **228**; Septic Arthritis **232**; Gout **234**; Multisystemic Autoimmune Diseases **236**; Systemic Lupus Erythematosus **238**; Scleroderma **240**; Sjögren's Syndrome **242**; Autoimmune Myositis **244**; Vasculitis **246**; Raynaud's Phenomenon **248**; Cryoglobulinaemia **249**; Carpal Tunnel Syndrome **250**; Collagen and Elastic-Tissue Diseases **252**; Back Pain **254**; Bone Cysts **256**; Sclerosis **257**

Neurology 259

Headache **260**; Acute Confusional State **264**; Coma **266**; Dementia **268**; Parkinsonism **270**; Chorea **272**; Dystonia **273**; Tremor **274**; Cerebellar Disease **276**; Blackouts **278**; Epilepsy **280**; Stroke **282**; Acute Weakness **284**; Guillain-Barré Syndrome **285**; Hand Wasting **286**; Walking Disturbance **287**; Myelopathy **288**; Anterior-Horn Cell Diseases **290**; ALS/Motor Neurone Disease **291**; Peripheral Neuropathy **292**; Neuromuscular Junction Disease **294**; Myopathy **296**; Acute Visual Loss **298**; Optic Atrophy **300**; Papilloedema **301**; Vertigo **302**; Deafness **303**; Facial Nerve Palsy **304**; Neurofibromatosis **306**; Neurocutaneous Diseases **307**

Endocrinology 309

Diabetes Mellitus – Causes **310**; Insulin – Physiology **311**; Diabetic Ketoacidosis **312**; Diabetes – HONK **314**; Diabetes – Lactic Acidosis **315**; Diabetes Mellitus **316**; Hypoglycaemia **324**; Hypopituitarism **326**; Hyperprolactinaemia **330**; Acromegaly **332**; Hypothyroidism **334**; Hyperthyroidism **338**; Goitre **342**; Thyroid Tumours **343**; Adrenal Insufficiency **344**; Cushing's Syndrome **346**; Hypermineralocorticoidism **348**; Steroid Synthesis **349**; Amenorrhoea **350**; Male Sexual Problems **354**; Male Infertility **355**; Precocious Puberty **356**; Delayed Puberty **357**; Neuroendocrine Tumours **358**; Carcinoid Tumours **360**; Multiple Endocrine Neoplasia **362**; Polyglandular Autoimmune Syndromes **363**

Clinical Chemistry 365

Acid–Base Balance **366**; Hyponatraemia **368**; Polyuria/Polydipsia **370**; Hypernatraemia **371**; Diabetes Insipidus **372**; Hyperkalaemia **374**; Hypokalaemia **375**; Hypocalcaemia **376**; Hypercalcaemia **378**; Osteomalacia and Rickets **380**; Osteoporosis **382**; Paget's Disease **384**; Hyperlipidaemia **386**; Porphyria **388**

Renal Medicine 391

Acute Renal Failure **392**; Chronic Renal Failure **394**; Haematuria **398**; Proteinuria **400**; Nephrotic Syndrome **401**; Renovascular Disease **402**; Glomerulonephritis **404**; Renal Tubular Disease **406**; Urinary Obstruction **408**; Urinary Retention **409**; Renal Stones **410**; Renal Enlargement/Renal Cysts **412**; Polycystic Kidney Disease **413**; Renal Cell Carcinoma **414**; Testicular Tumours **416**; Ovarian Tumours **418**

Haematology   421

Anaemia **422**; Bone Marrow Failure **424**; Aplastic Anaemia **425**; Haemolytic Anaemia **426**; Sickle Cell Anaemia **430**; Thalassaemia **432**; Folate and Vitamin B12 Metabolism **434**; Megaloblastic Anaemia **436**; Lymphadenopathy **438**; Splenomegaly **439**; Leucocytosis **440**; Acute Leukaemia **442**; Chronic Myeloid Leukaemia **446**; Polycythaemia/PRV **448**; Chronic Lymphocytic Leukaemia **450**; Hodgkin's Lymphoma **452**; Non-Hodgkin's Lymphoma **454**; Multiple Myeloma **456**; Paraproteinaemia **458**; Hyperviscosity **459**; Amyloidosis **460**; Hyposplenism **462**; Immunodeficiency **464**; Haemostasis **468**; Platelet Disorders **470**; Purpura **472**; Thrombosis **474**; Disseminated Intravascular Coagulation **476**; Haemophilias **478**; Blood Transfusion Complications **480**

Glossary   483

Index   493

Introduction

The purpose of this book is two-fold: firstly, to inject an air of amusement and refreshing jollity into one's academic studies; secondly, to highlight an important point about how (rather than what) we should be studying.

With hope, the light-hearted aspect of the book will be immediately appreciated – punchy and practical mnemonics, entertaining pictures, sprinklings of humour, and a general feeling of novelty and variety – at least relative to the average medical textbook. At the same time, weighty, wearisome text has been dispensed with as far as possible, to enable the salient points of each subject to stand out.

The serious side of the book, however, begins with the question of what does it take to memorize medicine? A large part of what it takes to be a good doctor undoubtedly depends on the skill of being able to recall large quantities of information. Hence the training of doctors should not merely involve exposing students to knowledge in a passive manner, but should actively incorporate methods that engender efficient memorization. Medical textbooks should not simply be catalogues of facts, or even distillers of information, but should potentiate factual recall at a later date.

There are three reasons why a book such as this needs to be written, and they all seem to grow increasingly more compelling as each year goes by:
- The amount of medical knowledge increases exponentially with time.
- Technological advances, e.g. the internet, expose us to an increasing amount of data despite our brains being fixed in the rate at which we can 'input' it.
- Neuropsychological advances increasingly inform us on the nature of memory. A sharp mind is cultivated not so much by 'sheer hard work' or 'burning the midnight oil' as opposed to adopting optimal strategies of learning.

The manner in which we are exposed to knowledge assumes that our brains are built in a simple, sequential fashion, like home computers: read a new fact, listen to a lecture – and this information gets stored as easily as one's own name. Yet, it is clear from each of our own experiences that human memory does not work this way. Facts are most efficiently memorized as visual images, chunks, acronyms, rhymes, webs, etc. and as we update our knowledge, we must first recall our pre-existing schema of the topic, and then peg the new data onto this internal structure.

Enlightened with basic psychological truths about what it takes to memorize efficiently, this book aims to 'rewrite' the classical medical textbook by taking the same information as before but setting it out in an original style that lends itself to effective learning. I hope it succeeds in leaving an imprint in your mind while at the same time not taking itself too seriously.

Examples of Effective Memorizing

Consider SF, an ordinary undergraduate who set himself the task of learning long lists of arbitrary numbers. Starting with the average person's digit recall of 7 numbers, he was able to build up his memory to a staggering 80, albeit over one-and-a-half years of regular training sessions. He was not explicitly given formal mnemonic strategies but simply devised his own as he went along. The methods he stumbled upon just so happened to be similar to those utilized by world memory champions, as well as, coincidentally, pigeons trained on a picture task.

When SF was read the numbers 34928931944, he recalled this as short 'chunks' and made real-life associations, e.g. 3 minutes 49 seconds point 2 – 'near world-record mile time'; 89.3 years old – 'very old man'; 1944 – 'near the end of World War II'. Furthermore, whether he used a 3- or a 4-digit chunk was based upon a higher order of structure – the chunks were themselves chunked into blocks e.g. 444 444 333 333 444 333. This way he could remember the order in which the chunks were arranged.

Learning medicine is not quite like learning random number sequences – and not just for the obvious reason of the relative utility that distinguishes the two. Factual knowledge, unlike number lists, is structured with interconnections and hierarchies. This enables each topic to be naturally fragmented into a few elementary chunks, each possessing a core fact surrounded by details; the first-order of details may themselves be subsequently chunked, etc., repeating the structure at different scales.

That this sort of structuring actually occurs in the accumulation of expert knowledge has been demonstrated in chess masters in their recall of game positions. By measuring the time interval between the recall of particular positions, it has been found that masters chunk their memory of positions into meaningful groups. The maximum number of chunks that can be stored at any one time (into short-term memory) is about 4, but cumulatively the total number of chunks that can be stored in long-term memory can reach 100 000 or so – similar to the vocabulary span of the average adult!

In a more recent experiment, world memory champions performed a memory task while the metabolic activity of the brain was observed using functional magnetic resonance imaging. Not only did these experts utilize methods that involved chunking and ordering chunks according to a spatial plan (the 'method of loci'), but the activated parts of the brain were those recognized to be involved in spatial memory and navigation. The experts were no more intelligent and had no differences in the structural appearance of their brains, relative to control subjects. The results suggest that skilled memory can be learnt through efficient methods rather than necessarily being a quality that one is born with.

References
Science 1980; **208**: 1181; *Nature* 1987; **325**: 149; *Memory* 2004; **12**: 232; *Nature Neurosci* 2003; **6**: 90

Book Guide

Sample page explained:

Asthma

Def | **Definition**

Episodic, reversible COAD, due to bronchial hyper-reactivity to various stimuli

Epi | **Epidemiology**

The order of facts is best remembered by recourse to the old mnemonic -

'In **A** **S**urgeon's **G**own **A** **P**hysician **M**ight **M**ake **P**rogress'

Incidence - and prevalence, **A**ge, **S**ex, **G**eographical (and ethnicity),
Aetiology, **P**redisposing factors, **M**acroscopic and **M**icroscopic pathology, **P**rognosis

Inc: Prevalence – Children – 5%; Adults – 2%
Age: Peaks at 5 years; most outgrow in adolescence
Sex: M:F = 1:1, except under 5, when boys predominate (3:2)
Geo: Western World
Aet: Acute phase: mast cell-Ag interaction; Late phase: T_{H2} cell $\rightarrow$ IL-3,4,5
Micro: Sputum contains mucus casts, eosinophils, Curschmann spirals

Causes   *A.S.T.H.M.A.*

Atopy, **S**tress, **T**oxins, **H**elminths, **M**alignancy - carcinoid, **A**utoimmune / **A**spergillosis

PC | **Presenting complaint**

For the purpose of memorization, this is sometimes meant loosely so as to
include symptoms, signs and abnormal investigations, e.g. LFT derangement.

1. Cough: often at night, tenacious yellow sputum
2. Wheeze: often post-exercise, early morning; relieved by empirical salbutamol Rx
3. SOB, or 'chest tightness'

O/E | **On Examination**

If there are multiple key signs, picture the order in which the examination is
normally performed.

General
Underweight

(hypermetabolic)

Chest
Inspection
Hyperexpanded, Harrison's sulci
Auscultation
– Widespread, polyphonic wheeze
– Often normal – as often episodic

<u>Ix</u> Investigations

If there are more than three crucial tests, use the mnemonic -

B.U.M.M.E.R.S.

Bloods — if there are multiple blood tests, split into the different departments
    1. Chemistry   *R.E.A.L.M.S.*
       Renal, **E**lectrolytes, **A**BGs, **L**FTs, **M**etabolic (glucose, lipids, TFT), **S**pecial
    2. Haematology
    3. Immunology

Urine

Microbiology 1. Blood – culture, serology
             2. Excretions – sputum, stool, urine, discharge
             3. Collections – CSF, joint, pleural or ascitic effusion, abscess, lymph node

Monitor   – e.g. PEFR ('peak flow'); oxygen; cardiac monitor

Electro - **E**CG ($\pm$ Echo), **E**EG

Radiology   1. Plain X-rays, e.g. CXR
            2. CT / MRI
            3. Radionuclide scanning

Surgical / '**S**cope / **S**pecial
            1. Surgical – e.g. biopsy
            2. 'Scope – e.g. bronchosopy
            3. Special – e.g. respiratory function tests

<u>Rx</u> Treatment

1. Divide into 3–4 main category types:
    Conservative; Medical (supportive / disease-modifying), Surgical
2. For emergencies, picture the patient lying in bed with the various
    investigation / treatments surrounding him/her in order of priority.

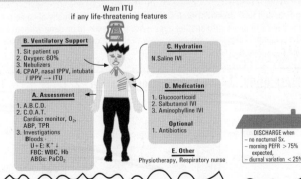

Warn ITU
if any life-threatening features

B. Ventilatory Support
1. Sit patient up
2. Oxygen: 60%
3. Nebulizers
4. CPAP, nasal IPPV, intubate / IPPV → ITU

C. Hydration
N.Saline IVI

A. Assessment
1. A.B.C.D.
2. C.O.A.T.
Cardiac monitor, O_2, ABP, TPR
3. Investigations
Bloods -
U + E: K^+ ↓
FBC: WBC, Hb
ABGs: $PaCO_2$

D. Medication
1. Glucocorticoid
2. Salbutamol IVI
3. Aminophylline IVI

Optional
1. Antibiotics

E. Other
Physiotherapy, Respiratory nurse

DISCHARGE when
– no nocturnal Sx.
– morning PEFR > 75% expected,
– diurnal variation < 25%

Memorizing Medicine – 6 Tips

One subject – one page

Have you ever tried to work out the route between two places using a map-book when the two places are on different pages? Similarly, if you sit down to learn a medical subject plot all the main headings on one piece of paper. It will also show you how much relative time to spend on each subheading. Never let a list run over 2 pages – you'll never remember it!

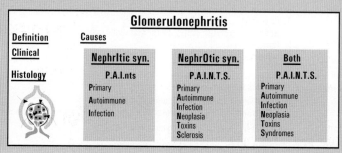

Glomerulonephritis

Definition

Clinical

Histology

Causes

NephrItic syn.	**NephrOtic syn.**	**Both**
P.A.I.nts	P.A.I.N.T.S.	P.A.I.N.T.S.
Primary	Primary	Primary
Autoimmune	Autoimmune	Autoimmune
Infection	Infection	Infection
	Neoplasia	Neoplasia
	Toxins	Toxins
	Sclerosis	Syndromes

Hierarchy

Every doctor should know that glomerulonephritis can result in nephritic syndrome, nephrotic syndrome, or both. Every general physician should know the main categories of causes. Every renal specialist should know the causes of each type of primary nephrotic syndrome. Therefore learning should proceed in this order. This is captured on the page by the size of the text.

NephrItic syndrome

Primary
    Proliferative glomerulonephritis
      Immune-complex
        - proliferation of endocapillary
        - Proliferative = sube**P**ithelial granular deposits
          ('starry sky')

NephrOtic syndrome

Primary
    Membranous glomerulonephritis
      - diffuse thickening of GBM
      - subepithelial immune-complex deposits
        ('silver spikes')
      - Epi: 40% adult; < 5% child nephrotic syn.

Both

Primary
    Membranoproliferative glomerulonephritis
      - mesangial proliferation ('mesangiocapillary GN')
      - diffuse thickening of GBM
      - types:
        1: mesan**N**gio = sube**N**dothelial and mesangial

Nesting

As you learn finer and finer details of each subject, the text will eventually become too small for the page! At this point, you'll need to move onto another page – but this needs to be done without breaking down the overall structure. The solution? Take those sub-headings with the greatest amount of extra information and cross-refer them to a new double page.

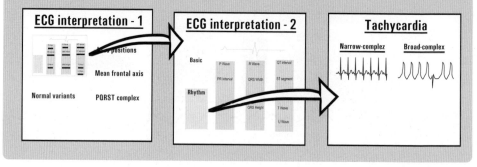

ECG interpretation - 1	ECG interpretation - 2	Tachycardia
positions	Basic	Narrow-complex Broad-complex
Mean frontal axis	P Wave / R Wave / QT Interval	
	PR Interval / QRS Width / ST segment	
Normal variants PQRST complex	Rhythm	
	QRS Height / T Wave	
	U Wave	

Logic

The first thing when learning a long list is to try breaking it down into categories that respect the underlying physiology or anatomy of the subject matter.

Jaundice		
Causes		
Pre-hepatic	Excess bilirubin production	
Hepatic	Unconjugated hyperBRaemia	Conjugated hyperBRaemia
Post-hepatic	Intrahepatic obstruction	Extrahepatic obstruction

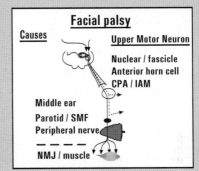

Facial palsy

Causes

Upper Motor Neuron

Nuclear / fascicle
Anterior horn cell
CPA / IAM

Middle ear
Parotid / SMF
Peripheral nerve

NMJ / muscle

Chunking

If a list doesn't easily lend itself to logical breakdown, then arbitrarily break the list down into bite-size chunks of 3, or possibly 4. This seems to be the maximum number of items the brain can remember at any one time. For example, in 'Facial palsy' above, see how the anatomical list of 8 is more easily remembered as 1 + 3 + 3 + 1 (conveniently, symmetric). Also -

Pneumonia - clinical features

chest pain, cough, dyspnoea, malaise, myalgia, fever, rigors, D + V, headache, confusion; PMH of pulmonary disease or immunocompromise, smoker, pets, travel
(extract from standard textbook)

→

Pneumonia - clinical features

1. **Specific** – chest pain, cough, dyspnoea
2. **Systemic** – myalgia, fever + rigors, D + V; headache, confusion;
3. **Other PC** – PMH (pulmonary disease or immunocompromise)

Mnemonics

1. Link

One of the main faults with mnemonics is remembering which mnemonic goes with which disease - so try to create ones with some meaningful connection.

Causes of hyperkalaemia

C.A.R.D.I.A.C.

2. Order

Try to make the order of the items within the mnemonic approximate the order of importance or the frequency of occurrence.

3. Consistency

Try to keep the same names between mnemonics to assist recalling what each letter stands for, e.g., use **T**oxins only, rather than sometimes **T**oxins and sometimes **D**rugs.

4. Bend rules

Let's face it - you can't always make mnemonics that adhere to all of the above, so you will need to exercise artistic licence... e.g. the 'B' for 'hepatitis B' in *T.A.B.O.O.S. (p. 152)*

Acknowledgements

I would like to thank Dr Michael Fertleman for suggestions and advice in the early development of this book, and Elliot Cravitz for the graphic design tutorials. Some of the images used in *Memorizing Medicine* are protected by copyright by 'New Vision Technologies Inc.'. All rights reserved.

Dedication

To Annie, Mia and Tess

Cardiology

Chest Pain

Causes

C.A.R.N.A.G.E.

Acute | Chronic

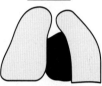
Cardio-
Thoracic

Cardiac
i) Ischaemia:
unstable angina,
myocardial infarction
ii) Peri-, myo-, endocarditis

Aortic: dissection

Respiratory:
i) Pleurisy, pneumonia, TB
ii) Pneumothorax
iii) Pulmonary embolism

Cardiac
i) Ischaemia: stable angina: inc.
ii) Aortic stenosis, HOCM
iii) Pulmonary hypertension

Aortic: Aneurysm / Aortitis

Respiratory:
i) Bronch. carcinoma, lymphoma
ii) Pleural plaques, mesothelioma
iii) Pulmonary hypertension

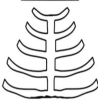
Chest wall
Mediastinal

Neuromuscular
i) Zoster: cutaneous rash
ii) Intercostal myositis:
coxsackie B5
(Bornholm disease)
iii) Intercostal muscle sprain

Arthritic-Orthopaedic
i) Rib: fracture, metastasis
ii) Joint:
costochondritis (Tietze's Dis.),
disc prolapse,
shoulder dislocation, bursitis

Neoplasia etc.
i) Thymoma
ii) Lymphoma (or TB, sarcoid
lymph nodes)
iii) Mediastinitis

Arthritic-Orthopaedic
i) Rib: osteomalacia
ii) Joint: spondylosis

Abdominal

Gastro-intestinal
Bowel
i) Perforation
• Esophagus (Boerhaave's syn.)
• Peptic ulcer
ii) Spasm, diffuse oesophageal
iii) Trapped colonic gas

Biliary–Pancreatic
i) Acute cholecyst-pancreatitis
ii) Sub-diaphragmatic abscess

Gastro-intestinal
Bowel
i) Inflammation:
• Reflux, hiatus hernia
• Peptic ulcer
ii) Carcinoma, lymphoma
iii) Irritable bowel syndrome

Biliary–Pancreatic
i) Chronic cholecyst-pancreatitis
ii) Biliary colic

Psychogenic

Excitement
Anxiety attack:
associated with mitral valve
prolapse, hyperventilation

Excitement:
Recurrent anxiety attacks

<u>History</u> Any symptom can be categorized exhaustively according to the following 4 logical categories,
each of which has 2 convenient subdivisions :

WHEN ⎯*F.O.P.P.*: First occurred (when + what were you doing then?)
Onset (rapid / slowly?)
Persistent (until present, or has now gone?)
Pattern (continuous / episodic?)
Ever had before? (first time or recurrent?)

WHERE⎯ Location
Radiation

XTER⎯ Type: e.g. pleuritic (sharp, localized, worse on inspiration); pressing; ache-burning
(character) Severity

XTRA ⎯ Aggravating / relieving factors
Associated symptoms

OTHER HISTORY: PMH e.g. arteriopathy (angina); immunodeficiency (pneumonia); SLE (PE)
DH: Thyroxine (angina), NSAIDs (gastritis). PH: smoking (angina)
FH: Angina. SH: Travel abroad (pneumonia)

<u>O/E</u>

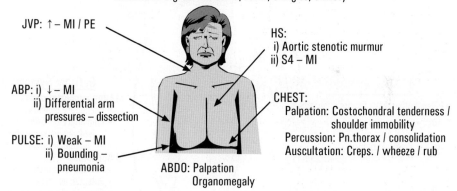

GENERAL: e.g. xanthelasma, fever, shingles, anxiety

JVP: ↑ – MI / PE

HS:
i) Aortic stenotic murmur
ii) S4 – MI

ABP: i) ↓ – MI
ii) Differential arm
pressures – dissection

CHEST:
Palpation: Costochondral tenderness /
shoulder immobility
Percussion: Pn.thorax / consolidation
Auscultation: Creps. / wheeze / rub

PULSE: i) Weak – MI
ii) Bounding –
pneumonia

ABDO: Palpation
Organomegaly

<u>Ix</u>

Blood: WCC (pneumonia, MI, cholecystitis);
CK, troponin I (MI); LFTs (cholecystitis)

Urine: Glucose (diabetes – angina); blood (SBE)

Micro: Blood, sputum cultures, inc. for AFB

ECG: Angina / MI / pericarditis

Radiology: CXR: pneumothorax / consolidation / dissection / pericardial effusion
V/Q scan or pulmonary angiography / liver USS / chest CT

Special: i) Exercise tolerance test / MIBI scan / stress ECHO
ii) Upper GI endoscopy / oesophageal manometry /
Bernstein's acid perfusion test (reproduces oesophageal pain)

Cardiology Examination

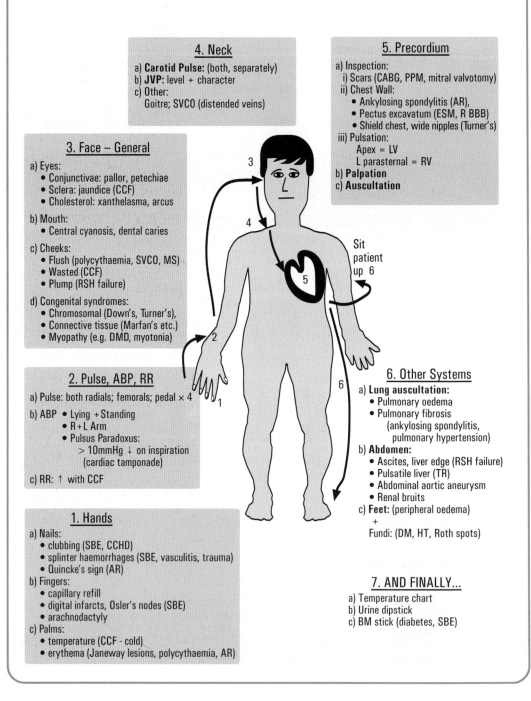

4. Neck
a) **Carotid Pulse:** (both, separately)
b) **JVP:** level + character
c) Other:
   Goitre; SVCO (distended veins)

5. Precordium
a) Inspection:
   i) Scars (CABG, PPM, mitral valvotomy)
   ii) Chest Wall:
   • Ankylosing spondylitis (AR),
   • Pectus excavatum (ESM, R BBB)
   • Shield chest, wide nipples (Turner's)
   iii) Pulsation:
      Apex = LV
      L parasternal = RV
b) **Palpation**
c) **Auscultation**

3. Face – General
a) Eyes:
   • Conjunctivae: pallor, petechiae
   • Sclera: jaundice (CCF)
   • Cholesterol: xanthelasma, arcus
b) Mouth:
   • Central cyanosis, dental caries
c) Cheeks:
   • Flush (polycythaemia, SVCO, MS)
   • Wasted (CCF)
   • Plump (RSH failure)
d) Congenital syndromes:
   • Chromosomal (Down's, Turner's),
   • Connective tissue (Marfan's etc.)
   • Myopathy (e.g. DMD, myotonia)

Sit
patient
up 6

2. Pulse, ABP, RR
a) Pulse: both radials; femorals; pedal × 4
b) ABP • Lying +Standing
      • R+L Arm
      • Pulsus Paradoxus:
         > 10mmHg ↓ on inspiration
         (cardiac tamponade)
c) RR: ↑ with CCF

6. Other Systems
a) **Lung auscultation:**
   • Pulmonary oedema
   • Pulmonary fibrosis
      (ankylosing spondylitis,
      pulmonary hypertension)
b) **Abdomen:**
   • Ascites, liver edge (RSH failure)
   • Pulsatile liver (TR)
   • Abdominal aortic aneurysm
   • Renal bruits
c) **Feet:** (peripheral oedema)
   +
   Fundi: (DM, HT, Roth spots)

1. Hands
a) Nails:
   • clubbing (SBE, CCHD)
   • splinter haemorrhages (SBE, vasculitis, trauma)
   • Quincke's sign (AR)
b) Fingers:
   • capillary refill
   • digital infarcts, Osler's nodes (SBE)
   • arachnodactyly
c) Palms:
   • temperature (CCF - cold)
   • erythema (Janeway lesions, polycythaemia, AR)

7. AND FINALLY...
a) Temperature chart
b) Urine dipstick
c) BM stick (diabetes, SBE)

Pulse

- **Rate:** Tachycardia (> 100); Bradycardia (< 60)
- **Rhythm:**
  - i) Regular
  - ii) Reg. irregular: Mobitz II Heart Block, ectopics
  - iii) Irreg. irregular: AF, frequent ectopics
- **Volume (felt at brachial or carotid):**
  - i) ↑ Bounding: hyperdynamic circulatn, AR, PDA
    - Wide pulse pressure: arteriosclerosis
  - ii) ↓ Thready: hypovol. shock, LVF, AS, MS, MR
  - iii) Differential volume of R vs L brachial:
    - dissection, atheroma
- **Character:**
  - i) Slow-rising: AS
  - ii) Collapsing: AR, PDA, bradycardia
  - iii) Double:
    - Bisferiens = Mixed AR + AS
    - Bigeminy = Regular VE's
    - Jerky = HOCM
    - Dicrotic = Hyperdynamic circulation
  - iv) Variable: Paradoxus (↓ es a lot on inspiration)
    - = Cardiac tamponade
    - Alternans = LVF
- **Delay:** R vs. L; Radio vs. Femoral = Coarctation

(curve labelled: p, d wave)

JVP

- **Level:** Normal: < 3 cm above sternal notch
  - Causes of raised JVP, may be classified
  - according to the response to inspiration:
  - 1. ↓ es on inspiration (normal response):
    - i) RSH failure / fluid overload
    - ii) Bradycardia
    - iii) Cardiac tamponade
  - 2. ↑ (Kussmaul's sign):
    - i) Constrictive pericarditis
    - ii) Restrictive cardiomyopathy
    - iii) Tricuspid stenosis
  - 3. None: SVCO
- **Character:**

  WAVES: a c   v   a: atrial systole
  c: TV closure
  v: ventricular filling

  DESCENT: x   y   x: ventricle systole
  y: TV opening

  1. **CANNON WAVES:** big a wave + big x descent
     = Atrial systole against closed TV
     Complete heart block
     Atrial flutter
     Nodal / ventricular rhythm (inc. pacemaker)
  2. **BIG A WAVES:** = RV filling ↓
     = pulmo. hypertension, tricuspid stenosis
  3. **CV (single) WAVES:** = Tricuspid regurgitation

Precordium – Palpation

- **Apex Beat Position:** Normal = Midclavic. line
  - Displaced: i) RV or LV enlargement
  - ii) Mediastinal shift
  - iii) Pectus excavatum, absent pericardium
- **Apex Beat Character:**
  - i) Heaving: Pressure overload = LVH, inc. AS, HT
    - Thrusting: Volume overload = AR, MR, VSD
  - ii) Knocking: MS (palpable S1)
  - iii) Dyskinetic, rocking: LV aneurysm
  - iv) Double or triple ripple: HOCM
  - v) Impalpable: fat, fluid (effusion), air (COAD);
    - CCF; dextrocardia
- **Heave:** at either sternal edge =
  - RVH or severe LA dilatation, e.g. MS
- **Thrill:** palpable murmur in location
  - of murmur radiation

Precordium – Auscultation

- **Heart Sounds**

  s4   *M1 T1*   *A2 P2*   *s3*
  Atrial systole   *Rapid LV filling*

  S1: Loud (MS); Soft (MR, heart block);
    Wide Split (normal at apex, heart block, VT)
  S2: Loud (HT, PHT); Soft (aortic sclerosis, PS);
    Wide Split (ASD – fixed; VSD, MR – variable)
  S3: Volume Overload: AR, MR, acute MI
  S4: Pressure Overload: AS, HT, HOCM; heart block

- **Added**

  E   P   L   O   P   K

  E: Ejection Click (bicuspid AV – non-calcific)
  P: Pericardial rub / Click (pericarditis)
  L: Late Systolic Click (mitral valve prolapse)
  O: Opening Snap: (MS, Prosthetic MV, TS, ASD)
  P: Plop (atrial myxoma)
  K: Knock (constrictive pericarditis)

- **Murmurs** (p. 6)

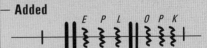

  Systolic   *Diastolic*

  Early Sys: VSD, Ebstein's anomaly (TR)
  Mid Sys (ESM): AS, PS, HOCM, coarctatn, ASD (flow)
  Pan Sys: MR; *Late Sys:* MVP with regurgitation
  Early Dias: AR, PR, Graha**M** Steel (PR 2° to **MS**)
  Mid Dias: MS, **A**ustin Fl**I**nt (**A**ortic Incomp.), MR (flow)
  Late Dias: MS (pre-systolic accentuation)

Murmurs

Aortic Stenosis

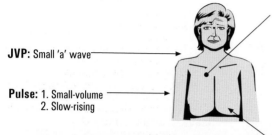

JVP: Small 'a' wave

Pulse: 1. Small-volume
2. Slow-rising

Auscultation:
1. Ejection systolic murmur:
   - aortic area → carotids
   - on sitting forward, on expiration
   - harsh
2. Ejection click: if pliable valves, e.g. bicuspid
3. S2: • single or reversed splitting S2
     (due to delayed AV closure)
   - silent A2: if calcified valve
   S4

Palpation:
1. APB (apex beat):
   Heaving, sustained, non-displaced
     = pressure-overload
2. Systolic thrill at aortic area,
   - on leaning forward, on expiration

Signs of Severity:
*1. **P**ulse pressure ↓ / ABP ↓*
*2. **A**pex beat: volume overload*
*3. **M**urmur: loud (thrill) or soft (CCF)*
*4. **S**2 becomes silent or single*

Aortic Regurgitation

Pulse: 1. Wide volume
   (*except in acute AR, CCF, or
   if hypertensive*)
2. Collapsing pulse
   or carotid shudder
3. Eponymous signs:-
   - Quincke's: Nail-bed pulsation
   - Corrigan's: Carotid pulsation
   - DeMusset's: Head nodding
   - Traub's: Pistol-shot femorals
   - Duroziez: To+fro femoral bruit

Auscultation:
1. Early diastolic murmur:
   - LSE 3rd–4th ICS →Tricuspid area
     (or RSE with dilated aortic root)
   - on sitting forward, on expiration
   - blowing = chronic; musical = perforation
2. Other murmurs: **A**ortic **I**ncompetence
   - Mid-diastolic murmur: 'Austin Flint'
     = anterior cusp of mitral valve
     hit by regurgitant stream
   - Forward-flow systolic murmur
3. S1: soft
   S2: soft, single (cf. Pulmo. Regurg. = S2 + loud P2)
   S3: ↑ LVEDP

Palpation:
1. APB: Thrusting, non-sustained, displaced
     = volume-overload
2. Diastolic thrill at LSE = Acute AR

Signs of Severity:
*1. **P**ulse pressure ↑ (but ↓es with coincident LVF or HT)*
*2. **A**pex beat displacement ↑es*
*3. **M**urmur: length ↑es (but ↓es with acute AR or CCF, due to*
*   LVEDP rising towards aortic pressure)*
*4. **P**ulmonary or peripheral oedema*

Mitral Stenosis

General:
1. Malar flush / cachectic
2. CVA or PVD 2° to AF
3. Mitral valvotomy scar

JVP: Prominent 'a'
(pulmo. hypertension)

Pulse: 1. AF
2. Small volume

Auscultation:
1. Mid-diastolic murmur
   - apex
   - lean to left, on expiratn., after exercise
   - rumble
2. Other murmurs: *Mitral Stenosis*
   - Early diastolic murmur: 'Graha**M-S**teel'
     = Pulmo. regurgitation loudest on inspiration
   - Pre-systolic accentuation: if sinus rhythm
3. Opening snap: if pliable valves
4. S1: if pliable valves
   S3: always absent

Palpation:
1. APB: Tapping S1, undisplaced
2. Parasternal heave (LAD / PHT)

Signs of Severity:
1. *P*ulse = AF, or systemic emboli
2. *O*pening Snap: *Severity inversely prop. to time between S2 and OS (↑ LAP / LVP)*
3. *M*urmur - length ↑ es *(except in CCF)*
4. *P*ulmonary oedema, or Pulmonary hypertension (RSH failure)

Mitral Regurgitation

JVP: Prominent 'a'
(pulmo. hypertension)

Pulse: 1. AF
2. Short, sharp
jerky

Auscultation:
1. Pan-systolic murmur:
   - blowing
   - apex → axilla (may be aortic area or spine)
   - lean to left, on expiration
2. Other murmurs: Forward-flow diastolic murmur
3. Mitral valve prolapse:
   = late systolic click + subsequent
   crescendo-decresc. murmur at LSE;
   make click louder + earlier by standing or Valsalva
4. S2: wide splitting
   S1: soft,
   S3: (↑ LADP)

Palpation:
1. APB: Volume-overload
2. Parasternal heave:
   = L atrial dilatation or Pulmo. hypertension
3. Apical thrill

Signs of Severity:
1. *P*ulse = AF
2. *A*pex beat displacement ↑ es
3. *M*urmur: becomes softer
4. *S*3 + Soft S1; S2 – Widely split
5. *P*ulmonary oedema, or Pulmonary hypertension (RSH failure)

N.B. Other Murmurs: 1. Pulmonary Hypertension (p. 98); 2. Congenital Heart Disease (p. 48)

Aortic Stenosis

Causes

Increasing Age

Congenital:
Presents in childhood; M:F = 4:1
- Valvar: 3, 2, or 1 Cusp
- Subvalvar : Congenital ring or HOCM
- Supravalvular : William's syn. = AS, Ca^{2+} ↑, elfin-like Face ↓IQ

Rheumatic fever
esp. females (*'tight-lipped' females*)
Rheumatoid arthritis: (rare) due to nodular thickening

Atherosclerosis
esp. FH homozygotes

Bicuspid AV calcification (40–60):
EPI: Commonest congenital anomaly (1%)
PATH: progressive mechanical stress leads to premature calcification
PC: Stenosis (1/3) + Mixed (1/3) + Asymptomatic (1/3)
ASSOC: i) Dissection; ii) Coarctation; iii) Turner's

Senile calcific degeneration (60+)
PATH: i) Initially, Aortic sclerosis: = Haemodynamically insignificant ring calcification
O/E: ESM only, no radiation
ii) Later: Cusp calcification, renders them immobile

C.R.A.B.S.

PC

1. ANGINA
   PROG: Survival = 2-3 yrs
   AET: due to O_2 demand ↑
   but O_2 supply ↓

2. ARRHYTHMIAS: • Stokes-Adams
   • Sudden death (8%)

1. EXERTIONAL SYNCOPE:
   i) Peripheral vasodilation
   ii) Cardiac reflex
   iii) Bradycardia / 3rd degree HB
2. EMBOLI, from calcified valve
   – TIA / CVA

1. Concentric LVH
2. LVF / RVF: Prognosis = 1–2 yrs

Ix

1. ECG:
   i) Pressure-overload LVH: lateral strain, LAD
   ii) P mitrale
   iii) Heart block: due to septal calcification
2. CXR:
   i) Calcified AV
   ii) Post-stenotic dilatation
   iii) LV prominence / LVF
3. ECHO:
   i) M-Mode: thickened cusps; LVH
   ii) 2D: Valve area
   iii) Doppler: peak jet velocity + pressure gradient
4. CATHETER:
   i) Pressure gradient
   ii) Angiography

Rx

1. Medical: Vasodilators contraindicated:
   • Nitrates
   • Ca antagonists
   • ACE inhibitors
2. SBE prophylaxis
3. Surgical:
   a) Valvuloplasty / valvotomy:
   IND = children; elderly
   b) Valve replacement: IND =
   • Symptomatic, esp. syncope
   • ECG: deteriorating
   • Valve area < 0.5 cm²
   • Systolic gradient > 55 mmHg
   N.B. Good pre-op nutrition / SBE prox.
   c) Myomectomy: Tunnel stenosis

Aortic Regurgitation

Causes

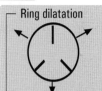

Ring dilatation
- a) Pressure: hypertension, aortic dissection, trauma
- b) Weak connective tissue:
    - Hereditary: Marfan's, osteogenesis imperfecta, Ehlers–Danlos syn.
    - Infection: Syphilis: cor bovinum

Cusp contraction
- a) Infection: • Infective endocarditis
    - • Rheum. fever (esp. males: *like to regurgitate on Saturday night!*)
- b) Autoimmune: • Seronegative arthropathies, e.g. ank. spondylitis, Reiter's
    - • SLE (Libman. Sacks endocarditis) / RA
- c) Toxins – cabergoline, pergolide

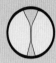

Poor fitting
- a) Bicuspid aortic valve disease
- b) Supracristal VSD

PC

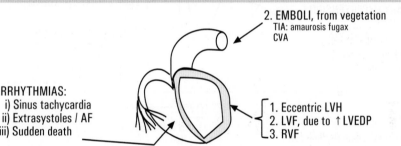

2. EMBOLI, from vegetation
TIA: amaurosis fugax
CVA

1. ARRHYTHMIAS:
  i) Sinus tachycardia
  ii) Extrasystoles / AF
  iii) Sudden death

1. Eccentric LVH
2. LVF, due to ↑LVEDP
3. RVF

Ix

1. ECG:
   Volume-overload LVH:
   Q waves anterolat / R6 + S1 > 35 mm
2. CXR:
   i) Proximal aorta dilatation
   ii) LV → LA dilatation
   iii) LVF
3. ECHO:
   i) M-Mode: dilated LV; flutter of anterior MV
   ii) 2D: Ejection fraction
      End-systolic volume
   iii) Doppler: Pressure half-time
4. CATHETER:
   i) Site + severity of AR
   ii) LV function
   iii) Angiography

Rx

1. MEDICAL:
   Nifedipine recommended, but avoid in heart failure
   ACE inhibitors
2. SBE prophylaxis
3. SURGICAL:
   Valve replacement:
   IND:
      i) Symptoms of heart failure
      ii) Pulse pressure > 100, or DBP < 40
      iii) Heart Size on CXR > 17 cm
      iv) ECG: lateral T inv: ST depression
      v) LV End-sys.volume > 5.5 cm
         Ejection fraction < 50%
   CONTRAIND:
      Dilated heart, as irreversible, and

Mitral Stenosis

Causes

> a) Congenital: Rare
> b) Rheumatic Fever (esp. Females)

PC

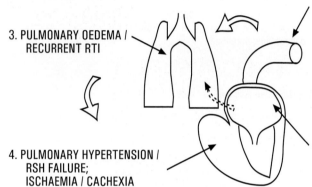

3. PULMONARY OEDEMA /
   RECURRENT RTI

2. EMBOLI
   Causes:
   • Mural thrombus forms on
     'McCallum's patch' above
     posterior MV cusp, or
   • Calcification of cusps
   Effects:
   TIA; CVA; PVD; Ischaemic colitis

4. PULMONARY HYPERTENSION /
   RSH FAILURE;
   ISCHAEMIA / CACHEXIA

1. LEFT ATRIAL ENLARGEMENT
   a) AF
   b) Hoarseness (Ortner's Syn. =
      L Recurrent Laryngeal N Palsy)
   c) Dysphagia
   d) L Bronchiectasis

Ix
1. ECG:
    i) P mitrale (with sinus rhythm) / AF
    ii) RHS strain (with RV hypertrophy)
2. CXR:
    i) LA enlargement:
       – *Loss of aorto-pulmonary concavity*
       – *Double R wall shadow*
       – *Splayed carina*
    ii) Pulmo. oedema ⇒ RV enlargement
    iii) Calcified MV
3. 2D-ECHO:
    i) Valve area: < 1 cm = severe
    ii) Rate of LV filling / regurgitatn (Doppler)
    iii) LA dilatation ± thrombus
    iv) RVH
4. CATHETER:
    i) Pressure gradient: > 20 mmHg = severe
    ii) Pulmonary vasc. resistance:
        > 8 Wood Units = High op. risk
        (Normal = 1)
    iii) LV Function / angiography

Rx
1. ANTI-COAGULATE:
   IND:
    i) Moderate – severe MS, with LA dilatation
    ii) Sx of systemic emboli
    iii) AF, even if paroxysmal

2. SBE PROPHYLAXIS
      Given to established MS, or
      Post-rheumatic fever < 25 yrs

3. SURGICAL
    i) Closed valvotomy:
       – Intercostal
       – Percutaneous transluminal catheter
         balloon dilatation
    ii) Open valvotomy
       – Median sternotomy
       – Allows ring insertion
    iii) Valve replacement
       – Indicated if partial mitral regurgitatn

Mitral Regurgitation

Causes

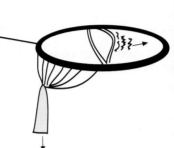

Ring dilatation

1. LV Dilatation:
   a) Volume overload: AR
   b) Pressure overload: AS, HT
2. Cardiomyopathy:
   HOCM, dilated, restrictive
3. Trauma /
   Mechanical valve leak

Cusp contraction

1. Infection:
   i) Rheumatic fever
   ii) SBE
2. Autoimmune:
   i) RA, SLE
   ii) Ank. Spond.
3. ASD, primum
4. Senile calcific degeneration

Subvalvular Apparatus Dysfunction

1. MI:
   a) Inferior: papillary muscle dysfunction ⟶ mild MR
   b) Anterior: papillary muscle rupture ⟶ acute, severe MR
2. Mitral Valve Prolapse: *M.V.P. S.I.N.*
   Def: Myxomatous degeneration of chordae tendinae
   Assoc: **M**arfan's + OI, ED, PXE
   VSD, ASD, PDA
   Polycystic kidney disease
   Straight back (loss of thoracic kyphosis)
   Ischaemic heart disease
   Neuroses / Women

PC

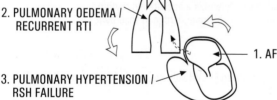

2. PULMONARY OEDEMA /
   RECURRENT RTI

1. AF

3. PULMONARY HYPERTENSION /
   RSH FAILURE

MVP

PC: 1. Chest pain – atypical
2. Palpitations / syncope
   (due to assoc. SVT, VT)
3. SOB, fatigue
COMPS:
1. Regurgitation (cord rupture)
2. Endocarditis / emboli
3. Death, sudden (VT)

Ix

1. ECG:
   i) P mitrale (with sinus rhythm) / AF
   ii) LHS strain (with RV hypertrophy)
   iii) MVP: Inferior T wave inversion
2. CXR:
   i) LA and LV enlargement
   ii) Pulmonary oedema
3. 2D-ECHO:
   i) Cause: thickened / flail valves / MVP / ASD
   ii) Volume overload of LV + LA
4. CATHETER:
   i) Distinguishes MR from LV muscle pump failure
   ii) LV function / angiography

Rx

1. ANTI-COAGULATE, if in AF

2. SBE PROPHYLAXIS, inc. for MVP

3. SURGICAL: Valve replacement
   IND: Deteriorating LV function
   (not asymptomatic pts, as the condition
   progresses slowly)

ECG Interpretation – 1

The ECG may be read either by instant pattern recognition (e.g. 'this shows fast atrial fibrillation; left bundle branch block; anterior infarction...'), or by adopting a systematic approach that includes all the sources of information an ECG trace carries. Novices to the ECG will have no choice but to use the systematic approach, but even when a learnt pattern 'jumps out' of a particular ECG, it is important to go over the ECG again, so as not to miss the smaller details.

ECG Interpretation – 2 (p. 4) takes the reader through a comprehensive ECG analysis in a logical order. A guide to the use of this double page is outlined below:

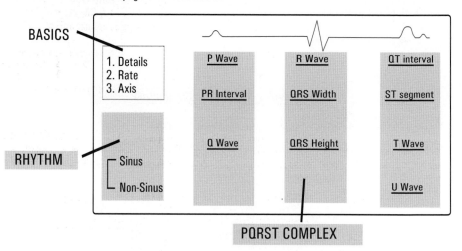

	P Wave	R Wave	QT interval
BASICS			
1. Details	PR Interval	QRS Width	ST segment
2. Rate			
3. Axis	Q Wave	QRS Height	T Wave
RHYTHM	Sinus		
	Non-Sinus		U Wave

PQRST COMPLEX

Tachycardias and Bradycardias (pp. 14–23) provides an overview of most ectopics and dysrhythmias.
Ectopics are beats that are interspersed randomly within a background rhythm.
When frequent, ectopics may degenerate into an abnormal rhythm of their own.

Normal Variants

Right:
R axis deviation; R bundle branch block; RVH in children (+ LVH voltage criteria in young or athletes); R-sided R wave dominance (i.e. R wave in V1)

Rhythm:
Sinus arrhythmia; nodal rhythm, wandering atrial pacemaker, esp. young, athletes
Extrasystoles: SV extrasystoles; any number acceptable; Ventricular extrasystoles < 10/hour.

PQRST complex:

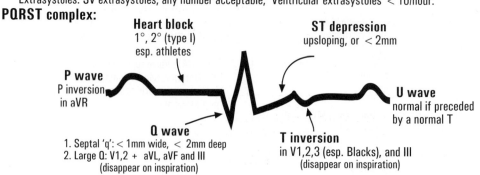

Heart block
1°, 2° (type I)
esp. athletes

ST depression
upsloping, or < 2mm

P wave
P inversion
in aVR

U wave
normal if preceded
by a normal T

Q wave
1. Septal 'q': < 1mm wide, < 2mm deep
2. Large Q: V1,2 + aVL, aVF and III
(disappear on inspiration)

T inversion
in V1,2,3 (esp. Blacks), and III
(disappear on inspiration)

Lead Positions

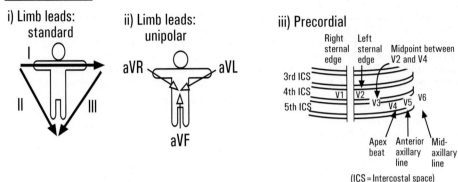

i) Limb leads: standard

I

II   III

ii) Limb leads: unipolar

aVR   aVL

aVF

iii) Precordial

Right sternal edge | Left sternal edge | Midpoint between V2 and V4

3rd ICS
4th ICS   V1 V2
5th ICS   V3 V4 V5   V6

Apex beat | Anterior axillary line | Mid-axillary line

(ICS = Intercostal space)

Mean Frontal QRS Axis

This can be estimated by noting the limb lead with the most positive complex, and reading off its 'viewing angle' as shown below. When two leads show equally positive vectors, average their corresponding angles. Leads with the smallest complexes lie at 90° to the axis, and leads showing negative complexes point 180° away from the axis:

aVR   aVL
I
III   aVF   II

-150°   -30°
0°
+120°   +60°

PQRST Complex   Normal ranges shown

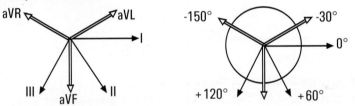

QRS width
(< 120 ms)

T wave

P wave   ST segment   U wave

J point

PR interval
(120–200 ms)

QT interval
(350–430 ms, at HR of 60 bpm)

Correct for heart rate of 60 bpm with Bazett's formula:

$$\text{Corrected Q-T Int.} = \frac{\text{Actual Q-T Int.}}{\sqrt{\text{R-R interval}}}$$

Scale

5 mm or
0.5 mV

200 ms   40 ms

ECG Interpretation – 2

P

Basics

1. Name, Age, Date, Lead Positions
2. Rate = 300 / R-R Interval (in big squares)
3. Mean frontal axis: *I.N.C.H.E.S.*:

CAUSES	R Axis Devtn > +90°	L Axis Devtn < −30°
Infarction	Anterolateral	Inferior
Normal	Tall, thin / dextrocardia	Fat, pregnant, COAD
Conduction △	L post. hemi blk. RBBB	L ant. hemi blk. WPW
Hypertrophy	RVH, PE	LVH
Extra:	Misplaced leads	Myotonia
Septal defect	ASD secundum	ASD primum

Rhythm

Classified by origin of depolarization:

Sinus
  i) Rhythm
  ii) Arrhythmia (varies with respiration: normal)
  iii) Tachycardia (> 100) or bradycardia (< 60)

Non-Sinus:
  Late Ectopics → Bradycardia
  ('Escape Beats')
    i) Atrial
    ii) Nodal
    iii) Ventricular (3° Heart Block)

  Early Ectopics → Tachycardia
  ('Extrasystoles')
    i) Atrial: Tachycardia, flutter, fibrillation
    ii) Nodal: Nodal tachycardia
        • Re-entry tachycardia (AVNRE, AVRE)
    iii) Ventricular:
        • Ectopics: benign or
            'R on T' phenomenon
        • Tachycardia
        • Fibrillation, torsades de pointes

P Wave

'P Mitrale' (Enlarged left atrium)
  Def: i) M-like P in II, ii) Biphasic P in V1
  Cause: Hypertension, aortic stenosis, mitral valve △

'P Pulmonale' (Enlarged right atrium)
  Def: i) Peaked P in II (> 2.5 mm); ii) Positive P in V1
  Cause: Pulmonary hypertension, COAD

PR Interval

Long:
  Heart block, i.e A-V conduction defect
Short:
  1. Accessory conducting pathways:
      A) Wolff–Parkinson–White syndrome
          PATH: Bundle of Kent connects atria to
              R (Type A) or L (Type B) ventricles directly
          ECG :
              i) δ waves = slurred   broad QRS
                  upstroke

                                          inverted T

              ii) R in V1; Q in III (Type A)
              iii) Paroxysmal SVT, esp. AVRT, AF
                  • DANGER! Rapid Ventricular Rate
      B) Lown–Ganong–Levine syndrome
          PATH: Fast pathway rejoins bundle of His directly.
          ECG: Short PR, no δ waves, paroxysmal SVT.
  2. Nodal rhythm
  3. Other: HOCM, Ia anti-arrhythmics

Q Waves

Significant Q waves =
  > 25% height of successive R (or > 2mm), or
  > 40 ms wide (i.e. > 1 mm wide)

Causes: *I.N.C.H.E.S.*
  Infarction, Infection (myocarditis)
  Normal: septal q, or disappear on inspiration
  Conduction △: L BBB, WPW
  Hypertrophy: LVH / RVH / HOCM
  Electrolytes: ↑ K$^+$
  Sarcoid + other infiltration

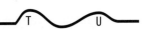

R Wave

The Transition Point of S → R waves in precordial leads (going from right to left) = V3/4
Causes of a dominant R wave in V1:
　　i) R BBB (+WPW Type A)
　　ii) RVH　(+ myotonic dystrophy)
　　iii) Posterior MI

QRS Width

The causes of a WIDE QRS are:
1. Ventricular initiation
2. Wolff–Parkinson–White syndrome
3. Intraventricular conduction defect:

　　a. RBBB:　　　　*'MaRRoW'*

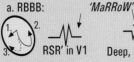

　　　　RSR' in V1　　Deep, slurred S in V6

　　b. LBBB:　　　　*'WiLLiaM'*

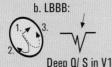

　　　Deep Q/ S in V1　　No Q in V6

CAUSES	RBBB	L BBB
Infarction	Inferior (RCA)	Inf. (RCA)
Normal	Pectus excavatum	Never normal
Conduction	anti-arrhythmics	
Hypertrophy	RVH, inc. PE	LVH, e.g. HT, AS
Electrolytes	K⁺ ↑	
Septal defect	ASD, Brugada syn.	
Syn., SAH,	SAH	

c. Fascicular block:
　　i) Unifascicular: most common =
　　　Left anterior hemiblock = L axis deviation
　　ii) Bifascicular = Unifascicular + R BBB
　　iii) Trifascicular = Bifascic. / LBBB + 1° HB

QRS Height

↑Voltage: i) LVH: S in V1 + R in V5/6 > 35 mm
　　　　ii) RVH: Dominant R in V1 (normal QRS width)

↓Voltage: i) Intervening tissue:
　　　　　Obesity, COAD, Effusion
　　　　ii) Heart muscle weakening:
　　　　　Dilated cardiomyopathy, myxoedema

QT Interval

LONG (> 430 ms): → VT
　　　　　　　　　　T.I.M.E.

Toxins:
　• Anti-arrhythmics: type Ia / III
　• Antibiotics: erythromycin, chloroquine
　• Antidepressants: TCA, phenothiazines
Inherited:
　• Romano Ward syn. (AD)
　• Jervell–Lange–Nielsen syn. (AR): + deaf!
Mitral valve prolapse
Electrolytes: HypO-Ca,-Mg,-K,-thermia:
　　　　　pr**O**long QT

SHORT (< 350 ms):
Digoxin, β-B, Phenytoin

ST Segment

ELEVATION:
1. Infarction/ischaemia
　A) Acute MI:
　　i) > 1 mm in 2 adjacent leads
　　ii) Convex upwards
　　ii) ST ↑ for < 24 hrs; T inverts EARLY
　B) Vasospasm
　C) Ventricular aneurysm
2. Peri-, Myocarditis:
　i) Concave upwards ('saddle-shaped')
　ii) ST ↑ for > 24 hrs; T inverts LATE
3. LBBB / LVH in V₁₋₂
4. Brugada syn. = blackouts or sudden death,
　　　　　due to inherited Na channelopathy
*N.B. Elevation not to be confused with
'Early take-off' in chest leads in Blacks*

DEPRESSION: (ST segment tries to *H.I.D.E.*)
　Hypertrophy ("strain pattern")
　Ischaemia (> 1mm at 80ms from J point)
　Digoxin ('Reversed tick' pattern)
　Electrolytes: Hypokalaemia

T and U Waves

Tented T: K⁺ ↑

Flattened inverted T:
　As for ST depression (*H.I.D.E.*) +
　Ventricular rhythm or WPW
U waves
　i) Normal, ii) Ischaemia, iii) K⁺ ↓

Tachycardia

Narrow-Complex = Supraventricular Tachycardia (SVT)

1. Sinus

Causes:
1. Shock
2. Haemodynamic circulation
3. Heart failure, inc. PE

regular PR interval
P embedded in preceding T

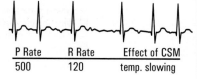

P Rate	R Rate	Effect of CSM*
100-180	100-180	temp. slowing

Rx:
Underlying cause,
e.g. atenolol for anxiety

2. Atrial

Fibrillation

Causes (p. 18):

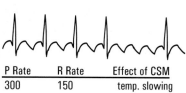

P Rate	R Rate	Effect of CSM
500	120	temp. slowing

Flutter

Causes: as for AF

P Rate	R Rate	Effect of CSM
300	150	temp. slowing

Rx:
1. Underlying cause
2. Rate control:
   digoxin
   verapamil
   beta-blocker
   RF ablation
3. Cardioversion:
   Amiodarone, sotalol
   DC 50–100 J
4. Anti-coagulation

Tachycardia

Causes: as for AF +
   COAD,

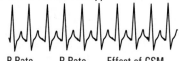

P Rate	R Rate	Effect of CSM
200	100	slows / terminates

3. Nodal

AVNRE (Atrio-Ventricular Nodal Re-Entry)

Causes:
Idiopathic (majority)
+ as for AF

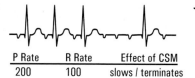

P Rate	R Rate	Effect of CSM
200	200	slows / terminates

P waves within / just after QRS
PR > RP' (slow anterograde–quick retrograde)

Rx:
1. Underlying cause
2. 1st-line (assists diagnosis):
   carotid sinus massage
   adenosine
   2nd-line:
   digoxin
   verapamil
   beta-blocker, esp sotalol
   amiodarone
3. DC 25–50 J +
   overdrive pace
4. RF ablation

AVRE

Cause:
Wolff–Parkinson-White syn.
(75% of SVTs in WPW)

Appears similar to AVNRE, although
QRS alternating amplitude at > 200 bpm.
WPW apparent from δ- waves in SR trace
Mechanism: depolarization spreads downwards via AVN,
and upwards via accessory pathway (orthodromic)

* Carotid Sinus Massage

<u>Broad-Complex = Ventricular or Supraventricular Tachycardia</u>

1. Ventricular

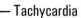 Tachycardia

Causes (p. 20):

Independent P wave activity

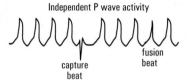

capture
beat

fusion
beat

Rx: 1. IV K$^+$, MgSO$_4$
2. Lidocaine
amiodarone
3. DC 100 J

Ventricular tachycardia: R-R rate: 100–250, usually regular
Accelerated idioventricular rhythm: R-R rate: 50–100: Cause = MI, post-thrombolysis

Torsades de pointes (Polymorphic VT)

Cause:
QT interval > 500 ms

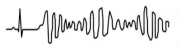

Frontal axis slowly rotates

Rx: 1. IV MgSO$_4$
2. Isoprenaline
beta-blocker (if congenital)
3. Pacing

Fibrillation

Causes:
VT,
QT interval > 500 ms

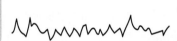

Rx: 1. CPR!
2. Epinephrine
3. DC 100–360 J

2. SVT

Intraventricular Block (R BBB or L BBB)

including K$^+$ ↑, subarachnoid haemorrhage

Rx: as for SVT

Pre-excitation (e.g. Wolff–Parkinson–White Syn.)

These SVTs are less commonly associated with WPW,
but potentially more dangerous due to ↑er risk of R-on-T, and VF

Pre-Excited AF (20%):
R-R rate 100, irregular

Pre-Excited AFlutter (3%):
R-R rate 250, regular

Antidromic AVRE (2%):
R-R rate 200, regular

Rx:
1. Drugs:
fleicanide
disopyramide
propranolol
2. DC 100 J
*N.B. avoid verapamil and digoxin
as blockage of AVN ↑ es
anterograde conduction down
bundle of Kent!*

Atrial Fibrillation

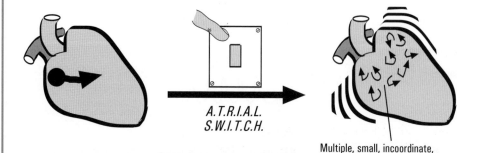

A.T.R.I.A.L.
S.W.I.T.C.H.

Multiple, small, incoordinate,
re-entrant circuits within the atria

Causes

Acute: PE, MI, infection, post-surgery

Thyrotoxicosis

Rheumatic heart disease

Ischaemic heart disease (via ischaemic cardiomyopathy or infarction)

ABP ↑ / Alcohol / **A**SD / **A**ortic regurgitation

Lung: bronchial carcinoma, PE

Sick sinus syndrome

Wolff–Parkinson–White syndrome

Inflammation: Pericarditis (± effusion), myocarditis, endocarditis

Toxin: digoxin toxicity

Cardiomyopathy: esp. infiltrative disease, e.g. sarcoid

Cancer: atrial myoxoma

Hypokalaemia

PATH: AF arises because parts of the atria lose their refractoriness before the end of atrial systole,
enabling recurrent but incoordinated atrial activation. This may be due to :
1. Atrial enlargement: e.g. CCF, rheumatic heart disease
2. Conduction velocity ↓ e.g. inflammation, fibrosis
3. Refractory period ↓ e.g. ischaemia, T4, sympathetic tone ↑

Management

Management is guided by 4 principles:-

1. Underlying Cause

e .g. anti-hypertensives, thyroidectomy

2. Rate Control

- Chemical: Digoxin, beta-blocker (e.g. sotalol), verapamil
- Radiofrequency catheter ablation of AV node
  induces complete heart block, and so requires a venticular pacemaker
- Pacemaker / Implantable atrial defibrillator
  INDICATIONS:
  Acute: • Reduces symptoms, LVF, ischaemia
  • Prepares for cardioversion by blocking AV junction and therefore
    decreases risk of atrial flutter with high ventricular response
  Chronic: • Pts who do not cardiovert

3. Cardioversion ⇒ Maintenance of sinus rhythm

- Cardioversion: Use either, or for a better result, both of:
  i) Antiarrhythmic (IV):
    Ia (quinidine); Ic (fleicanide); III (amiodarone)
  ii) Electrical: 100–200 J DC shock
    N.B. 1: If antiarrhythmic used, first gain rate control due to risk of
      converting AF into atrial flutter or tachycardia with ↑ AV conduction
    N.B. 2: If AF present for > 48 hrs, must first anti-coagulate for 4 weeks
- Maintenance of sinus rhythm:
  i) Antiarrhythmic: • Type III – amiodarone / sotalol
    • Type Ic – propafenone / fleicanide
    • Type Ia – quinidine
  ii) Surgery: Maze operation – strategic atrial incisions prevent AF re-entrant rhythms

  INDICATIONS:
  There is no difference in mortality rate between rate-control and cardioversion,
    but the following groups are selected for cardioversion:
    • Acute: for cardiovascular compromise
    • Elective: good chance of cardioverting: young, normal heart size, first episode

4. Anti-coagulation

Warfarin: INR range 2–3
  INDICATIONS:
  • Cardioversion: 1 month before and 1 month after
  • Chronic AF: If > 45 years; dilated atrium; thrombus seen on ECHO

Ventricular Tachycardia

Appearance

Broad-Complex
Tachycardia:
usually regular and
monomorphic

Independent P
wave activity

Capture Beat:
= Normal QRS complex
  occurring earlier than
  expected ventricular beat

Fusion Beat:
Ventricle activated from 2
different foci – one of
which is ventricular

Rate and Duration

Ventricular tachycardia:	R-R rate: 100–250
Accelerated idioventricular rhythm	R-R rate: 50–100

Ventricular ectopics, ventricular bigeminy	1–2 beats
Non-sustained VT	3 beats–30 s
Sustained VT	> 30 s

Distinguishing features from SVT

Atrio-ventricular dissociation:
  Independent P waves / Retrogradely conducted P waves
  On Exam: cannon waves; variable S1

Bundle branch block:

Left BBB
(commonest)   V1 ⎯╲╱⎯   broad R
notched S   V6 ⎯╱╲⎯ Q wave

Right BBB   V1 ⎯╱╲╱⎯   R > R'   V6 ⎯╲╱⎯ deep S wave

Concordance: in precordial leads

Duration of QRS complex: > 140 ms (> 160 ms if LBBB)

Extreme **LE**ft axis deviation: with LBBB
    or **LE**ft axis deviation: with RBBB

Fusion or capture beats

History of ischaemic heart disease

Intervention: Carotid sinus massage and adenosine do **NOT** terminate
        (Verapamil may induce VF if actually in VT !!)

Causes

I.'M. Q.V.I.C.K.

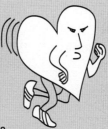

Infarction (esp. with ventricular aneurysm); ischaemia

Myocarditis

QT interval ↑

Valve abnormality: mitral valve prolapse, aortic stenosis

Iatrogenic – digoxin, antiarrrhythmics, catheterization, surgery

Cardiomyopathy, esp. dilated

K$^+$ ↓, Mg^{2+} ↓, O$_2$ ↓, Acidosis

Rx

— **Acute, unstable (hypotensive):**
  1. Precordial thump
  2. Synchronized DC shock 200J → 200J → 360J

— **Acute, stable:**
  1. K$^+$ – IV (to keep levels between 4.5 and 5.5)
     Mg^{2+} – IV 8mmol bolus over 5 min → 60 mmol in 50 ml 5% dextrose over 24 hrs
  2. Chemical cardioversion:
     a) Sotalol IV 20–60 mg slowly → PO 80–160 mg bd (or IV lignocaine)
     b) Amiodarone IV 300 mg /1 hr, followed by 900 mg /23 hrs – via CVP line
             PO 200 mg od
             (or load orally: 200 mg tds x 1 week → bd x 1 week → od)
  3. Synchronized DC shock 100 J → 100 J → 200 J

— **Ventricular premature beats (VPBs or ectopics):**
  IND for Rx = Ischaemic heart disease +
  i) VPBs: > 10 / hr; ii) Salvos of 3 +; iii) multifocal; iv) R on T phenomenon

     a) Beta-blockers, disopyramide – if good LV function
     b) Amiodarone   – if poor LV function

Bradycardia

Sinus or Junctional Rhythm

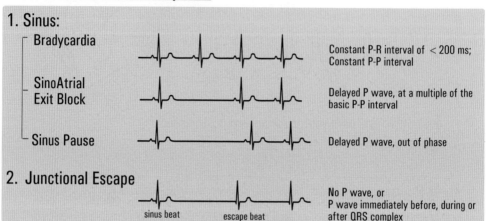

1. Sinus:

⌐ Bradycardia

Constant P-R interval of < 200 ms;
Constant P-P interval

└ SinoAtrial
Exit Block

Delayed P wave, at a multiple of the
basic P-P interval

└ Sinus Pause

Delayed P wave, out of phase

2. Junctional Escape

sinus beat   escape beat

No P wave, or
P wave immediately before, during or
after QRS complex

Heart Block = AV Conduction Defect

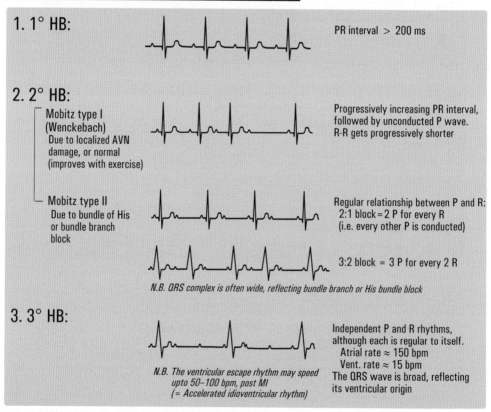

1. 1° HB:

PR interval > 200 ms

2. 2° HB:

⌐ Mobitz type I
(Wenckebach)
Due to localized AVN
damage, or normal
(improves with exercise)

Progressively increasing PR interval,
followed by unconducted P wave.
R-R gets progressively shorter

└ Mobitz type II
Due to bundle of His
or bundle branch
block

Regular relationship between P and R:
2:1 block = 2 P for every R
(i.e. every other P is conducted)

3:2 block = 3 P for every 2 R

N.B. QRS complex is often wide, reflecting bundle branch or His bundle block

3. 3° HB:

*N.B. The ventricular escape rhythm may speed
upto 50–100 bpm, post MI
(= Accelerated idioventricular rhythm)*

Independent P and R rhythms,
although each is regular to itself.
Atrial rate ≈ 150 bpm
Vent. rate ≈ 15 bpm
The QRS wave is broad, reflecting
its ventricular origin

<u>Causes:</u> The rates are *D.I.V.I.S.I.O.N.S.* of the usual sinus rhythm:

Drugs   - **A**ntiarrhythmics (type Ia, amiodarone), **B**eta-Blockers, **C**a^{2+} antags., **D**igoxin

Ischaemia / Infarction
- Inferior (right coronary artery), or anteroseptal MI (if large)

Vagus hypertonia:
- Athletes, vasovagal syncope, hypersensitive carotid sinus syndrome

Infection
- Typhoid, brucella (sinus bradycardia)
- Rheumatic fever
- Endocarditis, esp. involving aortic root
- Myocarditis (heart block)

Sick sinus syndrome = ' Tachy–Brady syndrome'
Path: Majority are due to senile amyloid or fibrosis of SAN, AVN and conducting tissue.
May also be due to other structural causes of bradycardia, e.g. ischaemia, infiltration
PC: Comprises combinations of the following brady-tachyarrhythmias:-
i) Any of the bradycardias shown opposite, esp. sinus pauses, sinoatrial or AV block
ii) SVT, esp. AF with slow ventricular response; VT or Torsades de Pointes

Infiltration - restrictive or dilated cardiomyopathy
esp. autoimmune, sarcoid, haemochromatosis, amyloid, muscular dystrophy

O: hyp**O**thyroidism, hyp**O**kalaemia (or hyperkalaemia),
hyp**O**thermia, **O**bstructive jaundice

Neuro: Raised intracranial pressure

Septal defect: ASD, primum; **S**urgery or catheterization (near AVN)

<u>Rx</u>

<u>Urgent</u>	<u>Elective</u>
1. Underlying cause	1. Permanent pacemaker insertion
2. Medical:	*Notation = Paced-Sensed-Response*
a) Atropine IV 0.6–3 mg	*VVI* when atrial rhythm unhelpful:
b) Isoprenaline	e.g. 3° Mobitz II HB, AF
3. Pacing:	*DDD* when atrial rhythm sometimes normal or
a) External transcutaneous	atrial systole needed for good cardiac output
• esp. if thrombolysis considered	e.g. sick sinus syn., LVF
b) Transvenous e.g.	*(DDD: If atrium triggers → Ventricle paced*
• MI with Mobitz II 2° or 3° HB	*If not → Both A + V paced*
(unnecssary in inf. MI unless CVS compromise)	*If AF → Ventricles paced steadily)*
	2. Amiodarone: SVT control in sick synus syn.

Acute Coronary Syndromes

Def: Acute coronary ischaemia due to unstable atheromatous plaque, classified according to:
1. Degree of myocardial damage: Ischaemia, or subendocardial or full-thickness infarction?
2. Treatment: Is thrombolysis indicated?

Acute Chest Pain
– radiating into arms
– N + V
– diaphoresis

Poor prognostic features
1. Faint: • hypotension
              • arrhythmia
2. SOB: pulmonary oedema
3. Age > 70 yrs, PMH of IHD

No ST elevation
(inc. ST depression, T inversion)

ST elevation
(or Posterior MI, or new LBBB)

Troponin −ve
Unstable Angina (UA)

Troponin + ve
NSTEMI

Troponin + ve
STEMI

Troponin −ve
Consider:
vasospasm, pericarditis

A.B.C. (O_2, IVI)

Analgesia ⟨**A**⟩ **A**rrhythmia-care

Aspirin + clopidogrel

A.B.C.D.
ACEI, Beta-blocker, + LMW Heparin (sc)
Cholesterol rx, DM   GTN (iv)
                          Ca antagonist

Low–mid risk
Investigate further
May require angiogram

High risk
GP IIb–IIIa antagonist
Angiogram < 48 hrs

A.B.C. (O_2, IVI)

Analgesia ⟨**A**⟩ **A**rrhythmia-care

Aspirin + clopidogrel

A.B.C.D.
ACEI, beta-blocker,
Cholesterol rx, DM

Thrombolysis

1° Angioplasty
GP IIb–IIIa antagonist

(p. 28)

(p. 29)

Non-Q Wave MI
(subendocardial)

Q Wave MI
(transmural)

Important trials
STEMI

Thrombolysis
1. Benefit:
   ISIS-2: streptokinase + aspirin (< 24 hrs pain): 20% ↓ + 20% ↓ = 40% ↓ in MR (i.e. additive effect)
2. Time:
   GISSI-1: benefit of thrombolysis inversely proportional to time from MI onset (benefit < 24 hrs)
3. Types:
   ISIS-3: no difference in MR between SK vs. rtPA vs. APSAC
   GUSTO-1: accelerated rtPA, (i.e. over 90 min) vs SK: 15% ↓ in MR with tPA relative to SK;
   the best response subgroups were < 70 years, anterior MI, treated < 4 h Sx.

1° Angioplasty
   STOPAMI: 1° PTCA + GP IIb-IIIa   vs. tPA: 70% ↓ in MR
   GUSTO-IIb: 1° PTCA + heparin   vs. tPA: 20% ↓ in MR

ACE Inhibitors
 a) With LVF:
      SAVE: Captopril, in pts with asymptomatic LVF: 20% ↓ in MR
      AIRE: Ramipril, in pts with clinical LVF (esp. anterior MI): 35% ↓ in MR
 b) Without LVF:
      ISIS-4: Captopril: 7% ↓ in MR
      GISSI-3: Lisinopril: 12% ↓ in MR

β-Blockers
      ISIS-1: Atenolol within 12 hrs: 15% ↓ in MR
      BHAT: Propranolol   30% ↓ in MR
      Norwegian timolol study: 40% ↓ in MR

Cholesterol
      CARE: 30% ↓ in MR or MI or CVA in pts with cholesterol < 6.2 mmol /l (mean 5.4)
      LIPID: pravastatin: 20% ↓ in MR, 30% ↓ in MI, CVA

Other
   Anti-arrhythmics:
      CAST, ISIS-4: fleicanide and Mg^{2+}, respectively, ↑ MR
      CAMIAT, EMIAT: amiodarone 13% ↓ in MR, esp. severe LVF, previous VT, > 10 VPBs / hr
   Anti-coagulation:
      GUSTO-1: IV heparin ↑ risk of haemorrhagic CVA, without ↓ MR

NSTEMI

GP IIb–IIIa Antagonist
   PURSUIT, PRISM, FRISC-II: ↓es MR / MI by 10–20%

Early Angioplasty
   TACTICS, FRISC-II ↓es MR / MI by 20%

All %s represent Relative Risk Reduction, and all figures refer to drug vs. placebo, unless stated.

Myocardial Infarction – Complications

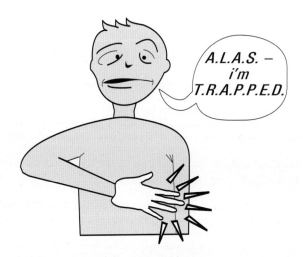

A.L.A.S. – i'm T.R.A.P.P.E.D.

Arrhythmias: esp. Post-Thrombolysis ⎤
LVF / RVF   ⎥ Occur acutely,
ABP ↑ (hypertension)   ⎬ and are the
Shock (esp. cardiogenic)   ⎦ most common

i'm

Thrombus: mural / DVT
Ruptured • Septum (VSD)
           • Papillary muscle / chordae tendinae (MR)
           • Wall (cardiac tamponade)
Aneurysm, ventricular
Pericarditis: early (< 1 week):   infarction
Pleuro-pericarditis: late (2–12 weeks): Dressler's syndrome
Extension of infarction
Death (e.g. due to VF, LVF, CVA):
     = 30% MR (of which half occur before hospital admission)

Arrhythmias / heart block

Tachycardias:
1. SVT:
  i) Sinus tachycardia - poor prognosis, if persists despite control of pain and heart failure
  ii) AF or AFlutter: assoc. with LVF
  iii) Accelerated junctional rhythm: esp. inferior MI
2. Ventricular:
  i) Ventricular ectopics:
    Frequent VPBs (> 10 / h) are seen in 70% of patients, in the first 3 days
    Rx: Do not treat, unless they become sustained. Maintain $K^+ > 4.5$, $Mg^{2+} > 2.0$ mmol/l
  ii) VT, VF:
    1° VF (i.e. within hours), due to reperfusion; carries a good prognosis if corrected
    2° VF (i.e. after days or weeks), due to extensive heart damage, carries a poor prognosis

Bradycardias:
  i) Sinus bradycardia - esp. inferior infarction, due to diaphragmatic / vagus stimulation
  ii) Ventricular bradycardia or Accelerated Idioventricular Rhythm - SAN, AVN damage
  iii) Heart block
    1°, 2° (Mobitz Type I), 3°   – associated with inferior MI (right coronary artery)
    2° (Mobitz Type II)   – associated with anterior MI (left coronary artery)

Left- or Right-sided heart failure

LVF = Anterior MI; RVF = Inferior MI

ABP ↑ : Hypertension

e.g. due to heart failure, tachycardia, pain

Shock (SBP < 100)

Causes: i) Myocyte loss (> 30%); ii) Arrhythmia; iii) Pain; iv) Diamorphine, nitrate, beta-blockers

Thrombus

a) Mural thrombi typically occur in a dyskinetic area of heart wall, or in AF $\rightarrow$ CVA / ARF / PVD
b) DVT may occur in any bed-bound patient

Rupture of septum, papillary muscle, wall

These typically occur after several days.
Both VSD and MR give a pan-systolic murmur. Ix = ECHO / catheter studies

Aneurysm, ventricular

a) A true aneurysm is a dyskinetic area of wall that becomes thin
b) A false aneurysm is a cardiac rupture with adherent blood clot

Pericarditis

a) Early pericarditis represents infarction of the pericardium
b) Dressler's syndrome is due to autoantibodies against sarcolemma + subsarcolemma of myocytes

Management of NSTEMI and UA

A.B.C.
(O$_2$, IVI)

Diamorphine + cyclizine **Analgesia**

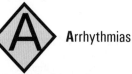

Arrhythmias

1. Admit to CCU to monitor
2. Anti-Arrhythmics:
   VT: Amiodarone, Mg
   SVT: Amiodarone, β-blocker

Aspirin + clopidogrel
300 mg stat   75 mg od
150 mg od

LMW Heparin: dalteparin 120 u/kg bd
GTN IV: titrate according to pain

PC: Pain ↑ing over 48 hrs; rest pain > 20 mins
O/E: HR ↑ or ↓ or ABP ↓: pulmonary oedema, MR
Ix: ST seg changes > 0.05 mv; TnI > 0.lng/mL

Low–Medium Risk

Tests
If the following test results are +ve, the patient should undergo in-patient angiography ± plasty:

a) Exercise Tolerance Test:
  • ST depression (down-sloping / horizontal) or ST elevation
  • Systolic BP drops or non-responsive
  • Arrhythmia: VT, sustained tachycardia

b) Myocardial perfusion scan:
  • Hypoperfusion in > 1 territory
  • Cardiac enlargement

c) Stress Echo
  • Resting ejection fraction < 35%
  • Wall motion score index > 1

High Risk

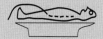

GP IIb–IIIa antagonists
Mechanism:
  Act against final common pathway of platelet activation
Types
  Monoclonal Ab (abciximab) or peptides (eptifibatide, tirofiban)

Early Angioplasty
i.e. < 48 hours

ACE inhibitor: ramipril 1.25 mg od
Beta-blocker: metoprolol 50 mg tds
Calcium antag.: diltiazem 90–120 mg bd , **Cholesterol:** pravastatin 40 mg od
Diabetes mellitus: sliding scale
Exercise: graded-rehabilitation; avoid driving, flying, work, for 1–3 months
Follow-up: Angiogram → Angioplasty / CABG

Management of STEMI

A.B.C.
(O$_2$, IVI)

Diamorphine + cyclizine **Analgesia** **Arryhthmias**

1. Admit to CCU to monitor
2. Anti-Arrhythmics:
   VT: Amiodarone, Mg
   SVT: Amiodarone β-blocker

Aspirin + clopidogrel 75 mg od
300 mg stat
150 mg od

Heparin: Use only if:
   i) tPA used: (IV heparin for 2 days); ii) bed-bound (SC LMW heparin)
GTN: avoid if hypotensive or inferior MI

< 24 hrs

Thrombolysis

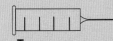

Types

a) Streptokinase: 1.5 Mu, in 100 ml N.Sal., 1 hr
b) tPA: accelerated regime:
   15 mg 0.75 mg/kg 30 min   0.5 mg/kg 60 min
   if < 50 yrs, Anterior MI, SBP < 140, Time < 4 hrs

Contraindications

The following argue *A.G.A.I.N.S.T.* giving:

Aortic aneurysm, dissection
GIT bleeding, active (or pancreatitis, liver failure)
ABP ↑ ↑ (malignant hypertension)
Iatrogenic: recent surgery, inc. tooth, ABGs
Neuro: CVA in last 2/12, brain tumour, aneurysm
Strepokinase within previous year (give tPA)
Trauma, inc. CPR / **T**hrombus – cardiac, aortic

1. Bleeding / Emboli (if cardiac, aortic thrombus)
2. Arrhythmia (esp. idioventricular rhythm)
3. Shock (kinin formation) / Hypersensitivity

1° Angioplasty

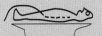

+ GP IIb–IIIa antagonist

Indications

1. Angioplasty should be offered if specialist centre is available, even if hospital transfer is required.
2. Use if contraindications for thrombolysis exist.
3. Can be used with any degree of ST elevation,
   (cf. thrombolysis: requires ST elevation in:
      2 contiguous leads,
      > 1 mm limb leads, > 2 mm chest leads)

1. Bleeding / Emboli (if cardiac, aortic thrombus)
2. Arrhythmia (esp. idioventricular rhythm)

A.B.C.D.E.F. – As for **NSTEMI**
except calcium antagonists not usually given

Shock

<u>Def</u>   Hypotension resulting in critical organ hypoperfusion.
Incipient shock may occur with normal blood pressure, but with tachycardia and narrow pulse pressure (esp. in young people).

Causes

Septic
Septicaemia,
    esp. lipopolysaccharide endotoxaemia

Hypovolaemia
1. Haemorrhagic (inc. aorta, GIT, placenta)
2. Inadequate input (fluid deprivation)
3. Excess output (diarrhoea, polyuria, burns)

Organ failure: hypovolaemia
1. Heart: chronic heart failure
2. Lungs: respiratory distress, e.g. asthma
3. Liver: failure, esp. if ascites
4. Pancreatitis

Cardiogenic
T.H.E. C.H.O.P. + M.E.A.T. (p. 35)

K anaphyla**X**is
1. Drugs, food
2. Bee-sting
3. C1-esterase inhibitor deficiency (hereditary angioedema)

Iatrogenic
1. Blood transfusion: haemolytic reaction
2. Anaesthesia: general, epidural, spinal
3. Drugs: beta-blockers, opioids, drug overdose

Neurogenic
Pain, stroke, seizure, autonomic neuropathy

Glands (endocrine)
1. Diabetes mellitus – DKA
    Diabetes insipidus
2. Addison's disease
3. Hypothyroidism

S.H.O.C.K.I.N.G.

<u>PC</u>   1. Non-localizing: Dizzy, weak, light-headed or syncope
2. Localizing, e.g.
   - Chest pain: MI, PE, aortic dissection, gastric perforation, anaphylaxis
   - Abdominal pain: bowel perforation, ectopic pregnancy, DKA
   - Back pain: aortic aneurysm, pyelonephritis

O/E

General
1. Pale, grey (hypovolaemia)
2. Fever, sweaty (sepsis)
3. Red face + eyes, urticaria, stridor (anaphylaxis)

JVP
1. ↓: hypovolaemia, septic
2. ↑: cardiogenic

ABP
1. Systolic
2. Pulse pressure
3. Differential R-L arm pressure
   (aortic dissection)

Pulse
1. Fast (except if bradycardia is
   cause of shock)
2. Small, thready (hypovolaemia)
   Bounding   (sepsis)

Hand
1. Poor capillary refill (hypovolaemia)
2. Erythema (sepsis, anaphylaxis)

Auscultation
1. New murmur
2. Chest: pulmonary oedema,
            pneumonia

Abdominal
1. Tender, guarding
2. PR: melaena
3. PV: tenderness, gravid uterus

Ix

Blood: U + E (pre-renal failure), LFT (liver failure), amylase (pancreatitis), troponin-I (MI)
         glucose (DKA), TFT; morning cortisol or short Synacthen test (Addison's)
         FBC (anemia – not acute blood volume loss); clotting; Group & Save
Urine: Volume (anuric, polyuric), glucose, ketones (DKA), β-HCG (pregnant, inc. ectopic)
Micro: Blood cultures
Monitor: ABP, temperature, fluid-balance chart
ECG (arrhythmia, MI), **ECHO** (MI, endocarditis)
Radiology: 1. CXR: pneumonia, pulmonary oedema, GIT perforation (erect CXR)
              2. CT–pulmonary angiogram: PE
              3. Abdo. USS: aorta, pregnancy
Special: e.g. OGD endoscopy

Rx

Septic: Broad-spectrum IV antibiotics; drain abscess;
               IV normal saline or colloid, epinephrine; activated protein C
Hypovolaemia: Haemorrhage: whole blood, packed RBC, FFP
               Fluid depletion: IV normal saline or colloid
               Haemodialysis may be required if acute tubular necrosis develops
Cardiogenic: Underlying cause, e.g. chemical or electrical cardioversion
K:anaphylaxis: O$_2$, IM epinephrine 0.5–1 mg, IV colloid;
               IV hydrocortisone 200 mg; IV chlorpheniramine 10 mg

Hypertension

<u>Causes</u>

P.R.E.D.I.C.T.I.O.N. (of arteriopathy)

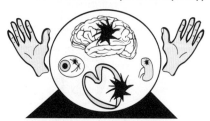

Primary
1. **Essential:** Risk Factors • Irreversible: Age, Genetic
   • Reversible: Exercise, Diet (salt, alcohol, weight)
2. **Isolated Systolic:** • Arteriosclerosis (elderly)
   • Hyperdynamic circulation, e.g. anxiety, pain

Renal
1. **Vascular** (e.g. renal artery stenosis, scleroderma, SLE)
2. **Glomerulonephritis, or tubulointerstitial nephritis** (e.g. pyelonephritis)
3. **Structural – APKD, tumour** (e.g. Wilms', periangiocytoma)

Endocrine
1. **Stress hormones** (in order of release, following acute stress):
   epinephrine (phaeochromocytoma); cortisol (Cushing's); GH (acromegaly); T4 ↑
2. **Hypermineralocorticoidism:**
   a) 1° HypERaldosteronism: • adrenal adenoma (Conn's) or carcinoma
      • glucocorticoid remediable aldosteronism (GRA)
   b) 2° HypERaldosteronism: • renin-secreting tumour, renal artery stenosis
   c) HypOaldosteronism: Liddle's syn, 'apparent mineralocorticoid excess' syn., DOComa
3. **Other:** somatostatinoma, hyperPTHism (hypercalcaemia), oral contraceptive pill

Drugs
   a) Drugs of abuse: alcohol, cocaine, amphetamines (inc ephedrine)
   b) Anti-Inflammatory: NSAIDs (renovascular dysfunction), steroids, cylosporin
   c) Other: 'Rebound effect': withdrawal of β-blockers or clonidine,
      'Cheese effect': MAO inhibitor

Intracranial pressure ↑ / Infarction, myocardial (acute)

Coarctation of aorta

Toxaemia of pregnancy = Pre-eclampsia

Increased viscosity: Polycythaemia

Overloaded with fluid (iatrogenic)

Neurogenic: Autonomic neuropathy: porphyria, lead poisoning, Riley–Day syndrome
   Injury: diffuse brain injury, spinal section, thalamic stroke ('diencephalic syn.')

<u>O/E</u>   <u>Basic Features, and Underlying Cause</u>

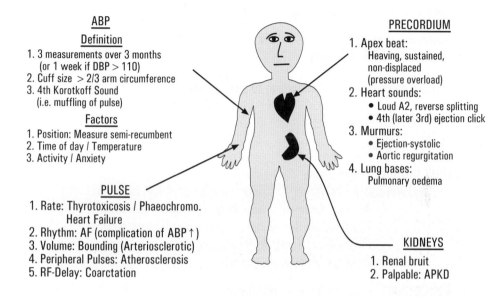

<u>ABP</u>

<u>Definition</u>
1. 3 measurements over 3 months
   (or 1 week if DBP > 110)
2. Cuff size > 2/3 arm circumference
3. 4th Korotkoff Sound
   (i.e. muffling of pulse)

<u>Factors</u>
1. Position: Measure semi-recumbent
2. Time of day / Temperature
3. Activity / Anxiety

<u>PULSE</u>

1. Rate: Thyrotoxicosis / Phaeochromo.
   Heart Failure
2. Rhythm: AF (complication of ABP ↑)
3. Volume: Bounding (Arteriosclerotic)
4. Peripheral Pulses: Atherosclerosis
5. RF-Delay: Coarctation

<u>PRECORDIUM</u>

1. Apex beat:
   Heaving, sustained,
   non-displaced
   (pressure overload)
2. Heart sounds:
   • Loud A2, reverse splitting
   • 4th (later 3rd) ejection click
3. Murmurs:
   • Ejection-systolic
   • Aortic regurgitation
4. Lung bases:
   Pulmonary oedema

<u>KIDNEYS</u>

1. Renal bruit
2. Palpable: APKD

<u>End-Organ Damage – *C.A.R.N.A.G.E.*</u>

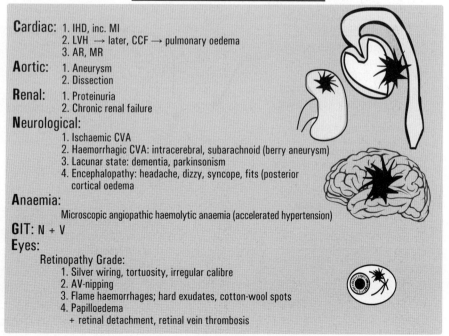

Cardiac: 1. IHD, inc. MI
2. LVH ⟶ later, CCF ⟶ pulmonary oedema
3. AR, MR

Aortic: 1. Aneurysm
2. Dissection

Renal: 1. Proteinuria
2. Chronic renal failure

Neurological:
1. Ischaemic CVA
2. Haemorrhagic CVA: intracerebral, subarachnoid (berry aneurysm)
3. Lacunar state: dementia, parkinsonism
4. Encephalopathy: headache, dizzy, syncope, fits (posterior
   cortical oedema

Anaemia:
Microscopic angiopathic haemolytic anaemia (accelerated hypertension)

GIT: N + V

Eyes:
Retinopathy Grade:
1. Silver wiring, tortuosity, irregular calibre
2. AV-nipping
3. Flame haemorrhages; hard exudates, cotton-wool spots
4. Papilloedema
   + retinal detachment, retinal vein thrombosis

Heart Failure

Def   Inability of heart to pump blood at a rate commensurate to the metabolic demands
of peripheral tissue, in the presence of normal filling pressures (cf. shock).

Epi   Prevalence: 2% at 50 years → 10% at 80 years
Mortality rate: 50% at 5 years

Causes   These can be classified according to pathophysiology:-

  ┌─ Fluid overload → LVF
  │   1. Iatrogenic
  │   2. Renal failure
  │
  ├─ High output → RVF, initially

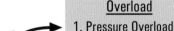

Hyperdynamic circulation – i.e. uses up a lot of A.T.P. moleculeS:
  Anaemia, **A**lcohol (Beri-Beri), **A**VM (e.g. Paget's), **A**ortic regurgitation
  Thyrotoxicosis, **T**emperature, **T**oxins (e.g. salbutamol, diuretics)
  Pregnancy (+infants); **P**roliferative: leukaemia, psoriasis; severe obesity
  Systemic: CO_2 retention, cirrhosis

  └─ Low output → LVF, or RVF if diastolic failure

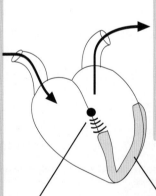

Diastolic Failure = Impaired Filling

1. Pericardial disease:
   effusion or constriction
2. Cardiomyopathy:
   restrictive or hypertrophic
3. Pulmonary hypertension:
   • Primary
   • Pulmonary embolism
   • Cor pulmonale
   • Mitral stenosis, myxoma
     Eisenmenger's syndrome
4. Ischaemic heart disease
   • MI (inf. or posterior)
   • LVF (↓RV filling)

Overload

1. Pressure Overload
   i.e. ↑ afterload
   • Hypertension
   • Aortic stenosis
   • HOCM
2. Volume Overload:
   • Aortic regurgitation
   • Mitral regurgitation
   • L-to-R shunt

Arrhythmia

1. Bradycardia, heart block
2. Tachycardia
3. Anti-arrhythmic e.g. beta-blocker,
                          verapamil

Myocardial Damage

1. Ischaemic heart disease / MI
2. Myocarditis
3. Cardiomyopathy: dilated
4. Elderly:
   35% myocytes lost from
   young adult to old age;
   > 40% causes heart failure

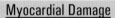

Causes - Cardiogenic Shock   The following may cause acute heart failure:

Tension pneumothorax
Hypovolaemia
Electrolytes: Ca^{2+}↑, K^+↓, acidosis

Cardiac tamponade
Hypothermia
Overdose / hyp**O**xia
Pulmonary embolism, massive

The causes of EMD

*T.H.E.
C.H.O.P.*

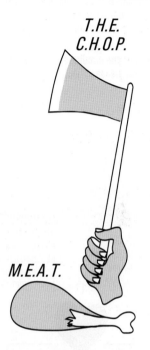

+

Myocardial infarction, esp:
- massive (> 40% heart)
- mitral regurgitation, VSD, haemopericardium

Endocarditis, myocarditis, septicaemia
Arrhythmia
Toxins: e.g. β-blockers, verapamil

M.E.A.T.

Pathogenesis of Low-Output Heart Failure

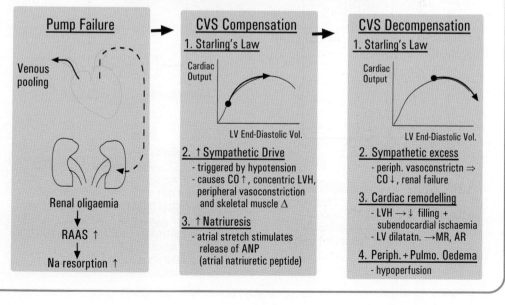

Pump Failure

Venous pooling

Renal oligaemia
↓
RAAS ↑
↓
Na resorption ↑

CVS Compensation

1. Starling's Law

Cardiac Output

LV End-Diastolic Vol.

2. ↑ Sympathetic Drive
- triggered by hypotension
- causes CO↑, concentric LVH, peripheral vasoconstriction and skeletal muscle Δ

3. ↑ Natriuresis
- atrial stretch stimulates release of ANP (atrial natriuretic peptide)

CVS Decompensation

1. Starling's Law

Cardiac Output

LV End-Diastolic Vol.

2. Sympathetic excess
- periph. vasoconstrictn ⇒ CO↓, renal failure

3. Cardiac remodelling
- LVH → ↓ filling + subendocardial ischaemia
- LV dilatatn. →MR, AR

4. Periph. + Pulmo. Oedema
- hypoperfusion

Cardiology Treatments

The following diagrams are aide-memoires for the choice and (approximate) order of drug initiation, in 3 main conditions.

Drugs used in cardiological treatment affect different parts of the circulation preferentially. These areas may be classified:

1. Cardiac:
i) β-Blockers
   – inhibit cardiac contraction AND angiotensin formation
ii) Digoxin

5. VenoDilators:
i) Nitrates
ii) K-channel opener – also arteriodilator and cardiac action

2. ArterioDilators:
i) Ca antagonists
ii) α_1 antagonists
iii) Centrally acting, e.g. moxonidine, methylDOPA

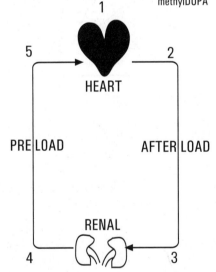

4. VenoDilators + Renal:
i) Diuretics

3. ArterioDilators + Renal:
i) ACE inhibitors
ii) Angiotensin-II receptor-1 inhibitors

Hypertension

Conservative
  Smoking; diet (weight, alcohol, salt, fish oil), exercise

Cause
  Identify + treat, e.g. adrenal adenoma (p. 32)

Comorbidity + Complications
  DM (treat BP more aggressively), cholesterol, TIA, angina (give aspirin)

Check: ABP regularly and appropriately
  i) Diagnosis based on average ABP > 140/90 on 3 readings over 3 months
  ii) Semi-recumbent; correct cuff-size
  iii) Variance: circadian / activity / anxiety

Rx

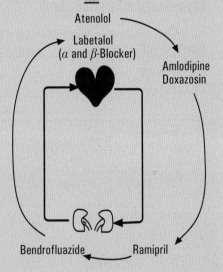

Notes:
a) In general: choose *AB / CD*
   ACE inhibitor or **B**eta-blocker AND
   Ca-antagonist or **D**iuretic
b) Aetiology, e.g.
   Young, WH**I**tes (**HI**gh renin)-ACEI, β-blockers
   Old, B**L**ac**k**s (**LO**w renin) – diuretics, arteriodilators
   Hyperaldosteronism – spironolactone, steroids
c) Co-existent diseases, e.g.
   Avoid β-Blockers in asthma, PVD

Heart Failure

Conservative
Smoking
Diet – reduce salt + fluid intake
Exercise – restrict in moderate heart failure;
hospitalize if severe heart failure

Cause
Identify + treat, e.g.
mitral valvotomy; anaemia; AF; T4 ↑

Comorbidity
e.g. pneumonia, arrhythmias

Check: fluid balance + weight

Rx

a) Carvedilol or metoprolol
(chronic, NOT acute LVF!)
b) Digoxin
c) IV dobutamine, dopamine

Isosorbide
mononitrate
(ISMN)

Hydralazine

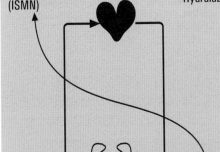
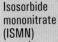
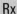

Bendrofluazide
Furosemide   Enalapril
Spironolactone

Intervention

a) Intra-aortic balloon counterpulsation
b) LV-assist device
c) Cardiac transplant

Angina

Conservative
Smoking
Diet (fish oil)
Exercise

Cause
Hypertension, hypercholesterolemia, DM

Comorbidity + Complications
e.g. arrhythmias

Check: ABP, glucose

Rx

Atenolol

GTN

Nifedipine
Diltiazem

ISMN
Nicorandil

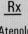
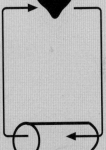

Anti-Thrombotic

a) Anti-Platelet: • aspirin
• dipyridamole, clopidogrel
• GP IIb–IIIa inhibitor: abciximab
b) Anti-coagulation: warfarin, heparin
c) Other: ACE inhibitors, statins

Intervention

a) Angioplasty ±
stent insertion (± tacrolimus-eluting)
b) Bypass graft (CABG)

Rheumatic Fever

Def Autoimmune response to *Streptococcus pyogenes* infection (β-haemolytic streptococcus), occurring typically 2-3 weeks after streptococcal pharyngitis

Epi **Inc:** Rare in West; common in 3rd world
Only 3% of population are susceptible
Half of previous sufferers will develop recurrences after streptoccocal outbreaks

Age: 3–30 (esp. 5–15 yrs)
Children more likely to develop **C**arditis + **C**horea + **C**utaneous rash
Adolescents + **A**dults develop **A**rthritis

Sex: M:F = 1:1
Women more likely to relapse, due to association with pregnancy and pill

Aet: Rheumatogenic (cf. nephritogenic strains of *S. pyogenes*)

PC Diagnosis made by Revised Jones Criteria:

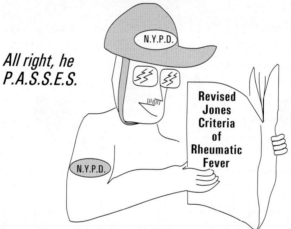

All right, he P.A.S.S.E.S.

Revised Jones Criteria of Rheumatic Fever

Pancarditis: pericarditis (chest pain), myocarditis, endocarditis
Arthritis: migratory polyarthritis
Subcutanous nodules
Sydenham's chorea: sufficient as a single major criterion
Erythema marginatum

⎫ **Major criteria**
⎬ (diagnosis requires
⎭ 2 Major,
or 1 Major + 2 Minor)

+

Streptoccocal infection in recent past   – necessary criterion

+

Extra symptoms: fever, arthralgia
ESR ↑ (or WCC, CRP ↑), ECG (PR int ↑)
Ever had rheumatic fever before?

⎫
⎬ **Minor criteria**
⎭

<u>PC</u> Major Criteria - explanations:

Pancarditis (60%)
1. Pericarditis:
   – chest pain
   – friction rub
2. Myocarditis:
   Path: Aschoff nodules = Granulomas
   – sinus tachycardia (nocturnal) or AV conduction block
   – cardiac failure
   – CK↑, T inversion
3. Endocarditis:
   Acute: • changing murmur
   • mitral valvulitis (Carey–Coombs murmur = Mid-diastolic murmur)
   Chronic: Valve disease may present up to 50 years after rheumatic fever:
   • mitral > aortic disease
   • women tend to get stenosis, men tend to get regurgitation of either valve
   men get drunk + regurgitate; women are tight- lipped (stenosis)

Arthritis (75%): Migratory polyarthritis
   – flits but persists symmetrically, esp. knees
   – effusions: painful, red, hot joints
   – Jaccoud's arthropathy (non-deformative subluxations)

Subcutanous nodules (10%): esp. on elbows

Sydenham's chorea
   – grimacing, clumsy, hypotonia - stops during sleep
   – chronic: Tourrette's syn – ADHD, Parkinsonism (post-encephalitic lethargicum)

Erythema marginatum
   – macules that extend centrifugally
   – trunk, thighs, arms (not face)

Streptoccocal infection in recent past
   1. Scarlet fever
   2. Throat swab: Culture +ve
   3. Serology: ASO or anti-DNase B titre – ↑ by 200 U / ml

<u>Rx</u>

Conservative
Bed rest until CRP normalized for 2 weeks (usually 3 months)
Immobilize inflamed joints
Medical
Penicillin: IM benzylpenicillin stat + PO penicillin V for 5 years,
due to risk of recurrence (or erythromycin)
+ pre-procedure antibiotics if permanent cardiac valve damage as endocarditis prophylaxis
Steroids: if severe
Symptomatic
Arthritis – high-dose aspirin, physiotherapy; pericarditis – aspirin; chorea – haloperidol

Infective Endocarditis

<u>Def</u>   Cardiac valves develop surface vegetations, that comprise bacteria and a platelet-fibrin thrombus

<u>Types</u>

Infective Culture +VE	Infective Culture −VE	Non-Infective (Marantic)

Infective Culture +VE

a) **Streptococci**
   S. viridans: oropharynx
   S. bovis, faecalis: bowel
   S. pneumoniae
b) **Staphylococci**
   S.aureus: IVDU,
            distant abscess
   S. epidermidis: prosthesis
   N.B. poor prognosis
c) **Gram Negatives**
   Pseudomonas

Infective Culture −VE

a) **Pre-treatment**
   with antibiotics
b) **Fastidious bacteria**
   Nutritionally-dependent strep:
   S. defectivus or *adjacens*
   CO_2-dependent HACEK orgs.
   Haemophilus, Actinobacillus
   Brucella
c) **Atypical bacteria / fungi**
   TB
   Chlamydia
   Coxiella
   Candida

Non-Infective (Marantic)

a) **Autoimmune**
   • SLE (Libman–Sacks)
   • Anti-phospholipid syn.
   • Rheumatoid arthritis
   • Rheumatic fever
b) **Neoplasia**
   • Adenocarcinoma
   • Atrial myxoma
c) **Other**
   • Thrombus on valve
   • Stitch on
     prosthetic valve

<u>Predisposing</u>

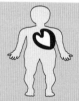   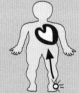

<u>Pre-Existing Cardiac Disease</u>

Usually SubAcute

a) **Congenital**
   VSD, PDA, MV Prolapse, HOCM
b) **Adolescent**
   Rheumatic heart disease
c) **Elderly**
   Degenerative valvulopathy
d) **Prosthetic heart valves**
   Early (< 1 yr):
      • *Staph. epidermidis, Candida*
        N.B. poor prognosis
   Late: (> 1yr):
      • *Strep. viridans*

<u>Haematogenous spread</u>

Usually Acute

a) **Infection elsewhere:**
   • Dental caries
   • Diverticulae, colon carcinoma (*S. bovis*)
   • Pneumonia, UTI
b) **Iatrogenic:**
   • Dental, ENT procedure, GIT or GU endoscopy
   • IV cannula, acupuncture
   • IUCD insertion, labour
c) **IVDU:**
   • *S. aureus* or *Candida*: Rt-sided endocarditis
d) **Immunocompromised:**
   • DM tend to get *S. aureus*

PC

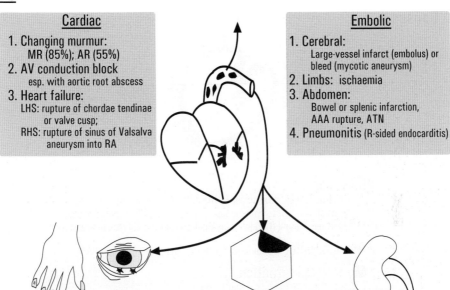

Cardiac

1. Changing murmur:
   MR (85%); AR (55%)
2. AV conduction block
   esp. with aortic root abscess
3. Heart failure:
   LHS: rupture of chordae tendinae
   or valve cusp;
   RHS: rupture of sinus of Valsalva
   aneurysm into RA

Embolic

1. Cerebral:
   Large-vessel infarct (embolus) or
   bleed (mycotic aneurysm)
2. Limbs: ischaemia
3. Abdomen:
   Bowel or splenic infarction,
   AAA rupture, ATN
4. Pneumonitis (R-sided endocarditis)

Peripheral

1. Hands:
   • Splinter haemorrhages
   • Osler's nodes:
     painful, purple papules on finger pulp
   • Janeway lesions: palmar macules
   • Clubbing
2. Eyes:
   • Conjunctival haemorrhages
   • Roth spots = retinal infarct + bleed

Constitutional

1. Fever
2. Splenomegaly
3. Weight loss
4. Arthralgia, myalgia,
   arthritis

Murmur, fever, splenomegaly, haematuria = most reliable signs

Renal

1. Microscopic
   haematuria
   – Due to proliferative
     glomerulonephritis
   – Also proteinuria,
     reversible renal failure

Ix

Blood: i) N.chromic N.cytic anaemia
   ii) ESR ↑, CRP ↑
Urine: Microscopic haematuria
   RBC casts
Micro: Blood cultures x 3
   Serology for atypical organisms
Monitor: temperature, murmur
ECG : heart block
ECHO: Trans-thoracic or TOE
   – detects vegetations > 3mm
Radio: CXR: cardiomegaly, pulmonary oedema
Special: catheter study

Rx

1. Antibiotics for 6 weeks:
   Blind or streptococci:
       benzylpenicillin + gentamicin (IV for 2 weeks)
   Staphylococci suspected:
       flucloxacillin + gentamicin
       (and / or vancomycin, rifampicin)
2. Surgery:
   IND: Acute heart failure, emboli, prosthetic valve

Prophylaxis

IND: pts with heart valve disease undergoing dental or
   other operative treatment
Choice: Amoxicillin ± gentamicin 1 hr pre-operative

Pericardial Disease

Causes

I. A.M. H.U.R.T.I.N.'

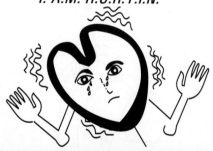

Infection:
1. Viruses, esp. coxsackie, ECHO, EBV, influenza, HIV
2. Bacteria: Strep. pneumoniae, mycoplasma, TB, rheumatic fever
3. Other: Fungal (Candida, aspergillosis), protozoal (toxoplasmosis)

Autoimmune: Rheumatoid arthritis, SLE, scleroderma, PAN

Myocardial Infaction:
1. Early: self-limiting
2. Late (2–12 weeks): 'Dressler's syn.': anti-myocardial Abs

Haemorrhage:
1. Clotting Δ
2. Aortic dissection
3. Rupture: trauma, MI, catheterization, cardiac surgery

Uraemia

Radiotherapy: Acute or chronic pericarditis

Thyroid ↓ / cholesterol ↑

Iatrogenic: Procainimide, hydralazine

Neoplasia:
1. Local: Lung cancer, thymoma
2. Systemic: metastases, leukaemia, lymphoma
3. Amyloid

Effusion types

Cholesterol – viral; Haemorrhagic – TB, uraemia, neoplastic
Constrictive Pericarditis (late fibrosis) – viral, TB, Rh. fever, post-haemorrhagic

Rx   1. **Conservative:** Bed-rest, avoid anti-coagulants
2. **Symptomatic:** NSAID: aspirin (900mg qds), indomethacin (25–75 mg qds)
                Prednisolone (20 - 80 mg od, as tapering course)
3. **Pericardiectomy** for multiple, recurrent episodes of pericarditis

PC I. Pericarditis

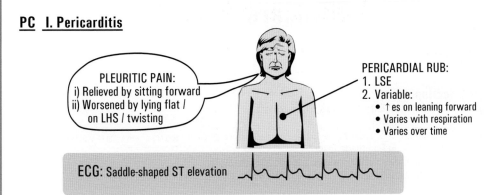

PLEURITIC PAIN:
i) Relieved by sitting forward
ii) Worsened by lying flat /
   on LHS / twisting

PERICARDIAL RUB:
1. LSE
2. Variable:
   • ↑ es on leaning forward
   • Varies with respiration
   • Varies over time

ECG: Saddle-shaped ST elevation

II. Pericardial Effusion → Cardiac Tamponade

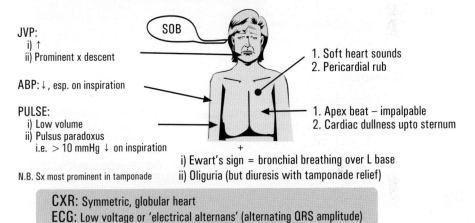

JVP:
  i) ↑
  ii) Prominent x descent

ABP: ↓, esp. on inspiration

PULSE:
  i) Low volume
  ii) Pulsus paradoxus
    i.e. > 10 mmHg ↓ on inspiration

N.B. Sx most prominent in tamponade

SOB

1. Soft heart sounds
2. Pericardial rub

1. Apex beat – impalpable
2. Cardiac dullness upto sternum

+
i) Ewart's sign = bronchial breathing over L base
ii) Oliguria (but diuresis with tamponade relief)

CXR: Symmetric, globular heart
ECG: Low voltage or 'electrical alternans' (alternating QRS amplitude)

III. Constrictive Pericarditis

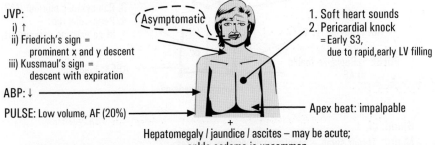

JVP:
  i) ↑
  ii) Friedrich's sign =
      prominent x and y descent
  iii) Kussmaul's sign =
      descent with expiration

ABP: ↓

PULSE: Low volume, AF (20%)

Asymptomatic

1. Soft heart sounds
2. Pericardial knock
   = Early S3,
      due to rapid,early LV filling

Apex beat: impalpable

+
Hepatomegaly / jaundice / ascites – may be acute;
ankle oedema is uncommon

CXR: Calcification of posterior border (lateral CXR) = TB
ECG: Low voltage and T inversion

Myocarditis

Causes

Infection
- 1. Viral: i) Enterovirus, esp. coxsackie B
         ii) HIV
- 2. Bacteria: i) *S. aureus* (complication of staphylococcal endocarditis: abscess of valve ring or septum)
         ii) Diphtheria toxin
- 3. Lyme disease: often requires a temporary pacemaker
- 4. Protozoa: i) Chagas'
         ii) Toxoplasmosis

Autoimmune
   Giant cell myocarditis: assoc. with SLE, thymoma, thyrotoxicosis

Iatrogenic
   Toxins, radiation, trauma

PC   Viral Myocarditis

i) Prodromal flu-like symptoms,
   e.g. fever, sore throat, myalgia ➡
ii) Contact with other cases (epidemic)

i) Chest pain
   (may co-exist with Bornholm disease)
ii) Arrhythmias, ↑ by exertion
iii) Heart failure:
   – acute
   – dilated cardiomyopathy (10%)
iv) MR < 1%

O/E

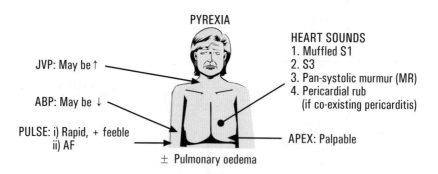

PYREXIA

JVP: May be ↑

ABP: May be ↓

PULSE: i) Rapid, + feeble
       ii) AF

± Pulmonary oedema

HEART SOUNDS
1. Muffled S1
2. S3
3. Pan-systolic murmur (MR)
4. Pericardial rub
   (if co-existing pericarditis)

APEX: Palpable

Ix   **B**lood: CK ↑
     Micro: Throat swab + stool sample virology cultures
     ECG: Widespread ST depression; T inversion
     ECHO

Rx   Symptomatic only

<u>Myxoma</u>

<u>Epi</u>

Inc: Commonest 1° cardiac tumour
Age: 50-60's (except familial syndromes: present < 30yrs)
Sex: Females: 70%
Assoc: Familial (AD) in 7%: The Carney Complex of Syndromes:
- **N**AME Syn.: **N**aevi, **A**trial myxoma, **M**yxoid neurofibromas, **E**phelides (facial freckles)
- **L**AMB Syn.: **L**entigines, **A**trial **M**yxoma, **B**lue naevi
- Multiple tumours

Path: i) Location: L atrium, in fossa ovalis - 90%
ii) Solitary
iii) Gelatinous, friable, attached by pedicle to fossa ovalis

<u>PC</u>

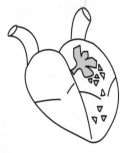

F.L.E.C.K.S. fall off

Failure, cardiac:
LHS or RHS failure, depending on site of tumour
LOC or sudden death:
due to prolapse via mitral valve / AF
Emboli:
i) CVA
ii) PVD, inc. aortic saddle embolus / Raynaud's
iii) MI
N.B. Tumour never grows at implanted site!
Clubbing
Koagulation Δ:
+ polycythaemia, thrombocytosis ⇒DVT, PE
Systemic: fever, LOW, myalgia

<u>O/E</u>

⎡ LA tumour: Signs are similar to Mitral Stenosis:

Similarities	Differences from Mitral Stenosis
1) Loud S1	1) Sinus rhythm
2) Mid-diastolic murmur	2) Postural changes affect murmur
3) Pre-systolic accentuation	3) Early diastolic plop: tumour prolapses via valve in place of opening snap

⎣ RA tumour - RV Failure

<u>Ix</u>

Bloods: i) ESR↑↑, Ig↑
ii) Albumin ↓
iii) WCC↑, Plts ↓or↑, Hb ↓(chronic disease or haemolytic)
Radio:
CXR: i) Small heart with LA appendage enlargement (± pulmonary oedema)
ii) Calcification of tumour (not MV)
ECHO: Multiple echos
Special: Histology

<u>Rx</u>

1. SURGERY with cardiopulmonary bypass ± atrial septectomy / interatrial patch
2. RECURRENCE IS VERY RARE!

Cardiomyopathy

<u>Def</u>   Structural pump failure due to primary myocardial damage

Hypertrophic – HOCM

Pathology and Causes

Hypertrophy: ASH = Asymmetric Septal Hypertrophy, or concentric LVH

Obstruction: SAM = Systolic Anterior Motion of anterior leaflet of mitral valve

Catecholamine and **C**alcium Excess = Causes

     i) Catecholamine: neural crest cell disorder: assoc. hypertension, lentigines, phaeochromocytoma

     ii) Calcium overload intracellularly → impaired relaxation and diastolic failure

Myosin: β-myosin heavy chain is commonest mutation (AD); also, troponin T: worst prognosis

PC

1. Angina
2. Arrhythmias:
     esp. AF,
       WPW,
       VT

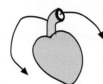

Exertional syncope, or sudden death, due to:
  i) Peripheral vasodilation
  ii) Catecholamine-induced outflow obstruction
  iii) Vagal-bradycardia / WPW / VT-VF

Diastolic Heart Failure, i.e. ↑ LVEDP

O/E

General: Friedrich's ataxia

JVP: Large a wave

ABP: ↓ on exercise

PULSE:
  i) Jerky
  ii) Small, collapsing
  iii) AF

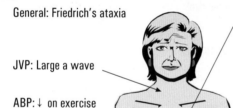

AUSCULTATION:
1. HS: i) 4th HS; ii) Single / reversed S2 splitting
2. Mid-late ejection systolic murmur, over LSE
3. Mitral regurgitation or stenosis-like murmurs

Manoeuvres that ↑ Murmur + ↑ Outflow Obstruction =		
↓ PRELOAD	↓ AFTERLOAD	↑ CONTRACTILITY
Valsalva	Standing	Exercise
Nitrate / Diuretic	Nifedipine / ACEI	Digoxin

PALP: i) Pressure overloaded APB
  ii) Double / triple impulse / LV lift
  iii) Systolic thrill

Ix

1. CXR: Normal / RA or LA dilatation
2. ECG:
     i) LVH / LAD / L-sided strain
     ii) Widespread Q waves
     iii) Pre-excitation
3. ECHO:
     i) ASH: Ground-glass appearance
     ii) SAM
     iii) Hypertrophied,
        dilated atria due to LVEDP ↑

Rx

1. Medical:
     i) −ve inotropes ↓ obstruction / diastolic failure:
       β-blockers, verapamil
       (AVOID nitrates, ACEI, diuretics, nifedipine)
     ii) Anti-Arrhythmics, esp. disopyramide, amiodarone
     iii) SBE prox.
2. Pacemaker DDD:
     Delays septal depolarization and ∴ ↓ obstruction
3. Surgery:
     Myomectomy/ MVR

Dilated

Causes:

Dystrophy: primary; muscular dystrophy, myotonic dystrophy, glycogen storage disease

Infection: sequela of myocarditis, esp. enterovirus

Late pregnancy: 3rd trimester – 6 months post-partum

Autoimmune: SLE

Toxin: i) Alcohol (thiamine deficiency), cocaine
ii) Doxorubicin, cyclophosphamide (and radiotherapy)

Endocrine: i) Dysthyroidism; ii) Acromegaly; iii) Addison's; iv) Diabetes

Diet: osteomalacia, selenium deficiency

D.I.L.A.T.E.D.

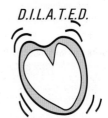

PC

  1. LVF:
- Pulmonary oedema
- Pleural effusion
- Renal failure

  2. RVF:
- Peripheral oedema
- Liver failure, ascites

  3. Arrhythmias

O/E

JVP: ↑ ↑
   cv wave (TR)

ABP: ↓ pulse pressure

PULSE:
Fast, thready;
pulsus alternans

AUSCULTATION:
1. HS: 3rd + 4th
   gallop
2. MR, TR

APEX:
Displaced, diffuse

Ix

  1. CXR: Dilated RV + LV
  2. ECG: T inversion, poor R wave progression,
     AF, VT
  3. ECHO: i) LVEDV ↑ ii) LV ejection fraction ↓ iii) LV thrombus
  4. CATHETER + Bx: myocardial fibre disarray

Rx

  1. Bed rest
  2. Medical:
    i) Diuretics, ACE, digoxin (not β-Blockers)
    ii) Anticoagulation
  3. Surgery: LV assist device / transplant

Restrictive

Causes

  Sarcoidosis / Systemic sclerosis
  Haemochromatosis: only reversible cause
  Amyloidosis
  Primary: endomyocardial fibrosis (esp. Uganda)
  Eosinophilia (Loffler's)
  Neoplasia: carcinoid (⇒ tricuspid, pulmo. stenosis), carcinoma, lymphoma

miS.S.H.A.P.E.N.

PC   Diastolic heart failure

O/E   *Similarities* to Constrictive pericarditis:-
    i) JVP + prominent x,y descents, Kussmaul's Sx.
    ii) Peripheral oedema, hepatomegaly, ascites
  Differences:
    a) Palpable apex beat
    b) MR / TR (sarcoid, amyloid)

Ix 1. CATHETER: Difference in LVEDP and RVEDP
    > 7 mmHg, at end-expiration (cf. constriction)
  2. Biopsy
  3. AMYLOID Ix: e.g. BJP, SEP, SAP-scan

Rx *AVOID* digoxin in amyloid heart disease

Congenital Heart Disease: Cyanotic

1. Fallot's Tetralogy

<u>EPI</u>
    i) Commonest congenital cyanotic heart disease presenting after 1 year
    ii) Age: > 3–6 months, although most are cyanosed at birth

<u>PATH</u>   Failure of bulbis cordis to rotate:-

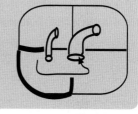

                         OVER - riding
1. **O**ver-riding aorta with wide aortic ring
    (aorta displaced anteriorly and rightwards)
2. **V**SD: Infundibular–subaortic
3. **E**xtra: e.g. right-sided aorta in 25%
4. **R**ight-ventricular outflow tract obstruction (RVOTO):
        → Right ventricular hypertrophy
        → Right – left shunting: cyanosis

<u>O/E</u>

General:
  1. Central cyanosis
    (growth delay, clubbing,
    stroke due to paradoxical
    embolism or abscess)
  2. Polycythemia
    (plethora, acne,
    gingivitis, gout)

JVP: Absent a
   (VSD)

Pulse: R > L strength
   (Blalock shunt)

HS: i) Pulmonary ESM (LSE ⟶ pulmo)
    - manoeuvre-dependent (see table)
  ii) Aortic ejection click
    AR murmur
    Single S2 (absent P2)
  iii) Continuous murmur at back:
      aortopulmonary collaterals

Palpation:
  i) Palpable A2 (anterior aorta)
  ii) Pulmonary thrill
  iii) RV heave

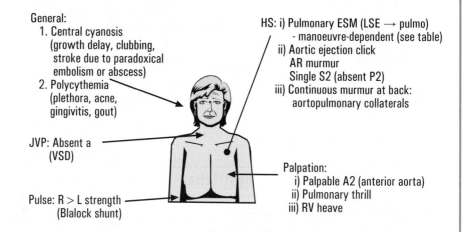

Murmur / Cyanosis Variability
    The murmur reflects flow through the pulmonary artery, so that:
        the louder the murmur, the less the cyanosis!

Mechanism	Murmur	Cause		
Shunting ↓ ∴ no cyanosis	Intensity ↑	Afterload ↑: squatting	Preload ↑: leg elevation	Cardiac Contractility ↓: beta-blockers
Shunting ↑ ∴ cyanosis	Intensity ↓	Afterload ↓: exercise, sepsis	Preload ↓: nitrates, ACE inhibitors	Cardiac Contractility ↑: digoxin

1. Fallot's Tetralogy – cont.

Ix

   1. CXR: i) Coeur en sabot
              ii) Pulmonary oligaemia / Absent L pulmonary artery
              iii) Large aortic knuckle
   2. ECG: i) RAD
              ii) R BBB
              iii) VEs, paroxysmal VT
   3. Catheter + Cineography

Rx

   1. Medical:
          Propranolol – Infundibular spasm
          Digoxin   – AF
          Amiodarone – VT
   2. Shunt:
          Blalock–Taussig: L saubclavian artery → pulmonary artery
   3. Pulmonary Valvuloplasty / Infundibular Resection

2. Eisenmenger's Syndrome

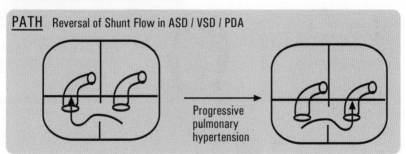

PATH   Reversal of Shunt Flow in ASD / VSD / PDA

Progressive
pulmonary
hypertension

3. Rarities

   1. TGA + essential shunt: Hyperdynamic circulation
   2. Corrected TGA
   3. TAPVD
   4. Tricuspid atresia / Ebstein's anomaly

Congenital Heart Disease: Non-Cyanotic

EPI: Congenital heart defects occur in < 1% live births, or 4% if mother had congenital heart disease.
Of these, 50% require medical / surgical intervention in infancy, and a further 30% in later life.

1. ASD: Atrial Septal Defect (30%)

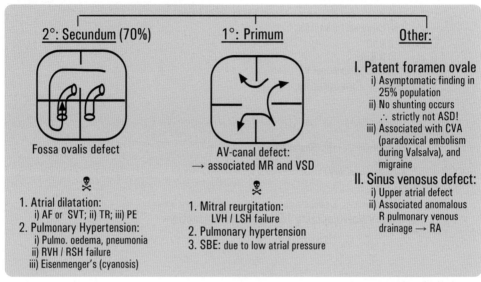

2°: Secundum (70%)

Fossa ovalis defect

☠

1. Atrial dilatation:
   i) AF or SVT; ii) TR; iii) PE
2. Pulmonary Hypertension:
   i) Pulmo. oedema, pneumonia
   ii) RVH / RSH failure
   iii) Eisenmenger's (cyanosis)

1°: Primum

AV-canal defect:
→ associated MR and VSD

☠

1. Mitral reurgitation:
   LVH / LSH failure
2. Pulmonary hypertension
3. SBE: due to low atrial pressure

Other:

I. Patent foramen ovale
   i) Asymptomatic finding in
      25% population
   ii) No shunting occurs
      ∴ strictly not ASD!
   iii) Associated with CVA
      (paradoxical embolism
      during Valsalva), and
      migraine

II. Sinus venosus defect:
   i) Upper atrial defect
   ii) Associated anomalous
      R pulmonary venous
      drainage → RA

O/E

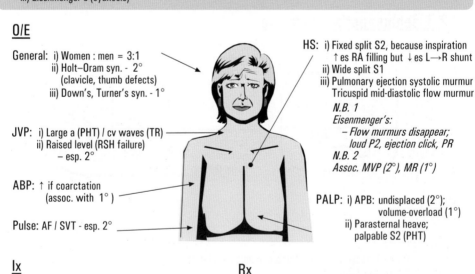

General: i) Women : men = 3:1
   ii) Holt–Oram syn. - 2°
      (clavicle, thumb defects)
   iii) Down's, Turner's syn. - 1°

JVP: i) Large a (PHT) / cv waves (TR)
   ii) Raised level (RSH failure)
      – esp. 2°

ABP: ↑ if coarctation
   (assoc. with 1°)

Pulse: AF / SVT - esp. 2°

HS: i) Fixed split S2, because inspiration
      ↑es RA filling but ↓es L→R shunt
   ii) Wide split S1
   iii) Pulmonary ejection systolic murmur
      Tricuspid mid-diastolic flow murmur
      N.B. 1
      Eisenmenger's:
      – Flow murmurs disappear;
      loud P2, ejection click, PR
      N.B. 2
      Assoc. MVP (2°), MR (1°)

PALP: i) APB: undisplaced (2°);
      volume-overload (1°)
   ii) Parasternal heave;
      palpable S2 (PHT)

Ix

1. ECG Long PR, R BBB, RAD (2°), LAD (1°)
2. CXR
   pulmonary plethora,
   prominent pulmonary arteries
3. ECHO (+ bubble injection)

Rx

Rarely close spontaneously
a) Closure: catheter-inserted device or surgical
   IND = P:S flow ratio > 1.5
   CI = Eisenmenger's (P:SVR > 0.7)
b) SBE prox. if MVP or MR

2. VSD: Ventricular Septal Defect (70%) = Maladie de Roger

<u>Types:</u>
1. Membranous: Commonest –
   closes spontaneously due to
   adjacent papillary muscle
2. Muscular: Post-MI, multiple –
   closes spontaneously
3. Infundibular: assoc. AR, Fallot's

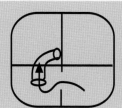

 ☠
1. LVH / LSH failure
2. PHT (as for ASD 2°)
3. SBE, R-sided →
   pneumonia / pleurisy

<u>O/E</u>

General: Scars:
- CABG scar
- Childhood correction

JVP: large a (PHT)

ABP: ↑ if coarctation – 1°

HS: i) Wide, but variable S2
   ii) PSM at LSE → Apex
   iii) Mitral mid-diastolic flow murmur
   iv) Eisenmenger's:
   - Single S2 (equal ventric. pressures)
   - Soft ESM at LSE, or no murmur
   - Loud P2 + ejection click + PR

PALP: i) APB: Volume overload
   ii) Parasternal heave
   iii) LSE thrill

<u>Rx</u> Often close spontaneously (50% by 10 yrs)
   a) Double clamshell device
   b) SBE prophylaxis

3. PDA: Patent Ductus Arteriosus (10%)

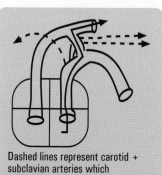

Dashed lines represent carotid +
subclavian arteries which
branch off before PDA

<u>Assoc:</u>
1. Fetal hypoxia
2. Maternal rubella
3. VSD, PS, coarctation

☠
as for VSD
+
aneurysm,
rupture

JVP:
Large a (PHT)

Pulse:
Bounding, collapsing

Differential cyanosis +
clubbing – in feet,
not hands
(reversed if TGA)

HS: i) Continuous machinery
   murmur + late sys.
   accentuation at L 2nd ICS,
   subclav. fossa + posteriorly

1   2   1
ii) Silent S2

PALP:
   i) APB: Volume overload
   ii) Parasternal heave
   iii) Thrill at L 2nd ICS

<u>Rx</u> a) Closure: ligation, catheter-placed device, indomethacin
   b) SBE prophylaxis

Respiratory Medicine

Respiratory Examination

4. Neck

a) Accessory muscles of respiration:
sternocleidomastoid, arm support, alae flaring
b) JVP: ↑ in: – Pulmonary hypertension
– SVCO (non-pulsatile), due to
bronchial ca. (90%), lymphoma,
Hodgkin's (8%)

3. Face - General

a) Eyes:
- Conjunctivae: pallor (anaemia)
- Sclera: jaundice (cor pulmonale, cystic fibrosis)
- Horner's syn. (Pancoast tumour)

b) Mouth:
- Central cyanosis

c) Cheeks, nose:
- Flushed (polycythaemia, SVCO, mitral stenosis)
- Rash (SLE, scleroderma, sarcoid, caricnoid)

d) General habitus:
- Obese (Pickwickian syn.)
- Cachexia (TB, ca., bronchiectasis)
- Marfanoid (pneumothorax)

2. Pulse, ABP, RR

a) Pulse: ↑ in PE, infection, severe asthma

b) ABP
- ↓ in PE, infection, severe asthma
- Pulsus paradoxus: > 10 mmHg ↓ on inspiration (severe asthma)

c) RR: rate and pattern (periodic?)
Measure surreptitiously, while appearing to take pulse, so as not to make patient self-conscious

1. Hands

a) Clubbing (ca., bronchiectasis)
b) Nicotine staining (actually due to tar)
c) Hand wasting: T1 wasting (Pancoast tumour)
d) Arthritis, sclerodactyly (fibrosis)
e) Hand flap: CO_2 retention

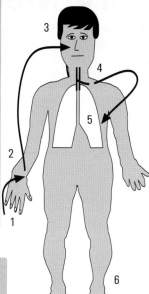

5. Chest

a) Inspection:
- Barrel chest, pectus carinatum
- Kyphosis: ankylosing spondylitis thoracic vertebral fracture (TB)
- Concavity: lobe- or pneumonectomy
- Scars: chest drain, thoracotomy, radiation marks

b) Palpation:
- Front: trachea + apex beat (mediastinal shift, LVF) parasternal heave
- Back: lymphadenopathy

c) Expansion:
↓ with most pathologies

d) Percussion:
Include clavicle + axillary areas

e) Auscultation:
- Air entry: intensity, quality
- Added sounds: creps, wheeze

f) Manoeuvres:
- Tactile vocal fremitus (TVF)
- Vocal resonance
- Whispering pectoriloqy

(For all: transmission
loud with consolidation,
soft with effusion, collapse)

Order

1. Recline patient at 45°
2. Stand back and get pt. to take 2 deep breaths in and out, while inspecting
3. Examine front; palpation, expansion...
4. Sit patient forward, inspect and palpate for cervical + axillary lymph nodes; then repeat palpation, etc.

6. Elsewhere

a) Ankle oedema (cor pulmonale)
b) Ascites, liver edge

7. And finally...

a) Talking in sentences?
– indicates severity of respiratory distress
b) PEFR; temperature charts
c) Surrounds: sputum pot

Patterns

1. Consolidation

a) Palpation: lymphadenopathy in TB, HIV
b) Expansion: ↓
c) Percussion note: dull
d) Auscultation: • air entry: ↓, bronchial breathing
 • added: coarse creps
e) Tactile vocal fremitus or vocal resonance ↑
 whispering pectoriloquy (whispering sounds loud + harsh)

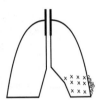

2. Pleural effusion

a) Palpation: mediastinum shifts away
b) Expansion: ↓
c) Percussion note: stony dull
d) Auscultation: • air entry: absent
 • bronchial breathing just above effusion
e) Tactile vocal fremitus or vocal resonance ↓
 egophony (patient's voice sounds like bleeting sheep just above effusion)

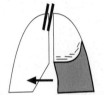

3. Collapse (or lobectomy, or pneumonectomy or thoracoplasty)

a) Palpation: mediastinum shifts towards
b) Expansion: ↓
c) Percussion note: • dull (collapse)
 • stony dull (pneumonectomy, due to fluid replacement)
d) Auscultation: air entry: ↓
e) Tactile vocal fremitus or vocal resonance ↓

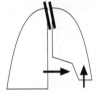

4. Fibrosis

a) Palpation: mediastinum shifts towards
c) Expansion: ↓
d) Percussion note: dull
e) Auscultation: • air entry: ↓, bronchial breathing
 • added: end-inspiratory fine or coarse creps,
 don't shift with coughing

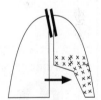

5. Pneumothorax

a) Palpation: mediastinum shifts away (with large or tension pneumothorax)
b) Expansion: ↓
c) Percussion note: hyper-resonant
d) Auscultation: air entry: ↓
e) Tactile vocal fremitus or vocal resonance ↓
 + Hamman's sign: systolic click, heard in time with heart (left-side pn.tx.)
 + coin sign (tap on coin placed on chest ⟶ ringing sound heard)

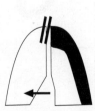

6. Bronchiectasis a) Clubbing, cyanosis; b) Coarse crepitations; c) Extra: fever, copious green sputum in pot

7. Pleural fibrosis a) Dull percussion note; b) Bronchial breathing; c) TVF ↑, but vocal resonance ↓

8. Cavity Amphoric breathing (like blowing over a bottle top)

Clubbing

O/E

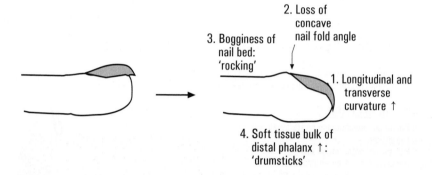

2. Loss of concave nail fold angle

3. Bogginess of nail bed: 'rocking'

1. Longitudinal and transverse curvature ↑

4. Soft tissue bulk of distal phalanx ↑: 'drumsticks'

Causes   *All the Cs*

Respiratory

1. **C**ancer:
   i) Bronchial, esp. squamous cell carcinoma
      - assoc. hypertrophic pulmonary osteoarthropathy (HPOA)
   ii) Mesothelioma (or asbestosis)
2. **C**ystic fibrosis + other **C**hronic suppurative disease:
   i) Lung abscess / bronchiectasis
   ii) Empyema – may occur within a few weeks
   iii) TB – uncommonly associated
3. **C**ryptogenic fibrosing alveolitis

Cardiac

1. **C**ongenital cyanotic heart disease
2. Infective endo**C**arditis
3. **C**ancer: Myxoma

GIT

1. **C**irrhosis
2. **C**rohn's
3. **C**oeliac
4. **C**ancer: GI Lymphoma

Other

1. **C**ongenital
2. T4
3. Local: Brachial AVM

Cyanosis

Def Blue discolouration of mucosal membranes / skin, caused when:

Mean Capillary Conc. of DeoxyHb > 5 g/dl
O_2 **Sats. $< 85\%$**
$PaO_2 < 8$ **kPa**
(or at lower O_2 concentration if anaemic)

Types: 1. Peripheral: Cold, blue peripheries, e.g. nail beds
2. Central: Blue tongue, lips; warm peripheries; digital pulses present

Causes   *Think of the path of O_2 from air to red blood cells:*

Atmosphere

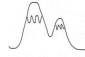

1. High-altitude acclimatization:
   i) ↑bicarbonate excretion: counters hypoxia-driven hyperventilation +respiratory alkalosis
   ii) ↑Hb 2,3–DPG ⟶ ↓affinity for O_2
   iii) polycythaemia
2. Nitrite-contaminated water
3. Cold exposure (peripheral cyanosis)

Respiratory

1. Ventilation ↓: COAD, musculoskeletal Δ
2. O_2 diffusion ↓ : Pulmo. oedema, pneumonia, fibrosing alveolitis
3. V/Q mismatch: PE, shunts: pulmonary AVM
   e.g. hereditary hemorrhagic telangiectasia, cirrhosis

Cardiac

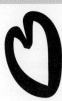

1. Congenital
   i) R→L shunt: Eisenmenger's (ASD, VSD, PDA), Fallot's
   ii) R+L mixing: - Transposition of Great Arteries
   iii) Pulmonary blood flow↓ : Pulmonary atresia
2. Cardiac output ↓
   i) Mitral stenosis
   ii) Systolic LVF
3. Vascular (peripheral cyanosis)
   i) Arterial obstruction: Raynaud's, thromboembolic disease
   ii) Venous obstruction: DVT, constrictive pericarditis
   iii) Shock: sympathetic redistribution

Red-Blood Cells

1. Hereditary low-affinity Hb:
   i) Hb Kansas
   ii) Methaemaglobinaemia =Cyt B5 reductase deficiency
2. Acquired low-affinity Hb:
   i) MetHbaemia
   ii) SulphHbaemia
   iii) CarboxyHbaemia: (CO poisoning): pt appears cherry red
3. Polycythemia (peripheral cyanosis):
   due to sluggish circulation

Respiratory Failure

<u>**Def**</u>   The respiratory system has 2 main functions + 2 associated consequences of failure:

Function	Effect of failure	Causes
O_2 Supply	$PaO_2 < 8.0$ kPa (Type 1 respiratory failure)	1. Diffusion failure 2. $\dot{V}/\dot{Q}$ mismatch (+ alveolar ventilation failure)
CO_2 Removal (acid-base balance)	$PaCO_2 > 6.5$ kPa pH < 7.35 (Type 2 respiratory failure)	1. Alveolar ventilation failure

<u>**Causes**</u>

Alveolar ventilation failure

PaO_2 ↓ $PaCO_2$ ↑ pH ↓
Alveolar–arterial grad. normal

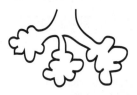

Obstructive

Small airway:
1. COAD
2. Asthma – severe
3. Bronchiectasis
4. Bronchiolitis

Large airway:
5. Intrathoracic: Ca., LN, FB
6. Extrathoracic: Ca., OSA, Epiglottitis

Restrictive

Extraparenchymal:
a) Neuromuscular:
  1. CNS Δ, sedatives
  2. High – cervical cord Δ
  3. Lower-motor neurone: MND, GBS, myasthenia
b) Structural:
  1. Ankylosing spondylitis + other skeletal Δ
  2. Pleural disease
  3. Obesity

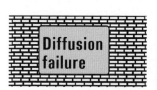

Diffusion failure

Fluid

a) Pulmonary oedema
b) Pneumonia
c) Infarction
d) Blood

Fibrosis

Both also cause $\dot{V}/\dot{Q}$ mismatch + alveolar ventilation failure, due to lung compliance ↓ ⇒ work of breathing ↑

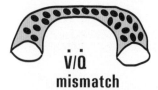

$\dot{V}/\dot{Q}$ mismatch

PaO_2 ↓ $PaCO_2$ ↓ pH ↑
Alveolar–arterial grad. ↑

Vascular
a) PE
b) PHT
c) Pulmonary shunt

Asthma – early

Atelectasis

Pneumothorax

<u>**PC**</u>	**PaO$_2$ ↓**	**PaCO$_2$ ↑ or pH ↓**

Acute	1. Cyanosis (deoxyHb $\geq$ 5 g/dl)
	2. Cardiac:
	   i) Angina, MI
	   ii) Arrhythmias, esp. VT
	3. Cerebral: encephalopathy
		1. Tachypnoea
		2. Cardiac:
		   i) Peripheral vasodilation (warm),
		     pulse volume ↑
		   ii) Arrhythmia, esp. sinus tachycardia, SVT
		3. Cerebral: encephalopathy, inc.:
		     asterixis, papilloedema, miosis, reflexes ↓

Chronic	1. Polycythaemia
	2. Pulmonary hypertension /
	   cor pulmonale
	3. Renal: ATN (vasoconstriction)
		Renal compensation: HCO$_3^-$ ↑
		
		          Cl$^-$ ↓

<u>**Ix**</u> 1. ABG:

   a) **pH / HCO$_3^-$**: Determines chronicity and whether renal compensation has occurred:

> Equivalent concentrations in acute respiratory disturbance
> | **PaCO$_2$** | : | **pH** | : | **HCO$_3^-$** |
> |---|---|---|---|---|
> | 13 | : | 1 | : | 50 |
>
> **Normal values: 5.3 kPa : 7.40 : 24 mmol/l**

     e.g. i) If Pa CO$_2$ = 7.9 kPa, then Pa CO$_2$ error = 7.9-5.3 = 2.6 kPa.
         ∴ Estimated pH Δ = 2.6 / 13 = 0.2 ↓ (i.e. Estimated pH = 7.40 - 0.2 = 7.20)
      ii) If actual pH Δ = 0.1 (i.e. pH = 7.30), then pH error = 0.2 - 0.1 = 0.1
         ∴ Estimated HCO$_3^-$ Δ = 0.1 x 50 = 5 mmol/l (i.e. Estimated HCO$_3^-$ = 24 + 5 = 29 mmol/l)

   b) **Alveolar - Arterial Gradient (PAO$_2$ –PaO$_2$)**

> **PAO$_2$ (Alveolar O$_2$) = 20 –(PaCO$_2$ x 1.25)**
>
> Normal A-a gradient = 2 kPa (50-yr-old, at sea-level, room air)
>
> Raised A-a gradient indicates Diffusion Failure or V̇/Q̇ Mismatch

  2. PEFR, spirometry, transfer factor

<u>**Rx**</u>

  Underlying Cause: e.g. BDZ's - Flumazenil; Opiates - Naloxone

  Oxygenation failure (PaO$_2$ < 8.0 kPa):
    1. Low / high-flow O$_2$, e.g. nasal cannulae, Venturi face-mask, reservoir bag
      ☠: Chronic Ventilatory Failure: ventilation depends on hypoxaemic drive!
    2. Continuous Positive Airway Pressure (CPAP) – tight-fitting mask (non-invasive)
    3. Mechanical Ventilation via Intubation or Tracheostomy

  Ventilatory failure (PaCO$_2$ > 6.5 kPa)
    1. CPAP
    2. Mechanical ventilation
    3. Respiratory stimulant, e.g. iv doxapram

Respiratory Function Tests: Spirometry

Obstructive

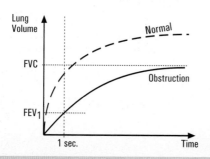

$$\frac{FEV_1}{FVC} < 0.6$$

$FVC \downarrow$

$TLC \uparrow, RV \uparrow$

$KCO \downarrow$ emphysema

FEV$_1$: Forced Expiratory Volume in 1 s
FVC: Forced Vital Capacity
TLC: Total Lung Capacity
RV: Residual Volume
PEFR: Peak Expiratory Flow Rate
KCO: Transfer factor (diffusion rate)

Causes

C.A.B.B.I.E. (typical smokers!)

Small Airways

1. **C**OAD, Irreversible:
   chronic bronchitis / emphysema
2. **A**sthma:
   peak flow depressed most at lower lung volumes
3. **B**ronchiectasis
4. **B**ronchiolitis

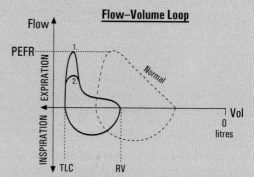

1. Volume-dep.collapse: early asthma, bronchitis
2. Pressure-dep. collapse: emphysema, bronchiolitis

Large Airways

5. **I**ntrathoracic: fixed obstruction
   • Bronchial carcinoma, lymph node, foreign body
   • Relapsing polychondritis: intermittent bronchial collapse

6. **E**xtrathoracic: collapse on inspiration only
   a) Laryngeal carcinoma, epiglottitis, tracheal stenosis
   b) Foreign body in throat
   c) Goitre, cervical lymph nodes
   d) Obstructive sleep apnoea:
      • Obesity: pharynx hypotonia during REM sleep
      • Acromegaly

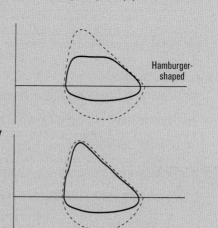

Hamburger-shaped

Restrictive

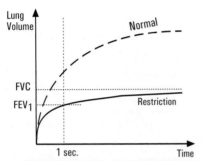

Lung Volume — Normal — Restriction
FVC
FEV₁
1 sec. — Time

Intraparenchymal	Extraparenchymal
$\dfrac{FEV_1}{FVC} > 0.75$	$\dfrac{FEV_1}{FVC}$ variable
FVC ↓↓	FVC ↓↓
TLC ↓, RV ↓	TLC ↓, RV ↑
KCO ↓	KCO normal

Causes

Flow–Volume Loop

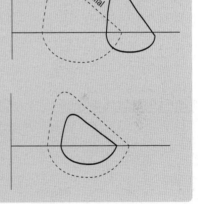

IntraParenchymal

1. Fibrosing alveolitis
2. Pulmonary oedema, severe
3. Pulmonary hypertension

ExtraParenchymal

= expiratory and inspiratory weakness

1. Neuromuscular:
   high spinal cord injury,
   Guillain–Barré syndrome, motor neurone disease
2. Chest wall:
   ankylosing spondylitis

Restrictive – Inspiratory Weakness Only

Causes

1. Neuromuscular: Isolated diaphragm paralysis
   a) Muscular dystrophy, acid maltase def., polymyositis
   b) Selective neuropathy: brachial neuritis, polio, zoster
2. Chest wall:
   a) Skeletal: thoracoplasty, kyphoscoliosis
   b) Pleural: asbestosis, thickening, mesothelioma
   c) Obesity–hypoventilation syndrome
      • Collapse of alveoli at end-expiration
      • Compliance ↓ due to weight of abdomen + chest wall
      • Central respiratory drive ↓

PC ↑ SOB + O_2 ↓ on lying down
due to pressure effect and
↑ V̇/Q̇ mismatch

Ix 1. Max. Insp. Pressure (MIP) ↓
and FVC ↓,
and are posture-dependent
(FEV_1 / FVC may be normal)
2. Fluoroscopy: diaphragm moves
upward on sniffing
3. Phrenic nerve conduction studies

<u>Chest X-Ray Patterns</u>

<u>Reticulo-Nodular Shadowing</u>

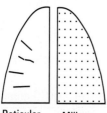

Reticular   Miliary
or linear   nodules
        (< 2mm)

= Interstitial disease

F.I.N.E. shadows

Fibrosis
   a) Upper zones:
       pneumoconioses, extrinsic allergic alveolitis
       seronegative arthropathies, TB, aspergillosis
   b) Mid zones: sarcoid
   c) Lower zones: SLE, CFA, asbestosis, radiotherapy, drugs

Infection
   a) Atypical pneumonia: psittacosis, Q-fever
   b) Viral, VZV pneumonitis: nodular

Neoplasia
   a) Lymphangitis carcinomatosis: reticular
   b) Thyroid carcinoma (follicular): "snowstorm" appearance
   c) Other: renal cell, melanoma, lymphoma: nodular

Edema
   a) Pulmonary oedema: Kerley B lines (horizontal, peripheral)
   b) Long-standing pulmo. oedema / haemosiderosis: nodular

<u>Coin Lesions, Cavities</u>

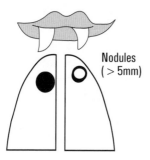

Nodules
(> 5mm)

F.A.N.G.S.

Fibrosis
   a) Upper zones:
       pneumoconioses (progressive massive fibrosis)
   b) Lower zones: rheumatoid arthritis

Abscess
   a) Bacterial: staphylococci, TB, Klebsiella
   b) Mycetoma, Aspergillus
   c) Hydatid cyst; amoebic cyst

Neoplasia
   a) 1°, 2°
   b) Benign: hamartoma, bronchial cyst

Granulomatous
   Rheumatoid arthritis, Wegener's

Structural
   a) AVM
   b) Pulmonary infarction
   c) Traumatic haematoma

Opacification

Consolidation: Air-Space Infiltration

Fluid: a) Oedema 2° to LVF or ARDS
b) Alveolar proteinosis

Cells: a) Neutrophils:
• Pneumonia: bacterial, viral, TB, PCP
• Infarction 2° to PE
b) Eosinophilis:
• Pulmonary eosinophilia, ABPA
c) Red blood cells (pulmonary haemorrhage):
• Goodpasture's, Wegener's
• Mitral stenosis, L → R shunt, e.g. VSD
• Idiopathic pulmonary haemosiderosis
d) Tumour:
• Bronchioalveolar cell carcinoma, Kaposi's sarcoma

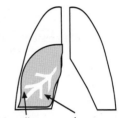

confluent   air
shadowing   bronchogram

Collapse

Lobar
Segmental atelectasis
Surgery: pneumonectomy, thoracoplasty (for TB)

Patterns observed with lobar collapse:

Upper lobe   Middle lobe / lingula   Lower lobe

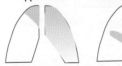

Pleural Disease

Effusion

Plaques: holly-leaf plaques or linear shadows
a) Asbestos exposure / mesothelioma (but not asbestosis)
b) TB
c) Old haemothorax

Mediastinal Mass

Thyroid (retrosternal goitre); **T**hymoma, **T**eratoma, **TB** (or sarcoid) lymph nodes
+ **T**errible diagnoses!!!: lymphoma or aneurysm/dissection!!!

Pneumonia – Clinical Features

PC   1. Specific: pleuritic pain, cough productive of rusty sputum, SOB

2. Constitutional: fever, rigors, malaise, myalgia,
D + V (esp. *Legionella*), headaches (esp. *Mycoplasma*)
confusion, falls

3. Other history: PMH: pulmonary disease or immunocompromised
PH: smoking,
pets (psittacosis),
travel (Legionnaire's, typhoid, TB)
SH: job, contacts

O/E

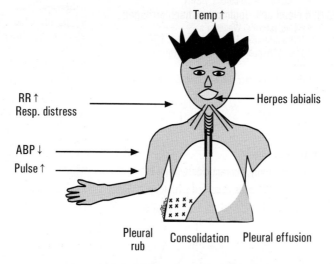

Temp ↑

RR ↑
Resp. distress

Herpes labialis

ABP ↓

Pulse ↑

Pleural
rub   Consolidation   Pleural effusion

Poor Prognostic Features
H.A.R.M.F.U.L.

History: age > 50, comorbidity (e.g. IHD, ca.)

Hypoxia: sats < 92%, PaO_2 < 8 kPa on room air

ABP: SBP < 90 mmHg, or DBP < 60 mmHg

RR: > 30/min

Mental confusion

Fluid: pleural effusion

Urea: > 7 mmol/l

Leucocytosis: WCC < 4 or > 20 x10^9/l

Lobar, multi-, appearance of CXR

Ix and Rx

B. Ventilatory Support

1. Sit patient up: aids respiration
2. Oxygen: 35–100% ,
   ± rebreath bag
3. Nebulizers: if COAD or wheeze
4. CPAP or intubate

WARN ITU
if still hypoxic or $PaCo_2$
> 6KPa

C. Hydration

e.g. N.saline IVI,
unless possibility of
pulmonary oedema

A. Assessment

1. A.B.C.D.

2. C.O.A.T.

Cardiac monitor,
O_2 stats, ABP, TPR

3. Investigations

Bloods
  ABGs:
  PaO_2 – index of severity
  $PaCO_2$ – should be low;
      if normal or high, suggests
      fatigue and need for ventilatn
  U + E: fluid depletion, *Legionella*
  LFT: *Mycoplasma, Legionella*
  FBC: Neutrophilia (not *Mycoplasma*)
  ESR, CRP: allows monitoring
  Clotting, FDP: DIC is complication
  Igs: is patient immunodeficient?
Urine
  Glucose; *Legionella* antigen serology
Micro
  Blood cultures
  Serology: *Mycoplasma, Legionella,
    Chlamydia, Coxiella* (4x↑over 10 days)
  HIV
  Sputum: Gram, silver, AAFB stains;
      ELISA
Monitor: PEFR, O_2
ECG: AF may occur
Radiology: CXR
Special: 1. Bronchoscopy:
      if PCP or carcinoma possible
    2. Pleural aspirate or biopsy
    3. Lung biopsy

D. Medication

Antibiotics:
selected according to likely organism:
      C.R.A.N.E.

Community-acquired:
    *S. pneumoniae, H. influenzae,
    Mycoplasma, Legionella*
    amoxicillin + erythromycin

Recent-flu:
    Staphylococcus
    above + flucloxacillin

Aspiration possible, e.g. alcoholic:
    Anaerobes, Gram –ves
    cefuroxime + metronidazole

Nosocomial:
    Gram –ves, MRSA
    cefotaxime ±
    vancomycin (if MRSA possible)

Extra:
    HIV *(consider PCP)*
      add co-trimoxazole
    TB: consider R.I.P.E.

Optional
1. Analgesics, e.g. NSAID if not
          asthmatic
2. Glucocorticoids if COAD

E. Other
Physiotherapy:
clear pooled secretions

On discharge

Follow-up
1. Advice smoking, pets, job
2. Isolate TB until smear –ve
3. Vaccine: pneumococcus,
   flu – in immunocompromised

Asthma – Chronic

Def Episodic, reversible COAD, due to bronchial hyper-reactivity to various stimuli

Epi

Inc: Children 5%; Adults 2%
Age: Peaks at 5 years; most outgrow in adolescence
Sex: M:F = 1:1, except under 5, when boys predominate (3:2)
Geo: Western World
Aet: a) Acute phase (30 min): Mast cell–Ag interaction $\rightarrow$ histamine $\rightarrow$ local axon + central reflexes
　　 b) Late phase (12 h): T_{H2} cell $\rightarrow$ interleukins-3,4,5 $\rightarrow$ mast cells, eosinophils, B cells
Micro: Sputum contains mucus casts, eosinophils, Curschmann spirals, Charcot-Leyden crystals

Causes   A.S.T.H.M.A.

Atopy

Def: Predisposition to allergic, or Type 1 hypersensitivity reactions, inc.
　　 allergic rhinitis, nasal polyps, urticaria, eczema, food poisoning

Aet: i) Polygenic: mutations in IgE receptor, $\alpha\beta$-TCR, IL-4; family Hx common .
　　 ii) Triggered by: dust, dust mite, dander (animals), pollen, food

Ix: i) Serum IgE $\uparrow$, blocking IgG $\downarrow$
　　 ii) Skin prick test: allergen induces Lewis's 'Triple Response'
　　 iii) RAST (Radio-AllergoSorbent Test): identifies specific Abs to Ags

Rx: i) Avoidance; ii) Disodium cromoglycate; iii) Desensitization (esp. in children)

Stress: exercise, emotion, viral URTI, cold, premenses, GO reflux

Aet: Idiosyncratic, non-allergenic mechanisms

Ix: Serum IgE and skin prick test – both negative

Toxins

Smoking, pollution
Allergens: i) Factory: epoxy resins, platinum, formaldehyde
　　　　　　 ii) Farming: cotton, red cedar wood
Drugs　　　 i) NSAIDs, esp. aspirin
　　　　　　 ii) β-blocker: inhibits bronchodilator β_2-receptor

Helminth: *Ascaris, Strongyloides, Toxocara*: migration phase

Malignancy: Carcinoid

Autoimmune

1. Churg–Strauss Syn. = PAN-like vasculitis + eosinophilia + p-ANCA
2. Addison's (may ppte. asthma in susceptible individual; Assoc.: eosinophilia)

Aspergillosis: allergic bronchopulmonary (ABPA)

Aet: Type I + III hypersensitivity reactions
PC: i) Upper lobe fibrosis; ii) Proximal bronchiectasis; iii) Lobar collapse

PC

1. **Cough:** often at night, tenacious yellow sputum
2. **Wheeze:** often post-exercise, early morning; relieved by empirical salbutamol Rx
3. **SOB**, or 'chest tightness'
    + **Failure to Thrive:** Children

O/E

General: Underweight
(hypermetabolic)

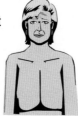

Chest:
  Inspection:
   i) Hyperexpanded
   ii) Harrison's sulci: indrawn subcostal margins
  Auscultation:
   i) Widespread, polyphonic high-pitched wheeze
      (small-airways obstruction)
   ii) Often normal – as characteristically episodic

Ix

Bloods: i) FBC: eosinophilia, ii) ANCA
Urine: glucose (if on chronic steroids)
Micro: i) Sputum – microscopy; ii) Serology: *Aspergillus, Ascaris, Strongyloides*
Monitor:

> **PEFR:** Varies according to sex, age, height (normal = 300 - 600 L / min)
>
> Characteristic Daily Pattern
> i) Early morning dips: may be fatal
>   despite normal daytime values
> ii) β_2-Agonist improves
> iii) 3-weeks prednisolone 30mg od:
>   improvement suggests COAD reversibility,
>   and hence utility of steroids
>
>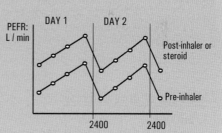

Radio: CXR: hyperexpanded
Special:

  a) **Spirometry**
     - FEV_1/FVC ↓ (20–40%, cf. 70–80%)
     - RV, and TLC ↑
     - Flow–volume loop: peak flow depressed most at lower lung volumes

  b) **Methacholine or histamine-inhalation challenge test**
       PEFR and FEV_1 dip at 30 minutes and 12 hours, consistent with 2-phase mechanism

  c) **Atopy tests:** see opposite

Asthma Management – General

Remember to T.A.M.E. your patient ....

Technique for inhaler use:

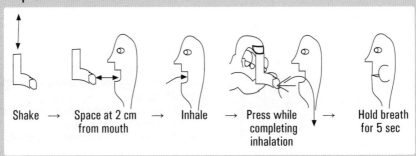

Shake → Space at 2 cm → Inhale → Press while → Hold breath
              from mouth   completing   for 5 sec
                                            inhalation

Avoidance: • Allergens: smoke, carpets, grass in Summer
                 • Prophylactic measures: dust covers, synthetic pillows

Monitor: • Peak flow monitor (2–4x / day) on chart → Adjust drugs accordingly

Educate: • Liaise with Specialist Respiratory Nurse and / or District Nurse
                 • Pt. to be able to assess severity based on symptoms and PEFR
                 • Reinforce need for compliance with Rx

Methods of drug delivery

1. Inhaler:
Metered-Dose Inhaler (MDI): Needs correct technique
Spacer + MDI: Spacer acts as a short-term reservoir for aerosol, and creates smaller particles for inhalation.
Advantage: – Better for children or elderly who cannot coordinate technique, and may be administered by carer.
Breath-Activated e.g. pressurized cylinder (Autohaler); dry-powder (Rotahaler)
– depends on pt.'s. effort

2. Nebulizer:
Mechanism: Finer particle size (3- 10 μm) allows tracheobronchial deposition
Advantage: Allows high-dose drug to be administered; coordination not required
Disadvantage: • Higher doses causes systemic effects
              • Over-reliance at home makes pts. delay seeking help or forget prophylactic Rx
              • Expensive + bulky

Drug ladder

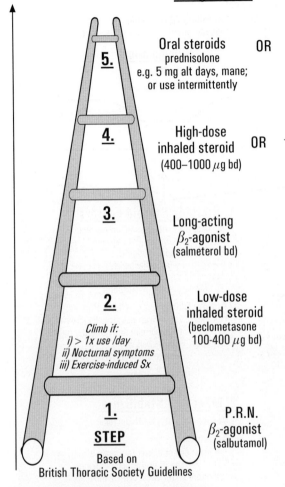

5. Oral steroids   OR   Steroid-sparer
prednisolone   e.g. methotrexate,
e.g. 5 mg alt days, mane;   cyclosporin
or use intermittently

4. High-dose   OR   { Oral long-acting β_2-agonist
inhaled steroid   Oral theophylline
(400–1000 μg bd)   Oral leukotriene receptor antagonist
     (montelukast, zafirlukast)

3. Long-acting
β_2-agonist
(salmeterol bd)

2. Low-dose
inhaled steroid
(beclometasone
Climb if: 100-400 μg bd)
i) > 1x use /day
ii) Nocturnal symptoms
iii) Exercise-induced Sx

1. P.R.N.
β_2-agonist
STEP (salbutamol)
Based on
British Thoracic Society Guidelines

Rules

1. Start on step commensurate with present severity.
2. Move up and down 1 step at a time.
3. Take each lower step medication in addition to medication of step currently on.

Brittle Asthma Rx

a) MedicAlert bracelet

b) Self-Medication in emergency:
 • Salbutamol nebulizer/SC
 • Prednisolone PO

c) Direct access to ITU if admitted

Asthma Management – Drugs

Pharmacology

Drugs can be classified depending on when they act :
a) Early Phase: Bronchodilators: immediate onset (mins)
b) Early AND Late Phases: Prophylactic: delayed onset (hours – days – weeks)

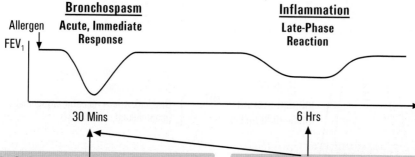

1. β_2-Agonists

Short-acting: Salbutamol (inhaler, nebulizer, IV)
Long-acting: Salmeterol (inhaler, PO – bd)

Action: cAMP ↑ + cGMP ↓

Reduces S.E.E.PA.Ge:
Smooth muscle: bronchospasm ↓
Epithelium: mucociliary clearance ↑
Endothelium: permeability ↓
PArasympathetic ganglia: vagal tone ↓
DeGranulation of mast cells ↓

   Onset = 3 min. Offset = 5 hr

2. Muscarinic Antagonists

Ipratropium bromide (inhaler, nebulizer)

Action: non-selective, but M3 receptor mediates:
   Smooth muscle: bronchospasm ↓
   Epithelium: submucosal gland secretion ↓
   Endothelium: permeability ↓

   More effective in COAD than in asthma

   Onset = 30 min. Offset = 6 hr

3. Methylxanthines

Theophylline, aminophylline (PO, IV)
(both caffeine-like adenosine analogues)

Action: Phosphodiesterase inhibition and
      P1 (A1) antagonist ⇒ cAMP ↑ ⇒
Smooth muscle: bronchospasm ↓
DeGranulation mast cell ↓
Noradrenaline release ↑
+ Anti-inflammatory effect at low-dose

   Onset = 2 hrs

1. Steroids/Steroid sparers

Inhaled: Beclomethasone (activated in lungs),
      budesonide, fluticasone
Systemic: Prednisolone PO,
      hydrocortisone IV
Steroid Sparers:
   Methotrexate, cyclosporin

Action: Blocks Early + Late Phases:-
• Early: Histamine, leukotrienes, prostaglandins,
        PAF (platelet activating factor)
• Late: Interleukins-3,4,5
       Upregulation of β_2-receptors

   Onset: 3–7 days

2. Mast Cell Stabilizers

Na Cromoglycate, Na Nedocromil

Action:
• Mast cell stabilizer (not main effect) ⇒
   release of preformed cytokines ↓
• Neuronal reflexes (central + axonal) ↓
• Substance P + PAF antagonist

3. Leukotriene Receptor Antagonists

Montelukast, zafirlukast

Action:
Competitive antagonists at cysteinyl-
leukotriene receptor (LTC4, D4, E4)

Effective for NSAID, allergen or exercise-
induced asthma

Side-Effects

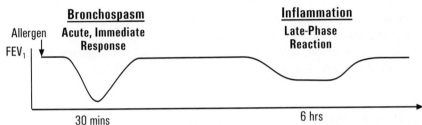

Bronchospasm
Acute, Immediate
Response

Inflammation
Late-Phase
Reaction

Allergen
FEV$_1$

30 mins

6 hrs

1. β_2-Agonists

Local:
   i) Rebound hyper-reactivity
   ii) Tolerance ($\downarrow$ ed by steroids)
   iii) Paradoxical bronchospasm
   iv) V/Q mismatch $\uparrow$ due to pulmonary vasodilation
   v) Long-term worsening $\uparrow$?
      (due to $\downarrow$ mast cell release of heparin
       that $\downarrow$ late-phase reaction)

Systemic:
   i) Fine tremor, muscle cramps, anxiety
   ii) Dysrhythmias
   iii) Periph. vasodilation: headache, flushing
   iv) K$^+$ $\downarrow$ ($\uparrow$ uptake of K$^+$ into skeletal muscle)

2. Muscarinic Antagonists

Local:
   i) Glaucoma, diplopia (with face-mask)
   ii) Dry mouth
   iii) Paradoxical bronchospasm
Systemic: Rare, as 4° NH$_4^+$ compounds
   e.g. urinary retention

3. Methylxanthines

Therapeutic Range (10–20 mg/l):
   i) Periph. vasodilation: headache,
      irritability, insomnia
   ii) GIT: N+V, constipation, G-O reflux
   iii) Diuretic (GFR $\uparrow$, tubular resorption $\downarrow$)

Toxic Range:
   i) K$^+$ $\downarrow$
   ii) Dysrhythmias (use ECG if IV)
   iii) Cerebral vasoconstriction:
      Fits, IQ $\downarrow$ in children

1. Steroids

Local:
   i) Oral candidiasis
   ii) Dysphonia (vocal cord myopathy)
Systemic (high-dose inhaled or oral):
   i) Osteoporotic-bone change /
      skin-thinning, bruising
   ii) Growth suppression in children
      (> 400 μg/day)
   iii) Adrenal suppression

Minimize by:
- Titrating dose upwards
- Using inhalers with high 1st-pass
  metabolism, e.g. budesonide (90%) or
  fluticasone (99%), esp. in children
- Steroid-sparing agents

2. Mast Cell Stabilizers

   i) Transient bronchospasm:
      give salbutamol 1st!
   ii) Minor URT irritation / cough
   iii) Hypersensitivity

3. Leukotriene Receptor Antagonists

   i) Dry mouth
   ii) URTI/flu-like symptoms
   iii) Unmasking of Churg-Strauss syndrome
      (by encouraging steroid reduction)

Acute Severe Asthma

<u>**Epi**</u> 75% hospitalizations could be avoided in that effective Rx should have begun 48 hours earlier

At-Risk Groups   *R.A.M.P.*

Recent deterioration: noctural symptoms, diurnal lability, ↓ing PEFR
Allergen exposure: pollen (e.g. Summer, holiday), storm, evening
Misjudged perception of severity; **M**eter use inadequate (PEFR); **M**iserly use of systemic steroids
Personal xteristics: **P**revious recent attacks, **P**sychiatric, **P**oor, **P**uberty, steroid or nebulizer use

PC

Respiratory Distress

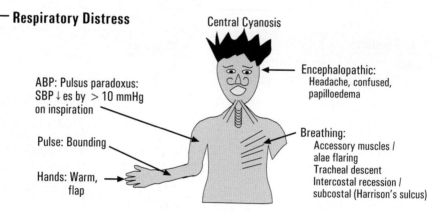

Central Cyanosis

Encephalopathic:
   Headache, confused,
   papilloedema

ABP: Pulsus paradoxus:
SBP ↓es by > 10 mmHg
on inspiration

Pulse: Bounding

Hands: Warm,
   flap

Breathing:
   Accessory muscles /
   alae flaring
   Tracheal descent
   Intercostal recession /
   subcostal (Harrison's sulcus)

Specific Markers of Severity

	Acute, Severe	**Life-Threatening**
Airway	PEFR < 50%	PEFR < 33%
Breathing	RR ≥ 25	Resp. effort ↓ , silent chest, central cyanosis
Circulation	Pulse > 110	Pulse < 60, hypotension
Disability	Can't complete sentence in 1 breath	Exhaustion / confusion / coma
Exchange, gas		PaCO$_2$ Normal or ↑ (> 5.0 kPa) PaO$_2$ ↓(< 8.0 kPa) pH ↓ (< 7.36)

Complications

A. Lung: i) Collapse: segmental / lobar
   ii) Pneumothorax / pneumomediastinum
   iii) Pulmonary oedema

B. Heart: i) Dysrhythmia (esp. due to O$_2$↓, and K$^+$, exacerbated by salbutamol or theophylline use)
   ii) Myocardial infarction

Ix and Rx

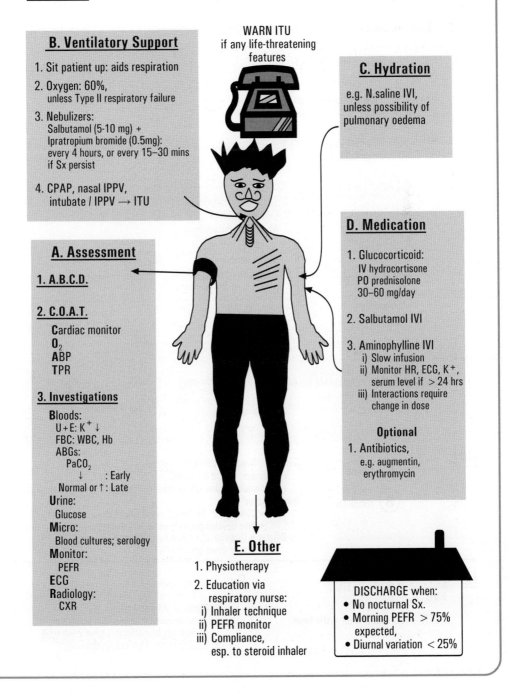

B. Ventilatory Support

1. Sit patient up: aids respiration

2. Oxygen: 60%,
   unless Type II respiratory failure

3. Nebulizers:
   Salbutamol (5-10 mg) +
   Ipratropium bromide (0.5mg):
   every 4 hours, or every 15–30 mins
   if Sx persist

4. CPAP, nasal IPPV,
   intubate / IPPV → ITU

WARN ITU
if any life-threatening
features

C. Hydration

e.g. N.saline IVI,
unless possibility of
pulmonary oedema

A. Assessment

1. A.B.C.D.

2. C.O.A.T.
   Cardiac monitor
   O$_2$
   ABP
   TPR

3. Investigations

   Bloods:
   U + E: K$^+$ ↓
   FBC: WBC, Hb
   ABGs:
   PaCO$_2$
   ↓ : Early
   Normal or ↑: Late
   Urine:
   Glucose
   Micro:
   Blood cultures; serology
   Monitor:
   PEFR
   ECG
   Radiology:
   CXR

D. Medication

1. Glucocorticoid:
   IV hydrocortisone
   PO prednisolone
   30–60 mg/day

2. Salbutamol IVI

3. Aminophylline IVI
   i) Slow infusion
   ii) Monitor HR, ECG, K$^+$,
   serum level if > 24 hrs
   iii) Interactions require
   change in dose

Optional
1. Antibiotics,
   e.g. augmentin,
   erythromycin

E. Other

1. Physiotherapy

2. Education via
   respiratory nurse:
   i) Inhaler technique
   ii) PEFR monitor
   iii) Compliance,
   esp. to steroid inhaler

DISCHARGE when:
• No nocturnal Sx.
• Morning PEFR > 75%
  expected,
• Diurnal variation < 25%

COAD

Chronic Bronchitis

Def **Productive Cough, 1**x / day (most days), of **3** months of the year, for at least **2** consecutive yrs

Epi
Inc: Prev = 15% of city-dwellers
Age: Middle-aged
Sex: Men
Geo: Urban: Pollution aggravates
Pre: i) Smoking = 4-10x ↑ Risk
ii) Childhood asthma
Aet:

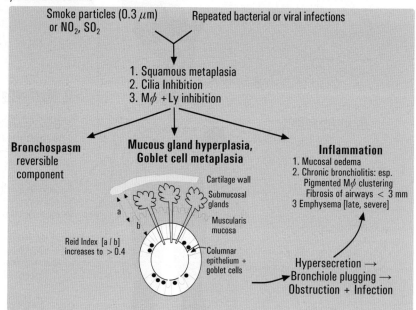

Smoke particles (0.3 μm)   Repeated bacterial or viral infections
or NO_2, SO_2

1. Squamous metaplasia
2. Cilia Inhibition
3. Mϕ + Ly inhibition

Bronchospasm
reversible
component

Mucous gland hyperplasia,
Goblet cell metaplasia

Cartilage wall
Submucosal
glands

Muscularis
mucosa

Reid Index [a / b]
increases to > 0.4

Columnar
epithelium +
goblet cells

Inflammation
1. Mucosal oedema
2. Chronic bronchiolitis: esp.
Pigmented Mϕ clustering
Fibrosis of airways < 3 mm
3 Emphysema [late, severe]

Hypersecretion →
Bronchiole plugging →
Obstruction + Infection

HPC

C hronic

B ronchitis

Cough with white, purulent sputum
+ Wheeze, esp. if 2° to asthma
+ exacerbations due to infection, pollution
"Blue Bloater":
Blue • Cyanosis 2° to Type 2 respiratory failure
• Also develop polycythaemia and respiratory acidosis
Bloater • Oedema 2° to RSH Failure (Cor Pulmonale)
• may develop acute CCF

Ix
$\dfrac{FEV_1}{FVC}$ < 0.6, TLC, RV ↑

PEFR – Normal / ↓ es with time

Rx 1. Conservative:
i) Stop smoking; ii) Pulmonary rehabilitation
2. Medical: As for Asthma, but
i) Ipratropium bromide more effective
ii) Steroids less effective (give 2-wk trial)
3. Venesection – for polycythaemia

Emphysema

Def 1. Permanent enlargement of air spaces, distal to terminal bronchiole ('Emphysema' = Inflation)
2. Alveolar wall destruction, without obvious fibrosis

Epi Inc: 50% post-mortem finding (5% cause of death)
Age: Older age (60-75)
Sex: Men
Geo: Urban: Pollution aggravates
Pre: i) Smoking = 4-10x ↑ risk
ii) Genetic: α_1- Anti-trypsin deficiency Prev: 1/7000

Aet:

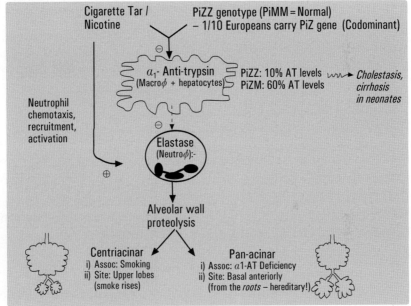

Cigarette Tar / Nicotine

PiZZ genotype (PiMM = Normal)
– 1/10 Europeans carry PiZ gene (Codominant)

α_1- Anti-trypsin
(Macroϕ + hepatocytes)

PiZZ: 10% AT levels ⟿ *Cholestasis, cirrhosis in neonates*
PiZM: 60% AT levels

Neutrophil chemotaxis, recruitment, activation

Elastase
(Neutroϕ):-

Alveolar wall proteolysis

Centriacinar
i) Assoc: Smoking
ii) Site: Upper lobes (smoke rises)

Pan-acinar
i) Assoc: α1-AT Deficiency
ii) Site: Basal anteriorly (from the *roots* – hereditary!)

HPC

Em Ⓟ hysema

'Pink Puffer':
• SOB, pursed lips (↑ Intrabronchial pressure → Bronchiolar closure ↓)
  Barrel chest, bent-over
• Type 1 respiratory failure (Type 2 occurs later)
• Cachexia

Ix as for Chronic Bronchitis, only
PEFR ↓ early

Rx As for Chronic Bronchitis, +
1. Oxygen more useful as pts are in type 1 failure
2. Surgery:
    bulla stapling; lobectomy; transplant
3. α_1-*AT Def.*: i) Danazol (↑es α_1-AT)
                          ii) α_1-AT concentrate

Fibrosing Alveolitis

Causes

P.E.N.T.A.-H.ouS.e

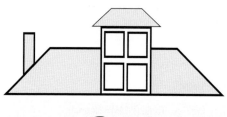

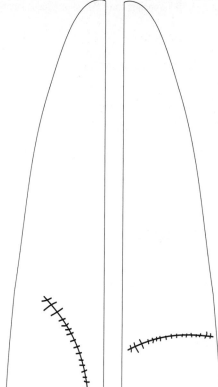

S.C.A.R.R.E.D.

Upper Zone

Pneumoconioses
- Coal-worker's; silicosis
- Berryliosis: electronics or nuclear power workers
- Siderosis (Fe), or stannosis (Sn) – metal workers

Extrinsic allergic alveolitis
- Chronic disease

Negative, sero-arthropathies
- Ankylosing spondylitis

TB

Aspergillosis: ABPA

Histiocytosis X

Mid Zone

Sarcoidosis

Lower Zone

Scleroderma, SLE, Sjögren's
+ Rheumatoid arthritis, polymyositis

Cryptogenic fibrosing alveolitis

Asbestosis

Radiotherapy

Renal failure

Rare syndromes:
- Atypical pneumonia: varicella, psittacosis,
- Pulmonary eosinophilia
- Neoplasia: lymphangioleiomyomatosis, amyloid
- Neurofibromatosis

Edema + other fluid:
- Oedema: Chronic mitral stenosis
- Blood: Goodpasture's, Wegener's
- Protein: Alveolar proteinosis
- Lymph: Lymphangitis carcinomatosis

Drugs: *B.A.N. M.E.:*
Bleomycin, busulphan, cyclophosphamide
Amiodarone
Nitrofurantoin
Methotrexate, **M**ethysergide
Environmental: paraquat

<u>Cryptogenic Fibrosing Alveolitis</u>

= Usual Interstitial Pneumonitis (UIP)

<u>Path</u>

1. Leaky alveolar-capillary membrane $\rightarrow$ Macrophage and neutrophil infiltrate
2. Antibodies to unknown antigen, e.g. viral
3. Macrophage –T cell interaction $\rightarrow$ IL-8, LT-B4, TNF $\rightarrow$ Fibrosis and lung destruction

<u>Epi</u>

1. Age: Middle age
2. Sex: M:F = 2:1
3. Assoc.: Autoimmune disease in 1/3

<u>HPC</u>

PC	1. **C**onstitutional: Malaise / LOW / arthralgia	
	2. **C**ough (Dry) / Progressive SOBOE (Acute form = Hamman–Rich syn.)	
O/E	1. **C**yanosed	
	2. **C**lubbed	
	3. **C**reps: Basal, fine end-inspiratory; best heard in axillae, pt. lying on side	
COMPS	1. **C**arcinoma, lung: 15%	

<u>Ix</u>

Bloods

1. ESR, immunoglobulins $\uparrow$
2. AutoAbs, e.g. ANA, RhF in 35%
3. ABG: $\downarrow O_2$, $\downarrow CO_2$

Radiology

1. CXR: Bilateral basal; diffuse reticulonodular shadowing: 'honeycombing'
2. High-resolution CT: Cystic spaces

Special

1. Spirometry: Restrictive picture with $\downarrow$ KCO
2. BAL: Neutrophils + Eosinophils (if Lymphocytes, then suggests Rx-responsive)

<u>Rx</u>

1. Immunosuppression:
   Prednisolone 60 mg od for 1–2 months, or
   Prednisolone 20 mg od + cyclophosphamide for < 6 months
2. Lung Transplant

<u>Prognosis</u>

1. 5 year SR = 50%: Highly variable -
           65% if steroid-responsive   (1/3)
           25% if steroid-unresponsive (2/3)
2. Life expectancy: 1–20 years

Occupational Lung Diseases
A. Pneumoconioses

Path

Inhaled inorganic dust is phagocytosed by alveolar macrophages, resulting in:
   i) Disruption of lysosomal membranes and release of proteolytic enzymes, e.g. elastase
   ii) Impaired immunity (also caused by defective ciliary flow)

Epi

a) Coal worker's pneumoconiosis (dust = coal + kaolin + mica + silica; anthracite mine dust is more antigenic)
      • 2% miners in developing world (rare where precautions heeded)
b) Silicosis: seen in other types of miners, quarryworkers, sandblasters, pottery man
c) Asbestosis: shipworkers; demolition or boilers; pipe-laggers; sputum reveals 'asbestos bodies' in macrophages

HPC

a) Acute (uncommon – usually silicosis or talcosis):
         i) Rapidly progressive SOB; ii) Respiratory failure; iii) Fever
b) Chronic (common):
         i) Slowly progressive SOB; ii) **C**ough (haem- or melanoptysis); iii) **C**yanosis, **C**lubbing, **C**repitations

CXR

a) Coal worker's pneumoconiosis

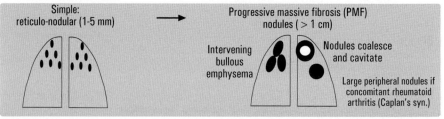

b) Silicosis

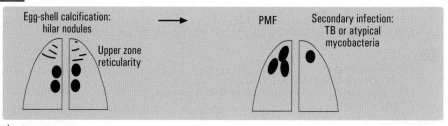

c) Asbestos exposure

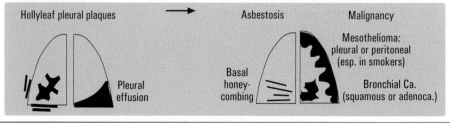

B. Extrinsic Allergic Alveolitis

Path
Inhaled organic dusts result in acute or chronic alveolar sensitization to particular antigen:
  i) Acute: type III hypersensitivity reaction (starts 4–8 hours post-exposure; lasts 1–2 days)
  ii) Chronic: type IV hypersensitivity reaction, with granulomas (starts after 5–20 years)

Epi
  a) Farmer's lung: antigen = *Actinomycetes* spores (thermophilic filamentous bacteria), found in moist hay;
          worsens in Winter (hay is moved); improves with smoking!
  b) Bird fancier's lung: antigen = serum proteins in bird droppings or feathers.
  c) Byssiniosis : antigen = cotton dust, flax, hemp;
          worst on 1st day of week, and improves as week progresses; worsens with smoking
  d) Other: baggasosis (sugar); mushroom-worker's; grain-worker's; ventilator's lung

HPC
  a) Acute:
      i) Flu-like (fever, myalgia);   ii) Cough (dry); iii) SOB
  b) Chronic:
      i) Constitutional (malaise, LOW); ii) Cough (dry); iii) SOB; iv) Fine creps or squeaks (*N.B. no wheeze!*)

Ix
  Bloods:
    i) Neutrophilia (N.B. Eosinophils normal)
    ii) ESR ↑
  Micro:
    Serum precipitins Farmer's Lung (ELISA): 80% sensitivity + 80% specificity
  Radio:

  CXR:

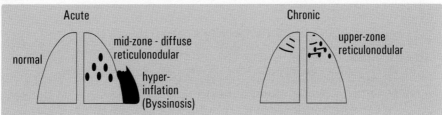

  Special:
      i) Spirometry: Restrictive / obstructive picture
                    ↓ KCO
      ii) BAL: Lymphocytes + mast cells
      iii) Intradermal skin test (6 hours)

Rx
  a) Avoidance
  b) Prednisolone – acutely / long-term
  c) Lung transplant

Sarcoidosis

Characterized by *G.R.A.N.U.L.O.M.A.S.*

General
1. Fever (Löfgren's syndrome = acute fever + arthralgia + cough + erythema nodosum)
2. Anorexia: weight loss, fatigue
3. Lymphadenopathy, hepatosplenomegaly

Respiratory
1. Upper tract: otitis, sinusitis, rhinitis, laryngitis
2. Lower tract: a) Bihilar lymphadenopathy (BHL): CXR = egg-shell calcification (stage 1)
                    b) Parenchymal infiltration: diffuse, miliary nodules   (stage 2)
                    c) Fibrosis: apical and perihilar linear streaks   (stage 3)
                    d) Complications: cavitation ± mycetoma; collapse, 2° to bronchial obstruction

Arthralgia
1. Painful joints more common than arthritis
2. Dactylitis, bony cysts, tufting + sclerosis of terminal phalanges
3. Soft tissue calcinosis

Neurological
1. Brain: diffuse, meningeal thickening: dementia, meningo-encephalitis
         focal granulomas: seizures, focal signs, hydrocephalus
2. Cord: transverse myelitis
3. Peripheral and cranial neuropathy, e.g. bilateral VII cranial nerve palsy
4. Myopathy

Urine
1. Polyuria, polydipsia (diabetes insipidus):
         due to neurohypophysis and tubular disease
2. Renal stones, nephrocalcinosis:
         due to hypercalcaemia: due to 1α–hydroxylase activity in lung lesions
         worse in Summer when light causes Vit D synthesis
3. Interstitial nephritis:
         due to hypercalcaemia and renal infiltration (tubulointerstitial nephritis + glomerulonephritis)

Liver
Causes cholestatic LFTs, but only rarely liver failure or cirrhosis

Ophthalmological
1. Lacrimal: xerophthalmia, Mikulicz's syndrome: enlarged lacrimal + 3 salivary glands
   'uveoparotid fever' (Heerfordt's syn.) = acute fever + Mikulicz's syn. + uveitis + Bell's palsy
2. Anterior: conjunctivitis (inc. due to sicca), band keratopathy, cataract, anterior uveitis, glaucoma
3. Posterior: posterior uveitis: perivascular cuffing of equatorial veins, optic atrophy

Myocardial
1. Restrictive cardiomyopathy, 2° to myocardial granulomas + fibrosis ⇒ 3° heart block / VT
2. Pericardial effusion

Amenorrhoea etc: hypopituitarism

Skin
1. Lupus pernio: raised, dusky-purple plaque on nose, cheeks, fingers
2. Boeck's sarcoid: purple-red nodules on face, back, extensor surfaces
3. Scar infiltration
4. Erythema nodosum: painful, erythematous nodules on legs, forearms

Epi

Inc: 10/100,000 p.a.
Age: peaks in 20s–30s, but can occur at any age
Sex: F > M
Geo: a) Blacks have 10x higher incidence, and have more severe disease
     b) Chinese: rarely occurs
Aet: a) Immune: • T cell function impaired, although
            CD4 T cells, activated macrophages, and soluble IL-2R levels ↑
           • B cell function ↑: hypergammaglobulinaemia
     b) Infection: unidentified mycobacteria ?, since similar immune response (granulomas, ↑ $\gamma\delta$ T cells)
         and PCR +ve in some cases

Ix

Bloods 1. Serum ACE ↑ (+ve in 75%; false +ves = atypical mycobacteria; leprosy; Gaucher's)
       2. Other: Ig ↑, ESR ↑, Ca^{2+} ↑
Urine: Ca^{2+} ↑
Radio: 1. CXR: see opposite
       2. Gallium scan: • Taken up by activated Macrophages in granuloma
               • 'Panda appearance' due to uptake in salivary + lacrimal glands
               • Can be used to monitor disease activity)
Special:
     1. Tuberculin skin test: –ve in sarcoid (cf. TB = +ve)
     2. Kveim test: intradermal injection of sarcoid-spleen suspension ⇒ skin biopsy at 6 weeks shows granulomas
     3. Lung function tests: – KCO ↓ (1st sign of parenchymal disease); restrictive picture (FVC ↓, FEV₁/FVC norm or ↑)

Microscopy: Non-caseating Granulomas

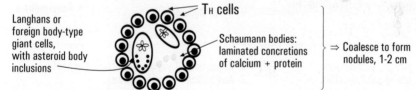

Langhans or foreign body-type giant cells, with asteroid body inclusions

T_H cells

Schaumann bodies: laminated concretions of calcium + protein

⇒ Coalesce to form nodules, 1-2 cm

Rx
          S.erum A.C.E.

1. **S**teroids: Prednisolone, 3 month course
    Indications: respiratory, cardiac, ophthalmic, neurological, renal disease, hypercalcaemia
2. **A**zathioprine / methotrexate / hydroxychloroquine: Act as steroid sparers / maintenance therapy
         • Need to check FBC (Aza, MTX) + LFT (MTX)
         • Need to check central visual field (Amsler Eye Test)
3. **C**alcium reduction: see p. 379
4. **E**ye drops: a) Cyclopentolate: mAch receptor inhibitor
           b) Fluorometholone: steroid with least tendency to ↑ intraocular pressure

Prognosis

70% recover within 1–2 years, _{esp. acute presentation e.g. Löfgren's syndrome, young, White}
25% relapses or chronic disease: _{more likely if insidious onset, e.g. lupus pernio, chronic uveitis, middle aged, Black}
5% death due to complications

Bronchiectasis

Causes

1. Chronic Infection – Inhalation
a) Bacterial: *S.T.I.N.K.* (see opposite)
b) Viral (measles, flu); pertussis
c) Aspergillosis (ABPA)
d) Toxic gas inhalation

2. Bronchial Obstruction
a) Foreign body
b) Tumour (esp. carcinoid); lymph node, e.g. sarcoid
c) Congenital: e.g. pulmonary sequestration

3. Host Defences ↓
a) Secretions:
  • Cystic fibrosis: ↑ Viscosity → Bronchial clogging
  • Yellow nail syndrome: ↓ Lymphatic drainage
b) Structural:
  • Kartagener's syndrome: Ciliary dyskinesia
    PC: Sinusitis, male infertility, dextrocardia
  • Marfan's syndrome: ↓ Bronchial elasticity
c) Immune:
  • Hypogammaglobulinaemia, HIV

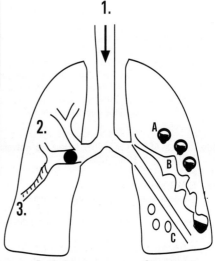

Pathology
A. Cystic: Blind-ending saccules with fluid levels

B. Varicose: Irregular beading

C. Cylindrical: 'Tram-tracks'

Complications
• Abscess
• Emphysema – Fibrosis
• Amyloidosis

PC
1. Cough: haemoptysis
2. Chest pain: pleuritic
3. Systemic: fever, weight loss

O/E
1. Inspection: Cyanosed, Clubbed, Cachectic
2. Auscultatn: Creps – coarse
   Clicks – inspiratory
   Wheeze
3. Sputum: Copious, purulent, bloody (cf. CFA – dry)

Ix
1. Culture: Sputum, BronchoAlveolar Lavage
2. X-ray: i) CXR: 'Tram-tracks', cystic cavities
   ii) CT: 'Signet-ring sign' = Large bronchiole + paired vascular bundle:
3. Special: Ciliary function studies / sweat test / *Aspergillus* precipitins etc...

Rx
1. Physiotherapy: Chest wall percussion with head-down postural drainage
2. O$_2$, long-term: to prevent cor pulmonale
3. Medical: i) Bronchodilators
   ii) Mucolytics (DNase) – degrade DNA released from neutrophils
   iii) Rotating courses of antibiotics , with staphylococcal + pseudomonal cover
4. Surgical: i) Resection; ii) Artery embolization (for hemoptysis); iii) Lung transplant

Lung Abscess

Causes *Sputum tends to S.T.I.N.K. (due to anaerobes)*

1. Infection

Staphylococcus aureus:
Risk: • Post-Pneumonia, e.g. post-Influenza
       • Haematogenous, e.g. IVDU, CVP line

TB:
Upper zone ± 2ndary *Aspergillus* infection

Intestinal bacteria:
Organisms:
    • Anaerobes: *Bacteroides, Actinomyces*
    • Coliforms
    • Enterococcus
Risk:
    • Dental caries / pharyngeal abscess
    • Aspiration pneumonia
    • Liver abscess via diaphragm:
Strep. milleri (anaerobic), *Entamoeba*

Nocardia

Klebsiella

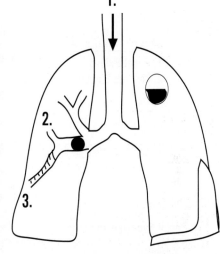

2. Bronchial Obstruction

Due to FB, tumour, lymph node
– mixed organisms

3. Host Defences ↓

AIDS, leukaemia,
chronic granulomatous disease

Location

Usually on R side,
as R bronchus is
shorter + more
vertical
(in the supine pt abscess develops
in apical lower lobe or posterior
upper lobe)

Complications

• **Empyema**
  If abscess
  progresses into
  interlobar fissures +
  pleural spaces

• **Broncho-Pleural
  Fistula:**
  Causes pyo-
  pneumothorax

PC   As for bronchiectasis   **O/E**   As for bronchiectasis +
Amphoric breathing = Breath sound,
                     like blowing over a jar, suggests air-fluid level

Ix   1. Culture – Sputum, blood, bronchoalveolar lavage
         2. X-ray: i) CXR (AP + lateral): cavity ± fluid-level
                   ii) CT

Rx   1. Physiotherapy
         2. Medical: IV benzylpenicillin + gentamicin + metronidazole
         3. Bronchoscopy: Repeated bronchoalveolar lavage
         4. Surgical: Resection

Cystic Fibrosis

<u>**Def**</u> Commonest **Autosomal Recessive** disease among Caucasians, caused by defective
Epithelial Chloride Channel (CFTR), resulting in excessively concentrated epithelial secretions.

PC

Nose – Sinuses
1. Nasal Polyps
2. Chronic Sinusitis

Lungs
1. **Recurrent Pneumonia**
   Staph. aureus; HiB; *Pseudomonas*, Burkholderia,
   aspergillosis; atypical mycobacteria / *E. coli*
2. **Bronchiectasis (asthma-like)**
   PC: Haemoptysis - 50%
   O/E: i) Clubbing, HPOA; ii) Wheeze / creps
   iii) ☠: abscess, fibrosis, emphysema, amyloidosis
3. **Atelectasis**: mucus plugging

Liver
1. **Portal Hypertension**
   due to
   - Periportal fibrosis (CAH)
   - Focal biliary cirrhosis
2. **Gallstones**

Bowel
1. **Meconium Ileus**
   in infants
2. **Meconium Ileus**
   Equivalent
   PC: i) Painful mass in RIF
   ii) Obstruction
   iii) Intussusception
3. **Rectal Prolapse**
   in children

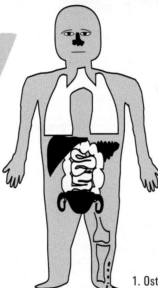

Pancreas
1. **Malabsorption**
   (exocrine):
   - diarrhoea
   - weight loss
2. **Diabetes mellitus**
   (endocrine): 30%

Other
1. Osteoporosis
2. Arthropathy
3. Rash, vasculitic

Sexual Organs
1. **Male Infertility**
   - Hypogonadism
   - Azoospermia
   - Vas deferens maldevelopment
2. **Female Infertility**
   Cervical mucus thickening
3. **Hazardous Pregnancy**

<u>Epi</u>

Inc: Carrier = 1/25 ; Disease = 1/2500 (in Caucasians)

Age: Neonatal presentation: meconium ileus; Guthrie heel-prick (serum trypsin ↑);
Childhood presentation: failure to thrive; asthma; diarrhoea

Sex: M:F = 1:1

Geo: Caucasians predominantly

Aet: **Law of 7s:**
1. Chromosome **7**p
2. **70**%: ΔF508 = Phenylalanine substitution or deletion
3. > **70** mmol/l: NaCl concentration in sweat test

Micro:

**Normal epithelial lumen,
e.g. pancreas, bronchus**

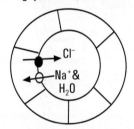

Cystic fibrosis

Cl⁻ channel (CFTR)
fails due to
• Intracellular
trafficking
defect
• Abnormal
functioning

Also:
Cl⁻ Influx ↓
⇒
NaHCO₃ and
Trypsin secretn ↓

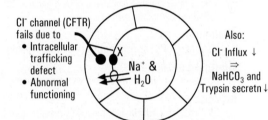

<u>Ix</u>

1. Sweat test: NaCl > **70** mmol/l (adults: > 90); fludrocortisone ↑ es sensitivity
2. Nasal transepithelial potential difference more negative than normal (< –35 mV)
3. Faecal elastase ↑

<u>Rx</u>

<u>Lungs</u>

1. Conservative: Physiotherapy (postural drainage), O₂, vaccinate
2. Medical: i) Mucolytic: DNase
    ii) Bronchodilators, inc. aminophylline; Steroids - for COAD
    iii) Antibiotics: e.g. flucloxacillin, piperacillin, gentamicin, ceftazidime,
        ciprofloxacin
3. Surgery: Lung Transplantation

<u>Liver</u>

1. Ursodeoxycholic acid
2. Injection sclerotherapy
3. Liver transplant

<u>Bowel</u>

1. Surgery

<u>Pancreas</u>

1. Oral pancreatin
2. Insulin

<u>Other</u>

1. Genetic counselling (screen family with gene probes)
2. Chorionic villous sampling for prenatal Dx, at 9–12 weeks
3. DEXA scan for osteoporosis; Rx with bisphosphonates

Pneumothorax

<u>Def</u> Accumulation of air in pleural space, with secondary partial collapse of lung

<u>Types</u> a) Closed = deficit reseals
b) Open = air moves in + out via broncho-pleural fistula, or traumatic external defect
c) Tension = air moves in, but not out, due to fistula or defect acting as one-way valve

<u>Causes</u> *S.T.R.I.P.*

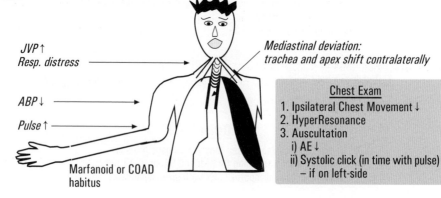

Spontaneous, associated with
a) **S**moking:
Causes bronchiolitis, peripheral hyperexpansion, subpleural bleb rupture
b) **S**tructural:
Congenital, apical bleb ruptures
Young, thin men (M:F = 6:1), esp. Marfan's syndrome
Recurrence common (unilateral): 25% if had one; 50% if had two
c) **S**udden aeroplane ascent
Trauma
blunt (e.g. CPR) or penetrating (e.g. stab wound)
Ruptured oesophagus
Boerhaave's syndrome (severe vomiting causing rupure) → hydropneumothorax
Iatrogenic
CVP line, esp. subclavian; positive-pressure ventilation; bronchoscopy, esp. w. biopsy
Pulmonary disease
a) Diffuse: • Obstructive: asthma, emphysema, bronchiectasis
• Restrictive: fibrosing alveolitis, sarcoid, rheumatoid arthritis, histiocytosis X
b) Focal: Infection, tumour, esp. secondaries, congenital

<u>PC</u> 1. Non-Tension: pain (sudden, pleuritic, radiates to shoulder); dry cough; SOB
2. Tension: acute respiratory distress; collapse; EMD

<u>O/E</u> *italicized signs are only present in tension pneumothorax*

JVP↑
Resp. distress

Mediastinal deviation:
trachea and apex shift contralaterally

ABP↓

Pulse↑

Marfanoid or COAD
habitus

Chest Exam
1. Ipsilateral Chest Movement ↓
2. HyperResonance
3. Auscultation
i) AE↓
ii) Systolic click (in time with pulse)
– if on left-side

Ix

1. CXR on expiration
   a) Translucency + collapse
      visible rim between lung and chest-wall > 2 cm $ = > 50\%$ lung volume loss
   b) Mediastinal shift
   c) Pneumomediastinum or surgical emphysema: air in local tissues
   d) Underlying lung disease
2. CT: distinguishes loculated pneumothorax from bullae

Rx

1. Small ($< 20\%$):
   Resorbs spontaneously $\longrightarrow$ Follow-up in 1–2 weeks

2. Large:
   a) Aspiration
      i) Remove < 2.5 litres or until resistance or excessive coughing
      ii) If 2.5 l reached and air is still readily evacuated, then suspect bronchopleural fistula
      iii) CXR after: if resolved, can be discharged; if not resolved, suspect bronchopleural fistula

   b) Intercostal drain:
      IND: Required if aspiration fails, or if severe (e.g. patient distressed, or in ITU)

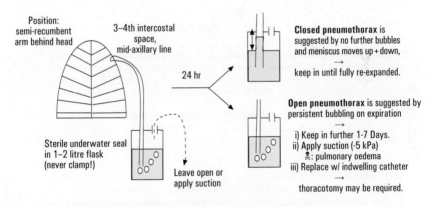

Position:
semi-recumbent
arm behind head

3–4th intercostal
space,
mid-axillary line

24 hr

Sterile underwater seal
in 1–2 litre flask
(never clamp!)

Leave open or
apply suction

Closed pneumothorax is
suggested by no further bubbles
and meniscus moves up + down,
$\longrightarrow$
keep in until fully re-expanded.

Open pneumothorax is suggested by
persistent bubbling on expiration
$\longrightarrow$
i) Keep in further 1-7 Days.
ii) Apply suction (-5 kPa)
☠: pulmonary oedema
iii) Replace w/ indwelling catheter
$\longrightarrow$
thoracotomy may be required.

3. Refractory or recurrent: lateral thoracotomy or thoracoscopy:
   IND: Required if no improvement with intercostal drain after 1 week, or if recurrent pneumothorax

   Method: i) Pleurodesis, e.g. tetracycline, bleomycin, talc injection
            ii) Pleural abrasion or pleurectomy
            iii) Bulla stapling or lasering

4. Tension pneumothorax
   a) Immediate insertion of wide-bore cannula into 2nd I/C sp. , mid clav. line (don't wait for CXR)
   b) Rapid insertion of chest drain

Pleural Effusion

Causes Categorized according to protein or LDH (lactate dehydrogenase) content of pleural fluid:

Transudate: redistribution of Starling forces across microcirculation (as for pulmo. oedema – p. 90)
protein < 30 g/l or pleural : serum protein $< \frac{1}{2}$ or pleural : serum LDH $< \frac{2}{3}$

Exudate: capillary permeability increases or lymph drainage decreases
protein > 30 g/l or pleural : serum protein $> \frac{1}{2}$ or pleural : serum LDH $> \frac{2}{3}$

C.H.E.S.T. I.N.S.U.L.A.T.I.O.N.

Transudate

Cardiac failure: LVF, RVF, pericardial effusion or constriction:
due to pulmonary (LVF) or bronchial (RVF) capillary hydrostatic pressure ↑

Hypoalbuminaemia – plasma oncotic pressure ↓ :
cirrhosis, nephrosis, malnutrition, malabsorption, protein-losing enteropathy (e.g. intestinal lymphangectasia):
- often R-sided effusion and concomitant ascites

Embolism, pulmonary: due to hydrostatic pressure redistribution

Superior vena cava obstruction (or inferior vena cava obstruction):
due to drainage of Bronchial Veins into SVC / IVC

Subclavian or jugular vein catheter misplacement with infusion of crystalloid, or
peritoneal dialysis in presence of congenital pleuro–peritoneal communication

Thyroid ↓ : due to myxoedema

Exudate

Infection: *Strep. pneumoniae, Mycoplasma*, TB, viruses (EBV, coxsackie), rheumatic fever:
may cause either a parapneumonic effusion or empyema (i.e. bacterial infection of pleural fluid)

Neoplasia: bronchial carcinoma, pleural mesothelioma or fibroma, breast, ovarian, lymphoma

Surgery or trauma: CABG, mastectomy, radiotherapy, lung contusion

Uraemia

Liver, pancreatic, ovarian disease:
subphrenic or hepatic abscess;
pancreatitis or pancreatic pseudocyst or carcinoma; pleural fluid amylase ↑
ovarian fibroma (Meigs' syndrome); ovarian hyperstimulation; pleural endometriosis

Autoimmune: SLE, rheumatoid arthritis, scleroderma, polyarteritis nodosa

Toxins: *B.A.N. M.E.* – **B**romocriptine, **A**miodarone, **N**itrofurantoin, **M**ethysergide, Environmental: asbestosis

Infarction: pulmonary (due to multiple PEs), myocardial (Dressler's syndrome)

Oesophageal rupture: pleural fluid amylase ↑

Nail syndrome, yellow: due to lymphatic hypoplasia, and also associated with pitting oedema and sinusitis

+ familial Mediterranean fever: periodic fever + pains in pleura, peritoneum and joints, due to pyrin mutation

PC

1. SOB, progressively worsening
2. Chest pain

O/E

1. Mediastinal shift contralaterally
   - Tracheal deviation
   - Apex beat displacement (if large)
2. Expansion ↓
3. Stony dullness
4. Absent AE

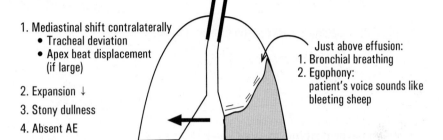

Just above effusion:
1. Bronchial breathing
2. Egophony:
   patient's voice sounds like bleeting sheep

Ix

Radiology
CXR: • Meniscus-shaped, rises towards axilla
  • Repeat after drainage to look for tumour / lymph nodes
USS: localizes small effusions, and allows their tapping
CT: allows underlying lung and mediastinum to be visualized

Pleural Fluid Aspiration
1. Appearance:
   a) Clear, straw-coloured: suggests transudate
   b) Turbid, green: indicates exudate (pus cells) or empyema (i.e. actual bacterial infection)
   c) Bloody (i.e. haemothorax) : tumour; pulmonary embolism; acute pancreatitis, trauma
   d) White (i.e. chylothorax = lymph): blocked thoracic duct, usually due to tumour
2. Analysis:
   a) Protein and LDH: determine whether transudate or exudate
      glucose: ↓ in most exudates
   b) Amylase: ↑ in pancreatitis, tumour, oesophageal rupture
   c) Microbiology, inc. AAFB staining and cultures
   d) Cytology

Rx

Underlying cause
Specific
1. Transudate: diuretics can result in rapid resolution
2. Exudate: • Repeated drainage (thoracocentesis): limit drainage rate to < 2 / 24 hr
   • Intrathoracic streptokinase via chest drain: lyses fibrinous adhesions
   • Pleural adhesion: tetracycline, bleomycin, talc
   • Decortication surgery

Pulmonary Oedema

Causes   May be classified in accordance with Starling's Forces:

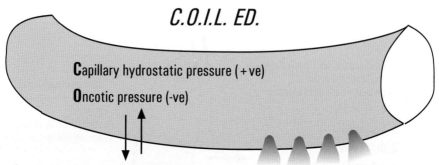

C.O.I.L. ED.

Capillary hydrostatic pressure (+ve)

Oncotic pressure (-ve)

Interstitial hydrostatic pressure (−ve)
    contributed to by alveolar air pressure   **ExuD**ate – Capillary permeability ↑

Lymph drainage (−ve)

Transudate

Capillary hydrostatic pressure ↑
  a) LVF
  b) PE
  c) Overhydration, e.g. with N.Saline

Oncotic pressure ↓
  a) Malnutrition, malabsorption, protein-losing enteropathy
  b) Cirrhosis
  c) Nephrosis

Interstitial negative hydrostatic pressure ↑
  a) Asthma: acute airway obstruction with high end-expiratory volume
        (more −ve pleural pressure required)
  b) Aspiration of pneumothorax or pleural effusion – if too rapid
  c) Altitude – unacclimatized athletes

Lymphatic drainage ↓
  a) Lymphangitis carcinomatosis
  b) Fibrosis, esp. secondary to silicosis
  c) Lung transplant

ExuDate

Capillary permeability ↑
  = A.R.D.S. (see opposite)
  Path: a) Diffuse endothelial + alveolar epithelial damage
      b) Acute inflammatory exudate: fibrin forms in airspaces ('hyaline membrane')
      c) Pulmonary thromboemboli

Adult Respiratory Distress Syndrome

<u>**Def**</u> Common inflammatory response to various lung insults, resulting in:

T.O.X.I.C.

Tachypnoea
Oxygen ↓ : progressive respiratory failure
X-Ray: bilateral pulmonary infiltrates
Interstitial fluid ↑
    1. Lung compliance (volume / pressure) ↓ ⇒ ∴ ↑ Positive End-Expiratory Pressure (PEEP) required
    2. V/Q mismatch: due to alveolar flooding + microvascular occlusion with platelets and neutrophils
    3. Fibrosis: > 4 weeks
Cardiac function is normal (i.e. normal left atrial pressure or PAWP)

<u>**Causes**</u>   *lungs get T.I.G.H.T. due to poor compliance*

Toxins: – Aspirated
           – Inhalation: smoke, paraquat, O_2
           – Systemic: opiates, barbiturates, anaesthesia, aspirin, heparin
Infection: – Pneumonia: bacterial, viral, PCP
             – Septicaemia, esp. acute pancreatitis
Gynaecological: Eclampsia, amniotic fluid embolism
Hypotension (shock): Hypovolaemic, anaphylaxis, anaesthesia /
                  massive transfusion, cardiopulmonary bypass,
                  cardioversion neurogenic: ICP ↑, e.g. SAH / status
Trauma: Lung contusion, DIC, fat embolism

<u>**Rx**</u> 1. Underlying cause
      e.g. antibiotics, pleural drainage
  2. Ventilation
    Aims: a) High PEEP: to recruit unused alveoli
           b) Low tidal volume: to avoid pneumothorax
           c) Low FiO_2 e.g. 0.6: to avoid O_2 toxicity + permissive hypercapnia
    ☠:   a) Pneumothorax: Due to high PEEP, high tidal volume, fibrosis
                  More apparent in lungs with near-normal compliance
        b) Nosocomial Infection: i) ventilator-assoc. pneumonia; ii) IV lines; iii) catheters
        c) Organ failure: i) Cardiac, renal, neuro: avoid by keeping tight fluid control
                    ii) GIT: enteral nutrition; H_2-antagonists, sucralfate
  3. Adjuvants
      a) Prone positioning: aerates better perfused dorsal lung segments
      b) Nitric oxide ± nebulized prostacyclin: vasodilate in vicinity of ventilated alveoli
      c) Corticosteroids: decrease fibrosis

Lung Carcinoma

PC + O/E   *Lung carcinoma may present at 4 different levels:*

1. Lung

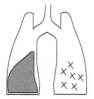

PC: a) SOB / cough (esp. haemoptysis) / chest pain
    b) Recurrent pneumonia

O/E: a) Quiet breath sounds
         tumour; lobar collapse; pleural effusion;
         elevatated hemidiaphragm (phrenic N. palsy)
     b) Crepitations:
         consolidation; bronchiectasis; (radiotherapy: fibrosis)
     c) Pneumothorax esp. pulmonary mets, e.g. osteosarcoma, Wilms'

2. Lymph nodes + Local compression

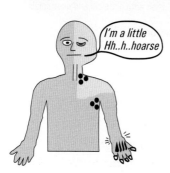

I'm a little Hh..h..hoarse

PC: a) Hoarseness: due to L recurrent laryngeal N. palsy
    b) Dysphagia, stridor

O/E a) Lymphadenopathy: supraclavicular, axillary
    b) Neuro: Pancoast tumour infiltrates T1 stellate ganglion →
         Horner's syn; wasting of intrinsic hand muscles; shoulder pain
    c) Hands: Clubbing; tender wrists = hypertrophic pulmonary
         osteoarthropathy; Hyperhidrosis; Tar Staining Fingers (smoker)
    d) Catastrophic:
       Superior vena cava obstruction (SVCO)
         PC: Headache, SOB
         O/E: Conjunctival oedema, plethora, vein dilatation
       Pericardial tamponade: JVP↑, ABP↓, Quiet HS

3. Metastases   *B.L.O.B.S*

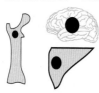

Bone pain
Liver, adrenal (Addison's)
Other lung, pleura, thoracic cage
Brain (stroke); spinal cord
Skin: slightly blue umbilicated lesions

4. Constitutional + Paraneoplastic

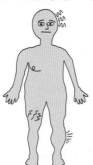

a) Constitutional:
    cachexia; leucoerythroblastic anaemia; immunocompromise, e.g. shingles

b) Neurological (assoc. with small–cell carcinoma):
    cerebellar degeneration; limbic encephalitis; peripheral neuropathy;
    dermatomyositis; Lambert–Eaton myasthenic syndrome

c) Endocrine: ectopic secretions (mostly assoc. with small cell ca.)
    ACTH: Cushing's; SIADH: confusion; β-HCG: gynaecomastia, body hair loss;
    PTHrp: hypercalcaemia (esp. squamous cell carcinoma)

d) Skin:
    dermatomyositis: acanthosis nigricans; erythema gyratum repens; pruritus
    (also radiotherapy marks; burns)

e) Hypercoagulable state (assoc. with adenocarcinoma)
    DVT, thrombophlebitis migrans, marantic endocarditis

<u>Types of lung neoplasia</u>

1°

1. Squamous Cell Carcinoma
Epi: 30% of all primary lung tumours, but decreasing incidence
Prog: relatively good prognosis if localized (5-yr survival rate ≈ 50%) – mets occur late
Histo: squamous metaplasia; keratin whorls
Xters: **C**entral location, **C**avitates, **C**lubbing (+HPOA); **C**alcium ↑(PTH-rp secretion)

2. Adenocarcinoma
Epi: 30%; increasing incidence, esp. women, less association with smoking
Prog: poor (1 year median survival) – metastases occur early
Histo: gland-like, mucin-secreting
Xters: peripheral location; pleural effusions; hypercoagulable state

3. Small cell carcinoma
Epi: 20%; strongest association with smoking
Prog: poor (1 year median survival) – metastases occur early
Histo: small APUD cells with neurosecretory granules; dark, oval nuclei, little cysts
Xters: central location; paraneoplastic syndromes common

4. Large cell carcinoma
Epi: 10%; Prog: poor – metastases occur early
Histo: giant cells; clear cells; anaplastic
Xters: Local invasion into mediastinum

5. Rare
a) Bronchoalveolar cell carcinoma
> Variant of adenocarcinoma that is associated with chronic lung inflammation, e.g. fibrosing alveolitis,
> rather than smoking. Prognosis relatively good
> Xters: Copious, clear mucoid sputum; SOB; recurrent bilateral pneumonia (cells carried in sputum)

b) Adenoma
> Majority are carcinoid tumours (APUDomas) that occur in young people and have good prognosis
> Xters: Haemoptysis, lobar collapse, wheeze; 2% develop carcinoid syndrome or acromegaly
> > Tumours occupy a central location, so often not visible

c) Hamartoma
> Benign tumour of older men, seen on CXR as a peripheral calcified mass, and consisting of disordered
> but differentiated smooth muscle and cartilage

2°

Breast
Oesophago/gastric/head – neck (+ colon if liver mets)
Melanoma
Bone, sarcomas
Endocrine: thyroid
Renal, prostate
Sex: ovary, choriocarcinoma, testes

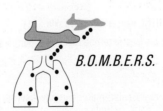

B.O.M.B.E.R.S.

<u>Rx</u>

a) **Non-Small Cell:** Surgical resection possible in a third. Adjuvant chemo/radiotherapy
b) **Small Cell:**   Radiotherapy + chemotherapy (etoposide + cisplatin)
            90% show limited regression

Obstructive Sleep Apnoea

Def

Obstruction: Obstruction of upper airway occurs at night with loss of muscle tone in sleep
Sleep: Sleep disruption, snoring, sleepiness during day
Apnoea: Apnoeic spells: O_2 ↓, patient awakes from sleep

Causes   *O.S.A.*

Obesity, central
a) The strongest risk factor for OSA is central obesity.
b) This is measured as Neck Circumference, and Waist/Hip Ratio (rather than Body Mass Index)
c) Pathogenesis: • Fat deposition around upper airway → airway narrowing and resistance ↑
                     • Abdominal fat → elevates diaphragm

Structural features of upper airway

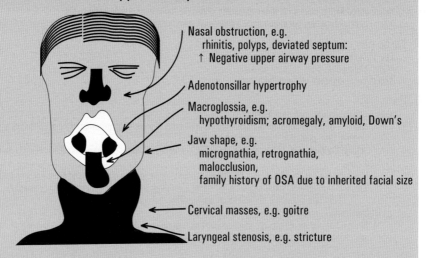

Nasal obstruction, e.g.
rhinitis, polyps, deviated septum:
↑ Negative upper airway pressure

Adenotonsillar hypertrophy

Macroglossia, e.g.
hypothyroidism; acromegaly, amyloid, Down's

Jaw shape, e.g.
micrognathia, retrognathia,
malocclusion,
family history of OSA due to inherited facial size

Cervical masses, e.g. goitre

Laryngeal stenosis, e.g. stricture

Smoking: exacerbates hypoxia
Sex: male (testosterone reduces upper airway tone)

Atony:
a) Neuromuscular: motor neurone disease, myopathy, myotonic dystrophy
b) CNS: CVA, multiple systems atrophy, encephalitis
c) Connective tissue laxity: Marfan's syndrome (also because of high-arched palate)

Alcohol: Acts as a sedative thereby reducing upper airway tone
            (same for anaesthetics, benzodiazepines)

PC

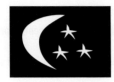

Nocturnal Sx.

1. Obstruction and apnoea
   - Snoring, choking, gasping
   - Awakening with nocturia
   - Uvula and soft palate appear red and oedematous from heavy snoring
2. Gastro-oesophageal reflux

Daytime Sx.

1. Morning headache
2. Daytime somnolence
3. Memory + attention ↓
   ⇒ accident risk!
4. Irritability, Depression

Complications

1. Cyanosis → polycythaemia
2. Systemic hypertension:
   (loss of normal nocturnal dipping)
3. Pulmonary hypertension: late
   (2° to chronic hypoxia)
   → cor pulmonale

Ix

Bloods: i) Causes: TFTs: hypothyroidism; LFTs: alcoholism
ii) Effects: Hb ↑; ABG: CO_2 ↑
Urine: Glucose (Type II DM assoc with obesity)
Monitor: Overnight oximetry
ECG: R sided strain
Radio: CXR: Cardiomegaly
Special: Polysomnography (overnight sleep study) –
i) Apnoea–Hypopnea Index: > 5/hr abnormal (except elderly)
ii) O_2 dipping: titrate nasal CPAP to ↑O_2
iii) EEG: categorizes apnoea as REM or NREM sleep predominant

Rx

1. Conservative: i) Weight loss
   ii) Avoid smoking, alcohol, sedatives
   iii) Sleep: Avoid supine position and sleep deprivation
2. CPAP (Continuous Positive Airway Pressure)
   Method: 4–20 cm H_2O for > 4 hr per night, via nasal mask, maintains upper airway patency
   Benefits: Reverses daytime Sx (inc. accidents); prevents complications; MR ↓
   Side Effects: Poor compliance due to encumberance; skin ulceration; rhinorrhoea, epistaxis; aerophagia
3. MAD (Mandibular Advancement Device):
   = Intra-oral device that ↑ A-P diameter of upper airway → ↓ Snoring + Apnoea
4. Surgery:
   i) Adenoidectomy (curative in children); ii) Uvulopalatopharyngoplasty (50% benefit);
   iii) Maxillomandibular osteotomy; iv) Tracheostomy if CPAP-intolerant

Pulmonary Embolism

Path a) Embolus originates from deep-vein thrombosis in proximal leg or iliac veins (peri-operative), renal vein or IVC (renal or pelvic tumour), or cerebral venous or SVC thrombosis.

b) Thrombosis gets dislodged following Valsalva manoeuvre, e.g. straining on stool.

c) Ultimately due to an underlying prothrombotic state, e.g. immobility, oral contraceptive pill.

Types PE may be classified according to size, with different pathologies and presentations for each:

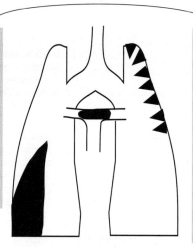

Small – Medium

Path:
1. Infarction
2. Haemorrhage

PC:
1. Pleuritic pain
2. Haemoptysis
3. Acute SOB

O/E:
1. Fever, low-grade
2. Tachycardia (inc. AF)
3. Pleural rub, wheeze

Multiple

Path:
1. Widespread infarction
2. Pulmonary hypertension

PC:
1. Cough, wheeze
2. Progressive SOB, due to subacute right-sided heart failure

O/E:
1. Respiratory distress, cyanosis
2. Pulmonary hypertension: JVP ↑, gallop rhythm (S3), loud P2

Large

Path: Pulmonary insufficiency due to occlusion of pulmonary trunk or main artery

PC: 1. Acute right-sided heart failure
2. Collapse, EMD, sudden death

Ix

Bloods: 1. ABGs: i) O_2 ↓; ii) CO_2 ↓; pH ↑ but ABGs may be entirely normal
2. D-Dimers (ELISA): 90% sensitive, but poor specificity (false +ves: MI, pneumonia)

ECG: 1. Sinus tachy., AF; 2. SI-QIII-TIII (R axis deviation); 3. R sided strain; R bundle branch block

Radio:
1. CXR: i) Normal; ii) Vascular markings or focal oligaemia; iii) Wedge-shaped infarct;
iv) linear atelectasis; v) small pleural effusion
2. V/Q isotope scan:
i) Ventilation phase = xenon or krypton; perfusion phase = IV albumin
ii) +ve = V/Q mismatch (cf. pneumonia: matched deficits)
iii) 50% sensitive, 90% specific
3. Spiral CT / MRA: sensitive for medium-large PE (ultimately, angiography may be needed)

Special:
1. Establish underlying cause: Doppler USS thigh, pelvis (+ve in 2/3); thrombophilia screen
2. ECHO: sensitive for pulmonary hypertension; large PE

Rx

WARN ITU
if any life-threatening
features

B. Ventilatory Support

1. Lie patient down: aids venous
   return
2. Oxygen: 100%
3. Intubate / IPPV → ITU
   (☠: hypotension with
   sedation)

C. Hydration

N. Saline, to avoid
hypotension

D. Medication

1. Analgesia
   i) Oral NSAID
   ii) Diamorphine + cyclizine
   (☠: hypotension)

2. Anti-coagulation:
   Mild–Moderate:
   LMW heparin, e.g. dalteparin
   10,000 units SC od
   (weight-adjusted)
   Severe:
   tPA or streptokinase via
   pulmonary artery catheter

3. Dobutamine if cardiogenic
   shock

A. Assessment

1. A.B.C.D.

2. C.O.A.T.

Cardiac Monitor
O_2
ABP
TPR

3. Investigations

See opposite

On discharge

Warfarin (INR 2–3)

Continue for 6 months, or
longer if recurrent; or
prothrombotic tendency

Surgery

Thrombendarterectomy
if life-threatening

Radiology

Inferior vena cava filter

IND: recurrent or chronic PE
☠ i) Recurrent PE
ii) IVC occlusion;
leg + genital oedema

Pulmonary Hypertension

Causes

Pulmonary Disease

1. **Cor Pulmonale:**
   Def: lung disease causes hypoxia and therefore pulmonary vasoconstriction,
   and eventually right ventricular hypertrophy and failure
   Examples: COAD, pulmonary fibrosis, obstructive sleep apnoea
2. **Recurrent PE**
3. **Primary pulmonary hypertension**
   Epi: rare (2 / million p.a.), middle-aged women (30–50s)
   Aet: i) Autoimmune ?
   ii) Genetic • 20% autosomal dominant
   • BMPR II (bone morphogenetic protein receptor)

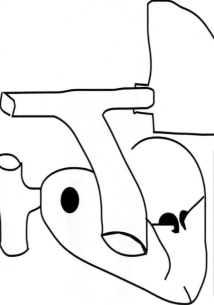

Systemic
1. **Autoimmune:**
   SLE, scleroderma
2. **Infection:**
   HIV
3. **Drugs:**
   dexfenfluoramine
   (amphetamine)

Mitral valve disease
Stenosis or regurgitation
O/E; pulmonary regurgitation
murmur
(GrahaM Steel murmur,
i.e. secondary to
Mitral Stenosis)

L-to-R shunt
(Eisenmenger's syndrome)

Path

Primary pulmonary hypertension and systemic causes are characterized by medial hypertrophy, concentric fibrosis, thrombosis and vascoconstriction of arterioles and venules.

PC

1. SOBOE – worsens with right ventricular failure
2. Syncope
3. Angina or myocardial infarction (right ventricle)

O/E

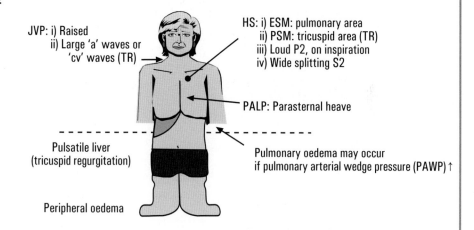

JVP: i) Raised
ii) Large 'a' waves or
'cv' waves (TR)

HS: i) ESM: pulmonary area
ii) PSM: tricuspid area (TR)
iii) Loud P2, on inspiration
iv) Wide splitting S2

PALP: Parasternal heave

Pulsatile liver
(tricuspid regurgitation)

Pulmonary oedema may occur
if pulmonary arterial wedge pressure (PAWP) ↑

Peripheral oedema

Ix

Bloods: 1. ABG: O_2↓ CO_2↓ ; respiratory alkalosis
ECG: 1. Sinus tachy., AF; 2. SI-QIII-TIII (R axis deviation); 3. R sided strain; R bundle-branch block
Radio: 1. CXR: large pulmonary arteries; clear lung fields
2. V/Q isotope scan: diffuse patchy filling defects (non-segmental, cf. PE = segmental)
3. Angio: risk of bradycardia (give atropine)
Special lung function tests – Mild restrictive picture; KCO ↓

Rx

1. Conservative: Avoid exercise
2. Drugs: a) Diuretics
b) Warfarin (INR 1.5 - 2.5)
c) Vasodilators: • nifedipine, diltiazem
• IV prostacyclin via indwelling central venous catheter:
☠: tolerance (need continuous dose titration);
flushing , jaw or headache, diarrhoea, hypotension, angina
3. Bilateral lung (± heart) transplantation

Prognosis

Survival: 3 years from diagnosis; 6 months from symptomatic heart failure (grade IV)

Gastroenterology

Abdominal Pain

<u>**Causes**</u>   *Abdominal pain has the P.O.T.E.N.T.I.A.L. for being serious*

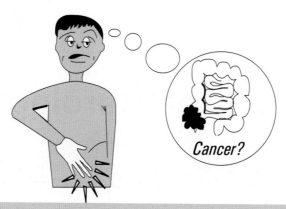

Cancer?

Peritonitis / **P**erforation (see opposite)
   Path: Inflammation of viscus with extension to local peritoneum
   PC: Constant, worsened by movement, patient tends to lie down and shallow breathe

Obstruction / c**O**lic (see opposite)
   Path: Colic suggests excessive contraction of viscus, e.g. due to obstruction or infection
   PC: Waxes and wanes, patient tends to writhe and move around

Toxins
   a) Food poisoning
   b) Drugs, e.g. opioid addiction, antibiotics, anticholinesterases; radiotherapy
   c) Poisons: chronic lead poisoning, black widow spider bite

Endocrine crises
   a) Diabetic ketoacidosis
   b) Addison's
   c) Hypermetabolic state: thyrotoxicosis, phaeochromocytoma, carcinoid

Neuro-psychiatric
   a) Functional: Irritable bowel, anxiety, conversion disorder, Munchausen's syndrome
   b) Radiculopathy: shingles; spondylosis. N.B. dermatomal pattern and hyperaesthesia
   c) Syphilis – 'tabetic crisis'

Thoracic origin (referred pain)
   Basal pneumonia, pulmonary embolism; myocardial infarction; pericarditis; thoracic radiculitis

Inherited
   a) Acute porphyria – colic
   b) C'1-esterase inhibitor deficiency: hereditary angioedema
   c) Familial Mediterranean Fever

Abdominal wall
   Rectus sheath haematoma (e.g. over-anticoagulation); myositis
   N.B. worsened by lifting head off pillow

Labour / abortion or other gynaecological disorder

Peritonitis

PC: a) Localized peritonitis: constant localized pain, worsened by movement, patient tends to lie down and shallow-breathe.
e.g. appendicitis: umbilical $\longrightarrow$ RIF pain, constipation, later faeculent vomiting (generalized peritonitis)
b) Sub-diaphragmatic: L shoulder-tip pain
c) Retroperitoneal origin: vague localization or back pain; patient tends to sit up or move around

O/E: • Inspection: scaphoid-like abdomen (concave); distended – perforation or generalized peritonitis;
flexed leg – retrocaecal appendicitis; Hippocratic facies (cold, moist, cyanosed) – generalized
• Palpation: abdominal rigidity; guarding (involuntary abdominal wall contraction); rebound (pain on release);
Murphy's sign (tenderness on inspiration); pain per rectum – retrocaecal appendicitis
• Auscultation: absent bowel sounds (paralytic ileus)

Ix: Erect CXR (air under diaphragm with oesophageal – bowel rupture); USS – free fluid in peritoneum or bowel

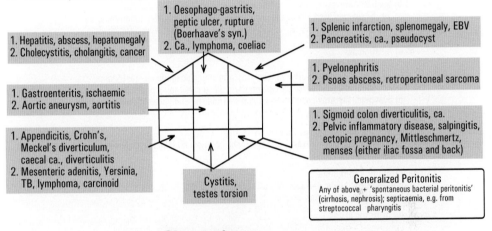

1. Oesophago-gastritis,
   peptic ulcer, rupture
   (Boerhaave's syn.)
2. Ca., lymphoma, coeliac

1. Hepatitis, abscess, hepatomegaly
2. Cholecystitis, cholangitis, cancer

1. Splenic infarction, splenomegaly, EBV
2. Pancreatitis, ca., pseudocyst

1. Pyelonephritis
2. Psoas abscess, retroperitoneal sarcoma

1. Gastroenteritis, ischaemic
2. Aortic aneurysm, aortitis

1. Sigmoid colon diverticulitis, ca.
2. Pelvic inflammatory disease, salpingitis,
   ectopic pregnancy, Mittleschmertz,
   menses (either iliac fossa and back)

1. Appendicitis, Crohn's,
   Meckel's diverticulum,
   caecal ca., diverticulitis
2. Mesenteric adenitis, Yersinia,
   TB, lymphoma, carcinoid

Cystitis,
testes torsion

Generalized Peritonitis
Any of above + 'spontaneous bacterial peritonitis'
(cirrhosis, nephrosis); septicaemia, e.g. from
streptococcal pharyngitis

Obstruction

1. Bowel

Mechanical

PC: a) Colic:
  • Umbilical: small bowel
  • Lower half; lumbar: large bowel
b) Constipation + vomit
c) May progress to bowel infarction
   and/or perforation, with peritonitis
O/E: a) Abdominal distension
b) Tinkling bowel sounds
c) Hyperperistaltic movements

Paralytic
PC: Constipation + vomit only
O/E: Absent bowel sounds

V.A.N.I.S.H.I.N.G. P.O.O. (i.e. constipated!)

Volvulus
Adhesions 2° to peritonitis, surgery
Neoplasia
Inflammation: Crohn's, ischaemia, diverticulitis
Strangulated **H**ernia
Intussusception: Meckel's diverticulum, polyp
Neonatal: imperforate anus
Gallstone ileus; faecal bolus, FB, bezoar

Pseudo-**O**bstruction: reflex atony:
post-surgery; trauma; retroperitoneal haematoma

2. Biliary: Cause: Calculi, ca. PC: colicky or constant; epigastric $\longrightarrow$ upper lumbar

3. Renal–bladder: Cause: Calculi, ca.
PC: Constant but migrates: loin $\longrightarrow$ flank $\longrightarrow$ suprapubic $\longrightarrow$ perineum

Diarrhoea

Def 1. Reduction in stool consistency: essential
2. > 3x bowel opening per day, or > 250 g stool per day: not essential

Causes   *S.O.I.L.I.N.G.S.*

Secretory – diarrhoea persists with fasting
   1. Infection:
     a) Food poisoning (toxin or organism pre-formed within food):
       • Toxin-mediated: *Staph. aureus, Clostridium perfringens*
       • Inflammation: *Salmonella, Camplylobacter*
     b) Gastroenteritis (i.e. organism colonizes and multiplies within bowel):
       • Toxin-mediated: cholera, *E. coli* (enterotoxigenic: traveller's diarrhoea)
       • Inflammation: *Shigella, E. coli* (enteroinvasive), *Clostridium difficile*, viral
   2. Endocrine:
     a) APUDomas:
       • Carcinoid
       • Islet-cell tumour (VIPoma, somatostatinoma, glucagonoma, gastrinoma)
       • Endocrine: medullary carcinoma thyroid (via calcitonin), phaeochromocytoma
     b) Systemic: thyrotoxicosis, hypoadrenalism (Addison's), hypopituitarism

Osmotic
   1. Malabsorption – diarrhoea relieved by fasting
     Causes: i) Wall disease; ii) Bile salt malabsorption; iii) Pancreatic disease
   2. Haemorrhage into bowel

Inflammation or **I**schaemia
   1. Inflammatory bowel disease: ulcerative colitis, Crohn's, microscopic colitis
   2. Ischaemia, inc. vasculitis

Laxatives or other drugs
   1. Laxatives: • Secretory: phenolphthalein-containing, e.g. senna, bisacodyl
             • Osmotic: Na, Mg or anion-containing
   2. Antibiotics, esp. erythromycin; prokinetics
   3. Radiation

Irritable bowel syndrome
   Rome criteria: a) Abdo–rectal pain: relieved by defaecation, radiates to thighs+back, bloating
              b) Stool frequency: > 3x/day or < 3/week
              c) Stool form: hard pellets, watery, mucus
              Exclusion criteria: onset > 40 yrs; bloody stool; wt loss, + normal sigmoidoscopy

Neuropathy, autonomic e.g. diabetes; multiple sclerosis

Gastrectomy + other surgery
   • Short-bowel syndrome: extensive bowel resection; dumping syndrome: gastrectomy
   • Fistulae, e.g. jejuno–ileal bypass; anal sphincter disturbance

Structural
   Rectal adenoma, neoplasia, diverticular disease

Special
   1. Alcohol, dietary indiscretion
   2. Overflow – faecal impaction

<u>Constipation</u>

<u>**Def**</u> 1. Bowel opening < 3x per week
2. Straining during defaecation > 25%

<u>**Causes**</u>   *O.P.E.N. I.T. W.I.D.E.*

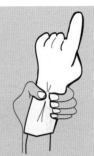

Obstruction
    a) Mechanical (colic) – see p. 103:
        volvulus, adhesions, neoplasia, inflammation, strangulated hernia,
        intussusception, gallstone ileus
    b) Pseudo-obstruction (reflex atony), e.g. post-surgery

Pain
    Anal fissure; 3° piles

Endocrine / **E**lectrolytes
    1. Endocrine: $T_4\downarrow$, DM (DKA, $\downarrow$gastrocolic reflex)
    2. Electrolytes: $Ca\downarrow$, $K\downarrow$, uraemia

Neurological
    1. Brain: PD, CVA, MS
    2. Spine: myelopathy, cauda equina, sacral plexopathy
    3. Neuropathy: botulism, Hirschsprung's disease, Chagas' disease (*Trypanasoma cruzi* – S.America)

Inflammation or Ischaemia
    IBD or diverticulitis, or ischaemia

Toxins
    Opioids, anticholinergics, nicotine (ganglion blocker), aluminium salt (antacid), iron

Wall disease
    Systemic sclerosis or visceral myopathy

Irritable bowel syndrome
    Or other functional: disobeying call to stool, depression, idiopathic megarectum or megacolon

Diet or **D**ehydration
    Inadequate roughage, diuretics, starvation

Elderly, pregnancy

<u>**Rx**</u> 1. Underlying cause
2. Laxatives: *B.O.S.S.E.S.*

    Bulking: faecal mass $\uparrow \longrightarrow$ peristalsis $\uparrow$: bran, ispaghula husk, methylcellulose
    Osmotic: fluidity of faeces $\uparrow$: lactulose (also probiotic), $MgSO_4$
    Stimulant: GIT motility and secretion $\uparrow$: senna, bisacodyl, dioctyl; ☠ colic, carcinoma ?
    Softeners: liquid paraffin
    Enemas: osmotic: PO_4, Na citrate; stimulant: Na picosulphate softener: arachis oil
    Suppositories: stimulant: glycerol

Nausea and Vomiting

Causes   *Too many G.I.N. & T.O.N.I.C.S.*

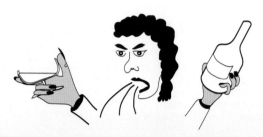

Gastrointestinal: Gastro-oesophageal: reflux, ulcer, pyloric stenosis
Pancreatic, liver, gall bladder disease
Obstruction
Peritonitis

Infection: GIT: gastroenteritis; hepatitis; visceral abscess
Systemic: RTI (esp. tonsillitis, otitis media); UTI; septicaemia

Neoplasia: GIT: oesophago–gastric–duodenal carcinoma; lymphoma; amyloid
Other: hypernephroma; hepatoma; ovarian
Paraneoplastic

Toxins: Chemotherapy, opioids
Antibiotics, aminophylline, antiarrhythmics (esp. digoxin), L-DOPA
Alcohol

Obstetric: Pregnancy

Ophthalmic: Acute closed-angle glaucoma

Neurology: Labyrinthitis, Ménière's, brainstem–cerebellar disease, e.g. MS
ICP ↑; meningo-encephalitis; tabetic crisis
Migraine; vasovagal syncope
Autonomic neuropathy: diabetes, acute intermittent porphyria
Psychiatric: bulimia or anorexia nervosa, psychogenic

Infarction   Myocardial - esp. posterior, transmural

Calcium ↑ / endocrine dysfunction:
DKA gastroparesis
Addison's crisis
Thyrotoxicosis

Systemic: Respiratory failure: acidosis
Cardiac failure, esp. right-sided: bowel oedema
Renal or liver failure: uraemia

Physiology

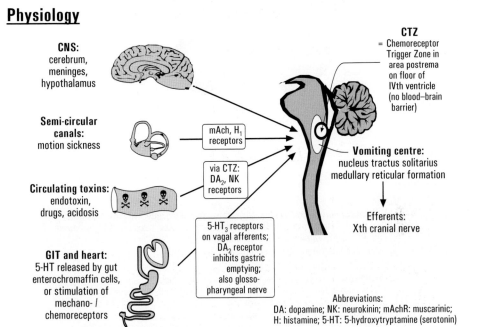

CNS:
cerebrum,
meninges,
hypothalamus

Semi-circular canals:
motion sickness

Circulating toxins:
endotoxin,
drugs, acidosis

GIT and heart:
5-HT released by gut
enterochromaffin cells,
or stimulation of
mechano- /
chemoreceptors

mAch, H₁ receptors

via CTZ:
DA₂, NK
receptors

5-HT₃ receptors
on vagal afferents;
DA₂ receptor
inhibits gastric
emptying;
also glosso-
pharyngeal nerve

CTZ
= Chemoreceptor
Trigger Zone in
area postrema
on floor of
IVth ventricle
(no blood–brain
barrier)

Vomiting centre:
nucleus tractus solitarius
medullary reticular formation

Efferents:
Xth cranial nerve

Abbreviations:
DA: dopamine; NK: neurokinin; mAchR: muscarinic;
H: histamine; 5-HT: 5-hydroxytryptamine (serotonin)

Rx

1. Underlying cause
2. Supportive: hydration (PO/IV), NaCl replacement
3. Anti-emetics: select according to receptor-type relevant to cause

A.1.2.3.

Muscarinic (Ach**) receptor antagonist:** hyoscine
 Indication: motion sickness, GIT causes
 ☠ : Sedation, dry mouth

Histamine type 1 receptor antagonist: cyclizine, cinnarizine, promethazine
 Indication: motion sickness, GIT, cardiac causes
 ☠ : Sedation, other anti-cholinergic side-effects

Dopamine type 2 receptor antagonist: metoclopramide, domperidone
 Indication: most causes, esp. gastro-oesophageal reflux (as pro-motility effect)
 ☠ : Sedation, extrapyramidal reactions (less likely with domperidone), diarrrhoea

5-HT type 3 receptor antagonist: ondansetron, granisetron
 Indication: most causes, esp. chemotherapy, post-surgery, neoplasia, MS
 ☠ : Headache, constipation

Others: • Steroids - for neoplasia
 • Nabilone (cannibinoid – acts on opiate receptors) – for chemotherapy, MS

Sore Throat

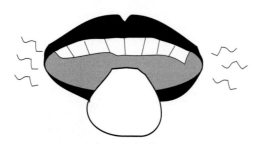

Causes

I.N.T.E.R.N.A.L.S.

Infection

1. Viral
a) Influenza or coryza (coronavirus, adenovirus, rhinovirus, enteroviruses, coxsackie)
b) Exanthems: rubella; measles; hand, foot and mouth disease: coxsackie A16, enterovirus 71
c) EBV: PC: pearly-white exudate + palatal petechiae
d) Other: parainfluenza, croup, haemorrhagic fever

2. Bacterial – localized
a) *Streptococcus pyogenes* (β-haemolytic; Lancefield group A);
    also causes tonsillitis and quinsy (peritonsillar abscess), and rheumatic fever
b) *Staphylococcus aureus*: facial erysipelas
c) *Haemophilus influenzae* type b – epiglottitis
d) Anaerobes: *Fusobacterium necrophorum* (necrobacillosis): Lemierre's disease;
    also causes jugular thrombophlebitis; lung and brain abscesses

3. Bacterial – general
a) Pneumonia: *Streptococcus pneumoniae*, *Mycoplasma*, *Chlamydia*, tularaemia, brucellosis
b) GIT: typhoid, leptospirosis
c) STD: gonorrhoea, 2° syphilis
d) Neurological:
    • Diphtheria (bull neck, stridor, brassy cough, palatal weakness, myocarditis)
    • Meningococcus, listeriosis (associated meningitis)

4. Fungal: oral candidiasis

Neoplasia
Carcinoma of oral cavity or pharynx

Toxins
1. Smoking, alcohol, pollution, e.g. H_2S
2. Drugs: thionamides (carbimazole, propylthiouracil) due to neutropenia; lamotrigine

Exogenous: radiotherapy-induced mucositis

Reflux, gastro-oesophageal

Nutritional
Vit B12, folate, iron deficiency – cause mucositis, glossitis, cheilitis

Autoimmune
Sjögren's syndrome: dry mouth

Long styloid process: chronic sore throat in children

Sinusitis, chronic: post-nasal drip

<u>Oral Ulceration</u>

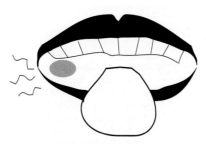

Causes   *I.N.T.E.R.N.A.L.*

Infection
1. Viral
a) Herpangina: enterovirus, coxsackie, echovirus – children
b) Herpes: HSV-1 (acute gingivostomatitis or recurrent); VZV; EBV
c) HIV: acute gingivitis, ulceration; glandular fever-like illness

2. Bacterial
a) TB: tip-of-tongue ulcers
b) STD: • Gonorrhoea
  • Syphilis (1°–chancre; 2°–snail-track ulcer; tongue; 3°–gumma)
c) Anaerobic:
  • Vincent's angina = symbiosis of Borrelia vincentii + Bacteroides
  • Actinomycoses: assoc. with tooth extraction or jaw fracture:
    inspection reveals yellow sulphur granules

3. Fungal
Histoplasmosis: ulcerative nodules, laryngitis, fever

Neoplasia
Carcinoma of oral cavity – raised edge

Toxins
1. Sulphonamides, chloramphenicol, cytotoxics: neutropenia
2. Stevens–Johnson syndrome, erythema multiforme

Exogenous: Trauma/dentures

Recurrent aphthous ulceration
Epi: 20% lifetime incidence; assoc. with stress, menses
PC: Painful, single or cluster of ulcers with grey base and red surround
Types: minor (1–5 mm); major (5–15 mm); herpetiform (200 x 1 mm)

Nutritional
1. Haematinics: Vit B, folate, Fe deficiency
2. Vit C deficiency
3. Malabsorption, e.g. coeliac

Autoimmune
Most are aphthous ulcers (i.e. painful, gray base, red surround)
1. Behçet'syn.: orogenital ulceration + anterior uveitis + arthritis
2. SLE
3. Seronegative arthropathies: IBD (esp. Crohn's); Reiter's syndrome
4. Pemphigus (ruptured bullae); pemphigoid (bullae); lichen planus (white striae)

Leukaemia, acute: esp. AMML, 2° to neutropenia

Dysphagia

Causes

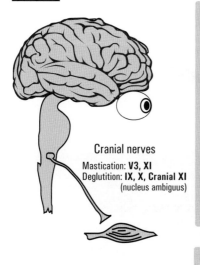

Cranial nerves

Mastication: **V3, XI**
Deglutition: **IX, X, Cranial XI**
(nucleus ambiguus)

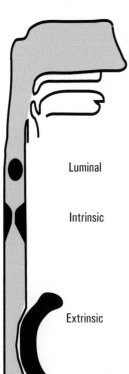

Luminal

Intrinsic

Extrinsic

Neuromuscular

Central
1. CVA: extensive small-vessel disease
2. Parkinson's, esp. progressive supranuclear palsy
3. Psychiatric 'globus pharyngeus'

Bulbar palsy (lower motor neurone)
1. Brainstem: syringobulbia, infarction (lateral medullary syn), MS
2. Motor neurone disease (partially upper-motor neurone), polio
3. Peripheral autonomic neuropathy:
    diphtheria, GBS, Chagas' disease

Muscular/myenteric plexus
1. NMJ: myasthenia, botulisim
2. Myopathy
3. Ganglion/peristalsis dysfunction:
    a) Scleroderma/C.R.E.S.T.
    b) Spasm: lower oesophageal (achalasia) or diffuse

Oral

Pharyngitis and oral ulcers cause painful swallowing
(odynophagia) with secondary dysphagia

Pharynx–oesophagus

Luminal
Foreign body, large bolus

Intrinsic
1. Upper:
    a) Pharyngeal pouch
    b) Post-cricoid web
2. Middle:
    a) Oesophagitis
    b) Oesophageal stricture
    c) Oesophageal carcinoma
3. Lower:
    a) Hiatus hernia
    b) Schatzki ring

Extrinsic
B.U.L.G.I.N.'
Bone: cervical spondylosis
U: dysphagia **LU**soria: vascular compression:
    aberrant R subclavian artery, aortic aneurysm,
    mitral stenosis (enlarged left atrium)
Lymphadenopathy
Goitre
Infection: retropharyngeal abscess
Neoplasia: pancreatic cancer

PC

Neuromuscular
1. Solids = liquids; nasal regurgitation
2. Aspiration occurs while attempting to swallow
3. Other: diplopia, ataxia

Oral
Odynophagia

Pharynx – oesophagus
1. Solids > liquids
2. Aspiration unrelated to swallowing
3. Other: chest pain; dyspepsia, hiccups (lower oesophagus)

O/E

Neuromuscular
Other neurological deficits e.g. ataxia, dysarthria, Horner's syndrome

Oral
Erythema, apthous ulcers, candida

Pharynx–oesophagus
1. Hoarse:
   - Laryngitis (gastro-oesophageal reflux)
   - Left recurrent laryngeal nerve palsy (carcinoma, lymph nodes)
2. Respiratory Sx:
   Right middle lobe consolidation (aspiration pneumonia);
   unilateral wheeze (main bronchus compression)

Ix

Neuromuscular
Videofluoroscopy: identifies weakness or incoordination

Pharynx–oesophagus
1. Barium swallow
2. OGD
3. Oesophageal motility + manometry studies

Specific causes

Neuromuscular
1. Psychiatric 'globus pharyngeus'
   - Pt. feels lump in throat at level of cricoid
   - Middle-aged female, depression
2. Achalasia: chest pain

Pharynx–oesophagus
1. Pharyngeal pouch: elderly
2. Post-cricoid web:
   occurs as part of Plummer–Vinson or Paterson–Brown–Kelly syndrome, also characterized
   by Fe-deficiency anaemia, koilonychia, glossitis, and risk of squamous cell carcinoma

Haematemesis

Causes

V.I.N.T.A.G.E.

Varices

Inflammation: Oesophago–gastro-duodenitis or peptic ulcer; PC: coffee-grounds vomit

Neoplasia: Oesophageal or gastric (carcinoma, polyp, leiomyoma, Menetrier's disease)

Trauma
  1. Mallory–Weiss tear
      • Mucosal break < 2 cm proximal to gastro-oesophageal junction
      • Due to forceful vomiting, esp. males drinking alcohol
  2. Surgery, ERCP (haemobilia), aorto-duodenal fistula, $2°$ aortic aneurysm / repair
  3. Hypovolaemic shock: ischaemic, stress ulcer in stomach

Angiodysplasia + other vascular anomalies
  1. Angiodysplasia
      Dilated vessel complexes in *clusters*
  2. Hereditary haemorrhagic telangiectasia
      • Dilated vessels over *entire* bowel wall
      • Autosomal dominant: endoglin mutation (TGF-receptor on endothelium)
      • PC: haematemesis, haemoptysis (pulmonary AVM), cerebral abscess, epistaxis
  3. Other
      • Dieulafoy lesion = protruding large submucosal vessel
      • Watermelon stomach = gastric antral vascular ectasia
      • Vasculitis, e.g. PAN

Generalized bleeding disorder
  1. Connective tissue defects: Ehlers–Danlos syndrome; pseudoxanthoma elasticum
  2. Coagulopathy, e.g. chronic renal failure, warfarin

Epistaxis; or
  Dental; oropharynx; epistaxis or haemoptysis (swallowed blood)

Exogenous
  Factitious

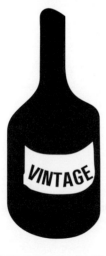

Ix for any GIT bleeding

Bloods
  1. U+E: urea $\uparrow\uparrow$ with upper GIT lesion; ARF
  2. FBC: chronic or acute
  3. Clotting times
      + group + save + X-match as appropriate

Radiology
  1. Barium enema $\pm$ follow-through
  2. Tc-labelling: (detects bleeding > 0.5 ml/min):
      colloid / autologous RBCs
  3. Selective mesenteric angiogram

Special
  1. Endoscopy: needs good bowel prep. (e.g. PO_4 enema)
  2. Laparotomy; investigative ileo-/colostomy

Rectal Bleeding

Causes   *D.R.I.P.P.I.N.G. T.A.P.S.*

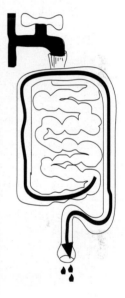

Diverticulae
    1. Colonic: diverticular disease
        PC: Pellety stool, pain, pr bleeding + diarrhoea
    2. Ileal: Meckel's diverticulum
        PC: Childhood bleeding
    3. Jejunal:
        PC: Usually present with malabsorption + Vit B12 deficiency
              due to bacterial overgrowth

Rectal
    1. Piles: PC: blood separated from stool; painless unless thrombosed
    2. Solitary rectal ulcer; proctitis, e.g. 2° to gonorrhoea

Infection
    1. Bacterial: *Salmonella, Campylobacter, E. coli,*
               pseudomembranous colitis, TB
    2. Other: HIV, CMV, *Candida*
    3. Parasite: amoebic dysentery, hookworm (melaena)

Polyps – Benign
        a) Hyperplastic, esp. rectal
        b) Hamartomatous, e.g. Peutz–Jeghers' syndrome
            PC: Obstruction, intussusception → strawberry-jelly stool

Polyps – Neoplastic
        Adenoma → carcinoma

Inflammation
    1. Ulcerative colitis: bloody diarrhoea
    2. Crohn's: ileal bleeding – uncommon

Neoplasia
        Carcinoma, lymphoma, Kaposi's sarcoma

Gastric-upper bowel bleeding
        PC: Melaena (black, tarry stool), or bloody, if rapid transit

Trauma
        Surgery, colonoscopy, e.g. polypectomy; radiation colitis

Arterial / **A**ngiodysplasia / **A**VM
    1. Ischaemic colitis
    2. Angiodysplasia
    3. AVMs, hereditary haemorrhagic telangiectasia

Pseudomembranous colitis / Parasites
    see under Infection

Systemic
    1. Coagulopathy
    2. Amyloid

Abdominal Examination

2. Face

a) Eyes:
- Conjunctivae:
  pallor – anaemia
- Cornea: jaundice
- Xanthelasma: lipids

b) Mouth:
- Pigmentation
  (Peutz–Jeghers' Syndrome
   Addison's)
- Telangiectasia
  (HHT, scleroderma)
- Glossitis, cheilitis
  (Vit B12 or Fe def.)
- Ulceration:
  Crohn's (also swollen lips),
  Candida (white plaques –
    check genitalia)
  Oral hairy leukoplakia
    (lymphoma, HIV)

c) Parotid enlargement:
   liver failure

3. Neck

a) JVP ↑: R-sided cardiac failure as a cause of cirrhosis
b) Lymphadenopathy:
- Lymphoma, TB, HIV
- Gastric cancer: supraclavicular LN = Troisier's sign

c) Goitre (dysphagia, T4-toxicosis causes diarrhoea)

4. Abdomen

a) Inspection of trunk and back
   i) Skin of trunk and back:
   - Stigmata of chronic liver disease:
     spider naevi, gynaecomastia,
     testis atrophy, sexual hair loss,
     caput medusa, dilated abdominal veins
   - Uraemic frost: brown-yellow tinge
   ii) Scars, stoma, sinuses, striae
   iii) Masses, e.g.
        Sister Joseph's nodule (umbilical 2°),
        hernia (on coughing and standing)
   iv) Peristalsis: obstruction

b) Palpation + percussion
   i) Peritonism   – see p. 103
   ii) Masses, organomegaly   – see opposite
   iii) Ascites: shifting dullness, fluid thrill
   iv) Pulsation: expansile (aneurysm)
                  transmitted (overlying mass)
                  liver (tricuspid regurgitation)

c) Auscultation
   i) Bowel
   - Tinkling or succussion splash (obstruction)
   - Hyperactive
   ii) Renal bruits
   iii) Liver bruit (hepatoma; portal hypertension)

d) Extras, where appropriate
   i) PR: for unexplained weight loss, anaemia,
      altered bowel habit, bleeding
   ii) PV: e.g. discharge, pelvic pain
   iii) Genitalia:
        e.g. unexplained abdominal pain (testes),
        signs of immunocompromise (HIV)

1. Hands

a) Nails:
- Clubbing (cirrhosis, colitis,
  coeliac, lymphoma)
- Leuconychia (hypoalbuminaemia)
- Sclerodactyly, telangiectasia
  (scleroderma)

b) Palms:
- Asterixis (liver failure)
- Dupuytren's contracture
  (alcoholism)
- Hyperkeratotic-oesophageal
  cancer (tylosis)

c) Forearms:
- AV-fistula thrill, excoriations:
  chronic renal failure
- Tattoos: hepatitis or HIV risk

Order:

1. *Examine JVP at 45° recline*
2. *Sit patient forward to
   examine back and palpate
   cervical lymph nodes*
3. *Lie patient completely
   horizontal*
4. *Palpate, first light, then
   deep, in clockwise fashion*

6. And Finally...

a) Temperature chart
b) Weight chart, abdominal girth
c) Urine dipstick, β-HCG test

5. Other Systems

a) Feet (peripheral oedema)
b) Fundi (hyperlipidaemia)
c) ABP, chest (renal failure)

Abdominal Masses

Hepatomegaly

Hepatomegaly
1. Diffuse liver disease:
   T.A.B.O.O.S. – see p. 148
2. Nodular:
   a) Cirrhosis, esp. due to alcohol
   b) Neoplasia – 2°, 1°
   c) Cysts
      • Benign, e.g. adult polycystic kidney disease
      • Abscess, inc. hydatid, gumma
      • Haemangioma (usually solid)
3. Riedel's lobe (apparent hepatomegaly)

Hepatomegaly and splenomegaly
   As for causes of splenomegaly (see opposite)

Palpable gall bladder:
   Courvoisier's Law: Jaundice + palpable gallbladder =
   cancer of pancreas, common bile duct, or duodenum,
   but **not** chronic cholecystitis as gall bladder is fibrosed

Splenomegaly

B.I.G. S.P.A.N.

Blood disorders:
   CML, CLL, myelofibrosis, myeloproliferative,
   haemolytic anaemia, ITP
Infection:
   hepatitis, EBV, CMV, endocarditis, HIV,
   malaria, toxoplasmosis, schistosomiasis
Granulomatous: sarcoid, primary biliary cirrhosis

Storage disease: Gaucher's, Niemann–Pick dis.
Portal hypertension, esp. 2° to cirrhosis
Autoimmune: rheumatoid arthritis, SLE, Graves'
Amyloid
Neoplasia: cysts, melanoma

Features:
1. Cannot get above
2. Superficial (dull on percussion)
3. Descends medially on inspiration
4. Medial notch

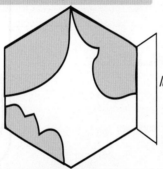

loin

Renal Enlargement

P.H.O.N.E. - shaped
Polycystic kidneys
Hypertrophy 2° to
   contralateral renal agenesis
Obstruction / occlusion:
   • Hydronephrosis
   • Renal vein thrombosis
Neoplasia:
   • Renal cell carcinoma
   • Myeloma, lymphoma
   • Amyloid
Endocrine:
   diabetes mellitus

Features:
1. Can get above
2. Deep (tympanic on percussion)
3. Does not descend on inspiration
4. Bimanually ballotable
*   i.e. freely moving*

Other Abdominal Masses

I.N.V.I.S.I.B.L.E. to the naked eye
Infection – abscess:
   appendicular, viral mesenteric adenitis, amoebic
   TB, Actinomyces, Yersinia (esp. RIF for all above)
Neoplasia:
   gastric, pancreatic cancer or pseudocyst (epigastrium)
   colorectal, carcinoid (esp. right iliac fossa)
Vessel: aortic or iliac aneurysm
Inflammatory: Crohn's (esp. RIF), diverticular (esp. LIF)
Sex: pregnancy, ovarian cyst or cancer
Bladder, pelvic kidney (e.g. transplant)
Lymphoma (esp. RIF, epigastrium)
Endocrine: adrenal mass

Oesophagitis

Causes

I.R.R.I.T.A.N.T.S.

Infection
- Herpes (HSV, CMV, VZV), HIV, Candida
- Usually only occurs in immunocompromised, e.g. HIV, lymphoma

Reflux, gastro-oesophageal (GOR) – 1: structural
Lower oesophageal sphincter weakness may be 1°, or due to:
1. Hiatus hernia
    EPI: 10% – of which 10% are symptomatic:
          presents in infancy (congenitally short oesophagus),
          middle-age or elderly; females:male = 4:1
    Types: a) Sliding (95%) = along axis of oesophagus
           b) Rolling (5%) = greater curvature rolls over
2. Pregnancy; multiparous women; obesity:
    - Pushes stomach up
    - Estrogen relaxes oesophageal sphincter
    - Abdominal wall weakness
3. Iatrogenic: cardia resection; nasogastric tube

Reflux, gastro-oesophageal (GOR) – 2: toxic
1. Smoking
2. Anti-cholinergics
3. Smooth-muscle relaxants:
    calcium antagonists, aminophylline, sildenafil

Inflammatory bowel disease – Crohn's

Toxins
1. Alcohol, hot tea, poisoning, e.g. caustic, corrosive
2. Drugs: Fe, aspirin, chemotherapy
3. Radiotherapy

Autoimmune
1. Vasculitis, inc. Behçet's
2. Pemphigus, pemphigoid, epidermolysis bullosa

Neurological
All cause disordered motility, inc. food stasis and reflux:
1. Achalasia causes food stasis
2. Scleroderma
3. Visceral myopathy

Trauma
Endoscopy / severe vomiting

Systemic
1. Uraemia
2. Hypothyroidism

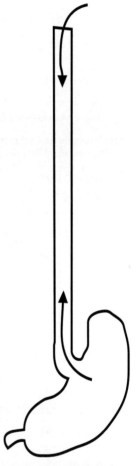

Lower Oesophageal Sphincter Mechanisms

1. *Oesophageal smooth muscle sphincter*
2. *Right crus diaphragm*
3. *Abdominal wall – increases intra-abdominal pressure*
4. *Acute angle of junction*
5. *Tall mucosal folds*

PC *B.U.R.N.S.*

Burning pain, heartburn
- Retrosternal or epigastric; radiates to arm + jaw
- Relieved by GTN (oesophageal spasm), sitting up, alkali (milk)

Ulceration
Haematemesis, melaena, Fe-deficiency anaemia

Reflux

Acid regurgitation, water-brash (sour taste), halitosis, dental caries

Neoplasia
1. Pre-malignant: Barrett's oesophagus = columnar metaplasia within normal stratified, squamous epithelium of lower oesophagus (appear as red-brown, velvety islands among pink oesophageal mucosa); develops in 10% GOR
2. Malignant: adenocarcinoma; develops in 10% Barrett's oesophagus

Stricture
Dysphagia

Spasm
Severe, acute, crushing (also caused by rolling hiatus hernia)

SOB, wheeze, palpitations, hiccoughs
Due to reflex bronchospasm, hiatus hernia, aspiration pneumonitis

Ix

Blood: FBC/ferritin: Fe-deficiency anaemia
Radio: 1. CXR: • Hiatus hernia seen as gas bubble and fluid level in chest
                • Aspiration pneumonitis, esp. right-middle lobe
        2. Barium swallow: reflux, spasm, mucosal irregularity
Special: 1. OGD + biopsy
        2. Oesophageal manometry: propulsive motion, sphincter tone
        3. Nasogastric tests:
            • Bernstein's test : 0.1M HCl via NGT – reproduces pain
            • 24-hour ambulatory pH: 2 x intraluminal electrodes records diurnal variation

Rx

Conservative: *S.O.S.*
    Smoking; **O**besity (+loose clothing around waist); **S**mall **S**nacks and **S**leep upright
Medical
    1. Mucosal protectants: antacids ± alginates (Gaviscon) – forms viscous 'raft' on gastric contents
    2. Secretion suppression: proton-pump inhibitor, e.g. omeprazole, ranitidine
    3. Pro-kinetic: domperidone or metoclopramide: ↑ LOS tone and gastric emptying
                ☠: extrapyramidal symptoms inc. acute dystonic reaction
Surgical
    1. Hiatus hernia repair
    2. Nissen fundoplication: gastric fundus mobilized and sutured around LOS,
                       so that gastic contraction closes LOS

Oesophageal Carcinoma

Epi   Inc: 1% of all cancers, but 5% of cancer deaths due to early spread to mediastinal structures
Age: elderly (squamous cell carcinoma); middle-aged (adenocarcinoma)
Sex: men > women, esp. adenocarcinoma
Geo: 1. Blacks (squamous cell carcinoma); Whites (adenocarcinoma)
2. China, Iran, South Africa

Causes – any cause of chronic oesophagitis or stricture:

Upper Oesophagus – Squamous Cell Carcinoma (10%)

1. Pharyngeal pouch
PC: Elderly person with dysphagia, regurgitation
2. Post-cricoid web (Plummer–Vinson syndrome)
PC: Middle-aged woman with chronic Fe-deficiency anaemia, dysphagia

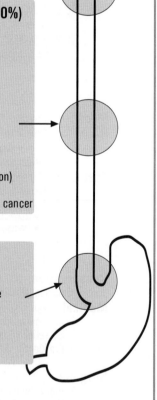

Middle Oesophagus – Squamous Cell Carcinoma (40%)

1. Toxins
   • Nitrites, nitrosamines – environment, food
   • Alcohol, smoking, hot liquids, caustics
   • Proton-pump inhibitor: i.e. *H. pylori* eradiaction
2. Nutrition
   Vit A, B, C, Zn deficiency; poor oral hygiene
3. Infection
   • *Aspergillus flavus* contamination of grain
   • Human papillomavirus
4. Inflammation
   • Coeliac, achalasia (food stasis leads to chronic inflammation)
   • Epidermolysa bullosa
   • Tylosis (palmar keratosis) – autosomal dominant: 40% get cancer

Lower Oesophagus – Adenocarcinoma (50%)

Gastro-Oesopohageal Reflux (GOR)
   • 'Barrett's oesophagus' refers to columnar metaplasia at the
      lower oesophagus
   • Metaplasia occurs in 10–15% of reflux patients
   • Adenocarcinoma occurs in 10% of metaplasia
   Predisposing: obesity, hiatus hernia, cardia surgery

Rare Oesophageal Tumours

1. Benign: mesenchymal leiomyoma, polyp, squamous papilloma
2. Malignant: metastases or direct invasion (bronchial, gastric); Kaposi's sarcoma

PC

**Polypoid or
Constrictive**

1. Pain: retrosternal, due to direct pressure
2. Obstruction:
   - Dysphagia (poorly localized), odynophagia
   - Anorexia: LOW, malnutrition
3. Regurgitation: heartburn, water-brash (sour taste),
   halitosis,dental caries, cough due to aspiration pneumonitis

Ulceration

1. Pain: mediastinitis; pleuritis
2. Haematemesis, melaena, Fe-deficiency anaemia;
   catastrophic exsanguination (aorto-oesophageal fistula)
3. Perforation; infection: mediastinitis, peritonitis

O/E

1. Cachexia
2. Pallor (anaemia
   of chronic disease)
3. Obstructive jaundice
   (lymph nodes at
   porta hepatis)

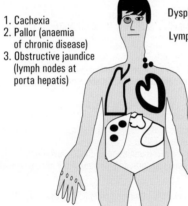

Dysphonia (L recurrent laryngeal nerve palsy)

Lymphadenopathy: cervical, supraclavicular

Cardiac
1. Pericarditis

Respiratory
1. Pneumonitis: direct spread, tracheal fistula
2. Lung metastases (via azygos or thyroid veins)
3. Pneumothorax (oesophageal rupture), pyothorax

Abdomen
1. Craggy epigastric mass
2. Portal hypertension: splenomegaly, ascites
3. Liver metastases (via L gastric vein)

Ix

Blood: FBC (Fe-deficiency anaemia); ESR; U+E (vomiting); LFT (biliary obstruction, liver metastases)
Urine or faeces: faecal occult blood
Radio: • CXR: aspiration pneumonia, thoracic invasion, pulmonary metastases
   • Ba swallow: irregular filling defect, stricture
   • CT, MRI
Special: OGD with biopsy: ulcerated mucosa, friable, oedematous, haemorrhagic

Rx

1. Curative: total or subtotal oesophagectomy
2. Palliative: if evidence of local or systemic spread
   a) Endoscopic pulsion intubation
   b) Endoscopic laser photocoagulation or alcohol injection

Prog

5-year survival rate = 5% due to early spread (75% if resected before it spreads)

Peptic Ulcers – Causes, Clinical

Locations

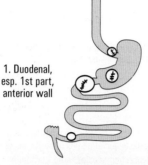

1. Duodenal, esp. 1st part, anterior wall

3. Oesophageal – secondary to Barrett's oesophagus

2. Gastric, esp. antrum and lesser curvature; greater curvature ulcer suggests carcinoma

4. Meckel's diverticulum

Locations listed in order of frequency

Causes   *G.I.T. S.C.A.R.S.*

Genetic
A family history often exists.
Mutations: blood group O (duodenal ulcers), interleukin-1β (gastric ulcers); non mps secretor status; heritable gastrin & H^+ hypersecretion status

Infection – *Helicobacter pylori*
Associations depend on location of infection:
    1. Antral–duodenum: duodenal ulcers (95% *H.pylori* +ve); gastric ulcers (70% *H.pylori* +ve)
    2. Diffuse gastritis: chronic gastritis; gastric carcinoma; MALTomas and Ménétrier's disease
Pathology:
    1. Antral infection: a) Inhibits somatostatin-secreting D-cells, which in turn disinhibits gastrin-secreting G-cells.
                  b) Bacteria produce urease that ↑es local ammonia, and ↑es mucosal IL-8 and TNF-α
    2. Duodenal infection: causes gastric metaplasia, inflammation and HCO_3^- secretion ↓
    3. Corpus infection: causes parietal cell atrophy, achlorhydria, and resultant chronic gastritis

Toxins
    1. NSAIDs – 25% of all drug side-effects, and 25% of all long-term NSAID users get PUs:
        inhibit COX-1 $\Rightarrow$ prostaglandins E_2, I_2 ↓ $\Rightarrow$ mucosal +HCO_3^- secretions ↓;
                                    HCl secretion ↑; mucosal blood flow ↓
    2. Chemotherapy, e.g. doxorubicin
    3. Smoking (duodenal ulcers); alcohol (acute gastritis and gastric erosions); salt

Surgery
    1. Antrectomy or gastro-enterostomy: causes duodeno-gastric reflux of bile salts
    2. Extensive small-bowel resection: disinhibition of gastrin secretion

Calcium ↑; Cirrhosis; CRF; COAD

APUDoma – gastrinoma
Zollinger–Ellison syndrome = non-islet cell pancreatic gastrinoma $\longrightarrow$ gastrin ↑
PC: a) Multiple, refractory peptic ulcers;
      b) Diarrhoea; steatorrhoea, malabsorption, inc. Vit B12 deficiency

Reflux, gastro-oesophageal

Stress – anxiety

'Stress ulcers' = ischaemia secondary to shock from sepsis, burns, intracranial pressure ↑

Epi
Inc: Life-time risk = 20% (males), 10% (females)
Age: 20–30s first presentation
Geo: Japan–China, South America: more common and higher risk of carcinoma

PC
Pain: • Epigastric–left upper quadrant, back, chest–shoulder, localized by fingertip
• Recurrent (every 2 months; lasts 2 months), but when occurs is constant and burning
• Relieved by milk or vomiting
• Assoc. bloating, abdominal distension, nausea + vomiting

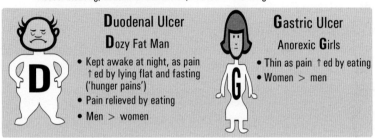

Duodenal Ulcer

Dozy Fat Man

• Kept awake at night, as pain ↑ed by lying flat and fasting ('hunger pains')
• Pain relieved by eating
• Men > women

Gastric Ulcer

Anorexic **G**irls

• Thin as pain ↑ed by eating
• Women > men

Comps *H.O.P.I.N.G. .... I won't have !*

Haemorrhage
• Acute: haematemesis, melaena, or chronic: Fe-deficiency anaemia

Obstruction
• Vomiting, copious, projectile, stale-food (i.e. non-bilious), tetany due to alkalosis
• Constipation
• Colic, visible peristalsis
• Distension, succussion splash

Perforation
• Acute abdomen due to peritonitis, or back pain due to retroperitoneal perforation

Infection: septic shock

Neoplasia: gastric carcinoma, esp. if chronic, atrophic gastritis

Gas: pneumatosis coli or pneumatosis cystoides intestinalis

Ix

Bloods: Hb ↓, MCV ↓; urea ↑ (haemorrhage); hypochloraemic alkalosis (obstruction)
Urine: paradoxical aciduria (pyloric obstruction)
Micro: a) *Helicobacter pylori* ELISA: 90% sensitive, 80% specific
        b) Urea-breath test: ingested ^{13}C-urea is catabolised by *H. pylori* urease to CO_2
Radio: barium swallow: 'hour glass' deformity due to fibrosis of lesser curvature
Special: 1. OGD–endoscopy:
            a) Brush cytology and biopsy of rim + base
            b) *H. pylori* urease test: gastric biopsy incubated with urea $\Rightarrow NH_4^+ \Rightarrow$ pH ↑
        2. Gastrin tests:
            a) Serum gastrin: fasting, post-prandial and post-secretin (gastrin ↓es in normals)
            b) Pentagastrin IV: measure hypersecretion of HCl

Peptic Ulcers – Treatment

Conservative

1. Avoid smoking, alcohol, caffeine, NSAIDs
2. Small and regular snacks; at night, take biscuits, milk or antacids to bed
3. GOR Rx for oesophageal ulcers: lose weight, Gaviscon, pro-motility drugs

Medical

1. *Helicobacter pylori* treatment

H. pylori eradicarion regime ('triple therapy') = 2 week course of:
P.A.C or R.A.C.:   **P**roton-pump inhibitor or **R**anitidine–bismuth citrate +
Amoxicillin,
Clarithromycin (or metronidazole)

2. Acid-suppression

Proton-pump inhibitors: omeprazole, lansoprazole
- Irreversible inhibitors of H^+–K^+–ATPase pump in apical parietal cell membrane
- Require acidification for activation (rabeprazole not as pH-dependent)
- Decreases *H. pylori* infection of antrum, but increase corpus–fundus infection
- ☠: Diarrhoea, N+V, gastroenteritis by decreasing gastric protection; transaminitis (esp. lansoprazole); anaemia; headache; potentiates warfarin, anti-convulsants (esp. omeprazole) theoretical: atrophic gastritis of corpus, and gastric ca., in *H. pylori* +ve pts.

Histamine (H2) receptor antagonists - ranitidine, cimetidine
- Competitive inhibitors of parietal cell H_2 receptor: H^+ and pepsin secretion ↓
- ☠ : Diarrhoea, bradycardia, gynaecomastia, impotence (esp. cimetidine)

Muscarinic (M1) receptor antagonists: pirenzepine

3. Mucosal protectant: *M.U.CO.S.A*

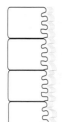

Misoprostolol = stable analogue of prostaglandin E_1
- Increases mucus and HCO_3^- secretion and mucosal blood flow; ↓es H^+
- Used as a prophylactic with long-term NSAID use
- ☠: Diarrhoea, hypotension

U: bism**U**th chelate
- Anti-microbial and a mucosal protectant by coating peptic ulcer, adsorbing pepsin, and increasing prostaglandin and bicarbonate secretion
- ☠: Black tongue and faeces; encephalopathy in presence of renal impairment

Carben**O**xolone: oesophagitis = deglycyrrhizinized liquorice

Sucralfate = **sucr**ose + **a**luminium + sul**fate**
- Coats peptic ulcer and increases prostaglandin release
- Used as stress ulcer prophylaxis in ITU
- ☠: Constipation, dry mouth, nausea; renal toxicity – due to aluminium

Antacids: $Al(OH)_3$, $MgSiO_3$, $NaHCO_3$ ± alginic acid (Gaviscon)
- Weak alkali inactivates pepsin; Al adsorbs pepsin ; anti-*H. pylori*
- ☠: Constipation (Al) or diarrhoea (Mg) – therefore used in combination; renal stones ($NaHCO_3$) due to precipitation of $CaPO_4$; fluid overload (Na); renal toxicity (Al)

<u>Surgical</u>

1. Truncal vagotomy

- Selective lesioning of L vagus and 'Nerves of Latarjet' that supply parietal cells of gastric fundus and body

2. Drainage procedure

- Required for gastric outlet or duodenal obstruction
- Types: a) pyloroplasty ± antrectomy (removes gastrin-secreting G-cells)
  b) gastro-jejunostomy:-

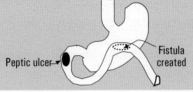

Peptic ulcer ➤ Fistula created

3. Gastrectomy

Billroth–1: for gastric ulcers

- Resect distal 1/2 to 2/3 stomach, and then anastamose proximal stomach with duodenum-part 1

Polya - for duodenal ulcers

- Resect distal 2/3 stomach, and then anastamose proximal stomach with jejenum, via one-way valve; duodenal ulcer allowed to heal in blind-ending stump

☠: *D.I.N.N.E.R.S.*

Dumping syndrome
    1. early – osmotic hypovolaemia
    2. late – rebound hypoglycaemia
Intestinal hurry: diarrhoea, malabsorption, wt. loss
Nutritional
    1. Fe deficiency – due to achlorhydria, malabsorption, ulceration
    2. vitamin B12 deficiency – due to intrinsic factor loss,
                         blind-loop syn. (bacterial overgrowth)
    3. vitamin D, calcium deficiency – due to malabsorption (rare)
Neoplasia of remnant
Epigastric fullness
Reflux, or bilious vomiting (improves with time)
Stricture, or obstruction of anastamosis
Stump leakage

Gastric Neoplasia

Epi   1% of all cancers, but 3% of cancer deaths due to gastric cancer presenting late

Causes

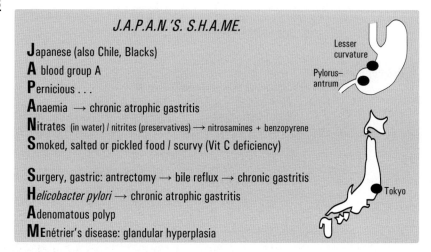

J.A.P.A.N.'S. S.H.A.M.E.

Japanese (also Chile, Blacks)
A blood group A
Pernicious . . .
Anaemia → chronic atrophic gastritis
Nitrates (in water) / nitrites (preservatives) → nitrosamines + benzopyrene
Smoked, salted or pickled food / scurvy (Vit C deficiency)

Surgery, gastric: antrectomy → bile reflux → chronic gastritis
Helicobacter pylori → chronic atrophic gastritis
Adenomatous polyp
MEnétrier's disease: glandular hyperplasia

Lesser curvature
Pylorus–antrum

Tokyo

Types

1. Malignant

a) Adenocarcinoma

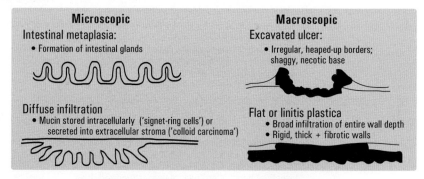

Microscopic

Intestinal metaplasia:
- Formation of intestinal glands

Diffuse infiltration
- Mucin stored intracellularly ('signet-ring cells') or secreted into extracellular stroma ('colloid carcinoma')

Macroscopic

Excavated ulcer:
- Irregular, heaped-up borders; shaggy, necotic base

Flat or linitis plastica
- Broad infiltration of entire wall depth
- Rigid, thick + fibrotic walls

b) APUDoma: gastrinoma (Zollinger–Ellison syndrome); carcinoid syndrome
c) Lymphoma
d) Secondaries: carcinoma, melanoma

2. Pre-Malignant
a) Adenomatous polyp: 30% have carcinoma within or in adjacent mucosa
b) Ménétrier's disease: rugal thickening due to glandular hyperplasia and mucin hypersecretion

3. Benign
Leiomyoma (mesenchymal)

PC

Anorexia, cachexia, dyspepsia, dysphagia (cardia cancer)

Projectile vomiting, stale-food (outlet obstruction – non-bilious), haematemesis

Pain: epigastric or back, early satiety

Obstruction: constipation, malnutrition
Haemorrhage: melaena, anaemia
Gastrocolic fistula: diarrhoea

O/E

1. Cachexia
2. Obstructive jaundice
   (lymph nodes at porta hepatis)

Virchow's node (Troisier's sign): spread via thoracic duct

Acanthosis nigricans

Tetany
(with prolonged vomiting)

1. Craggy epigastric mass
2. Obstruction:
   • Visible peristalsis
   • Succussion splash
3. Portal hypertension: splenomegaly, ascites
4. Transcoelomic spread:
   a) Sister Joseph's nodule: umbilical mass
   b) Krukenburg tumour: bilateral ovarian cancer, mucin-producing, signet-ring cells
   c) Pouch of Douglas mass (PR exam)

Metastases: Left hepatic lobe ⟶ bone, lung

Ix

Bloods 1 FBC, Ferritin: Fe-deficiency anaemia, ESR ↑
2. U + E: pre-renal renal failure; hypochloraemic alkalosis (vomiting)
3. LFT: biliary obstruction, liver metastases
Urine + faeces: aciduria (with outlet obstruction); faecal occult blood
Radio: 1. CXR: aspiration pneumonia, lung metastases
2. Barium meal + double contrast: i) ulcers; ii) polyp; iii) generalized narrowing (linitis plastica)
3. CT / MRI: staging
Special: 1. OGD + brush cytology + biopsy: lesser > greater curvature stomach
2. Endoscopic ultrasound: allows staging (**T**umour, **N**odes, **M**etastases in liver)
3. Laparoscopy / laparotomy

Rx

1. Curative: radical gastrectomy, node removal and adjuvant chemotherapy
   a) Polya-type gastrectomy (distal 3/4) for antral cancer
   b) Total gastrectomy and distal oesophagectomy for gastric body cancer
2. Palliative: If evidence of local or systemic spread:
   gastrectomy, gastroenterostomy (for pyloric obstruction), Celestin tube (for cardia obstruction),
   endoscopic laser photocoagulation, alcohol injection

Prog

5-year survival rate = 10% (95% if detected + resected early, e.g. by screening, as in Japan)

Inflammatory Bowel Disease – 1

Epi

	Ulcerative colitis	Crohn's disease
Inc	10/100,000 p.a.	5/100,00 p.a. (rising)
Age	Bimodal: 20s and 60s	Bimodal: 20s and 60s
Sex	Females predominantly	Males predominantly
Geo	Ashkenazi Jews ↑; Africans + Asians ↓	As for UC

Aet	Genetic: MZ concordance = 10%	1. Genetic: MZ concordance = 70%
		2. Infection:
		  • *Mycobacterium paratuberculosis*?
		  • MMR vaccine ?

Pre	Smoking *protects*	**C**igarettes and **C**ontraceptive pill **C**ause **C**rohn's Appendicectomy *protects*

Path

	Ulcerative colitis	**C**rohn's disease
Macro	Restricted: always in the following order: rectum ⇒ colon ⇒ terminal ileum (proctitis) (colitis) ('backwash ileitis')	Global, but occurs as 'skip lesions' anywere between mouth ⇔ anus
Micro	Restricted: **U**lcers limited to m**U**cosa **U**ndermining ulcers	Transmural: **C**lefts + fissures **C**obblestone appearance non-**C**aseating granulomas ⇒ lymphadenopathy

LUMEN

Cryptitis and crypt abscesses

MUSCULAR WALL

Inflammatory pseudopolyp

Fibrosis, stricture, adhesions, fistula

PC

	Ulcerative colitis	Crohn's disease
Abdomen	**Colon–rectum** 1. Diarrhoea 2. Blood or mucus PR 3. Tenesmus; faecal urgency Less common: constipation, pain, abdominal distension (colon)	**Mouth** Aphthous ulcers, glossitis, cheilitis, granulomatous swollen lips **Ileum** Diarrhoea, colic, flatus **Terminal ileum** RIF pain, mass **Colon–rectum** As for UC **Anus** Piles, tags, fissure, fistula, dusky, blue coloration

Abdomen complic-ations	*A.B.C.*
	Acute colitis
	• PC: toxic megacolon
	• ☠: mortality rate: 10%, or
	  50% if bowel perforates
	Bleeding – massive
	Carcinoma:
	• Ascending colon commonest site
	• Risk = 10% every 10 years
	• Dep. on a) age at onset < 25 yrs
	    b) unremitting Sx
	    c) pancolitis (40% risk)
	
	+ less common:
	Obstruction: benign strictures of
	      sigmoid–rectum
	Protein-losing enteropathy
		F.O.A.M.
		Fistula
		• Entero-enteric or colonic: PC: Diarrhoea
		• Vesical: PC: Frequency, pneumaturia
		• Vaginal, perianal, abdominal wall skin
		Obstruction
		• Benign strictures anywhere in GIT
		Abscess
		• Bowel, psoas, subclinical perforation
		• PC: Diarrhoea
		Malabsorption
		• Fat: steatorrhoea; gall, renal stones,
		• Protein: oedema (also 2° protein loss)
		• Vit B12: megaloblastic anaemia
		• Vit D: osteomalacia
		
		+ less common
		Acute colitis or ileitis: ⇒
		    toxic megacolon + perforation
		Bleeding – massive
		Carcinoma / lymphoma

Extra-Abdominal	*S.C.A.R.E.D. S.L.O.U.C.H.E.R.S.* (p. 229), esp. **S**pondylosis **A**rthritis **S**ystemic: fever, weight loss, anaemia of chronic disease, DVT, AA amyloid **L**iver: sclerosing cholangitis, cholangiocarcinoma, chronic active hepatitis **O**phthalmological: iridocyclitis, phylectenular conjunctivitis, episcleritis **U**lcers: aphthous; urethritis **H**aematology: anaemia of chronic disease, DVT **S**kin: pyoderma gangrenosum; erythema nodosum or multiforme; vasculitis	

Inflammatory Bowel Disease – 2

Ix

Blood   1. Biochemistry:
U&Es: urea ↑, Na ↓, K ↓, Ca ↓, Vit D ↓, Mg ↓
LFT: ALT ↑, ALP ↑, PT ↑, albumin ↓
ABG: metabolic acidosis, HCO_3 ↓

2. Haematology:
Hb: microcytic anaemia; WCC: neutrophils ↑; ESR, CRP: ↑

Urine   MSU: faecal flora if entero-vesical fistula

Micro   1. Blood culture
2. Stool culture: exclude *Campylobacter*, *Salmonella*, amoebiasis ('hot' specimen)
3. Crohn's disease: exclude infectious causes of right-iliac fossa mass:
TB, *Yersinia*, actinomycosis (biopsy + stain)

Monitor 1. Tachycardia, temperature, tenderness (> 5 days)⎫
2. Stool count, daily (> 6 BO at day 3)   ⎬ *Indications for*
3. CRP (> 45 at day 3), albumin (< 30 g/l)   ⎭ *colectomy*

Radio   1. Erect CXR: a) Perforation; b) Upper zone fibrosis
2. PAXR: a) Transverse colon dilatation:
perform daily during flare-up; width > 6 cm requires surgery
b) Sacro-iliitis
c) Biliary or renal stones (Crohn's disease)
3. Barium enema (Crohn's: barium meal and follow-through) – see below
4. Radiolabelled-WBC scan

Special Endoscopy + mucosal biopsies:
UC: granular mucosa; superficial ulcers; pseudopolyps; Crohn's; granuloma
UC: perform annual check-up > 10 years disease to detect dysplasia or neoplasia

Ulcerative colitis

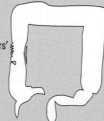

Rough appearance
- Irregular edge: 'granular'
- Double-contour 'undermined ulcers'
- Swollen islands 'pseudopolyps'
- Neoplasia: 'apple-core' lesions

Ileum
- Backwash ileitis
- Distended ileum

Smooth appearance
- Loss of haustrae: 'hosepiping'
- Shortened colon
- Megacolon: > 6 cm dilatation

Rectum
- Distensibility ↓
- Retrocaecal space ↑

Crohn's disease

Rough appearance
- Deep linear clefts – 'cobblestoning'
- Ulcers – 'rose-thorn' 'collar-stud'

Narrow appearance
- 'Eccentric luminal narrowing 2° to wall thickening, strictures and spasm (Kantor's string sign)

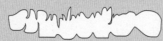

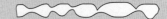

Fistulae

<u>**Rx**</u>   *S.N.A.C.K.S.*

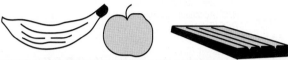

Supportive
1. Anti-diarrhoeal and anti-motility Rx:
   - Mebeverine, propantheline, codeine
   - Cholestyramine, hydrophilic colloid preparation (for bile-salt malabsorption in Crohn's)
2. Smoking (Crohn's only): stopping causes 30% ↓ in risk of relapse over 5 years

Nutrition
1. Nutrient replacement:
   protein; vitamins and haematinics (esp. Crohn's); TPN if obstruction
2. Fish oils; short-chain or medium-chain triglycerides, plus low-fat diet
3. Crohn's:
   a) Acute relapse: give liquid-formula diet to 'rest' bowel :
      elemental (amino acids); oligomeric (peptides); polymeric (protein)
      course =4–6 weeks as sole nutrition (as effective as steroids)
      ☠: Unpalatable (can use NGT / PEG); high relapse rate afterwards
   b) High-carbohydrate refined sugars; avoid dairy products (lactose-intolerant)

Aminosalicylates
   Mesalazine, olsalazine, sulphasalazine (more side-effects)
   - Activated by colonic bacteria: use laxatives to ↓faecal loading of colon
   - Oral (ileum – colon); retention enema (desc. colon): suppository (proctitis)
   - Indications: i) Acute disease if mild; ii) Chronic disease: maintains remission
   - ☠: Headache, abdo pain, diarrhoea, rash, interstitial nephritis, megaloblastic anaemia

Corticosteroids/other immunosuppressants
1. Steroids:
   Systemic: prednisolone: 30–60 mg od, ↓ 5 mg / week; IV hydrocortisone
   Topical: hydrocortisone by retention or foam enemas
            budesonide PO: minimal absorption; high 1st-pass metabolism; activated in ileum–colon
2. Cyclosporin (IV or enema), tacrolimus, mycophenolate – acute relapses
3. Methotrexate, azathioprine, thalidomide – chronic disease, esp. perianal Crohn's
4. Infliximab: mouse–human chimeric anti-TNFα monoclonal antibody:
   - Used for refractory disease (65% improve) or fistulae; good in Crohn's and maybe UC
   - ☠: Headache, SLE-like syn.; lymphoma; obstruction due to rapid healing with fibrosis

Kill bacteria – antibiotics
   UC: cefuroxime + metronidazole: acute
   Crohn's: metronidazole ± ciprofloxacin: chronic disease, esp. perianal or post-operative

Surgery
   UC: *30% require at some time*:
   - Types: panproctocolectomy, permanent ileostomy, and ileoanal anastomosis with ileal pouch
   - Indications:toxic megacolon; steroid-resistant disease; chronic (> 10 yrs) or dysplasia
   Crohn's: *70% require at some time*:
   - Types: limited resection; endoscopic balloon dilatation; abscess drainage
   - Indications: resistant disease; stricture, fistula, tumour
   - ☠: Recurrence occurs in 50% by 10 yrs

Colorectal Carcinoma

<u>Aet</u>   Most colorectal cancers arise from adenomatous polyps, via a succession of mutations:

K-**ras** proto-oncogene ⇒ *APC* (Adenomatous Polyposis Coli) gene ⇒ *p53* tumour-suppressor gene
DCC (Deleted in Colon Cancer) gene

<u>Assoc</u>   *Colorectal cancer is often H.I.D.D.E.N.*

Hereditary
The lifetime risk of developing colorectal cancer is 10% if one first-degree relative < 50 yrs is affected, and 5% if one first-degree relative > 50 yrs is affected. The background risk is 2%.

Familial Syndromes (all autosomal dominant)
1. Hereditary polyposis coli:
    a) Adenomatous polyposis coli (APC, or familial adenomatous polyposis):
        • 100% patients get carcinoma by 40 yrs old
        • Due to tumour-suppressor gene (5q–),
            involved in sporadic cases of adenomatous polyp transformation
    b) Gardner's syndrome:
        PC: Colonic polyps + bone tumours (osteomas; sarcomas) +
            soft tissue tumours (lipomas, sebaceous cysts, dermoid cysts)
    c) Turcot's syndrome:
        PC: Colonic polyps + brain tumours
2. Hereditary non-polyposis colon cancer (HNPCC) = Lynch syndrome
        Def = 3 cases colorectal cancer over 2 generations with at least 1 case < 50 yrs old
            Type 1 = colorectal cancer only: < 50 yrs old; usually R-sided; good prognosis
            Type 2 = colorectal, gastric, ovarian, endometrial cancer
        • 5% of all colorectal cancer; 1/200 population
        • Due to mismatch repair gene mutation ⟶ microsatellite instability
3. Hamartomatous polyps syndromes: polyps affect entire bowel + stomach
    a) Juvenile polyposis: = assoc. various congenital abnormalities
    b) Peutz–Jeghers' syndrome: = mucocutaneous pigmentation
        Complications: Obstruction, intussusception ⟶ PR bleed, adenoma ⟶ carcinoma

Inflammation
1. Ulcerative colitis – 10% per 10 years; 30% lifetime risk   (Crohn's disease = less risk)
2. Coeliac
3. Infection: *Streptococcus bovis* endocarditis or septicaemia

Diet
1. High-fat, low-fibre diet: (↑ in Western countries; ↓ Africa) – ↑ anaerobic flora
2. Vegetables protect

Diversion, urinary
Ureterosigmoidostomy

Endocrine
1. Acromegaly
2. Estrogen: HRT protects; women less at risk for rectal cancer

Nicotine: smoking ↑es colonic adenomas, not carcinoma

No physical activity: exercise protects

NSAIDs: aspirin and COX-2 inhibitors protective (prostaglandins required for cell synthesis)

PC Relative incidence in each site indicated:

Constitutional
weight loss

Transverse + Desc. Colon (15%)
1. Abdominal pain, lower:
   - Constant, gnawing: invasion
   - Colic: obstruction
2. Obstruction
3. Perforation → peritonitis
   (stool solidifies + ∴ gets stuck)

Sigmoid (30%)

Rectum (40%)
1. Bowel habit alteration
   and narrowing of stool caliber
2. Tenesmus (rectal discomfort,
   'incomplete emptying')
3. Rectal bleeding:
   Bright = distal colon–rectum
   Dark = proximal colon
4. O/E: PR mass (rectal–anal cancer)

Caecum + Asc. Colon (15%)
Iron deficiency anaemia
- Fatigue, palpitations,
  angina (stool is liquid
  + ∴ slips past luminal
  narrowing)

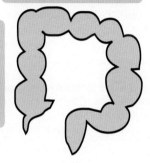

Anus (2%)
Painful mass, pruritus, bleeding

Complications
1. Fistula, e.g. colonic–vesical, colonic–vaginal
2. Metastases: liver, bone, lung

Ix **B**lood: FBC: Hb ↓, ferritin ↓, ESR ↑

Urine + faeces: Faecal occult blood: poor sensitivity (intermittent bleeding) + poor specificity (benign polyps)

Monitor: Plasma CEA (carcinoembryonic antigen): increases on tumour recurrence

Radio: 1. Double-contrast barium enema: annular, constricting 'apple-core' lesion
2. CT pneumocolon: non-invasive alternative to colonoscopy
3. CT, liver USS: staging

Special: • Proctosigmoidoscopy (< 60 cm) + biopsy
  • Colonoscopy + snare-biopsy: > 95% sensitivity + specificity
  • Entire colon must be visualized due to risk of > 1 polyp

Dukes' staging	5-year mortality rate	Polyp transformation risk
A : Limited to bowel wall	90%	1. Sessile > pedunculated
B : Crosses bowel wall	60%	2. Villous > tubular
C : Local lymph nodes	30%	3. Multiple > single
D : Liver metastases	1%	

Rx 1. Surgery: a) Anterior resection: proximal tumours: colorectal anastomosis with staple gun
          b) Abdominoperineal (AP) resection: distal tumours: end-sigmoid colostomy fashioned
2. Radiotherapy: given pre-operatively in rectal cancer (recurrence ↓; survival rate ↑)
3. Chemotherapy: a) 5-fluorouracil + folinic acid: given for Dukes' C: stage: mortality rate ↓ by 30%
          b) Alternatives: methotrexate and irinotecan (topoisomerase-I inhibitor)
4. Palliative: laser therapy, radiotherapy, chemotherapy

Malabsorption

Causes

Wall Disease

C.R.A.G.G.Y.

Coeliac disease / **C**rohn's disease
- Other autoimmune: collagenous sprue; scleroderma

Radiation enteritis

Arterial / venous
- Arterial: mesenteric ischaemia, e.g. AAA, vasculitis
- Venous hypertension: CCF, constrictive pericarditis

Giardiasis / **G**astroenteritis, other
- Salmonella, HIV, TB, protozoa
- Whipple's disease (lymphatic infection)

Genetic
- Brush-border disaccharidase deficiency (lactase, maltase)
- Agammaglobulinaemia

Y
- Am**Y**loid; eosinophilic enteritis; mastocytosis
- l**Y**mphoma (inc. coeliac disease); α-heavy-chain disease
- l**Y**mphangectasia

Bile Salt Circulation ↓

Bile salts combine with fatty acids to form micelles that are essential for fat absorption

1. Liver disease
a) Hepatocellular failure
b) Cholestasis; biliary fistula

2. Bacterial overgrowth
(bacteria deconjugate bile salts)

a) Structural Δ:
- Strictures, adhesions, fistulae, e.g. Crohn's, ischaemia
- Small bowel diverticulae
- Pneumatosis cystoides intestinales
- Blind loops, e.g. gastrojejunostomy

b) Motility ↓ : e.g. scleroderma

c) Defence impairments:
- Achlorhydria (e.g. long-term PPI)
- Nodular lymphoid hypoplasia
- Agammaglobulinaemia

3. Terminal ileal disease
Crohn's, TB, radiation

+ Drugs
cholestyramine, neomycin, $CaCO_3$

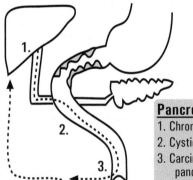

Pancreatic Disease
1. Chronic pancreatitis
2. Cystic fibrosis
3. Carcinoma of the pancreas, surgical resection

Other

1. Endocrine
a) Gastrinoma, or other APUDoma
- H^+ ↑↑ inactivates pancreatic lipase
- Rapid intestinal transit
b) Systemic:
hyper- or hypoT$_4$ism, Addison's, DM

2. Diarrhoea
Any cause of rapid transit, e.g.
a) Gastroenteritis
b) Drugs: laxatives
c) Surgery: gastrectomy, duodeno-jejuno-ileal bypass

PC   1. Malabsorption symptoms: carbohydrate, fat, protein, haematinics, vitamins (see p. 132)
2. Symptoms associated with cause: e.g. abdominal pain due to chronic pancreatitis or strictures

Ix   **Bloods**

1. U&Es: Ca, PO_4, Mg, Vit D ↓
2. LFT: alk phos ↑, albumin ↓, PT ↑
3. Glucose ↑: pancreatic or coeliac disease (assoc. DM)
4. FBC: micro- or macrocytic anaemia
   Film: megaloblastosis; hyposplenism (e.g. Howell-Jolly bodies) - coeliac disease
   Haematinics: ferritin ↓, Fe ↓, TIBC ↑
                            folate ↓ (↑ in bacterial overgrowth due to bacterial synthesis)
                            Vit B12 ↓: bacterial overgrowth; terminal ileal or pancreatic disease
5. Special: amylase ↑ : pancreatic disease; anti-endomysium – coeliac; serum electrophoresis

Urine – faeces

1. Hyperoxaluria: bile salt malabsorption
2. Faecal fat estimation: > 6 g / day (pre-treat with 100 g fat / day for 2 days)

Micro   Exclude *Giardia*: i) Stool cysts, faecal antigen; ii) Duodenal aspirate: trophozoites

Monitor   Weights, vitamins

Radiology

1. Bone X-ray: Looser's zones (OM); subperiosteal erosions (2° hyperPTHism)
2. Small-bowel enema: • jejunal dilatation + flocculation ('snowflakes')
                                    • blind loops; strictures – bacterial overgrowth
3. AXR, CT, USS, ERCP – pancreatic disease

Special

Wall disease

1. Biopsy, duodenal–jejunal, via OGD, or push enteroscopy
   • Sub-total villous atrophy present in most wall diseases, bacterial overgrowth, gastrinoma
   • Other: amyloid; Whipple's (PAS + ve macrophages)

2. Absorption tests
   • Administer oral D-xylose, lactose or ^{14}C-labelled triolein (triglyceride)
   • Measure urine xylose; exhaled H_2 (↑ in lactase deficiency) or CO_2 (↑ in lipase deficiency)

Bile salt circulation ↓

1. Breath tests
   a) ^{14}C-labelled-glycholate bile salt breath test:
      • Small-bowel bacteria deconjugate glycholate, with resultant CO_2 detectable in breath
      • Terminal ileal disease: bile salt not absorbed; ∴ colonic bacteria deconjugate it to CO_2 in faeces
   b) H_2 breath test: bacterial overgrowth: ↑ with fasting; oral glucose: early peak

2. Duodenal–jejunal aspirate: shows > 10^5 microorganisms/ml and polymicrobial flora
3. Empirical antibiotics: tetracycline, ciprofloxacin, metronidazole

Pancreatic disease

1. Urine tests
   a) Pancreolauryl or PABA tests
      fluorescin dilaurate cleaved by pancreatic cholesterol esterase ⟶ urine fluorescein
      PABA (*para*-aminobenzoic acid) cleaved by pancreatic chymotrypsin ⟶ urine PABA
   b) Dual-labelled Vit B12 Schilling test
2. Duodenal aspirate tests: i) Lundh test (500 ml meal); ii) Secretin (± CCK)

Coeliac Disease

Epi Inc 1 / 2000, ↓ing due to later introduction of cereals
Age: Any age, but esp. 1–5 yrs and 20–30 yrs
Sex: F > M
Geo: Common in West Ireland (1/300); rare in Blacks and Japanese
Aet: 1. Genetic: HLA-B8, DR3 in 80% (cf. 20% general population)
    2. Enzyme deficiency: pancreatic peptidase; brush border membrane disaccharidase
    3. Mucosal absorption deficit

PC

Anti-G.L.I.A.D.I.N.S.

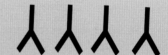

Gastrointestinal: malabsorption
    1. Carbohydrates:
        • N + V; watery diarrhoea
        • Abdominal distension + colic
        • Flatus, borborygmi (lactose intolerance)
    2. Fat: due to ↓ bile salt secretion (as cholecystokinin ↓) and bile salt malabsorption
        • Steatorrhoea
        • Renal stones (hyperoxaluria)
    3. Protein: due to peptidase deficiency, malabsorption, protein-losing enteropathy (ulcerative jejuno-ileitis)
        • Oedema, ascites
        • Weight loss, muscular atrophy
        • Leuconychia
    4. Haematinics: • Folate, Fe: dimorphic anaemia (Vit B12 deficiency – only occurs late)
        • Epithelial atrophy (cheilitis, glossitis, gastric atrophy, koilonychia, alopecia, pruritus)
    5. Vitamins: • Vit D, Ca, Mg: tetany, osteomalacia, osteoporosis
        • Vit A: night blindness
        • Vit K: petechiae
        • Vit B1 (thiamine): Wernicke's encephalopathy; niacin: pellagra

Lymphoma and carcinoma
    1. Lymphoma: small bowel > other MALToma > extra-intestinal
    2. Adenocarcinoma: small or large bowel; breast
    3. Squamous cell carcinoma: oesophageal, oropharynx

Immune abnormalities
    1. IDDM (type 1 DM), rheumatoid arthritis, thyroiditis
    2. Infertility: amenorrhoea, impotence
    3. Inflammatory bowel disease (UC), PBC, PSC

Anaemia
    1. Micro- or macrocytic anaemia + reticulocytosis
    2. Splenic atrophy: blood film shows Howell–Jolly bodies, acanthocytes, target cells, siderocytes

Dermatological
    1. Dermatitis herpetiformis (IgA deposits in upper dermis and dermo–epidermal junction)
    2. Follicular hyperkeratosis, pigmentation, aphthous ulcers, clubbing

Ig A mesangial nephropathy (and IgA deficiency)

Neurological
    Cerebral calcification (epilepsy), spinocerebellar degeneration, peripheral neuropathy

Systemic: Fatigue – 90%

Ix

Bloods: 1. Biochemical: *R.E.A.L.M.S.*
   a) **R**enal; b) **E**lectrolytes: Ca, PO_4, Mg, Vit D ↓; c) **A**BG; d) **L**FT: ALP ↑, albumin ↓, PT ↑;
   e) **M**etabolic: Glu (DM); f) **S**pecial: haematinics: ferritin ↓, Fe ↓, TIBC ↑, folate ↓

   2. Haematological: a) FBC: Micro- or macrocytic anaemia
      b) Film: features of hyposplenism (e.g. Howell-Jolly bodies)
      c) ESR ↑ or normal

   3. Immune: a) Anti-endomysium: 99% sensitive; 100% specific
      Anti-reticulin: 60% sensitive; 100% specific
      Anti-gliadin: 95% sensitive: poorly specific (also +ve in Crohn's)
      False −ve: IgA deficiency, adoption of gluten-free diet
      b) IgA: majority ↑ (may be ↓); IgM ↓

Urine: 1. Haematuria: IgA mesangial glomerulonephritis
   2. Hyperoxaluria: bile salt malabsorption

Micro: Exclude *Giardia*: a) Stool cysts, faecal antigen; b) Duodenal aspirate: trophozoites

Monitor: Weight; new bowel symptoms (risk of neoplasia)

Radio: 1. Bone X-ray: Looser's zones (osteomalacia); subperiosteal erosions (2° hyperPTHism)
   2. Small-bowel enema: jejunal dilatation + flocculation ('snowflakes')

Special: 1. OGD-endoscopy:
   'scalloping' of duodenal valvulae coniventes; loss of Kerkring's duodenal folds
   2. Small-bowel biopsy (via OGD; push-enteroscopy or Crosby capsule)
   subtotal / total villous atrophy, reversible after 3–6 month gluten-free diet

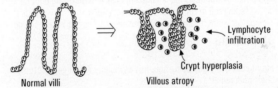

Lymphocyte infiltration

Crypt hyperplasia

Normal villi   Villous atropy

   + permeability test, tissue transglutaminase, disaccharidase activity
   3. Pancreatic function tests deranged; bacterial overgrowth test normal

Rx

1. Gluten-free diet: AVOID flour from: ACCEPTABLE (prescribable on NHS):

   BROW   **B**arley (hordein)   *MORE*   **M**aize
      Rye (secalin)   **O**ats (some tolerated)
      Oats (avenin)   **R**ice
      Wheat (α-gliadin)   **E**xtra: • Fibre
                  • Vitamins, Ca, Fe, folate

   Failure to respond (Ix: Repeat Bx after 3 months)
   a) Non-compliance (lesions return within 8-12 hrs of gluten-diet resumption)
   b) Resistant coeliac
   c) Complication: lymphoma, ulcerative jejuno-ileitis, intestinal stricture
   d) Wrong diagnosis, e.g. hypolactasia

2. Corticosteroids, azathioprine: for pts who have a poor response to gluten-free diet
   Dapsone: for dermatitis herpetiformis; ☠ headache; haemolysis; methaemoglobinaemia

3. Surgery: for lymphoma or ulcerative jejuno-ileitis

Acute Pancreatitis

Path

1. Pancreatic duct blocks off, causing activation of proteases and lipases within pancreas.
2. Histology shows oedema, fat necrosis and haemorrhage.

Causes

A.G.I.T.A.T.E.S. M.E.

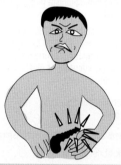

Alcohol
- Increases viscosity of pancreatic juice, thereby forming inspissated protein plugs in ducts
- Can occur with chronic consumption or one-off binge

Gallstones
- Large stones (wide cystic duct) block common biliary–pancreatic duct
- Stones may be recovered in faeces, several days after
- So-called 'idiopathic' pancreatitis may be caused by transient biliary sludge

⎫
⎬ 80%
⎭

Iatrogenic or trauma
- ERCP
- Surgery: may occur after any operation, but especially Polya gastrectomy
- Trauma: blunt abdominal

Triglyceridaemia, hyper-
- Triglycerides > 10 mol/l, inc. DM

Autoimmune or Arterial
- Autoimmune: vasculitis, Sjögren's
- Arterial: atherosclerosis, hypotension

Toxin
- Azathioprine, anti-HIV, tetracycline, valproate

Electrolytes
- Hypercalcaemia

Strucural
- Pancreatic carcinoma, sphincter of Oddie dysfunction, pancreas divisum

Mumps
- Or viral hepatitis, EBV, CMV, enteroviruses, mycoplasma

Estrogens – oral contraceptive pill

PC

P.A.N.C.R.E.A.S.

Pain
   a) Acute, severe, epigastric pain, radiates to back
   b) Relieved by sitting up and flexing trunk
   c) Assoc. N+V, abdominal distension, jaundice (pancreatic head compresses bile duct)

ABP ↓
   a) Third-space sequestration: blood and plasma protein accumulate retroperitoneally
   b) Vasodilator release: kinins, proteases, lipases
   c) Septic shock: coliforms, *Candida*
   d) Haemorrhage: gastritis, varices from portal vein thrombosis, DIC

Necrosis
   a) Pancreatic necrosis
      • Cullen's sign = faint blue umbilicus (haemoperitoneum)
      • Grey-Turner's sign = purple-brown flanks due to catabolism of tissue Hb
   b) Panniculitis = subcutaneous nodules due to fat necrosis

Calcium and Cardiac arrhythmias, due to Ca↓, 2° to fat necrosis

Renal: acidosis, ARF

Respiratory: hypoxia, left-sided pleural effusion, ARDS

Retinopathy or encephalopathy

Endocrine: DM, hyperlipidaemia

Abscess or pseudocyst
   a) Occurs after 4 weeks
   b) Pseudocyst = necrotic fluid in lesser sac (fistula with pancreas)
   c) Complications: rupture (MR = 15%) or haemorrhage (MR = 60%)

Stricture

Ix

1. Bloods: a) amylase > 1000 iU/l: non-specific and may normalize after few days
            b) pancreas-type isoamylase, lipase, trypsin elevation:
               more specific and remain high for weeks
2. Radiology: contrast-enhanced CT

Poor Prognostic Features

A.C.U.T.E.

ABGs: pO_2 < 8 kPa	**A**lbumin < 30
Ca^{2+} < 2 mmol/l	**C**RP > 150; WBC ↑↑
Urea > 16 mmol/l	**U**rine output < 50 ml/hr
Transaminases (AST > 200)	**T**rypsinogen activation pepetide (urine) ↑
Elderly, obese	**E**xtra: LDH, haematocrit ↑

Rx

1. Routine: a) NGT + IVI: 'Drip + Suck'; b) IV Cef. + metronidazole; c) Analgesics
2. Surgical debridement: for necrosis
3. For pseudocyst: s/c octreotide; drainage (internal or external)

Chronic Pancreatitis

Path

1. Caused by recurrent clinical or subclinical episodes of acute pancreatitis.
2. Similar causes to acute pancreatitis, **except that** gallstones do not cause it because cholecystectomy is normally performed after 1st attack!

Causes

A.G.I.T.A.T.E.S.

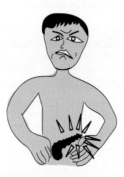

Alcohol

Genetic
- Hereditary pancreatitis (autosomal dominant)
- Cystic fibrosis
- Haemochromatosis
- a_1-antitrypsin deficiency

Iatrogenic
- Gastrectomy

Triglyceridaemia, hyper-

Autoimmune

Toxin
- Excess cassava (tropical)
- Protein–calorie malnutrition

Enzyme deficiency, isolated
- Trypsinogen, enterokinase, lipase, amylase
- Result in specific nutrient malabsorption

Strucural
- Stricture
- Pancreatic or duodenal neoplasia
- Congenital: pancreas divisum, choledochal cyst

PC   1. Abdominal pain
    a) Timing: intermittent (due to duct obstruction) or
               constant (due to inflammation or duodenal ulcers secondary to ↓ HCO$_3$ secretion)
    b) Location: epigastric radiating to back; may present as chest or flank pain
    c) Severity: may be severe enough to result in opiate abuse
    d) Exacerbation: ↑ by fatty food or alcohol (therefore encouraging anorexia)
  2. Steatorrhoea
    a) Pale, offensive, bulky, doesn't flush
    b) Profuse: > 35 g/day (cf. coeliac: 20–30 g/day; normal < 6 g/day)
    c) Malabsorption of fat-soluble vitamins + protein less problematic

O/E

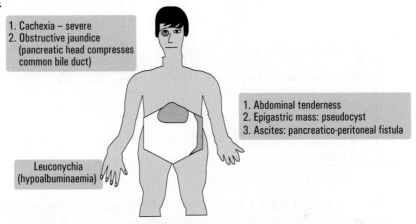

1. Cachexia – severe
2. Obstructive jaundice
(pancreatic head compresses
common bile duct)

1. Abdominal tenderness
2. Epigastric mass: pseudocyst
3. Ascites: pancreatico-peritoneal fistula

Leuconychia
(hypoalbuminaemia)

Ix

Bloods: a) Serum trypsinogen < 20 ng/ml (amylase ↑ only if pancreatic pseudocyst)
        b) CRP, WBC, ALT ↑ ↑

Urine or faeces
        a) Urine: pancreolauryl or PABA tests for malabsorption
        b) Faeces: faecal elastase < 100 mμ/mg stool; faecal fat collection > 6 g / day

Radiology
        a) PAXR, USS: calcification
        b) CT: pseudocyst
        c) ERCP: differentiates pancreatitis from carcinoma but 3% risk of acute pancreatitis!

Special: duodenal aspirate following 'Lundh meal' or secretin stimulation

Rx

  1. Diet: a) Low-fat; high-carbohydrate; protein supplements; fat-soluble vitamins
            b) Alcohol abstinence
  2. Medical: a) Pancreatic enzyme supplements
            b) Proton-pump inhibitor – due to risk of duodenal ulcers
            c) Oral hypoglycaemics or insulin
  3. Surgical: a) Sphincteroplasty
            b) Lateral pancreatico-jejunostomy
            c) Pancreatectomy – distal or Whipple's, with coeliac ganglion block

Jaundice

Causes

Pre-hepatic

Excess bilirubin production

1. Haemolytic anaemia
2. Inefficient erythropoiesis, e.g. pernicious anaemia, thalassaemia
3. Haematoma

Hepatic

Unconjugated hyperBRaemia

1. ↓ **Bilirubin uptake**
   a) Hereditary: Gilbert's syn. (AD)
      EPI: 5% pop., esp. young men
      PC: Malaise on fasting or illness
      Rx: Phenobarbitone (liver inducer)
   b) Fasting, acidosis
   c) Toxins: rifampicin, aspirin

2. ↓ **Conjugation**
   (BR-UDP-glucuronyl transferase ↓)
   a) Children:
      Crigler–Najjar syndrome:
      type I severe (AR); II mild (AR)
   b) Neonates / breast milk
   c) Hypothyroidism

Conjugated hyperBRaemia

1. ↓ **Bilirubin excretion**
   a) Hereditary
      i) Dubin–Johnson syndrome (AR):
         • Canalicular membrane carrier defect
         • Black liver due to catecholamine metabolite accumulation
         • PC: recurrent jaundice, asymptomatic
      ii) Rotor syndrome (AD):
         • Decreased uptake, storage, conjugation
         • Normal liver colour
         • Much rarer
   b) Diffuse hepatocellular disease
      (can also cause unconjugated hyperBRaemia)

Post-hepatic

Intrahepatic obstruction

I.N.T.R.A.H.E.P.A.T.i.C.

Infection: systemic, HIV, abscess
Neoplasia: 1° or metastases
Toxins:
   chlorpromazine (+tricyclic antidepressants),
   chlorpropamide, carbimazole,
   Ca-antagonists, carbamazepine,
   cloxacillin (+erythromycin estolate,
      augmentin, rifampicin),
   cyclosporin (+azathioprine)
Roids – steroids:
   anabolic steroids, contraceptive pill
Autoimmune: PBC, UC, coeliac

Hepatitis – icteric stage
Endocrine: thyrotoxicosis / DM
   obesity / malnutrition / TPN
Pregnancy
Amyloid
Transplant
Cholangitis, sclerosing

Extrahepatic obstruction

Biliary system

1. Stricture:
   post-cholecystitis
   (Mirizzi's syn.) or ERCP
2. Carcinoma
   • Cholangiocarcinoma, inc.
     Klatskin ca. (bifurcation
     of common hepatic duct)
   • Gall bladder carcinoma
3. Calculus
4. Congenital:
   • Choledochal cyst
   • Caroli's disease

Stomach–duodenum

1. Gastric
   carcinoma
   porta hepatis
   lymphadenopathy
2. Ampullary /
   duodenal
   carcinoma

Pancreas

Other
Retroperitoneal fibrosis

1. Carcinoma
2. Pancreatitis or
   pseudocyst

Physiology

Normal bilirubin (BR) = 3–17.   Jaundice occurs with levels > 51 μmol/l (i.e. 3x ULN)

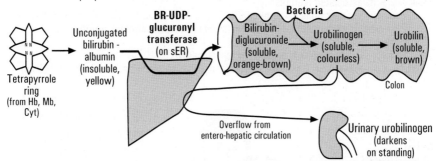

PC

	Urine	Stool	Other
Pre-hepatic	Dark: • Urobilinogen ↑ • Haemoglobinuria (if intravascular haemolysis)	Dark: urobilin ↑	Pale conjunctivae; leg ulcers
Hepatic	Dark: conjugated BR ↑ *(not Unconjugated hyperBRaemia)*	Pale: urobilin ↓ due to partial cholestasis	Portal hypertension: varices, ascites, encephalopathy
Post-hepatic	Dark: conjugated BR ↑	Pale: urobilin ↓ fat malabsorption (steatorrhoea)	Pruritus; abdominal pain

Ix

	Urine	LFTs	Other
Pre-hepatic	BR nil ('acholuric') Urobilinogen ↑ Intravascular haemolysis: • Haemoglobinuria • Haemosiderinuria • Methaemalbuminuria	BR unconjugated ↑ AST ↑ LDH ↑	FBC and film Reticulocytes: normal: 1–2% a_2-haptoglobin (intravascular) Causes: • Hb electrophoresis • Direct Coombs test
Hepatic	BR ↑ Urobilinogen ↓ Unconjugated hyperBRaemia: as for 'Pre-hepatic', except urobilinogen ↓	BR conjugated ↑ ALT ↑↑ ALP ↑ icteric stage GGT ↑↑ Function: Alb ↓, PT ↑ Unconjugated hyperBRaemia: BR unconjugated ↑	Anaemia: normocytic, -chromic Film: target, spur, burr cells Causes: MCV ↑; paracetamol levels; anti-LKM, ANA, ANCA; serology; liver USS + Doppler; a_1-AT, caeruloplasmin, ferritin
Post-hepatic	BR ↑ Urobilinogen ↓	As for 'Hepatic', except ALP ↑↑ greater than ALT ↑	Abdominal USS, ERCP, CT AMA, ANCA

Liver Failure

PC

1. Jaundice + its associated features:
   Hepatic: dark urine (conjugated BR ↑), pale stool (urobilin ↓ due to partial cholestasis)
   Post-hepatic: dark urine, pale stool-steatorrhea (fat malabsorption), pruritus
2. Portal hypertension:
   varices, ascites–peripheral oedema, encephalopathy
3. Underlying cause features: e.g. nausea, fever (hepatitis); paraesthesia, delusions (alcoholism)

O/E

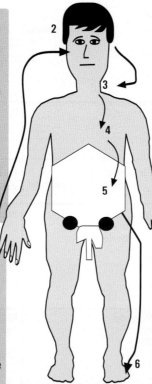

2. Face

1. Eyes:
   a) Jaundiced sclerae
      (BR > 50 μmol/l)
   b) Pallor:
      • Varices, marrow aplasia
      • Haemolysis
        (lemon-yellow facies)
   c) Hyperlipidaemia:
      xanthelasma,
      arcus cornealis,
      tendinous xanthomas

2. Parotid enlargement

3. Breath: hepatic fetor:
   sweet + sickly smell

3. Neck

JVP ↓ : hypovolaemia
      ↑ : cardiac cause

4. Trunk

1. Spider naevi:
   • Central arteriole that blanches
     ands fills from centre;
   • > 7 in SVC distribution
   • Skin appears 'paper-money' thin
2. Demasculinization
   a) Gynaecomastia
      = breast tissue around nipple
   b) Testicular atrophy
   c) Loss of 2° sexual hair
      (axillary; pubic; legs)
   • All due to testosterone ↓, oestrogen ↑,
     sex hormone binding globulin ↑
   • Also haemochromatosis (hypogonadism)
3. Scratch marks

1. Hands

1. Nails:
   a) Clubbing: cirrhosis
   b) Leuconychia:
      hypoalbuminaemia

2. Palms:
   a) Dupuytren's contracture
   b) Palmar erythema:
      due to estrogen ↑, SHBG ↑

3. Hand flap (asterixis):
   early Sx of
   hepatic encephalopathy

5. Abdomen

1. Hepatomegaly
2. Portal hypertension
   i) Dilated superficial abdominal veins,
      caput medusa, venous hum
   ii) Ascites
   iii) Splenomegaly
   iv) Encephalopathy:
      visuospatial deficits + apraxia

6. Feet

1. Oedema: due to:
   - hypoalbuminaemia;
   - 2ndary hyperaldosteronism
2. Peripheral neuropathy,
   esp. ↓ ankle jerks,
        ↓ vibration sense
3. Gout (esp. 1st MTP)
   due to alcohol, acidosis

7. And Finally...

1. Temperature:
   • Pneumonia, TB, meningitis (strep.)
   • Peritonitis (coliforms)

2. Weight chart:
   • Salt retention (ascites, oedema)

3. Urine dip: haematuria:
   • UTI, ATN, coagulopathy

<u>Ix</u>

Bloods

Biochemistry: *R.E.A.L.M.S.*

Renal: urea ↓, creatinine ↑
  Hepato-renal syn.: due to impaired prostaglandin synthesis and over-activation of sympathetic system,
    RAAS and ADH ⇒ renal vasoconstriction and pre-renal ARF
  Precipitants: i) Drugs: NSAIDs, diuretics; ii) Hypovolaemia, e.g. haemorrhage

Electrolytes:
  1. Na^+ ↓, K^+ ↓ : secondary hyperaldosteronism due to hypovolaemia
  2. Ca^{2+} ↓, Mg^{2+} ↓, Vit D ↓ : due to i) Vit D malabsorption; ii) ↓ 25-α-hydroxylation of cholecalciferol
  3. Ammonium (uncuffed) ↑ : encephalopathy
  4. Uric acid ↑ : due to acidosis; purine metabolism ↑

ABGs: 1. Metabolic acidosis, esp. with alcoholism, due to:
    i) $NADH / NAD^+$ ↑ ⇒ pyruvate converts to lactate, ii) Hypoglycaemia ⇒ lipolysis ⇒ ketoacidosis
  2. Hypoxia, due to pulmonary shunts ⇒ TLCO ↓

LFTs: BR↑, ALT↑, ALP↑, GGT↑, Alb ↓

Metabolic:
  1. Glucose ↓, due to:
    i) Glycogen storage ↓; ii) Gluconeogenesis ↓ (esp. alcoholism: $NADH / NAD^+$ ↑); iii) Malnutrition
  2. Cholesterol ↑   : cholestasis
    Triglycerides ↑ : alcoholism, hepatitis, due to
    i) Zone 3 necrosis; ii) LCAT and TAG lipase ↓; iii) Abnormal LDL (lipoprotein X) – cholestasis

Special: 1. AFP↑: hepatoma
  2. Causes of liver failure:
    a) Toxicology screen, esp. paracetamol; save serum; urine; gastric aspirate
    b) Transferrin saturation ↑ (haemochromatosis), caeruloplasmin ↓ (Wilson's), α_1-AT ↓

Haematology

Hb: ↓ + macrocytosis + film: target cells, acanthocytes, spur cells, ringed sideroblasts:
    anaemia due to: a) Marrow suppression + erythropoeitin insensitivity
                    b) Haemolysis: hypersplenism; alcohol ↑ es cholesterol in RBC membrane
                    c) Fe or folate deficiency: e.g. varices, malnutrition
WBC: ↓ frequent infections: – pneumonia, TB, spontaneous bacterial peritonitis
Plts: ↓ due to hypersplenism, ITP (also, abnormal platelet function)
PT: ↑ due to: i) Vit K deficiency; ii) Synthesis ↓ + activation ↓; iii) DIC
G&S; X-match: if anaemic; varices; liver biopsy

Immunology: ANA, Rh Factor, AMA, LKM – autoimmune hepatitis

Urine 1. Na ↓↓ ⎱ suggest hepato-renal syndrome
  2. Urine / plasma osmolality < 1.15 (cf. dehydration) ⎰

Micro 1. Blood cultures; ii) MSU; iii) Sputum; iii) Ascitic tap; iv) LP (stain for AAFB, for all)
  2. Serology: HBV, HCV, HDV

Monitor 1. Glucose: 4 hourly if encephalopathic
  2. Daily weights

ECG 1. Sx. of hypokalaemia
  2. ECHO: right-sided heart failure

Radiology 1. CXR: pneumonia or TB; pulmonary oedema; cardiomegaly (RSH failure)
  2. USS: cirrhosis; hepatoma; ascites

Special 1. Endoscopy: varices
  2. EEG: high voltage, slow waveform
  3. Liver biopsy: i) PT must not be > 3 s from control; ii) G&S; iii) Vital signs every 15 min

Liver Failure – Management

A. Airway - breathing

1. Airway:
   - Clean vomit, loose teeth
   - Cuffed endotracheal tube,
   - Nasogastric tube if vomiting
2. Oxygen: 60%
3. Ventilation if comatose

1. Urgent endoscopy if varices suspected
2. ITU transfer if:
   - Drowsy or comatose
   - Major haemorrhage
3. Liver transplant

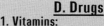

C. Hydration

1. **Salt restriction and depletion:**
   a) Fluid intake < 1 l/day
   b) Spironolactone, furosemide
   c) Low-dose dopamine or haemodialysis if ARF
2. **Fluids:**
   a) Dextrose 5–50%, depending on BM, + KCl
   b) Salt-free albumin if ABP ↓
   c) Packed red cells, platelets, FFPs - if haemorrhage
   d) Mannitol – cerebral oedema

B. Assessment

1. The Three Gs

Glasgow coma scale
Glucose – BM stick
Group and save, Hb, PT

2. C.O.A.T.

Cardiac Monitor
O$_2$ sats
ABP, CVP line
TPR

3. Investigations

Bloods: e.g. K$^+$ ↓, ABGs
Urine: Na, osmolality ↓
Micro: blood cultures; serology
Monitor fluid balance: daily weights, girth, urine catheter, NG–aspirate, ascitic taps
ECG
Radiology: CXR, abdominal USS
Special: OGD, EEG, liver biopsy

D. Drugs

1. **Vitamins:**
   a) thiamine (B1) - esp. alcoholics
   b) Vit B12, C – esp. alcoholics
   c) Vit K, FFP – for coagulopathy
2. **Laxatives:**
   a) Lactulose: lowers NH$_4$
   b) MgSO$_4$ enemas: aim for 2 soft stools / day
3. **Ulcer prophylaxis:** omeprazole; sucralfate NGT

$\pm$

1. **Broad-spectrum antibiotics:** e.g. ampicillin+ gentamicin + metronidazole
2. **Anti-convulsants:** diazepam; phenytoin
3. **Steroids:** based on Madri index: i.e. give if bilirubin and PT ↑↑

E. Specific

Toxin overdose: paracetamol – N-acetylcysteine
Autoimmune: steroids, AZA
B: HBV, HCV – Interferon-α
Occlusive anti-coagulation
Syndromes:
- haemochromatosis – venesection
- Wilson's – penicillamine

At home

1. Avoid alcohol; refer for counselling
2. Avoid: NSAIDs, sedatives, high-protein meals

<u>Liver Transplant</u>

<u>Indications</u>

General

1. End-stage liver failure must be apparent, despite best medical therapy:
   a) Cholestasis: pruritus, osteomalacia
   b) Portal hypertension: varices, ascites
   c) LFTs: BR $>$ 150 μmol/l, albumin $<$ 30 g/l, PT $>$ 5
2. No other organ failure – i.e. patient survival is good if liver corrected.
      Hence, pts with acute liver failure who are systemically unwell have
      a poorer 2-year survival rate (acute 70%, cf. chronic 90%)
3. Cause of liver failure does not predispose to recurrence in graft

Specific

Toxins:
   1. Drugs: e.g. paracetamol overdose, isoniazid or halothane idiosyncratic reactions
   2. Chronic alcoholism, if:
      a) Child's grade C cirrhosis
      b) abstinent for $>$ 6 months, and from stable socio-economic background

Autoimmune:
   good survival rate due to disease not recurring (CAH) or uncommonly recurring (PBC)

B: Infections: Hep B ,C, D:
   1. Hep B: poor success rate (50%) due to extrahepatic replication and graft infection;
         must be e Ag –ve and HBV DNA –ve, and pre-treat with IFN + lamivudine
   2. Hep C: good success rate due (90%) to recurrence of hepatitis being only mild
   3. Hep D: intermediate success rate as Hep D prevents Hep B re-infection

Occlusive venous disease: Budd–Chiari syndrome

Obstetric: fatty liver of pregnancy

Obstruction: primary sclerosing cholangitis, biliary atresia:
   PSC has poor success rate due to infection and recurrent bile duct strictures

Oncology: hepatoma:
   • Poor success rate due to tumour recurrence
   • Indications: a) Fibrolamellar variant (metastasize late); b) Tumour size $<$ 5 cm; c) AFP –ve

Syndromes: *W.A.T.C.H.*
   Wilson's; α_1-**A**nti-trypsin def., **T**yrosinaemia, galactosaemia, glycogen storage disease
   Cystic fibrosis; **H**aemochromatosis (latter two are not cured by liver transplant)

<u>Complications</u>

1. Graft failure
   a) Primary: poor donor organ; hepatic vessel thrombosis $<$ 2 days: Rx = re-transplantation
   b) Acute: immune   5–30 days: Rx = ↑immunosuppression
   c) Chronic: shrinking bile ducts   1–3 months: Rx = re-transplantation
2. Infection
   a) Opportunistic (from immunosuppression), e.g. PCP, *Candida*
   b) CMV or HSV reactivation from donor / host: use prophylactic ganciclovir and aciclovir
3. Recurrence of underlying condition: esp. infective hepatitis, hepatocellular carcinoma

Portal Hypertension

Def　Resting Portal Venous Pressure > 12 mmHg (may be upto 50 mmHg)

Causes

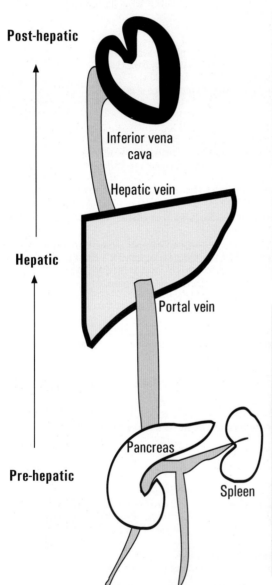

Post-hepatic

Inferior vena cava

Hepatic vein

Hepatic

Portal vein

Pancreas

Spleen

Pre-hepatic

1. **Right-sided heart failure**
   + a) Constrictive pericarditis
   b) IVC web – congenital
2. **Budd–Chiari Syndrome**
   (hepatic venous thrombosis)
3. **Granulomas in hepatic veins**
   a) Schistosomiasis ('Banti's syn.')
   b) TB
   c) Sarcoidosis

1. **Cirrhosis or fatty infiltration**
   (e.g. alcohol)
2. **Acute liver failure**
3. **Hepatocellular carcinoma**

Portal Vein Thrombosis due to:
P.I.N.C.H.E.S.
Pancreatic
　chronic pancreatitis, pseudocyst
　carcinoma
Inflammation
　diverticulitis, appendicitis
　colitis, haemorrhoids
Neoplasia
　GIT, pancreas, cholangiocarcinoma
Congenital
　atresia, AVM
Haematological
　prothrombotic state
Exogenous
　trauma, surgery

Splenomegaly, massive
　due to excess blood flow

PC

Varices + other porto-systemic collaterals

1. Oesophageal varices
- Occur in 2/3 of cirrhotics; 50% will die of them
- Due to dilated venules between:
  oesophageal ($\longrightarrow$ azygos v.) and
  left, and short gastric veins ($\longrightarrow$ portal v.)

2. Haemorrhoids
- Worsens existing piles, but does not cause
- Due to dilated venules between inferior, middle
  rectal (systemic) and superior rectal veins (portal)

3. Caput medusa
- Dilated venules emerge radially from umbilicus,
  superficial abdominal veins enlarge,
  venous hum (Cruveilhier–Baumgarten syndrome)
- Due to dilated venules between superficial
  epigastic, lateral thoracic (systemic) and
  umbilical (portal) veins

4. Surgical bleeding risk increased
- Due to dilated venules between retroperitoneal,
  and diaphragmatic veins (systemic) and
  portal vein

Encephalopathy

Cause
Diversion of GIT toxic metabolites, e.g.
NH_4^+, cyclic amino acids, mercaptans, indoles
away from liver into IVC directly

Precipitants: *H.E.I.G.H.T.e.N. risk*
Haemorrhage, e.g. varices (+ Rx of it with shunt)
Electrolytes: $Na^+ \downarrow$, $K^+ \downarrow$
Infection: spontaneous bacterial peritonitis
Glucose $\downarrow$, inc. low-calorie diet
Toxins: diuretics, sedatives, anaesthetics, alcohol
Neoplasia: hepatocellular carcinoma

PC *F.A.C.E*
Flap (myoclonus), dystonia
Ataxia, dysarthria, ophthalmoplegia
Confusion, **C**onstruction Apraxia, inverted sleep pattern
Epilepsy; o**E**dema, cerebral

Ix 1. EEG: high-voltage, slow-wave form
2. Plasma $NH_4^+ \uparrow$ (uncuffed)
3. Plasma bile acid $\uparrow$

Rx 1. Remove cause, e.g. IV glucose if hypoglycaemic;
IV colloid if hypovolaemic; IV antibiotics if sepsis
2. Lactulose: replaces aminogenic bacteria with
acidogenic types
3. $MgSO_4$ PR or PO: $\downarrow$ absorption of bowel toxins
4. Liver transplant

Ascites + other oedema

1. Ascites, due to:
   a) Back-pressure $\Rightarrow$
      fluid exudation
   b) Hyperaldosteronism,
      due to hypoalbuminaemia
      and reduced aldosterone
      catabolism
   c) Eicosanoid activation

2. Pleural effusion,
   esp. on R side

3. Ankle oedema

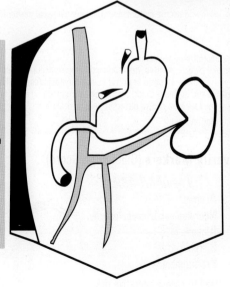

Splenomegaly

Due to back-pressure
(congestive) or
functional hypersplenism
(i.e. cause of portal HT)

Hepatomegaly

If post-hepatic venous
obstruction or
hepatic inflammation or
hepatic infiltration

Oesophageal Varices

Def   Dilated venules between oesophageal (systemic) and gastic (portal) veins, due to portal hypertension (see p. 156, for causes)

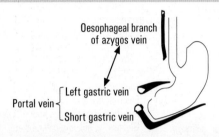

Oesophageal branch of azygos vein

Portal vein { Left gastric vein

Short gastric vein

PC   1. Asymptomatic, e.g. screening by endoscopy or barium meal
2. Massive haematemesis, hypovolaemic shock:
   precipitated by erosion; food bolus; vomit; rise in portal venous pressure
3. Hepatic encephalopathy: precipitated by GIT haemorrhage

Ix   **B**loods
- U+E: urea ↑ (blood digestion), creatinine ↑(ARF),
  Na ↓ (RAAS activation), K ↑(ARF)
- LFT / clotting: risk indicator (see below)
- FBC: Hb ↓ Plt ↓
- ABGs: lactic acidosis
- Glucose ↓

Urine
- Na ↓ : hepato-renal syndrome

Micro
- Blood, urine and ascitic culture: spontaneous bacterial peritonitis (Gram −ve)

ECG
Radio:
- CXR – aspiration pneumonitis
- Abdominal USS: – Ascites, hepatomegaly, hepatocellular carcinoma
  – Hepatic or portal vein thrombosis (use duplex USS)
- Tc-scintigram: in Budd–Chiari Syndrome liver shows ↓ activity, except in the central caudate lobe due to different venous drainage

Special: OGD endoscopy

Severity Markers (Child-Pugh Score)

I need AN ABP:

Ascites
Neurological: encephalopathy
Albumin ↓
Bilirubin ↑
Prothrombin time ↑

Used to assess operative risk

<u>Rx</u>

A. Airway – Breathing

1. Airway:
   - Clean vomit, loose teeth
   - Cuffed endotracheal tube,
   - Nasogastric tube,
     if vomiting
2. Oxygen: 60%
3. Ventilation if comatose

1. Urgent endoscopy, if:
   - varices suspected
2. ITU transfer, if:
   - Drowsy or comatose
   - Major haemorrhage
3. Liver transplant

B. Assessment

1. The three **G**s

Glasgow coma scale
Glucose – BM stick
Group and save,
   X-match 4 units

2. C.O.A.T.

Cardiac monitor
O2 sats
ABP, CVP line
TPR

3. Investigations

Bloods: inc. FBC, clotting,
   urea↑, K^+↓, ABGs
Urine: Na, osmolality
Micro: cultures; serology
Monitor fluid balance:
   CVP: aim for 5–15 cm H_2O
   UO: aim for > 30 ml/hr
ECG
Radiology: CXR,
   Abdominal USS
Special: OGD

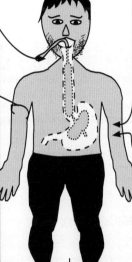

C. Hydration

1. Dextrose 50%, 50 ml if 'hypo'
2. Colloid, preferably salt-free
3. Packed red cells:
   Initially: O Rhesus −ve
      or grouped blood
   later: X-matched blood
   ☠: Ca↓, K↑, pH↑, temp.↓
4. Fresh frozen plasma (2 units),
   platelets (5 units),
   Vit K (10 mg iv)

D. Drugs

1. **Splanchnic vasoconstrictor**
   a) Terlipressin (glypressin) iv or
      vasopressin iv:
      mortality rate ↓es by 1/3
      ☠: coronary vasospasm, skin or
      gut necrosis, hypertension
      (for vasopressin: use GTN patch)
   b) Octreotide iv = (somatostatin
      analogue)
2. **Laxatives**
   - lactulose (laxative + probiotic) +
     $MgSO_4$ (oral + enemas) +
     neomycin (↓es NH_4^+ formation)
   - all ↓ 'blood meal' +
     encephalopathy
3. **Metoclopramide 20 mg iv,**
   ranitidine, PPI or sucralfate
   Metoclopramide ↑es lower
   oesophageal pressure
   and ↓es azygos blood flow
4. **Antibiotics:** ceftriaxone iv
5. **Thiamine**

E. Specific

Endoscopy: injection
   sclerotherapy;
   ethanolamine or thrombin
Balloon tamponade:
   < 12 hrs to avoid ischaemia
Radiological embolization
T.I.P.S.S.: transjugular
   intrahepatic
   porto-systemic shunt
Surgical: transgastric
   oesophageal stapling;
   distal oesophagectomy

Prophylaxis

1. **Propranolol or**
   octreotide SC:
   reduce portal pressure by
   more than systemic
2. **Endoscopy:**
   rubber-band ligation
3. **Surgery:**
   gastric vein ligation;
   porto-caval shunt

Ascites

Causes

P.A.T. P.I.N.T.S.

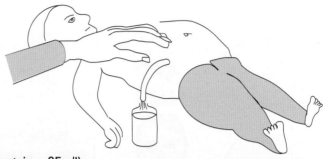

Transudate (protein < 25 g/l):

Portal hypertension
  a) Pre-hepatic: right-sided heart failure, schistosomiasis
          (N.B. Budd–Chiari syndrome: exudate!)
  b) Hepatic: cirrhosis, acute liver failure
  c) Pre-hepatic: pancreatic disease, inflammation, neoplasia, congenital

Albumin ↓
  a) Malnutrition, malabsorption, protein-losing enteropathy
  b) Cirrhosis
  c) Nephrosis
Thyroxine ↓

Exudate (protein > 25 g/l, plus WBCs, RBCs):

Pancreatitis
  a) Acute pancreatitis: bloody and yellow-white flecks of fat necrosis
  b) Chronic pancreatitis: purulent
  Ix: Amylase ↑

Infection
  a) TB (high protein content)
  b) Peritonitis (purulent)
  Ix: Culture +ve, lactate ↑, glucose ↓

Neoplasia
  a) 1° Peritoneal: mesothelioma, pseudomyxoma peritonei
  b) 1° Visceral:
      • Colonic or ovarian cancer, ovarian fibroma (Meig's syndrome)
      • Hepatoma
  c) 2°, e.g. breast
  Ix: Cytology +ve

Thrombosis, hepatic vein: Budd–Chiari syndrome
  Ix: Venography or Tc-scintigraphy showing caudate lobe sparing

Severe pain: ectopic pregnancy, abdominal aortic aneurysm, trauma
  Ix: Bloody tap on all of 3 attempts

PC
1. Weight + girth ↑
2. Peritonitis: Gram −ve, esp. if protein < 10 g/l

O/E
1. Abdominal circumference
2. Shifting dullness
3. Fluid thrill

Ix
Blood: Na, albumin ↓ (may precede oedema)
Urine: Na ↓
Monitor: Daily weights
Micro: 1. Ascitic tap culture;
       also send for:
         • Chemistry: protein, glucose, lactate, amylase
         • Cytology
     2. Mantoux test
     3. Blood cultures
Radio: 1. USS – confirm diagnosis and allow drain site to be marked
     2. CXR
     3. MRI, MRV, hepatic and portal venography

Rx
1. General
   a) Conservative:
     • Salt (fluid) restrict
     • Bed rest
   b) Diuretic:
     Spironolactone ± loop
   c) Drain (paracentesis)
     + IV salt-free albumin replacement

2. Specific
   a) Portal hypertension:
     TIPSS: transjugular intrahepatic porto-systemic shunt
   b) Malignant ascites:
     • Intraperitoneal bleomycin
     • Le-Veen shunt: subcutaneous catheter connects to internal jugular vein, via
      1-way valve

Acute Liver Failure – Causes

T.A.B.O.O.S. !

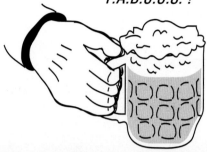

Toxins
1. Alcohol, and other poisons
2. Drug overdose
3. Idiosyncratic

Autoimmune hepatitis
1. Classical lupoid
2. LKM+ve
3. SLA +ve

B: hepatitis B virus + other infections
1. Virus: hepatitis A–G, herpes group (esp. EBV, CMV), measles, yellow fever
2. Bacteria: leptospirosis
3. Protozoa: malaria, toxoplasmosis

Occlusion / obstruction
1. Hepatic vein thrombosis: Budd–Chiari syndrome
2. Ischaemic hepatitis: hepatic artery thromboembolism, or profound hypotension
3. Obstructive jaundice

Obstetric
1. Acute fatty liver of pregnancy
2. Cholestasis of pregnancy
3. HELLP syndrome (Haemolytic anaemia + Elevated Liver enzymes + Low Platelets)

Oncology
1. Massive malignant infiltration
2. Lymphoma

Syndrome / **S**torage disease
1. Reye's syndrome
2. Wilson's disease

Toxins

1. Alcohol, and other poisons
   - Herbal tea
   - CCl_4, trichloroethylene, yellow phosphorus (zone 1 necrosis)
   - *Amanita phalloides* (Death cap mushrooms)
2. Drug overdose
   - Paracetamol: saturation of conjugation reactions $\longrightarrow$ P450 oxidation to NABQI $\longrightarrow$ glutathione consumption
   - Aspirin
   - Iron sulphate (zone 1 necrosis)
3. Idiosyncratic – *M.A.I.N.*

    Methotrexate + NSAIDs, esp. indomethacin, ibuprofen

    Amiodarone + other cardiac: methyl-dopa, Ca antagonists, enalapril,

    Isoniazid, esp. in fast acetylators, e.g. Inuits, other inducer, women > 50

    + other antibiotics: nitrofurantoin, flucloxacillin, AZT, fansidar, keto-/fluconazole

    Neuro / psychiatric / anaesthetic:
    a) Anticonvulsants (phenytoin, CMZ, valproate)
    b) Antidepressants (TCA / MAOI / chlorpromazine – cholestasis)
    c) Psychostimulants: ecstasy, cocaine, glue-sniffing (trichloroethylene, toluene)
    d) Halothane

Budd–Chiari Syndrome

Causes

1. Thrombophilic state, esp.
   myeloproliferative disorders (60%), paroxysmal nocturnal haemoglobinuria,
   antiphospholipid syndrome, ulcerative colitis, oral contraceptive pill
2. Local tumour:
   hepatocellular carcinoma, renal cell carcinoma, adrenal carcinoma
3. Congenital:
   membranous obstruction of inferior vena cava (commonest cause in Japan)
4. Exogenous:
   azathioprine, radiation, bone-marrow transplant,
   herbal bush teas (pyrrolidizine alkaloids = bush tea disease),
   trauma, hydatid cyst

PC
1. Abdominal pain – right upper quadrant (stretching of Glisson's capsule)
2. Jaundice, liver failure
3. Ascites (exudate!)

Ix
1. Duplex scan: cavernous transformation
2. Colloid scan: ↑ uptake caudate lobe
3. Venography with retrograde CO_2 portography
4. Liver Bx: centrilobular congestion / sinusoidal dilatation /
   haemorrhagic necrosis / fibrosis

Rx
Anticoagulation, providing clotting initially normal

Chronic Liver Disease – Causes

T.A.B.O.O.S. !

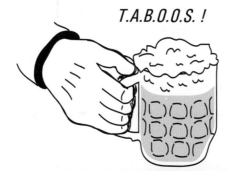

Toxins
   1. Alcohol, and other poisons
   2. Idiosyncratic

Autoimmune hepatitis
   1. Classical lupoid
   2. LKM + ve
   3. SLA + ve
   4. Other: sarcoid, inflammatory bowel disease, coeliac, diabetes –
         all show mild impairment of LFTs

B: hepatitis B virus + other infections
   1. Virus: hepatitis B, C, D, G, herpes group (esp. EBV, CMV), measles, yellow fever
   2. Bacteria: Brucella, syphilis
   3. Nematode: hydatid disease,
         schistosomiasis (pipe-stem fibrosis, pre-sinusoid portal hypertension)

Occlusion / obstruction
   1. a) Hepatic vein thrombosis: Budd–Chiari syndrome or IVC web
     b) Hepatic vein congestion: right-sided heart failure, constrictive pericarditis
   2. Hepatic ischemia: sickle cell anaemia
   3. Obstructive jaundice: primary biliary cirrhosis, sclerosing cholangitis, biliary atresia

Oncology
   1. Hepatoma
   2. Graft-versus-host-disease (GVHD)

Storage diseases, and other genetic diseases:
W.A.T.C.H.
   1. Wilson's disease
   2. α_1-antitrypsin deficiency
   3. Tyrosinaemia, galactosaemia, glycogen storage disease, fructose intolerance
   4. Cystic fibrosis
   5. Haemochromatosis
   6. Hereditary haemorrhagic telangiectasia

Surgical: Biliary atresia; small bowel resection; jejuno-ileal bypass

<u>Histology</u>

1. Chronic persistent hepatitis (CPH):
   lymphocytic infiltrate + fibrosis of portal tracts > 6 months
2. Chronic active hepatitis (CAH):
   piecemeal, bridging necrosis centred on portal tracts
3. Cirrhosis:
   fibrosis + nodular regeneration + distorted lobular architecture

<u>Toxins</u>

Drugs may induce a wide range of liver diseases:

1. Hepatitis – cirrhosis:
   a) Alcohol, and other poisons:
   - Alcohol: fatty change → hepatitis → cirrhosis
   - Vinyl chloride
   - Arsenic (e.g. psoriasis treatment)
   b) Idiosyncratic: *M.A.I.N.*
   Methotrexate + other NSAIDs, e.g. diclofenac
   Amiodarone + other cardiac: methyl-dopa
   Isoniazid (esp. fast acetylators) +
   nitrofurantoin, minocycline (+ isotretinoin)
   Neuro / psychiatric / anaesthetic:
   - Anticonvulsants: valproate, phenytoin, carbamazepine
   - Dantrolene
2. Fatty change:
   i) Valproate; ii) Amiodarone; iii) Asparaginase; iv) Tetracycline
3. Hypersensitivity and granulomas:
   i) Carbamazepine; ii) Allopurinol; iii) Phenylbutazone; iv) Sulphonamide
4. Veno-occlusion:
   azathioprine, radiation
5. Tumour:
   androgens, oral contraceptive pill
6. a) Biliary cholestasis:
   androgens, oral contraceptive pill, rifampicin, gold
   b) Calculi:
   ceftriaxone
   c) Sclerosing cholangitis:
   fluorodeoxyuridine

Infective Hepatitis

Types

	Spread	Virus type	Associated cause	Incubation (months)
A	FO	RNA ss+ve	**A**broad (esp. seafood); **A**utumnal peaks	1 (< 2)
B	IV	DNA ds	**B**lood; **B**ody fluids; **B**abies (vertical transmission)	3 (< 6)
C	IV	RNA ss+ve	As for Hep B, but ↑er blood and ↓ vertical risk	2 (< 6)
D	IV	RNA ss+ve	**D**ependent on prior Hep B as envelope-**D**eficient	3 (< 6)
E	FO	RNA ss+ve	**E**conomically-poor countries e.g. post-flood	1 (< 2)

FO: faeco-oral; IV: parenteral

Epi   Hep B: Mediterranean, Far East – 30% carriers; Hep C: Middle East – 15% carriers

PC

Prodrome

Hep A associated with small-joint Arthritis
Hep B has a particulary Bad prodrome: high fever, flu-like, angioedema, arthritis

PC 1. Fever, flu-like symptoms, headache, arthralgia
    2. Lymphadenopathy, hepatosplenomegaly

Acute Hepatitis

Hep A > B > C : in order of frequency of jaundice: 99%, 75%, 25%

PC 1. Hepatitis:
      • Cholestasis (dark urine, pale stool) may precede jaundice by 5 days
      • Fulminant hepatic failure: occurs in < 1%; more in Hep D and E
    2. Immune-complex reactions   *S.N.A.G.S.:*
      Skin: Hep A: pruritus, urticaria, papular
             Hep B, C: vasculitis (PAN, cryoglobulinaemia), lichen planus, porphyria cutanea tarda
      Neurological: peripheral neuropathy, transverse myelitis
      Aplastic anaemia
      Glomerulonephritis, membranous or membranoproliferative
      Systemic: pancreatitis, myocarditis, pneumonitis, thyroiditis
N.B. Infectivity begins from 3 days pre-jaundice and lasts until 2 weeks post-jaundice

Chronic

Hep C and Childhood Hep B are most Chronic, but Hep A may cause symptoms for < 1 year

Carrier is defined for: Hep B as: sAg +ve > 6 months, or eAg +ve > 2 months
                       Hep C as: HCV RNA or ALT ↑ > 6 months
Risks:
  1. **C**arrier: Hep B: 10% (↑ed if eAg +ve)   Hep C: 80%
  2. **C**hronic active hepatitis: Hep B: 10%   Hep C: 60%
  3. **C**irrhosis: Hep B: 5% (↑ed by Hep D)   Hep C: 20%
  4. **C**arcinoma (HCC): most pts with cirrhosis develop (10–30 years post-infection)

Serology

Hep A

> 1. **Anti-HAV:** IgM occurs from 1–3 months post-infection; IgG predominates > 3 months

Hep B

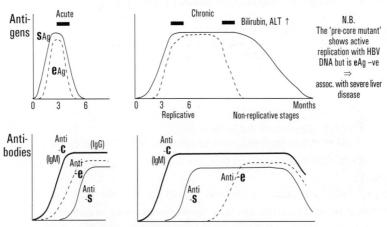

N.B. In acute infection, order of antibody appearance is alphabetic;
in chronic infection, anti-e appears late

> 1. **sAg** = acute infection; reactivation; chronic carrier
> 2. **Anti-c:** • **IgM** acute infection   *N.B. may be +ve even when*
>   • **IgG** reactivation or past infection   *HBsAg −ve and so more sensitive!*
> 3. **eAg** = high level of virus r**e**plication (also indicated by HBV DNA and pre-S1, S2 proteins)
>   **Anti-e:** **-ve** = high infectivity; **+ve** = low infectivity
> 4. **Anti-s:** past infection or immunized

Hep C

> 1. **Anti-HCV:** pre-clinical (anti-C22 or C33); clinical (anti-C100-3)
> 2. **HCV RNA PCR:** infectivity index

Rx   Liver support: no aspirin or alcohol; manage liver failure (lactulose, low-protein diet)
Anti-viral: 1. IFN-α : Indications: recently acquired chronic infection (6 months–2 years);
                                   low HBV DNA or HCV RNA, mild hepatitis on biopsy
                            Response: Hep B = 40% seroconvert; Hep C = 10% seroconvert
              2. Nucleotide analogues: Hep B: lamivudine; Hep C: ribavirin
Steroids: Indications: prolonged cholestasis (esp. Hep A); Prior to anti-viral (Hep B, C)
Transplant liver

Prox   1. Safe sex, needle exchange (Hep B,C); hygiene precautions (Hep A, E)
2. Vaccine: HAV; HBV sAg; human immunoglobulin

Primary Biliary Cirrhosis

Epi
1. Middle-aged Caucasian women
2. Predisposing:
    a) HLA-B8, -DR8
    b) Autoimmunity:
        • Scleroderma, dermatomyositis, rheumatoid arthritis, Sjögren's (in 80%)
        • Addison's, coeliac, vitiligo, Hashimoto's, pulmonary fibrosis

Path
Non-suppurative destructive cholangitis
        Stages   1. **G**ranulomas (may also occur in other tissues)
                     2. **P**roliferation or disappearing bile ducts
                     3. **B**ridging septa + fibrosis
                     4. **C**irrhosis

PC

P.B.C.

Pruritus: excoriations, due to cholestasis.
        Also pale stool, dark urine, steatorrhoea, but jaundice occurs late

Pigmentation: melanosis of face; Kayser–Fleischer rings may also occur in cornea

Bones: osteomalacia, osteoporosis – due to poor Vit D absorption; also arthralgia
Big organs: hepatosplenomegaly; lymphadenopathy, inc. at porta hepatis

Cirrhosis: clubbing ,varices, ascites
Cholesterol ↑ : xanthomata

50% are asymptomatic at presentation (abnomal LFTs); but 50% of these have cirrhosis!

Prognosis

Normal LFTs   = 12 yrs
Abnormal LFTs   = 10 yrs
Symptomatic   = 8 yrs
Cirrhosis   = 4 yrs
Bilirubin > 150 μmol predicts 18 months median survival

Ix
1. Anti-mitochondrial Abs: esp. PDH, E2 and E3 binding protein on inner mitochondrial membrane (95%)
2. Other autoantibodies: anti-smooth muscle, ANA, ANCA; IgM ↑ ↑
3. Liver biopsy: copper load – assoc. with good prognosis; differentiates from CAH (absent Cu)

Rx
1. **Supportive:** a) Pruritus • Cholestyramine, ondansetron, naltrexone, naloxone, barbiturates
                              • UVA, plasmapharesis, haemoperfusion, bile diversion
            b) Nutritional: Vit A, D, E, K, Ca, medium-chain triglycerides
2. **Disease-modifiying:**
            a) Penicillamine, colchicine (no effect on life expectancy)
            b) Azathioprine, cyclophosphamide, methotrexate
               (not steroids – worsen ostodystrophy)
            c) Ursodeoxycholic acid: slows disease progression
3. **Liver transplant:** disease may recur

Chronic Autoimmune Hepatitis

Epi
1. Middle-aged Caucasian women (ANA + ve)
   Equal sex ratio and occurs more commonly in children (LKM + ve)
2. Predisposing:
   a) HLA-A1, B8, DR3 occurs in 40%, and is associated with more severe disease
      (ANA + ve)
   b) Autoimmunity common in patient and family (any form)
   c) Hepatitis C (LKM + ve)

Path
1. Piecemeal bridging necrosis, and lymphocytic infiltrate, centred on portal tracts
2. Present for > 6 months
3. LE cells in 10%

PC

C.A.H.

Early:
   Constitutional: fatigue; nausea; pruritus
   Cushingoid: striae, hirsute, acne
   Amenorrhoea
   Arthralgia: may also develop rheumatoid or migratory arthritis
   Hepatitis: recurrent jaundice
   Hepatosplenomegaly: tender; lymphadenopathy

Complications:
   Cirrhosis
      • Present in 70% at presentation; esp. LKM + ve
      • Spider naevi, palmar erythema, purpura (PT ↑)
   Autoimmune
      Colitis, ulcerative; **C**holangitis, sclerosing; **C**onjunctivitis or uveitis
      Acidosis, renal tubular
      Hyperthyroidism (thyroiditis); **H**yperglycaemia – type 1 DM (LKM + ve)
   Haematological
      • Normocytic anaemia; Coomb's + ve haemolysis
      • Pancytopenia due to hypersplenism

Ix

Auto-Antibody patterns

1. ANA + ve (homogeneous immunofluorescent staining pattern):
   may occur with anti-dsDNA, anti-mitochondrial, anti-smooth muscle, p-ANCA
2. LKM Ab + ve (liver and kidney microsomal antigen = cytochrome P450)
3. SLA Ab + ve (soluble liver antigen = glutathione-S-transferase)

Rx
1. **Immunosuppression**
   Prednisolone 60 mg od: titrated according to ALT; can also use azathioprine
   Response better for no autoAbs > ANA + ve > LKM + ve
2. **Liver transplant:** disease does not recur in graft

Haemochromatosis

Epi **Inc:** Prevalence: 1 / 3000, although 10% of population are gene-carriers
Age: Onset 40–60 years
Sex: Women present 10 yrs later due to menses
Geo: Celtic origin
Aet: 1°: *HFE* gene (esp. C282Y mutation), results in:
   a) Increased divalent-metal transporter (DMT-1) expression on brush border of enterocytes
   b) Reduced hepcidin expression in liver (hepcidin inhibits Fe absorption from gut)
   ∴ Fe intake increases from 1 to 4 mg / day, and total body Fe increases from 4 to 25 g
  2°: Haemolytic anaemia, aplastic anaemia, sideroblastic anaemia, due to
  ineffective erythropoiesis and Fe release, increased Fe absorption, blood transfusions

PC   *Iron M.E.A.L.S.*

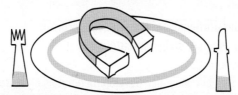

Myocardial: arrhythmias, heart block, dilated or restrictive cardiomyopathy
Endocrine: Pancreas – diabetes (in 2/3);
    Pituitary – amenorrhoea, infertility;
    Parathyroid – hypocalcaemia; hypothyroidism
Arthritis: 2nd + 3rd metacarpophalangeal joints, knees (X-ray: hooked osteophytes, cysts),
    chondrocalcinosis, acute pseudogout (calcium pyrophosphate)
Liver: Chronic active hepatitis, cirrhosis, hepatocellular carcinoma (in 1/3 if untreated)
    abdominal pain, hepatomegaly
Skin: Slatey-grey shins (due to melanosis and Fe), porpyria cutanea tarda
Systemic: Fatigue + **S**curvy (bruising, gum bleeding) as Fe oxidizes ascorbic to oxalic acid

Ix **B**loods: 1. Transferrin sat. ↑ (> 60%); TIBC ↓; plasma Fe ↑; ferritin ↑
    2. Genotype
Urine: 24-hr urinary Fe ↑ (post-desferrioxamine injection)
ECG, Echo
Radio: Liver CT or MRI – detects increased Fe stores
Special: Liver biopsy: dry weight > 2%: iron in hepatocytes

Rx 1. Iron removal: a) Venesection: initially, 1–2x per week for 1–2 years; then once every 3 months
         b) Desferrioxamine
    2. Liver transplant
    3. Family screening and treatment

Wilson's Disease

Epi **Inc:** Prevalence: 1 / 50,000

      Age: Presents between childhood and 30; never after mid-50s

      Aet: Reduced copper excretion from hepatic lysosome into bile, due to mutant Copper-Transporter
           ATPase 7B (chromosome 13; autosomal recessive)

PC   *C.L.A.N.K.I.N.G.*

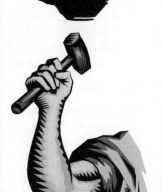

copper

Corneal / **C**ataracts
    1. Kayser–Fleischer rings:
        grey-green copper deposits around rim of cornea
    2. Sunflower cataracts

Liver
    1. Acute: hepatitis, fulminant hepatic necrosis
    2. Chronic: fatty liver, chronic active hepatitis, cirrhosis

Arthritis
    1. Chondrocalcinosis
    2. Osteoporosis

Neurology
    1. Parkinsonism; tremor (intention, postural) / chorea / tics
    2. Spasticity, pseudobulbar dysarthria and dysphagia
    3. Dementia, psychosis – mania, headache

Kidney
    Renal tubular acidosis / Fanconi's syn., resulting in osteomalacia

Negative, Coombs' – haemolytic anaemia

Growth failure (puberty)

Gynaecological – amenorrhoea, abortions

Ix   **Bloods:** 1. Serum caeruloplasmin ↓ (< 20 mg/dl); serum Cu-free ↑ (but total ↓)

        Urine: 24-hr urinary Cu ↑ (esp. post-penicillamine)

        Special: 1. Slit-lamp exam for Kayser–Fleischer rings:
               sensitivity = 70%; false +ves in primary biliary cirrhosis
            2. Liver biopsy: dry Cu weight increased: false +ve = primary biliary cirrhosis

Rx   1. Copper-chelators:
        a) Penicillamine: • Take for 2 years
                   • Adjuvant vitamin B6 and zinc ± steroids, e.g. for ITP, arthralgia
        b) Trientine: if penicillamine worsens neuro Sx or intolerance
        c) Dimercaprol
    2. Plasmapharesis
    3. Liver transplant: curative

Liver Tumours

Primary Hepatocellular Carcinoma

Causes   T.A.B.O.O.S.

Toxins
alcohol (most common), vinyl chloride, thorotrast (radioactive contrast agent)

Aflatoxin B1
derived from *Aspergillus flavus* in contaminated nuts + grain

B:hepatitis and hepatitis C
assoc with HBV eAg: IFN-α reduces risk

Oxytestosterone, Oral contraceptive pill, other androgens (danazol)

Orientals (South China), Africans
due to HBV, HCV, Aflatoxin B1

Storage disease / syndrome:
haemochromatosis, alpha-1 anti-trypsin deficiency, hereditary tyrosinaemia

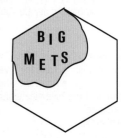

PC   **A**bdominal pain; **A**scites, blood-tinged; **A**cute decompensated liver failure (encephalopathy)

O/E   Abdominal mass; Liver bruit, friction rub

Comps   1. Paraneoplastic: glucose ↓, cholesterol ↑, PTH-rp: calcium ↑, polycythaemia, DIC
         2. Metastases: bone, lung

Ix   1. AFP ↑ ↑ (> 500 μg/l); ALP ↑ ↑
      2. USS or CT: satellite lesions may be present
      3. Angiogram + ^{131}I-lipiodol pre-injection: selectively retained within tumour
         (avoid biopsy due to vascularity, coagulopathy + risk of spread along needle tract!)

Rx   1. < 5 cm: a) Hepatic artery embolization: gel foam; alcohol; doxorubicin
                  b) Liver transplant: risk of recurrence if metastasized
      2. > 5 cm: Resection

Prog   Median survival: 4 months; prognosis better in fibrolamellar variant (no underlying cirrhosis)

Secondary: Metastases

Breast; **B**ronchus
Intestinal: colorectal, carcinoid, pancreas
Gastro-oesophageal

Melanoma
Endometrial
Testis
Special: lymphoma

BI**G**
ME**T**S

Pancreatic Tumours

Exocrine – Ductal Adenocarcinoma (90%)

Causes   *S.I.N.S.*

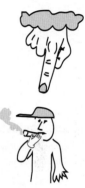

Smoking
  Risk increases three-fold

Inflammation
  Chronic pancreatitis, esp. hereditary pancreatitis

Nutrition
  High calorie intake, obesity, diabetes mellitus

Surgery
  Partial gastrectomy leads to biliary reflux into stomach, and secondary cholecystokinin release

PC   **A**bdominal–back pain
     Anorexia–weight loss
     Altered stool colour: pale (obstructive jaundice); silver (ampullary carcinoma)

O/E 1. Abdominal mass: • Umbilical mass due to tumour
                • Gall bladder due to bile duct compression (also causes jaundice)
                • Splenomegaly, and umbilical mass due to portal vein compression
     2. Lymphadenopathy: Troissier's sign (supraclavicular)

Comps 1. Local compression: obstructive jaundice, portal hypertension, IVC obstruction
       2. Pancreas failure: diabetes mellitus
       3. Paraneoplastic: • Thrombophilia causes migratory thrombophlebitis (Trousseau's sign)
                     • Panniculitis: fat necrosis
       4. Metastases: liver

Ix   1. Bloods: a) Amylase ↑ ; b) CEA, CA 19-9; c) FBC (anaemia), ESR ↑, LFT and clotting Δ
     2. Radio: a) CT; b) Angiography
     3. Special: a) ERCP or endoscopic USS; b) biopsy, via USS or CT guidance

Rx   1. Surgery (in only 10%): Whipple's procedure: pancreatico-duodenectomy
     2. Radiotherapy + 5-fluorouracil 'sensitizer': ↑es survival pre-operatively
     3. Chemotherapy: gemcitabine – for palliative use only

Prog Median survival = 6 months if inoperable

Endocrine – islet cell APUDomas (10%)

α: Glucagonoma; β: Insulinoma; δ: Somatostatinoma, **G**astrinoma, VIPoma; PPoma

Gallstones

Physiology

Normal bile content =

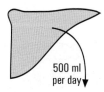

500 ml per day

10%: Bile salts (cholic and chenodeoxycholic acid) = *stone-preventing*
conjugate with glycine or taurine

5%: Phospholipid

1%: Cholesterol
1%: Conjugated bilirubin ⎫ **Stone-forming**
  also protein, drugs

Types

Mixed Cholesterol (75%)

Composition: monohydrate cholesterol (70%) + variable calcium salts (only 10% show on X-ray)+ bile acids
Cause: bile becomes supersaturated with cholesterol, relative to bile salt, due to:
  a) Excess hepatic secretion, e.g. HMG CoA reductase activity ↑
  b) Gall bladder concentration

Predisposing: *A.F.F.L.I.C.T.S.*

Age (20% of females over 40)
  + Americans (native USA, Chile)

Females (3:1 ratio), Fertile (multiparous)
  + Femodene (i.e. oral contraceptive pill, or HRT)

Fat + Fatty foods

Family history

Liver disease, chronic: bile salt production ↓

Ileum, terminal disease : Crohn's, lymphoma: bile salt recycling ↓

Congenital: choledochal cyst, cystic fibrosis

Toxins: clofibrate, ceftriaxone, cholestyramine + octreotide

Surgery: vagotomy: gall bladder contraction ↓
Somatostatinoma: gall bladder contraction ↓

Pigment (25%)

Composition: calcium bilirubinate + PO_4, CO_3 salts
Cause:
  1. Haemolytic anaemia: sickle cell, hereditary spherocytosis, malaria
    Path: Excess RBC turnover ⇒ black stones

  2. Helminths: • Nematodes – *Ascaris lumbricoides* (human roundworm)
         • Trematodes – *Clonorchis sinensis* (liver fluke; esp. Japan)
    Path: Supervening *E. coli* infection produces β-glucuronidase, which deconjugates
       bilirubin diglucuronide (soluble) to bilirubin (insoluble) ⇒ brown stones

PC Gallstones solely within the gall bladder fundus are asymptomatic – problems arise when they move out!
Presentation subsequently depends on site of gallstone occurrence:

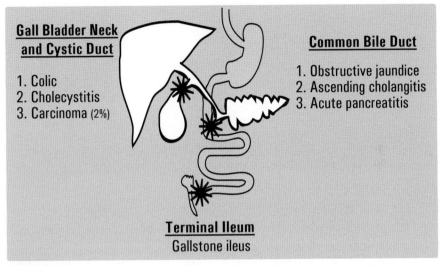

Gall Bladder Neck and Cystic Duct

1. Colic
2. Cholecystitis
3. Carcinoma (2%)

Common Bile Duct

1. Obstructive jaundice
2. Ascending cholangitis
3. Acute pancreatitis

Terminal Ileum
Gallstone ileus

Cholecystitis
Acute:
  Path: Sustained blockage of gall-bladder neck or cystic duct +
    secondary bacterial infection of stagnant gall bladder fluid (enterococci, coliforms)
  PC: Acute abdomen or chest pain, N + V, septic shock
  O/E: Right-upper quadrant tenderness + guarding, mass;
    Murphy's Sx (tender on inspiration); Boas' Sx (R loin hyperaesthesia)
  Ix: USS, ERCP – cholangiography
  Rx: NBM + IV hydration; IV cefuroxime + metronidazole; early or late cholecystectomy
Chronic:
  Path: Fibrous contraction of gall bladder following repeated bouts of gall bladder neck blockage
    and failure of gall bladder to concentrate fluid and contract
  PC: i) Episodic biliary colic; ii) Flatulent dyspepsia; iii) Fat intolerance
  Rx: i) High-dose bile salts; ii) Cholecystectomy
Complications:
  1. Empyema (pus collection); 2. Mucocoele (mucus collection); 3. Gangrene ⇒ Perforation

Obstructive Jaundice
Usually painless, unless stone is at sphincter of Oddie

Ascending Cholangitis
PC: Charcot's triad = fever + colic + jaundice
Complications: Liver abscesses, septicaemia, ARF

Gallstone Ileus
Stone erodes through gall bladder wall ⟶ penetrates duodenum ⟶ travels via small bowel to terminal ileum,
i.e. narrowest point

Infectious Diseases

Infectious Organisms – 1

Multicellular: invertebrates

Helminths (Worms)

Arthropods

Nematodes
= roundworms

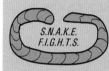

S.N.A.K.E.
F.I.G.H.T.S.

Cestodes
= tapeworms

Scolex = head with suckers | Proglottids = reproductive segments

P.h.D. P.E.T.S.

Trematodes
= flatworms

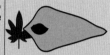

S.C.O.F.F.s HE.M.P.

Insect

1. Fleas
   Siphonaptera
2. Flies (Diptera):
   Anopheles
   Tsetse
   Midges
   Gnats
3. Lice, bugs
   Pediculus
   (hair + body)
   Phthirus pubis
   (pubic: 'crabs')

Intestinal

Strongyloides stercoralis

Necator americanus/

Ancylostoma duodenale
(human hookworm)

Ascaris lumbricoides
(human roundworm)

K: anisa**K**iasis, capillarious

Enterobius vermicularis
(threadworm)

Extra: whipworm –

Trichuris trichuria

Intestinal

Pork and beef tapeworms
= *Taenia solium* and
T. saginata

Hymenolepis:
1. *H. nana* (dwarf):
   human-limited
2. *H. diminuata*
   • Rodent-spread
   • Young children

Diphyllobothrium latum:
PC: • Diarrhoea, wt. loss
     • Vit B12 deficiency
     • Cholangitis /
       cholecystitis

Blood–veins

Schistosomiasis: ova
have characteristic
shapes and organ sites

Schistosoma mansoni:
colon, brain

Dorsal spine:
Charles Manson's
Knife!

S. japonicum: ileum, cord
Japanese small
willy!

S. haematobium: bladder
Terminal spine:
terminal like
the bladder

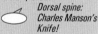

Arachnida

1. Spiders,
   scorpions
2. Ticks
3. Mites
   = Microscopic
   a) *Sarcoptes scabiei*
      (scabies)
   b) Chigger: red larvae

Tissue

Filariasis
 – *Onchocerca volvulus*:
   river blindness
 – *Wuchereria bancrofti*:
   elephantiasis
 – *Loa loa*
 – *Brugia malayi*

Guinea worm:
   Dracunculus medinensis

Toxocara canis

Trichinella spiralis

Skin: hookworm:
cutaneous larva migrans:
1. Animal hookworm, e.g.
   Ancylostoma brasiliense
2. Human hookworm
   PC: Serpiginous rash

Tissue

Pork tapeworm:
T. solium =
'cysticercosis'
PC: brain and cord
inflammation ⇒
epilepsy, hydrocephalus

Echinococcus granulosus:
'hydatid disease'
PC: Lung + liver cysts

T. solium (cysticercosis)

Spirometra: 'sparganosis'
PC: Subcutaneous tissue and
orbital swelling and
destruction

Liver

Clonorchis sinensis
Opisthorchis
Fasciola hepatica

Intestine

Fasciolopsis buski
HEterophyes heterophyes
Metagonimus yokogawai

Lung

Paragonimus westermani
PC: Cutaneous nodules,
epilepsy

Unicellular: eukaryotes (organelles, nucleus)

Fungi / yeasts
(rigid cell wall)

Protozoa

Superficial

1. Dermatophytes:
ringworm = tinea:
Trichophyton, Microsporum
PC: • Tinea capitis,
corporis, cruris or
pedis: athlete's foot
• Onychomycosis

2. *Malassezia furfur*
= *Pityrosporum orbiculare*
PC: 'Pityriasis versicolor';
seborrhoeic dermatitis;
dandruff

3. Subcutaneous:
Madura foot (mycetoma),
sporotrichosis,
chromoblastomycosis

Superficial + Deep

Candida albicans:
1. Thrush: oral, genital
2. Systemic (in
immunocompromised)
PC: • Meningitis
• Endophthalmitis
• Osteomyelitis
• Liver, spleen, kidney
• Endocarditis

Deep

1. Pneumonia:
• PCP (AIDS)
• *Aspergillus* (neutropenics)
**2. Pneumonia and / or
meningitis:**
• *Cryptococcus* (AIDS)
• *Histoplasma capsulatum*
(endemic S. USA)
• *Coccidioides immitis*
• *Blastomyces*
3. Retro-orbital:
• Mucormycosis (DM)

Sporozoa
= intracellular

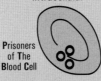

Prisoners
of The
Blood Cell

Plasmodium–malaria:
spread by *Anopheles*
mosquito

Types:
• *P. falciparum*: severe
• *P. vivax / ovale*: benign,
tertian
• *P. malariae*: benign,
quartan

Toxoplasma gondii:
spread from cat and
animal faeces
PC:
• Acute: lymphadenopathy
• Chorioretinitis
• Cerebral mass lesion
• Fetal malformation

Babesia – babesiosis:
• Spread by ixodid tick
• Similar to malaria
Types:
B. divergens: cattle
B. microti: rodents

Cryptosporidium +
• *Microsporum*
• *Isospora belli*
PC: Chronic gastroenteritis
in AIDS

Amoeboid
= simple

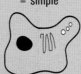

*Entamoeba
histolytica*
PC:
• 'Amoebic dysentry',
i.e. colitis
• Amoebic cyst

*Acanth***amoeba**
PC:
• Contact-lens keratitis
• Cerebral abscess

Naegleria fowleri:
found in swimming pools
contaminated with soil
e.g. Roman baths
PC: Meningoencephalitis

Flagellate
= has flagellum

Looks like
T.a.G.L.iaT.elle

Trypanosoma brucei
– *gambiense* (W.Africa)
– *rhodesiense* (E. Africa)

spread by *Glossina*, the
'Tsetse fly'

PC: 'Sleeping sickness' –
• Fever + lymphadenopathy
• Encephalopathy

EASt form: **A**cute, **S**evere
West form: chronic, mild

Trypanosoma cruzi –
autonomic neuropathy:
spread by reduviid bug in
South America
PC: 'Chagas' disease' –
• Myocarditis
• Achalasia
• Megacolon, constipation

Giardia lamblia
PC: duodeno-jejunitis

Leishmania: spread by sandfly
Types:
• Cutaneous –oriental sore:
L. mexicania or *L. tropica*
• Nasal mucosa – 'espundia':
L. brasiliensis
• **V**isceral – 'kala-azar':
*L. dono**V**ani*

Trichomonas vaginalis
PC: Vulvo-vaginitis

 Ciliate   The only pathogenic ciliate is *Balantidium coli*,
which causes an amoebic dysentry-like picture

Infectious Organisms – 2

Unicellular: prokaryotes (1 circular chromosome; no organelles)

Bacteria
(cell wall)

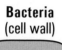

Mycoplasma/ Ureaplasma
(no cell wall)

Obligate intracellular parasites

Host Cell

Typical bacteria (p. 172)

	Gram +ve	Gram –ve
Cocci	●	○
Rods (bacilli)	▬	▭
	Anaerobes	

Mycobacteria (pp. 202–4)

- Weakly-staining Gram +ve rods
- Facultative intracellular parasites

T.A.X. S.L.U.M.

Tuberculosis
Avium intracellulare (MAI); *cheloni*
Xenopi; *kansasii*
Scrofulaceum
Leprae: leprosy
Ulcerans: Buruli ulcer
Marinum: fish-tank granuloma

Spirochaetes (pp. 206–8)

Helical-shaped

BO.L.T.

Borrelia:
1. Lyme disease: *B. burgdorferi*
2. Relapsing fever:
   B. recurrentis: louse-borne (epidemic)
   B. duTToni: Tick-borne (endemic)
3. Vincent's angina: *B. vincentii* – necrotizing gingivitis

Leptospira interrogans: Weil's disease

Treponema:
1. Syphilis: *T. pallidum*
2. Yaws: *T. pertenue*

Mycoplasma

M. pneumoniae: atypical pneumonia
M. hominis: UTI

Ureaplasma

U. urealyticum: UTI

N.B.
1. Smallest free-living organism
2. Small genome – limits biosynthesis and in vitro culture
3. No cell wall – so penicillins and cephalosporins are ineffective!

Rickettsiae (p. 210)

- Characterized by mammalian reservoirs and arthropod vectors
- All are small gram –ve bacilli

Q.ua.R.T.i.L.E.S.

Q-fever (*Coxiella burnetii*):
  Epi: No vector required: spread by aerosol from uterus or mammary glands of peripartum farm animals, pets
  PC: Atypical pneumonia

Rocky-mountain spotted fever:
  caused by *Rickettsia rickettsii* (tick-borne)

Tick-borne typhus – other:
  - *Ehrlichia chaffeensis*: monocytes
  - *E. phagocytophilia*: granulocytes
  - 'Mediterranean spotted fever' *Rickettsia conorii*

Louse-borne:

Epidemic and endemic typhus:
  - 'Epidemic typhus' caused by *Rickettsia prowazekii* humans are only host
  - 'Endemic murine typhus' caused by *Rickettsia typhi*:

Scrub typhus: *Orientia tsutsugamushi* (chigger-borne)

Chlamydia

1. *C. pneumoniae* / *C. psittaci*: atypical pneumonia

2. *C. trachomatis*:
   - PID / urethritis
   - Lymphogranuloma venereum
   - 'Trachoma': keratitis

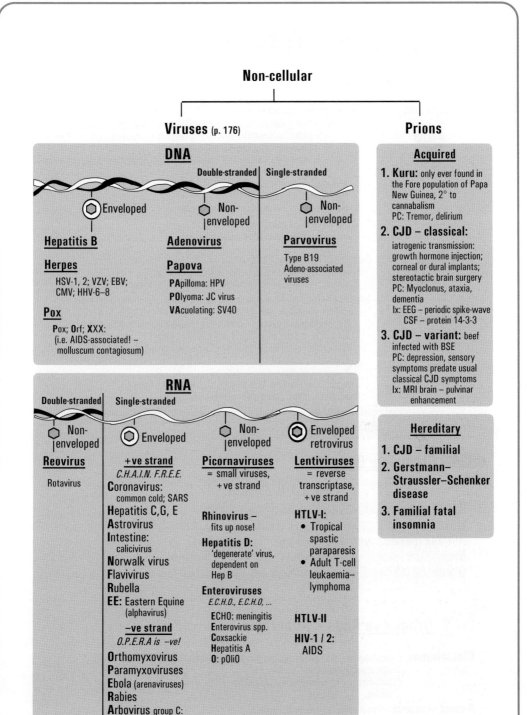

Non-cellular

Viruses (p. 176)

DNA

| Double-stranded | Single-stranded |

Enveloped

Hepatitis B

Herpes

HSV-1, 2; VZV; EBV;
CMV; HHV-6–8

Pox

Pox; Orf; XXX:
(i.e. AIDS-associated! –
molluscum contagiosum)

Non-enveloped

Adenovirus

Papova

PApilloma: HPV
POlyoma: JC virus
VAcuolating: SV40

Non-enveloped

Parvovirus

Type B19
Adeno-associated
viruses

RNA

Double-stranded | **Single-stranded**

Non-enveloped

Reovirus

Rotavirus

Enveloped

+ve strand
C.H.A.I.N. F.R.E.E.
Coronavirus:
common cold; SARS
Hepatitis C,G, E
Astrovirus
Intestine:
calicivirus
Norwalk virus
Flavivirus
Rubella
EE: Eastern Equine
(alphavirus)

–ve strand
O.P.E.R.A is –ve!
Orthomyxovirus
Paramyxoviruses
Ebola (arenaviruses)
Rabies
Arbovirus group C:
Hantavirus

Non-enveloped

Picornaviruses
= small viruses,
+ve strand

Rhinovirus –
fits up nose!

Hepatitis D:
'degenerate' virus,
dependent on
Hep B

Enteroviruses
E.C.H.O., E.C.H.O, ...

ECHO: meningitis
Enterovirus spp.
Coxsackie
Hepatitis A
O: p**O**li**O**

Enveloped retrovirus

Lentiviruses
= reverse
transcriptase,
+ve strand

HTLV-I:
• Tropical
spastic
paraparesis
• Adult T-cell
leukaemia–
lymphoma

HTLV-II

HIV-1 / 2:
AIDS

Prions

Acquired

1. **Kuru:** only ever found in
   the Fore population of Papa
   New Guinea, 2° to
   cannabalism
   PC: Tremor, delirium

2. **CJD – classical:**
   iatrogenic transmission:
   growth hormone injection;
   corneal or dural implants;
   stereotactic brain surgery
   PC: Myoclonus, ataxia,
   dementia
   Ix: EEG – periodic spike-wave
   CSF – protein 14-3-3

3. **CJD – variant:** beef
   infected with BSE
   PC: depression, sensory
   symptoms predate usual
   classical CJD symptoms
   Ix: MRI brain – pulvinar
   enhancement

Hereditary

1. **CJD – familial**

2. **Gerstmann–
   Straussler–Schenker
   disease**

3. **Familial fatal
   insomnia**

Bacteria

 ## Gram +ve Cocci

Staphylococcus — ***aureus*** (coagulase +ve): *S.T.A.P.H.*

Microscopy:
clusters of grapes

    Skin: • Boil (furuncle / carbuncle): becomes walled off due to coagulase
          • Cellulitis, impetigo, necrotizing fasciitis
    Toxin: • Gastroenteritis: heat-stable toxin
          • Toxic shock syndrome: septic shock; desquamation of palms + soles
          • Scalded skin syndrome
    Arthritis / osteomyelitis
    Pulmonary: lung abscess
    Heart: acute endocarditis / **H**epatic: abscess

— ***epidermidis*** (coagulase –ve):
    iatrogenic infection: line-associated sepsis

Streptococcus   *α*-**haemolytic**: Plate appears green
    S. viridans, e.g. *S. bovis*, *S. mitior*: subacute endocarditis
    S. pneumoniae (diplococci): pneumonia, endocarditis, meningitis, otitis media

Microscopy:
long chains

  β-**haemolytic**: Cause complete haemolysis: plate has 'punched-out holes'
    Group A: *S. pyogenes*: *S.T.R.E.P.*
      Skin: cellulitis, impetigo – spreads due to streptokinase and hyaluronidase
      Tonsillitis: quinsy, pharyngitis, otitis media, sinusitis
      Rheumatic fever; **R**enal: proliferative glomerulonephritis ⎱ immune
      Erythema nodosum   ⎰ phenomena
      Puerperal sepsis; wound infections
    Group B: *S. agalactiae*: puerperal sepsis, neonatal meningitis
    Group G: *S. milleri*: abscesses - cerebral, liver, lung

  Enterococci: endocarditis, peritonitis, UTI : non-haemolytic, lactose-fermenting
  Anaerobic: endocarditis

⬛ Gram +ve Rods

B.L.A.N.D. bacteria

Bacillus *cereus*: food poisoning from reheated Chinese food
Listeria *monocytogenes*: meningoencephalitis, miscarriage, septic shock in immunocompromised
Anthrax (*Bacillus anthracis*): cutaneous – eschar; pneumonia
Nocardia: 'No heart' – occurs with heart transplant / immunosuppressed
Diphtheria (*Corynebacterium diphtheriae*): pharyngitis ('bull neck'), myocarditis, bulbar palsy

- -

 ## Gram +ve Rods – Anaerobic

Clostridium: *C. perfringens*: food poisoning, gas gangrene, puerperal sepsis
              C. botulinum: botulism
              C. difficile: pseudomembranous colitis
              C. tetani: tetanus
Actinomycosis: dental-cervical; ileocaecal abscess
          Path: Form yellow sulphur granules, granulomas

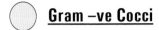 ## Gram –ve Cocci

Neisseria   – *meningitides:* bacterial meningitis (types A,B,C)
             – *gonorrhoeae:* urethritis, arthritis, pharyngitis
Moraxella catarrhalis: community-acquired pneumonia

Gram –ve Rods

S.P.Y.. S.E.E.K.s. G.B.H. , P.V.C. + L.eather!

Enterobacteria: all cause gastroenteritis (except where indicated)

Non-lactose fermenting (plates contain lactose + pH indicator that turns pink):
  Salmonella / **S**higella: bacillary dysentery
  Proteus mirabilis: UTI
  Yersinia enterocolitica or *pseudotuberculosis*: ilieocaecal mass / Y. pestis: plague

Lactose-fermenting ('coliforms'):
  Serratia
  Escherichia coli
  Enterobacteria spp.
  Klebsiella: UTI; neonatal meningitis, severe, nosocomial pneumonia
  Shigella sonnei: only *Shigella* sp. that ferments lactose

Parvobacteria (small size – **all end in 'ella', except** *Haemophilus*):
  Gardnerella vaginalis: vaginitis
    +*Francisella tularensis*: tularaemia: ulcers, lymphadenopathy, pneumonia – from rabbits, deer
    +*Pasteurella*: localized or systemic infection from animal-bite
  Brucella melitensis / abortus: pneumonia, meningitis, endocarditis – contracted from farm animals
    +*Bordetella pertussis*: whooping cough
    +*Bartonella*: cat-scratch disease (B. henselae), Oroya fever, bacillary angiomatosis
  Haemophilus influenzae: pneumonia, epiglottitis, meningitis / H. ducreyi: chancroid

Other:
  Pseudomonas aeruginosa: P.S.E.U.D.O.
    Pneumonia in cystic fibrosis or ITU; **S**epticaemia; **E**cthyma gangrenosum in immunocompromised;
    UTI; **D**ermatological – wound infection; **O**phthalmology – endophthalmitis 2° to trauma
    + *Burkholderia pseudomallei* (related bacteria): melioidosis; glanders – pneumonia
  Vibrio cholerae: cholera / V. parahaemolyticus: food-poisoning
  Campylobacteria jejuni: bloody diarrhoea
  Legionella pneumophila: atypical, severe pneumonia

Gram –ve Rods – Anaerobic

Bacteroides: • B. fragilis: peritonitis 2° to bowel / gynaecological disease
             • B. oralis / Fusobacteria: dental abscess-gingivitis / Lemierre's disease

Helicobacter pylori: peptic ulcer, gastric carcinoma, gastic MALToma

Antibiotics

Choice

Gram+ve Cocci

Staphylococci:
 1. Beta-lactams: flucloxacillin, co-amoxiclav
2. Glycopeptides: vancomycin, teicoplanin
3. Oxazolinedione: linezolid

+ Special circumstances:
a) Osteomyelitis: clindamycin, fusidic acid
b) Endocarditis: gentamicin

+ Penicillin-allergic: macrolide –
erythromycin

Streptococci:
Beta-lactams:
1. Penicillins
  • Benzylpenicillin, 'Pen G' (IV)
  • Phenoxymethylpenicillin, 'Pen V' (PO)
  • Amoxicillin, ampicillin
2. Cephalosporins:
  • 1°: cefaclor, cefalexin (PO)
  • 2°: cefuroxime (IV)
3. Carbapenems: meropenem, imipenem
  + cilastin

+ Penicillin-allergic: macrolide: –
erythromycin

Gram +ve Rods: *L.A.N.D.*

Listeria: ampicillin+gentamicin
Anthrax: penicillin / ciprofloxacin
Nocardia: cotrimoxazole
Diphtheria: anti-toxin

- -

▨ Gram+ve Anaerobes

Clostridia botulinum / perfringens:
benzylpenicillin, clindamycin, metronidazole
Clostridium difficile: metronidazole, vancomycin
Actinomycoses: co-amoxiclav

◯ Gram –ve Cocci

Meningococci:
1. Penicillins: benzylpenicillin
2. Cephalosporin, 3°: ceftriaxone, cefotaxime
3. Penicillin-allergic: macrolide – erythromycin

Gonococci:
1. Amoxicillin, ampicillin
2. Cephalosporins: 2°, 3°
3. Quinolone: ciprofloxacin
+ Penicillin-allergic: macrolide – erythromycin

Gram –ve Rods

Enterobacteria – e.g. *Salmonella, E. coli*
1. Trimethoprim
2. Aminoglycosides: gentamicin, amikacin
3. Quinolone: ciprofloxacin

Parvobacteria – e.g. *Haemophilus*, pertussis
1. Amoxicillin; ampicillin
2. Cephalosporins: 2° , 3°

Pseudomonas aeruginosa
1. Beta-lactams:
  • Ticarcillin, piperacillin
  • Ceftazidime
  • Aztreonam (monobactam)
2. Aminoglycosides: gentamicin, amikacin
3. Quinolone: ciprofloxacin

Brucella: doxycycline + gentamicin/rifampicin
Francisella: streptomycin
Legionella: erythromycin + rifampicin

- -

▭ Gram –ve Anaerobes

Bacteroides: metronidazole
Helicobacter: metronidazole or clarithromycin,
plus amoxicillin

Atypical Bacteria

Mycoplasma, Spirochaetes, Rickettsia, Chlamydiae:
1. **Macrolides**: erythromycin, azithromycin, clarithromycin
2. **Tetracyclines**: tetracycline, oxytetracycline

Mycobacteria:
1. **TB**: R.I.P.P.E.R.S. (p. 203)
2. **Leprosy**: rifampicin, clofazimine, dapsone
3. **Atypical**: rifampicin, clofazimine, macrolide

Sites of Action

Peptidoglycan cell-wall

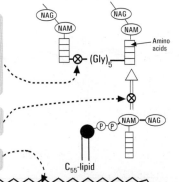

NAG: N-acetylglucosamine
NAM: N-acetylmuramic acid

1. **Beta-lactams:**
   - Binds to penicillin-binding protein
   - Inhibit transpeptidation cross-link between peptide backbones
   - Inhibit autolysis inhibitor: osmotic pressure ruptures plasma membrane
2. **Cycloserine:** inhibits addition of final 2 Alanine amino acids

3. **Glycopeptides, bacitracin**
   Inhibits release of peptidoglycan building block from lipid carrier

4. **Polymixin:** cationic detergents disrupt lipid bilayer

Cell wall
Lipid bilayer

DNA / RNA synthesis

1. **Quinolones (ciprofloxacin):**
   - Inhibit DNA relaxation prior to transcription or replication
   - Inhibit DNA coiling prior to cell division

2. **Metronidazole:**
   - Fragments DNA via free-radicals
   - Inhibits nucleic acid synthesis
   - Inhibits reductase enzyme in anaerobic respiratn pathway

3. **Rifampicin:** Inhibits prokaryote RNA polymerase

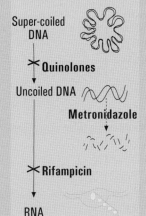

Super-coiled
DNA

✕ **Quinolones**

Uncoiled DNA

Metronidazole

✕ **Rifampicin**

RNA

Protein synthesis

1. **Tetracyclines:**
   - Selective uptake into bacteria
   - Competitive inhibitors with incoming tRNA for amino site

2. **Aminoglycosides:**
   - Selective uptake
   - Causes misreading of codon (mRNA) anticodon

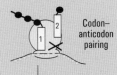

Codon–anticodon pairing

3. **Chloramphenicol, clindamycin:** inhibit transpeptidation

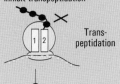

Trans-peptidation

4. **Macrolides, fusidic acid:** inhibit translocation

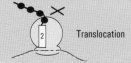

Translocation

Folate synthesis

1. **Sulphonamides:**
   competitive inhibitors of dihydropteroate synthetase

2. **Trimethoprim:**
   competitive inhibitor of bacterial DHFR (dihydrofolate reductase)

PABA
(*para*-amino benzoic acid)

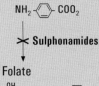

$NH_2 \!\!-\!\!\langle\rangle\!\!-\!\! COO_2$

✕ **Sulphonamides**

Folate

OH
$N\!\!-\!\!CH_2\!\!-\!\!NH\!\!-\!\!\langle\rangle\!\!-\!\!CO. Glu$
H_2N

✕ **Trimethoprim**

Tetrahydrofolate polyglutamate

<u>Viruses</u>

DNA

Double-stranded | Single-stranded

◉ Enveloped   ⬡ Non-enveloped   ⬡ Non-enveloped

<u>Hepatitis B</u> (p. 152)

<u>Herpes</u> (pp. 193–5)
1. HSV-1:
   - Labial herpes
   - Encephalitis
2. HSV-2:
   - Genital herpes
   - Meningitis, recurrent
3. VZV:
   - Chicken pox (varicella)
   - Zoster
   - Brainstem encephalitis, myelitis
4. EBV:
   - Glandular fever
   - Lymphoma (esp. Non-Hodgkin's)
   - Nasopharynx carcinoma
5. CMV:
   - Retinitis
   - Colitis / hepatitis
   - Pneumonitis
     (disease only occurs in
     immunosupressed,
     esp. AIDS and organ transplant)
6. HHV-6:
   - Roseola infantum
     (exanthema subitum)
   - Meningoencephalitis
7. HHV-7
8. HHV-8:
   - Kaposi's sarcoma

<u>Pox</u>
Pox:
  - Cowpox (vaccinia)
  - Smallpox (variola)
    both eradicated by vaccination
Orf:
  - Pustules, acquired from sheep
XXX (assoc. with HIV) –
  molluscum contagiosum
  - Pearly, umbilicated pustules

<u>Adenovirus</u>
1. Types 1–30:
   - Pharyngitis – bronchitis
   - Conjunctivitis
   - Meningitis
2. Types 40, 41:
   - Diarrhoea

<u>Papova</u>

<u>PA</u>pilloma:

Human papillomavirus (HPV)
Types 6, 11:
  - Warts, condylomata
    acuminata
Types 16, 18:
  - Carcinoma of cervix, vulva,
    penis, rectum

<u>PO</u>lyoma

JC virus:
  - Progressive multifocal
    leucoencephalopathy (PML)
  - Occurs in AIDS or pts. given
    integrin inhibitors, e.g. as Rx for
    multiple sclerosis

BK virus

<u>VA</u>cuolating, e.g. SV40:
  - Used in recombinant
    genetic engineering

<u>Parvovirus</u>
1. Type B19: (p. 193)
   - Erythema infectiosum
     ('slapped cheek syn.'
     or 'fifth disease')
   - Aplastic anaemia crisis
     esp. in hereditary
     haemolytic anaemias,
     e.g. sickle cell disease

2. Adeno-associated
   viruses

RNA

Double-stranded | **Single-stranded**

Non-enveloped | Enveloped | Non-enveloped | Enveloped retrovirus

Reovirus:

Rotavirus
• Infantile gastroenteritis

+ve strand
C.H.A.I.N. F.R.E.E.

Coronavirus:
• Common cold; SARS

Hepatitis:
• Hep C, G (flavivirus-like)
• Hep E   (calicivirus-like)

Astrovirus:
• Gastroenteritis

Intestinal, other:
• Calicivirus
• 'small-round structured viruses'

Norwalk virus

Flavivirus:
• Yellow fever
• Dengue haemorrhagic fever

Rubella

EE: Eastern equine encephalitis, Ross River virus (alphaviruses)

N.B. Flaviviruses, rubella and alphaviruses are part of Togavirus family

---

–ve strand
O.P.E.R.A is –ve!

Orthomyxovirus:
• Influenza A–C

Paramyxoviruses:
• Parainfluenza
• RSV
• Measles
• Mumps

Ebola virus other arena viruses, e.g. Lassa fever

Rabies (rhabdovirus)

Arbovirus group C:
• Hantavirus

Picornaviruses
= small viruses, +ve strand

Rhinovirus:
fits up nose!

Hepatitis D:
'degenerate' virus, dependent on Hep B

Enteroviruses
E.C.H.O., E.C.H.O, ...
ECHO: meningitis
Enterovirus spp.
Coxsackie
A: • Meningitis
   • Conjunctivitis (A24)
   • Hand, foot & mouth disease (A16)
   • Herpangina
B: • Myopericarditis
   • Bornholm disease
Hepatitis A
O: pOliO

Lentiviruses
= reverse transcriptase +ve strand

HTLV-I:
• Tropical spastic paraparesis
• Adult T-cell leukaemia- lymphoma

HTLV-II:
• Hairy cell leukaemia?

HIV-1 / 2:   (p. 196)
• AIDS

N.B. These viruses infect non-dividing cells: therefore slow replicators ('lenti')

Pneumonia – Pathogens

Community-Acquired

Typical

Lobar

Streptococcus pneumoniae:
    Epi: Recent viral upper-respiratory tract infection, winter
    PC: **R**apid onset, offset; **R**usty sputum; **R**igors (septicaemia); pleural, pericardial effusion; MR = 20%
  Gram –ves: *Haemophilus influenzae* type b (rods) or *Moraxella catarrhalis* (cocci)
    Epi: COAD, elderly, infants, septicaemic
    PC: insidious onset; purulent sputum; cor pulmonale

Cavities and empyema – *patients are pretty SicK*

Staphylococcus aureus:
    Epi: Influenza; measles; intravenous drug abusers; cystic fibrosis; MR = 30%
Klebsiella (short, plump, capsulated, Gram –ve bacilli):
    Epi: Alcoholics, diabetes mellitus, COAD; S.Africa
    PC: Bloody sputum; CXR – bowing of fissures; reduced lung volume; sputum microscopy +ve for organism

Atypical – 1

Constitutional symptoms with normal chest auscultation, but CXR shows consolidation

Mycoplasma pneumoniae
    Epi: Winter epidemics every few years; young adults, esp. in army or college
    PC: *F.A.S.C.I.N.A.T.E.*
         Flu-like: fever; **A**rthralgia, arthritis; **S**kin: erythema multiforme, Raynaud's (cold agglutinins);
         Cardiology: pericarditis, myocarditis; **I**ntestinal: D + V, pancreatitis;
         Neurological: headache common; Guillain–Barré syndrome, myelitis, meningo-encephalitis, cerebellar ataxia;
         Anaemia: cold agglutinin haemolytic anaemia; jaundice (N.B. normal white-cell count);
         Throat, sore, injected; laryngitis or tracheitis – dry or mucoid cough; **E**arache – bullous myringitis

Legionella pneumophila
    Epi: Outbreaks, esp. on contact with stagnant fresh-water supply, air-conditioning, humidifiers, whirl-pools;
             summer; mediterranean-travel; middle-age, obese, alcoholic, smokers, diabetes
    PC: *P.A.N.I.C.K.E.R.*
         Pyrexia, esp. > 40°C (with relative bradycardia); may be self-limiting without pneumonia ('Pontiac fever');
         Arthralgia, inc. marked pleuritic chest pain; **N**eurological: headache; encephalopathy;
         Intestinal: D + V, abdominal pain; **C**oagulopathy (DIC), CK↑; **K**idney: proteinuria, haematuria, renal failure;
         Electrolytes: Na ↓, PO4 ↓, ALT↑, albumin ↓; **R**espiratory failure, lung abscess

Chlamydia pneumoniae / psittaci
    Epi: *C. pneumoniae* – person-to-person spread; *C. psittaci* – parrots; sheep, turkey, duck, pigeon (ornithosis)
    PC: • *C. pneumoniae* – pharyngitis; otitis; dry or mucoid cough occurs late
          • *C. psittaci* – headache, myalgia; severe cough, haemoptysis, 2° bacterial infection; endocarditis

Coxiella burnetti (Q-fever)
    Epi: Sheep, goats, cattle-rearing areas, e.g E. Canada, NW Spain; contact with dairy products or faeces
    PC: Abrupt onset of flu-like illness; meningitis; endocarditis; hepatitis

Atypical – 2

  Bacteria: • TB: Epi: Alcoholics, debilitated, Indian; PC: Insidious symptoms – chronic cough, haemoptysis, weight loss
              • Meliodiosis (*Pseudomonas pseudomallei*); *Actinomyces israelii*; tularaemia; plague; anthrax
  Viruses: • Adenovirus, influenza, parainfluenza, RSV, measles – mainly children; causes interstitial pneumonitis
              • Hantavirus: rodents, deer in USA
  Fungi: • Histoplasmosis – Mid West or SE USA: bats, soil; coccidioidomycosis – SW USA deserts; blastomycosis;
              • Cryptococcosis – pigeon droppings

Nosocomial

Def: Pneumonia acquired in hospital ≥ 2 days after admission

Causes: *C.I.R.C.U.L.A.R... like the treatment of them*
         Contact with other patients
         Immunocompromise
         Recumbency (basal atelectasis)
         Catheters, inc. **U**rinary, **L**ines and ET tubes
         Antibiotic **R**esistance

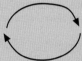

Organisms:

 Gram +ves (30%)   **Gram −ves (50%)**

Staphylococcus aureus, esp. MRSA   **P**seudomonas aeruginosa – tubes
Streptococcus faecalis   **A**cinetobacter
    inc. vancomycin-resistant   **L**egionella – nebulizer, ventilators
       enterococci (VRE)   Enterobacteria: *Proteus, Serratia, Enterobacter*
Streptococcus pneumoniae

        Anaerobes: *Bacteroides, Fusobacterium*
        Fungi

Immunocompromised

Innate

    1. Aspiration – e.g. alcoholics, drug overdose, bulbar weakness inc. stroke, seizure:
           anaerobes, e.g. *Bacteroides, Streptococcus milleri*
    2. Cystic fibrosis: *Haemophilus, Staphylococcus, Pseudomonas aeruginosa / cepacia*
    3. Bronchial obstruction – e.g. foreign body; carcinoma; lymph node, bronchopulmonary sequestration:
           anaerobes, e.g. *Bacteroides, S. milleri*
    4. Neutropenia: Coliforms, *S. aureus, Aspergillus*

B-cell – e.g. splenectomy, hypogammaglobulinaemia:
                  S. pneumoniae, Haemophilus (both encapsulated bacteria), *Mycoplasma*

T-cell e.g. AIDS:

    1. Bacterial: • Community-acquired pneumonia – occur early in AIDS; more severe
                • TB, MAI
    2. Fungi: PCP – 80% develop without prophylaxis; *Cryptococcus* – mild pneumonia
    3. Viruses: herpes viruses: CMV, EBV, HSV, VZV, HHV-8 (Kaposi's sarcoma)
    4. Toxoplasmosis

B- + T-cell – e.g. post-transplant immunosuppression:

    1. Nosocomial, e.g. *Legionella*
    2. *Nocardia* (esp. heart transplant): PC: Pleurisy, cavitates, metastases; Ix: Acid-fast hyphae
    3. *Candida; Aspergillus*
    4. CMV: systemic disease

Food Poisoning

Def 1. Caused by bacteria or toxin residing in food source
2. Derives from infection within animal, or contamination during food storage or preparation

Causes Classified by:
Cause: pre-formed toxin vs bacterial multiplication (often with toxin secretion)
Incubation time: hours (pre-formed toxin)–days (bacterial multiplication within gut)

Pre-Formed Toxin: 1–6 hrs   *S.iC.k*

Staphylococcus aureus: heat-**ST**able enterotoxins A–E
Food: Contaminated dairy or meat; septic lesion on hand of food-handler
PC: Vomiting (± diarrhoea)
Rx: Flucloxacillin if bacteria isolated

Clostridium botulinum: heat-labile toxin (blocks pre-synaptic release of Ach)
Food: Tinned foods kept in anaerobic conditions, esp. home-canners, canned fruit
PC: Vomiting (± constipation); descending paralysis (ophthalmoplegia, ptosis, bulbar weakness)
Rx: Anti-toxin; nerves resprout in 2–3 months

Toxin / Cell Multiplication: 8–24 hrs   *S.iC.k*

Special foods:

Seafood, raw – *Vibrio parahaemolyticus*:
Micro: Forms blue–green colonies on thiosulphate agar
PC: Vomiting; diarrhoea; abdominal pain
Rx: Tetracycline

Soups–sauces; or reheated, fried rice – *Bacillus cereus*:
Micro: Forms 'curled hair' colonies on agar
PC: Early vomiting (rice); diarrhoea, abdominal pain (soup, sauce)

Clostridium perfringens (heat-labile toxin + bacterial multiplication):
Food: Reheated meat, e.g. meat pies, mincemeat, stew
Micro: Nagler reaction detects toxin (half the plate has anti-toxin, which inhibits growth)
PC: Colic (gas-producing –same organism as in gas gangrene!)

Cell Multiplication: 1-10 days   *S.iC.k*

Salmonella spp. (2000 serotypes, inc. *S. enteritidis* phage type 4):
Food: Eggs, chicken, milk stored at room temp. / nursing home outbreaks
Micro: • Non-lactose-fermenting on MacConkey medium
• Serotyped by antigens O (lipopolysaccharide) and H (flagella)
PC: 1. Vomiting; diarrhoea (profuse, watery ± blood in 25%); abdominal pain
2. Fever; septicaemia, due to invasion of wall; esp. immunocompromised, *S. virchow*
3. Asymptomatic carriage
Rx: Ciprofloxacin or amoxicillin – only if septicaemia due to risk of prolonged carriage

Campylobacter jejuni (cholera-like heat-stable toxin):
Food: Cooked meat, heated milk
Micro: Motile, curved spiral-shaped rods - like 'seagulls'
PC: 1. Prodrome: fever, vomiting, headache, generalized aches
2. Profuse watery, bloody diarrhoea (± mucus, pus); abdominal pain
Rx: Erythromycin (decreases excretion rate), ciprofloxacin

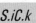

Gastroenteritis

<u>Def</u> 1. Bacteria spread between people, via faecal–oral route, e.g. food handling by case; in water supply
2. Bacteria cause colitis – except for *Vibrio cholerae* and *Salmonella typhi*, which cause ileitis

<u>Causes</u>   *V.E.R.Y. S.iC.k*

Vibrio cholerae

Escherichia coli: *P.I.T.H.y:*
    Pathogenetic – **P**aediatric (neonatal and infantile gastroenteritis)
    Invasive (*Shigella*-like dysentery)
    Toxicogenetic – **T**raveller's diarrhoea (cholera-like)
    Haemorrhagic – **H**aemorrhagic colitis / **H**aemolytic–uraemic syndrome

Rotavirus, and other viruses:
    Rotavirus (esp. group A) – double-stranded RNA:
        Epi: • Occurs in infants or elderly in institutions (outbreaks), esp. in Winter
                • Spread via respiratory secretions, as well as faecal–oral route
        PC: May cause respiratory symptoms, as well as D+V+abdominal cramps + fever
        Electron microscopy: Spherical particles with spoke-like surface
    Astrovirus, calicivirus, Norwalk-like viruses – single-stranded +ve RNA:
        Epi: Outbreaks among children (esp. caliciviruses) or families
        Electron microscopy: 6-pointed star, small-round structured viruses (SRSVs)
    Adenovirus (esp. serotypes 40, 41) – DNA virus:
        Epi: Endemic, due to prolonged faecal excretion by cases
        Electron microscopy: Icosahedral symmetry with round capsomeres
    CMV – DNA virus:
        Epi: Immunocompromised, e.g. HIV

Yersinia enterocolitica / pseudotuberculosis

Salmonella typhi: 'typhoid fever'

Shigella dysenteriae: 'bacillary dysentry'

Clostridium difficile: 'pseudomembranous colitis'
    Also *Clostridium septicum*: neutropenic enterocolitis

Cryptosporidium, and other protozoa:
    Sporozoa: *Cryptosporidium, Microsporidium, Isospora belli* – HIV-related
                Plasmodium – malaria
    Amoeba: *Entamoeba histolytica* – 'amoebic dysentry'
    Flagellate: *Giardia lamblia*
    Ciliate: *Balantidium coli*

Gastroenteritis – Ileal-Based

Salmonella – 'Typhoid' or 'Enteric Fever'

Bacteria

Salmonella typhi – severe; *S. paratyphi* – asymptomatic or mild, and less carriership

Epi

1. Spread by cases < 2 months post-infection, OR chronic carriers (2%), who excrete bacteria indefinitely; Carriage assoc. with elderly women, gallstones, *Salmonella* Vi antigen +ve (capsule)
2. Medium of spread: water supply (excreted by faeces, urine), or carriers' hands on meat, eggs, milk
3. Sporadic: 3/4 in UK acquired abroad; OR outbreaks, e.g. Croydon 1937; food-borne, e.g. Typhoid Mary
4. Risk factors: achlorhydria ↑ es risk; sickle cell: ↑ septicaemia

Path

Bacteria **cross** ileal epithelium (cf. *Shigella* – remains *within* colonic epithelium)

Weeks 1–2
Lumen of ileum / appendix

- Binds to mannose
- Distorts microvilli - 'actin splash'
- Transcytosis via endosome
- Transient bacteraemia

Weeks 2–3 +

- Proliferates in lamina propria
- Spreads to lymph nodes

- Multiplies within macrophages of reticuloendothelial system

Bacteraemia

Chronic cholecystitis – reinfects bowel in Peyer's patches

PC

G.O. S.A.L.M.O.N.E.L.L.A

GIT: 1st week: constipation; abdominal pain, distension
3rd week +: infectious diarrhoea
Complications: GIT haemorrhage; ileal ulceration, perforation

Organomegaly: hepatosplenomegaly

Systemic: fever (transient bacteraemia) / **S**kin: rose spots

Arthralgia, arthritis; myalgia, myositis, necrosis

Lungs: pneumonitis / URTI symptoms common: e.g. sore throat, epistaxis

Myocarditis: bradycardia common

Osteomyelitis

Neurological: headache common, meningo-encephalitis

Nephritis – glomerulonephritis, pyelonephritis

Extra: DVT

Lymphocytes ↑ ; WBC ↓

LAte: mortality 10% without Rx; 0.1% if treated

Ix

1. Culture: • 1st 10 days: blood or bone marrow culture; 2nd 10 days: stool or urine culture
   • Non-Lactose-fermenting on MacConkey medium
2. Serology: Widal test: diluted patient's serum (Ig) + killed test bacteria → visible clumps

Rx

1. Amoxicillin, trimethoprim, ciprofloxacin, ceftriaxone (IV) – resistance common
2. Cholecystectomy: cures carriage in 75%, but small risk of death
3. Vaccine: killed monovalent IM or Vi-capsular polysaccharide Ag, live oral – 3 years' protection

Cholera

Bacteria

Vibrio cholerae: • Type 01; biotype classical (severe); serotype Ogawa, Inaba, Hikojima, ...
• Type 01; biotype El-Tor (mild)

Epi

1. Spread by cases, and asymptomatic carriers that occur commonly in outbreaks
2. Medium of spread: water supply, seafood, flies – but cooking destroys bacteria
3. Risk factor: achlorhydria; epidemics and pandemics

Path

Bacterial toxin binds to ganglioside receptors, in ileum, via B ('binding') subunit

Subunit A enters cell and permanently activates Gsα via ADP-ribosylation

Adenylate cyclase activated thereby ↑ing cAMP, and leading to isotonic loss of water, NaCl, KCl, HCO$_3^-$

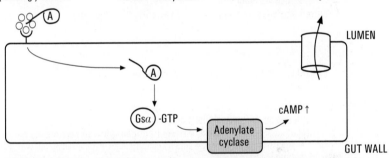

PC

Incubation period: 5 hours – 5 days

D + V:
• Profuse, 'rice-water' stool (turbid, due to flecks of mucus and shed epithelium)
• Severe dehydration: 'choleraic facies' = sunken eyes and cheeks; hypovolaemic shock, acute tubular necrosis

Ix

1. Bloods: • Na$^+$ normal; K$^+$ ↓ (muscle cramps)
• Metabolic acidosis
2. Stool microscopy / cultures:
• No WBCs or RBCs seen
• Culture: sucrose-fermenting
• Bacteria appear as small curved, comma-shaped , motile Gram –ve rods
3. Type: e.g. 01; biotype: classical or El-Tor; serotype: slide agglutination; phage type

Rx

1. Tetracycline (PO/IV): ↓ fluid loss and ↓ infectivity
2. Killed vaccine: only protects 50% (not 0139)

Bacterial Gastroenteritis – Other

Escherichia coli

Types

P.I.T.H.Y.

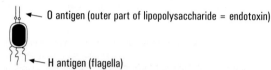

← O antigen (outer part of lipopolysaccharide = endotoxin)

← H antigen (flagella)

Paediatric:
1. EnteroPathogenetic: infantile gastroenteritis (0–2 years)
   Epi: • Sporadic, or outbreaks in nurseries and 3rd World
   • Breast-feeding protects
   Path: Acts by combination of invasion and toxins
   PC: • Profuse watery diarrhoea, dehydration, metabolic acidosis
   • High mortality rate
2. Entero-aggregative: neonatal gastroenteritis (0–6 months)

Invasive:
EnteroInvasive
   Epi: All ages
   Path: Shiga-like toxin causes *Shigella*-like dysentry in colon
   Ix: Stool microscopy: RBCs and WBCs

Traveller's diarrhoea:
EnteroToxicogenic: travellers' diarrhoea
e.g. O6 type (local *E. coli* possess different antigen types to commensal bacteria)
   Epi: • Adults recently arrived in foreign country ingesting contaminated water / food
   • Infants in 3rd World
   Path: • 'Colonization factor antigen' = special fimbriae or pili that allow ileal adherence
   • Heat-labile toxin or heat-stable toxin (activates guanylate cyclase)
   PC: • Cholera-like: profuse watery diarrhoea, vomiting, abdominal pain, mild fever
   • Lasts for a few days, or rarely weeks
   Rx: Doxycycline or ciprofloxacin in severe cases

Haemorrhagic:
EnteroHaemorrhagic (VerocYtotoxicogenic):   • haemorrhagic colitis
   • haemolytic-uraemic syndrome
e.g. O157 antigen type, H7 serotype (as in the USA hamburger outbreak)
   Epi: • All ages susceptible, but children and elderly most at risk
   • Sporadic (through contact with cattle that act as carriers), or
   • Outbreaks: e.g. undercooked hamburgers, unpasteurized milk, nursing homes
   Path: • 'Attachment–Effacement (eae)' gene = pilus that allows colonic binding via mannitol
   • 'Verocytotoxins' (VT1,2) = Shiga-like toxins
   PC: a) Haemorrhagic colitis:
   • Profuse bloody diarrhoea with red and white blood cells in stool
   • Thrombotic thrombocytopenic purpura
   • Usually apyrexial
   b) Haemolytic–uraemic syndrome (in 10%):
   • Haemolytic anaemia or thrombocytopenia
   • Uraemia (red blood cells crenate and block glomeruli)
   • 5% die!
   Rx: Fosfomycin?

Shigella: 'bacillary dysentery'

Bacteria (in order of decreasing severity):

S.dysenteriae   ⟶   S. flexneri / S. boydi   ⟶   S. sonnei

(epidemics)   (endemic in 3rd World)   (UK nursing home outbreaks)

Epi   **F**ood (cool, moist); **F**omites (towels, toilets); **F**lies; **F**ornication (anal intercourse, AIDS: *S. flexneri*)
        N.B. only a small infective dose is required, and cases continue to excrete several months after infection

Path   Infection confined to epithelium of terminal ileum and colon (as opposed to *Salmonella*)

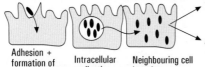

                                 Shiga toxin: inhibits ribosomal function and protein synthesis

                                   Apoptosis: epithelial sloughing, ulceration and haemorrhage
                                            (sigmoidoscopy: denuded mucosa)

Adhesion +   Intracellular   Neighbouring cell
formation of   replication   Invasion
'actin splashes'

PC   Incubation period: 1–7 days

S.H.I.G.A.

Systemic: • Abrupt fever
           • Septicaemia in 10%, esp. with *S. dysenteriae* in immunocompromised

Headaches: meningism (but sterile CSF)

Intestinal:
           • Diarrhoea – frequent, but scanty volume, with multiple white and red cells and mucus
           • GI haemorrhage
           • Abdominal pain and cramps

Glomerulonephritis: haemolytic–uraemic syndrome

Arthralgia: inc. Reiter's syndrome

Ix   Bloods: haemolytic–uraemic syndrome; Na ↓, glucose ↓
       Stool: • Microscopy: ↑ ↑ WBC (cf. amoebic dysentry), ↑ RBC, ↑ mucus
              • Culture: non-lactose-fermenting (except *S. sonnei*)

Rx   Amoxicillin, trimethoprim, ciprofloxacin; avoid anti-diarrhoeals

Yersinia enterocolitica / pseudotuberculosis

Epi: Milk, unpasteurized cheese, tofu; Fe-overload, e.g. thalassaemia, haemochromatosis; pets act as reservoirs
Path: Terminal ileitis with local mesenteric adenitis (right iliac fossa mass)
PC: Early diarrhoea (incubation period 1–7 days); immune reactions (erythema nodosum, Reiter's);
      S.A.L.M.O.N.ella-like systemic (**s**kin – cellulitis, **a**rthralgia, **l**ung, **m**yoendocarditis, **o**steomyelitis, **n**eurological).
Rx: Tetracycline, ciprofloxacin (PO); ceftriaxone or gentamicin (IV)

Clostridium difficile: 'pseudomembranous colitis'

Epi: Antibiotic therapy: within 24 hours starting–6 weeks after stopping; elderly, debilitated
Path: Proctitis, later colitis; may progress to toxic magacolon with perforation; toxin-mediated
PC: Abdominal pain, tenderness; profuse diarrhoea; fever; neutrophilia
Rx: Vancomycin or metronidazole (PO)

Protozoal Gastroenteritis

Sporozoa: intracellular organisms

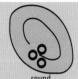

round,
circular
organisms

1. *Plasmodium falciparum* – acute malaria
2. Cryptosporidia; Microsporidia; *Isospora belli*

   PC: a) Immunocoompetent — self-limiting diarrhoea
   b) Immunocompromised, inc. AIDS – chronic diarrhea
   — wasting ('Slim Disease' in Africa)

   Ix: a) Fresh stool microscopy: — Ziehl-Nielsen staining (Cryptosporidia)
   — electron (Microsporidia)
   b) Bowel biopsy: — lieal (Cryptosporidia)
   — jejunal (Microsporidia)

   Rx: a) Chemotherapy: paromomycin (Cryptosporidium), albendazole (Microsporidium)
   b) Supportive: rehydration, electrolyte correction

Amoebae: simple unicellular organisms

Entamoeba histolytica: 'amoebic dysentry'

Path:

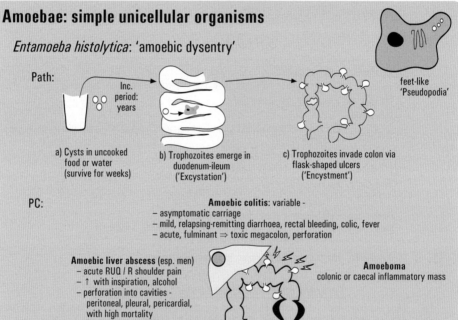

feet-like
'Pseudopodia'

Inc.
period:
years

a) Cysts in uncooked
food or water
(survive for weeks)

b) Trophozoites emerge in
duodenum-ileum
('Excystation')

c) Trophozoites invade colon via
flask-shaped ulcers
('Encystment')

PC: **Amoebic colitis**: variable -
— asymptomatic carriage
— mild, relapsing-remitting diarrhoea, rectal bleeding, colic, fever
— acute, fulminant ⇒ toxic megacolon, perforation

Amoebic liver abscess (esp. men)
— acute RUQ / R shoulder pain
— ↑ with inspiration, alcohol
— perforation into cavities -
peritoneal, pleural, pericardial,
with high mortality
— diarrhoea in only 10%

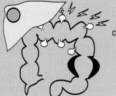

Amoeboma
colonic or caecal inflammatory mass

Ix: **B**loods – Serology: Immunofluorescence or ELISA +ve in 90%
WBC ↑ (not eosinophilia); LFT- normal unless abscess causes cholestasis
Micro – Fresh stool micro.: cysts, trophozoites found in < 40%; WBCs less than in bacillary dysentry
Radio – USS or CT abdomen: liver abscess - esp. right lobe
Special – Colonoscopy: ulcer biopsy

Rx: 1. Metronidazole (tissue amoebicide) – first 10 days; diloxanide (luminal amoebicide) – second 10 days
2. Carriers: diloxanide alone
3. Abscess: aspiration - fluid appears like anchovy sauce!

Flagellata: motile unicellular organisms

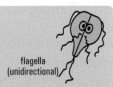

flagella
(unidirectional)

Giardia lamblia (also called *G. intestinalis*): Giardiasis

Path:

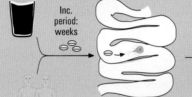

Cysts in unboiled water
(tropical or temperate
zones;
survive for 2 months)

Inc.
period:
weeks

a) Faeco-oral contact
  – homosexual men
  – nurseries
b) Immunodeficiency
  – achlorhydria
  – hypogammaglobulinaemia

Trophozoites emerge in
duodenum-jejunum
('Excystation')

Malabsorption due to:
1. functional disaccharidase
   and bile salt deficiency
2. sub-total villous atrophy
   and mucosal inflammation

PC: Patient may carry asymptomatically or present with malabsorption
  a) anorexia, weight loss
  b) epigastric cramps, flatulence
  c) chronic diarrhoea: pale stool, steatorrhoea

Ix: a) Stool – fresh microscopy: – cysts or trophozoites: 75% sensitivity if sample repeated
              – no WBCs or RBCs
  b) Stool antigen test (ELISA): sensitivity 90%, specificity 99%
  c) Duodenal aspirate and/or biopsy: demonstrates trophozoites with 90% sensitivity
      N.B. treatment is often given empirically without need for +ve microscopy, on basis of travel history

Rx: a) Avoid milk
  b) Metronidazole 2g (x 3 days) or tinidazole (2g single dose), or mepacrine, albendazole

Ciliate: motile unicellular organisms

Balantidium coli 'Balantidiasis'

Epi: Transmitted from pigs
PC: Resembles amoebic colitis
Ix: Fresh stool microscopy;
  – may also be visible with hand-lens or naked eye!
Rx: Tetracycline

cilia
(multidirectional)

**Largest protozoan
pathogen
(100-200 μm)**

Genital Discharge

Causes   The following cause **urethral** or **vaginal discharge**:

G.U.C.C.I.'S. V.A.G.I.N.A.

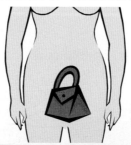

Gonorrhoea

Ulcers: e.g. HSV, syphilis chancre

Chlamydia

Candida

Infections – other:
UTI – Mycoplasma, Ureaplasma, enterobacteria, inc. 2° to pyelonephritis

Staphococcus aureus ('toxic shock syndrome');
Streptococcus pyogenes (scarletina vulvovaginitis)

Vaginalis, Trichomonas = flagellate protozoa:
O/E: Frothy green discharge, strawberry spots in vagina, vulval excoriation

Allergy, foreign body

Gardnerella vaginalis = Gram –ve bacillus (women only)
O/E: Thin grey discharge, with fish-like odour after sex

Inflammatory: Crohn's fistula

Neoplasia:
- Carcinoma of vulva, vagina, cervix / penile
- Wart (HPV)

Age (physiological):
1. Sexually active women:
   - Ovulation, menstruation, pregnancy, esp. in presence of ectropion (secretory mucosa moves out on cervix)
   - Contraception (OCP, tail of IUD)
2. Sexually active men:
   - Sexual stimulation
   - Spermatorrhoea or prostatorrhoea: normal on micturition or defaecation
3. Post-menopausal: atrophic vaginitis

Gonorrhoea *(Neisseria gonorrhoeae)*

Epi   Women > Men (5:1)

PC

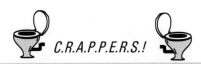

C.R.A.P.P.E.R.S.!

Conjunctivitis
Rash:
- Maculopapular; vesicular; haemorrhagic; vasculitic–necrotic
- Limbs, esp. on same limb as arthritis

Arthritis (septic or reactive): migratory polyarthritis, or monoarthritis, tenosynovitis, e.g. wrist extensors
Pharyngitis
Penis – Prostatitis: urethral gland and vesiculitis infection → discharge or stricture
Pelvic inflammatory disease – bartholinitis: often asymptomatic, and so in women, initial infection goes untreated and so septicaemia is more likely
Epididymo-orchitis
Rectum: asymptomatic; painful defaecation; bloody–purulent discharge
Septicaemia: meningitis; perihepatitis with adhesions; carditis

Chlamydia *(Chlamydia trachomatis)*

Epi   Men > Women

PC   Reiter's syndrome + features of seronegative arthropathies (p. 229)

a real G.O.A.

Genital: • urethritis (discharge); prostatitis
              • pelvic inflammatory disease; cervicitis

Ophthalmic: • conjunctivitis; anterior uveitis

Arthritis: • lower limb; mono- or oligoarthritis

+ S.C.A.R.E.D. S.L.O.U.C.H.E.R.S.

Spondylosis	**S**ystemic: fatigue, low-grade fever, anorexia – weight loss
Chest: thoracic spondylosis	**L**iver: Fitz-Hugh–Curtis syn. (perihepatitis + pleural effusion)
Arthritis	**O**phthalm. conjunctivitis, iridocyclitis, episcleritis
Respiratory: pulmonary infiltrates	**U**lcers: orogenital, inc. circinate balanitis
	Cardiac: aortic root fibrosis and regurgitation; pericarditis
Enthesopathy	**H**aem. anaemia of chronic disease
Dactylitis	**E**xtra: meningo-encephalitis, peripheral neuropathy
	Resp. chest wall ankylosis, apical fibrosis
	Skin: keratoderma blenorrhagicum; nail ridging, onycholysis

Genital Ulceration

S.H.A.G.G.I.N.' S.C.A.R.S.!!

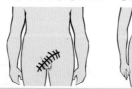

Syphilis *(p. 206)*
1. Primary chancre — single, painless ulcer
2. Secondary — multiple, painful ulcers
3. Gumma (latency stage between 2° and 3°) – single, painless ulcer

Herpes simplex virus -2 / (rarely - VZV)

Autoimmune
1. Behçet's syndrome
   PC: orogenital ulcers, uveitis, CNS disease
2. Reiter's:
   PC: G.O.A. – genital (circinate balanitis – single, painless ulcer), ophthalmic, arthritis
3. Crohn's - single, painless ulcer

Gonorrhoea, Chlamydia, Candida, Trichomonas – causes of urethritis

Granuloma inguinale, and other granulomatous:
1. Granuloma inguinale ('Donovanosis') – *Calymmatobacterium granulomatis*
   – tropical infection (esp. Papua New Guinea, Durban): solitary or multiple painless ulcers
2. Lymphogranuloma venereum – *Chlamydia trachomatis*
   – tropical infection (esp. Africa, Carribean): painless anal ulcer, with inguinal lymphadenopathy
3. Tuberculosis – single, painful

Injury: trauma

Neoplasia: squamous carcinoma
   – associated HPV; single, painless

Scabies, pubic lice; pediculosis; tinea cruris

Chancroid: *Haemophilus ducreyi*
   – tropical infection, causing multiple, painful ulcers, and inguinal lymphadenopathy ('buboes')

Allergy e.g. drug reaction, erythema multiforme, Stevens-Johnson syndome
   contact dermatitis - history of particular soap or underwear

Rash: dermatological
   1. Lichen sclerosus et atrophicus / Leukoplakia - painless
   2. Lichen planus: itchy mauve papules or annular lesions
   3. Psoriasis: red + shiny patches, or scaly
   4. Seborrhoeic dermatitis: - scalp, nose, chest also involved

Staphylococcus
   – folliculitis, impetigo, *Borrelia vincentii*

Herpes simplex virus -2

Types:
- – 1° infection: extensive lesions, fever, malaise, meningism
- – recurrence: milder and shorter course; no systemic symptoms; due to stress, illness, menses

PC: – prodromal symptoms: tingling 1–2 days before painful ulcers appear
- – superficial dyspareunia: cervical and vulval lesions
- – dysuria → urinary retention: urethral; sacral autonomic plexus lesions
- – painful defaecation → constipation: ano-rectal lesions

O/E: – erythema → pustular vesicle in centre → wet ulcer → dry crust
- – inguinal lymphadenopathy

Rx: – warm saline baths
- – antibiotics for 2° bacterial infection
- – aciclovir - effective only in 1st week

Granuloma inguinale and other tropical genital ulcers

Granuloma inguinale ('Donovanosis') – *Calymmatobacterium granulomatis* = intracellular Gram -ve rod
PC: genital, anal, inguinal ulceration:
  deep red ' beefy', contact bleeding, well-circumscribed, painless

Lymphogranuloma venereum – *Chlamydia trachomatis* = obligate intracellular bacteria
PC: – commonly presents as painful inguinal lymphadenopathy ('buboes'),
  with 'groove sign' due to inelastic Poupert's ligament
- – haemorrhagic proctitis, stricture or fistula
- – conjunctivitis, meningoencephalitis

Chancroid: *Haemophilus ducreyi*
PC: tender, sharply demarcated ulcer, usually on prepuce or coronal sulcus in men, or
  fourchette or labia majora in women

Scabies and other infestations

Scabies: *Sarcoptes scabiei*
PC: intense itching, worse at night
O/E: red papules, scaling, ulceration, bleeding
Ix: scrape a burrow with a scalpel blade → 10% KOH → microscopy to look for mite
Rx: BHC (Benzene HexaChloride); malathion; permethrin

Pubic Lice / Pediculosis *(Phthirus pubis)*
PC: itch, but no direct rash
Ix: hand lens
Rx: BHC, Carbaryl shampoo

Tinea cruris (Fungus: *Trichophyton / Epidermophyton*)
PC: erythematous, scaly rash with distinct margin, in groin of men
Ix: scrapings under microscope reveal mycelium
Rx: benzoic acid ointment, clotrimazole cream

Lichen sclerosus et atrophicus / Leukoplakia

PC: – white-purple plaques on thin, shiny, atrophic skin, with skin contraction
- – Men BXO: 'balanitis xerotica obliterans': urethral pain; phimosis; urinary obstruction
- – Women pruritus vulvae; superficial dyspareunia
- – complication: squamous cell carcinoma

Ix: skin biopsy
Rx: potent corticosteroid cream;
  surgery, e.g. meatal dilatation, circumcision

Viral Exanthema and Related

Measles

PC   Incubation period: 2 weeks   *M.E.A.S.L.E.S.*

Mouth:
- Koplik spots – day 2: salt-grain spots on buccal mucosa opposite molars
- Stomatitis (primary or secondary to herpes), gingivitis, cancrum oris

Eye:
- Ketaroconjunctivitis - glassy red eye, swollen semilunar folds (Meyer's sign)
- Corneal scarring, xerophthalmia, Vit A deficiency

Abdomen:
- Gastroenteritis: D + V
- Malabsorption from villous atrophy, esp. protein and energy

Skin (day 4):
- Maculopapular rash: post-auricular→ face → descent over trunk until 7th day
- Confluent, blotchy; stains, doesn't blanch; peels with healing
- DIC: purpura – rare complication
- Coincides with peak fever (40°C)

Lung:
- Bacterial pneumonia, esp. staphylococcal, pneumococcal, due to lymphopenia
- Giant-cell pneumonitis: high mortality

Ears:
- Sinusitis, otitis media

SSPE etc.
- Acute meningo-encephalitis: autoimmune demyelination post-infection (0.1%)
      PC: Deafness; cognitive impairment in 25%; death in 10%
- SSPE – subacute sclerosing panencephalitis: due to persistent viral replication (rare)
      PC: 3–12 years post-infection: cognitive impairment, ataxia, myoclonus, seizures

Speculative:
- Crohn's, Paget's, congenital infection – fetal malformation

Mumps

PC   Incubation period: 2–3 weeks   *M.U.M.P.S.*

Mouth: bilateral parotitis
Uro-genital: orchitis, oophoritis (both associated with infertility), mastalgia
Meningo-encephalitis (lymphocytic CSF), deafness, otalgia
Pancreatitis, or just elevated serum amylase
Severe: myocarditis

Rubella

PC   Incubation period: 2–3 weeks   *R.U.B.E.L.L.A.*

Rash
- Discrete, pink, punctate macules that become confluent; spread from face to trunk
- Purpura: due to thrombocytopenia

Unnoticed: often asymptomatic, or only mild 'cold'-like symptoms in children
Babies – congenital infection: cataracts, cardiac, deafness, microcephaly
Eyes – conjunctivitis; pharyngitis – usual first symptoms
Lymphadenopathy: suboccipital
Arthralgia: rheumatoid pattern

Varicella (Chicken Pox)

PC Incubation period: 2 weeks

S.O.R.E.

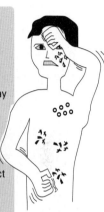

Skin: vesicular rash:
- Day 0: sparse, erythematous, maculopapular rash;
    coincides with low-grade pyrexia
- Day 2: central distribution of itchy, elliptical vesicles and pustules
    in 'crops', i.e. different areas at different stages of
    development
- Day 5: crusts – separates from lesion without scarring by 10th day
    temperature recedes
- Complications: haemorrhagic rash
    scarring due to scratching or
    secondary staphylococcal infection

Oral ulcers: pharynx and oesophagus: dysphagia

Respiratory: pneumonitis: due to ulcers spreading to upper respiratory tract
    PC: • Acute: severe pulmonary oedema, chest pain, haemoptysis
        • Chronic: lung fibrosis (CXR: diffuse nodular opacification)

Encephalitis, meningo:
- May just present as headache (common)
- Associated with cerebellar ataxia that recovers

N.B. More severe in adults, neonates and immunocompromised

Rx 1. Supportive: avoid scratching; daily chlorhexidine washes; flucloxacillin if spots are infected
2. Aciclovir or famciclovir: for adults or infants, within 24 hours of rash
3. VZV Ig: for exposed non-immune pregnancies and to subsequent newborns; immunocompromised

Parvovirus B19 (Erythema Infectiosum)

Epi 1. Occurs in 2-yearly epidemics, every 4 years, during winter–spring
2. Immunity occurs in 70% of population (one attack confers lifelong immunity)

PC Incubation period: 2 weeks

F.A.C.E. ('slapped cheeks')

Fever, mild and 'cold'-like symptoms during 1st week of infection
Arthralgia - commonest symptom in adults, esp. women; lasts weeks
Cheeks: 'Slapped-cheek' syndrome, – lacy, reticular erythema over face
Extreme:
    a) Aplastic crisis or chronic anaemia:
        • Esp. in sickle cell disease, thalassaemics, immunocompromised
        • Due to viral replication in erythroid progenitor cells
        • Rx: IVIg
    b) Miscarriage or hydrops fetalis if acquired in utero:
        • Rx: intrauterine blood transfusion

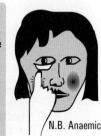

N.B. Anaemic

Herpes Simplex Virus

<u>**PC**</u>　　　　　　　　*G.O. S.O.O.N.*

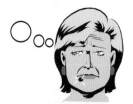

Genital / anal, cervical ulcers usually HSV-2 (unless oral sex with HSV-1 carrier) – see p. 191

see p. 191

Oral: usually HSV-1
1. Herpes labialis ('cold sore'):
Path: Virus resides in trigeminal dorsal root ganglion; reactivation causes centrifugal migration to skin
Epi: Recurrence assoc. with stress, menses, infections (e.g. pneumococcus, malaria), UV–light
PC: Prodrome of skin tingling 1–2 days pre-eruption
2. Gingivostomatitis:
Epi: Children - severe disease; adults - mild
PC: Sore throat $\rightarrow$ drooling; perioral vesicles; fever, lymphadenopathy
O/E: Extensive ulcers with yellow slough over entire oral cavity

Skin
1. Herpetic whitlow:
Epi: children, medical personnel (due to excretion from ill patients)
PC: - minor trauma to hand results in painful, red finger; vesicles; fever, lymphadenopathy
 - may recur with pain and oedema
2. Herpes gladiatorum:
Epi: Contact sports players
PC: Virus pressed into skin by force, similar to whitlow
3. Eczema herpeticum, or superinfection of other skin disease (e.g. burns):
Epi: Children or immunosupppresssed (inc. steroid Rx)
PC: Extensive, painful vesicles occur on eczema
4. Erythema multiforme
Ophthalmic
Keratoconjunctivitis:
PC: • Acute: painful, red eye; lacrimation, photophobia; chemosis (subconjunctival oedema)
 • Chronic: corneal 'dendritic' ulcers (appear as many branches under fluorescein staining)

Organs: Pneumonitis, hepatitis, oesophagitis, DIC – in immunocompromised
Neurological:
1. Encephalitis:
Epi: Occurs sporadically without apparent risk factors
Path: Haemorrhagic necrosis of temporal lobes, orbitofrontal cortex, due to HSV-1
PC: Fever, headache, N + V; complex partial seizures; confusion; coma
Ix: MRI – temporal lobe oedema; CSF – lymphocytes, PCR; EEG – periodic lateralized discharges
Rx: IV aciclovir; carbamazepine or other AEDs
2. Meningitis:
Types: 1. Occurs as part of 1° HSV-2 infection with genital ulcers
 2. Recurrent, mild, self-limiting, Mollaret's meningitis (probably HSV-2-mediated)
3. Bell's palsy

Epstein-Barr Virus

PC   *G.O.E.S. S.L.O.W.L.Y.*

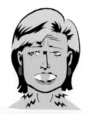

Glandular fever =

Oral: pharyngo-tonsillitis: pearly, white **E**xudate, with petechiae at junction of hard and soft palate
(oral hairy leukoplakia - white plaques that form on side of tongue in AIDS)

Systemic: fever

Skin • Maculopapular rash - esp. if patient inadvertently given amoxicillin (90% pts. get in this case)
• Periorbital oedema

Lymphadenopathy: generalized

Organomegaly: hepatosplenomegaly (± splenic rupture)

White blood cell count:
1. Lymphocyotsis: WCC = 10-50 x 10^9/l
2. 'Atypical lymphocytes' on blood film – also seen in:
   • Other infections: CMV, hepatitis A, HIV, rubella, brucella, toxoplasmosis
   • Non-infective: CLL, mycosis fungoides; drug reaction)

Liver: hepatitis (jaundice may occur due to both hepatitis and haemolytic anaemia)

Y: c**Y**topenias
1. Thrombocytopenia - due to splenomegaly
2. Autoimmune haemolytic anaemia (IgM cold agglutinins)

m**Y**elitis, transverse + other neurological:
Menigoencephalitis; peripheral neuropathy; Guillain-Barré syndrome

ps**Y**chiatric
Prolonged malaise for several months post-infection, or rarely, 'chronic fatigue syndrome'

m**Y**ocarditis, pericarditis, pneumonitis

l**Y**mphoma: associated with EBV: esp. Burkitt's lymphoma (occurs in African children
immunosuppressed with malaria. PC: jaw mass)
EBV is also associated with nasopharyngeal carcinoma

Ix

Heterophile antibodies e.g. Monospot – relies on differential absorption of antibodies by different
test cells:

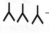   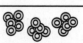

Patient's   Guinea-pig kidney: Ox RBCs:
serum   don't absorb Abs   do absorb Abs

(also seen in: rubella, malaria; hepatitis; SLE; lymphoma, adenocarcinoma)

HIV – Pathogenesis

Path
1. The RNA genome of HIV is converted to dsDNA within the host cell, and is there integrated within the host genome to form a DNA 'provirus'.
2. This may later be transcribed and translated back to form numerous virions.
3. The genome codes for 3 structural / enzyme proteins and 3 regulatory proteins:-

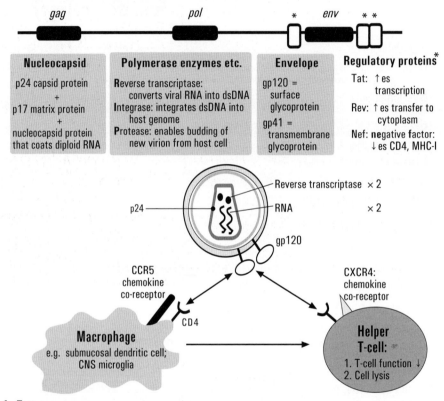

| | *gag* | | *pol* | | * | *env* | * * |

Nucleocapsid	**Polymerase enzymes etc.**	**Envelope**	**Regulatory proteins**[*]
p24 capsid protein + p17 matrix protein + nucleocapsid protein that coats diploid RNA	**Reverse transcriptase:** converts viral RNA into dsDNA **Integrase:** integrates dsDNA into host genome **Protease:** enables budding of new virion from host cell	gp120 = surface glycoprotein gp41 = transmembrane glycoprotein	Tat: ↑es transcription Rev: ↑es transfer to cytoplasm Nef: **n**egative **f**actor: ↓es CD4, MHC-I

Reverse transcriptase × 2

p24 — RNA × 2

gp120

CCR5
chemokine
co-receptor

CD4

CXCR4:
chemokine
co-receptor

Macrophage
e.g. submucosal dendritic cell;
CNS microglia

**Helper
T-cell:**
1. T-cell function ↓
2. Cell lysis

1. Entry:
- Virus enters macrophages or helper T-cells via gp120–CD4 interaction, facilitated by co-receptor
- HIV genome evolves to use CXCR4 co-receptor more efficiently, during course of infection

2. a) Integration:
- RNA homes in on nucleus via nuclear transport signals, e.g. p17
- Integration of viral RNA into host genome enabled via viral 'integrase', even in cells not actively dividing

b) Latency: viral DNA remains inactive for a variable period, depending on immune surveillance

3. Transcription – translation:
- Cellular DNA polymerase begins transcription of 'instability' sequences that code for Tat regulatory protein
- Tat re-enters nucleus and binds to specific 'Tat-responsive elements', which amplifies transcription

4. Capsid assembly – budding:
- Proteins assembled on rough ER and free ribosomes before being packaged
- Incorporates host protein called 'cyclophilin' (essential for replication); protease required for budding

HIV – Natural History

1. Inoculation:

↓ *3 weeks – 3 months*

2. Seroconversion (70% are symptomatic): *G.A.I.N.*

Glandular-fever-like: maculopapular rash, sore throat, aphthous ulcers, fever, lymphadenopathy
Arthralgia, myalgia
Intestinal: diarrhoea, weight loss
Neurological: meningo-encephalitis, retro-orbital pain, peripheral neuropathy, myelopathy

Ix: p24 antigenaemia, lymphopenia (initially all lymphocyte types; later CD4↓, CD8↑)

↓ *90% enter asymptomatic stage; 10% progress immediately and rapidly*

3. Latency stage

↓

4. Persistent generalized lymphadenopathy (PGL):

enlarged lymph node (> 1 cm), in 2 or more extrainguinal sites for > 3 months, without obvious cause

AIDS-related complex (ARC) – early symptomatic disease: *G.O.S.H.*

General: wasting, fever, diarrhoea
Oral: Candida, oral hairy leukoplakia (EBV), aphthous ulcers
Skin: molluscum contagiosum, shingles, HSV, seborrheic dermatitis, psoriasis, condylomata accuminatum
Haematology: ITP (assoc. anti-gp120), anaemia

↓

5. AIDS

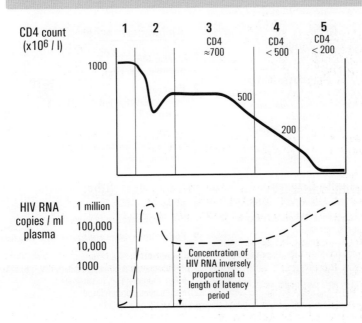

HIV – Clinical

PC

Neurological – Ophthalmological

1. **CNS:**
   - Meningitis: HIV ('aseptic') – at seroconversion or during early AIDS
     Cryptococcus, TB, histoplasmosis, coccidioidomycosis, syphilis
   - Mass lesion: toxoplasmosis, lymphoma, Kaposi's sarcoma, tuberculoma, cryptococcoma
   - Cerebral atrophy: HIV-dementia complex in 25% AIDS
   - White-matter: progressive multifocal leucoencephalopathy (PML): polyoma JC virus
   - Cord: HIV vacuolar myelopathy (dorsal columns), HTLV-I, HSV, VZV, CMV, syphilis, TB

2. **PNS:**
   - Roots: CMV polyradiculopathy – esp. lumbosacral: sacral pain, incontinence, paraparesis
   - Peripheral nerves: Guillain–Barré syn.; glove and stocking or mononeuritis multiplex due to HIV
   - Myopathy

3. **Retinitis:**
   - HIV 'cotton wool spots'; CMV retinitis – 'cheese + tomato pizza'; HSV, VZV – necrosis
   - Toxoplasmosis, *Pneumocystis carinii*, *Candida*, syphilitic papillitis

Respiratory

1. **Bacterial:** • Community-acquired pneumonia, sinusitis
   - TB, multidrug-resistant TB, MAI
2. **Fungal:** • *Pneumocystis carinii* Pneumonia (PCP) – 80% develop without prophylaxis
   - *Cryptococcus, Candida, Histoplasma, Aspergillus*
3. **Viral:** CMV; HSV, VZV, EBV - lymphocytic pneumonitis
4. **Neoplasm:** Kaposi's sarcoma (HHV-8), lymphoma
5. **Pulmonary hypertension**

Cardiac

1. **Pericardial effusion**
2. **Myocarditis**
   - Due to HIV or Cryptococcus
   - Results in arrhythmias, dilated cardiomyopathy
3. **Marantic endocarditis**

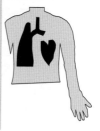

GIT

1. **Mouth:** Aphthous ulcers, HSV, VZV
2. **Oesophagitis:** *Candida*, CMV, HSV, VZV
3. **Gastroenteritis (esp. in homosexuals):**
   - HIV enteropathy = diarrhoea > 1 month, no other cause
   - *Cryptosporidium / Microsporidium / Isospora belli*
   - *Entamoeba histolytica / giardiasis*
   - *Shigella, Salmonella, Campylobacter*, atypical TB (MAI)
   - CMV colitis
4. **Neoplasia:** Kaposi's sarcoma (HHV-8), lymphoma

Abdominal - other

1. **Liver – MAI**
   Hepatitis; Alk. Phos. ↑
2. **Pancreas**
   Acute pancreatitis (often 2° to Rx, e.g. ddI)
3. **Renal**
   Focal glomerulosclerosis – nephrotic syndrome

Skin / Genito-Urinary

1. **Skin:**
   Viral: • VZV: severe chickenpox, multifocal zoster
   - HHV-8: Kaposi's sarcoma
   Bacteria: *Bartonella henselae* – bacillary angiomatosis
   Fungi: umbilicated rash (cryptococcosis), tinea
2. **Mucosa:** penis–vagina, cervix, anus:
   - HSV, HPV: cervical or anal carcinoma - esp. invasive
   - Other STDs: *Candida, Chlamydia, Trichomonas*

Other

1. **Arthritis**
   HIV; Cryptococccus, reactive, Sjögren's
2. **Endocrine:** primary weight loss, hypogonadism
3. **Cytopenias:** – due to:
   - Bone marow suppression due to HIV, TB, MAI
   - Autoimmune: ITP, haemolysis
   - Lymphoma, drug-related

<u>Rx</u>

Highly-Active Anti-Retroviral Therapy (HAART)

1. NARTIs: nucleoside analogue reverse transcriptase inhibitors:
Drugs: zidovudine (AZT); didanosine (ddI), zalcitabine (ddC); lamivudine (3TC), stavudine
Mechanism: are phosphorylated to triphosphate, and are then incorporated into growing DNA chain, thereby blocking further chain extension.

2. NNARTIs: non-nucleoside-analogue reverse transcriptase inhibitors:
Drugs: nevirapine; efavirenz
Mechanism: do not require phosphorylation

3. PIs: protease inhibitors
Drugs: indinavir, ritonavir, saquinavir
Mechanism: prevent viral budding

Combination: [2 NARTIs and 1 NNARTI] or [2 NARTIs and 1 or 2 PIs]

Indications: 1. Primary infection: within 6 months of contracting
2. CD4 count $< 500/\mu l$, or viral load $> 30{,}000$ copies/ml
3. Symptoms, esp. dementia
4. Pregnancy: ↓ risk of transmission (also use Caesarean, formula-feed)

Side-effects: *A.N.G.R.Y.*
Anaemia macrocytic (+ other cytopenias); **A**cidosis, lactic
Neurological: peripheral neuropathy, myopathy (lamivudine), cognitive (efavirenz)
GIT: anorexia, N+V, diarrhoea (ritonavir); renal stones (indinavir); pancreatitis (ddI)
Resistance: with NNARTI cross-resistance occurs between drugs
Reconstitution: immune syndrome – flare-up of subclinical infection on starting or on withdrawal, e.g. Hep B with lamivudine
Y: lipod**Y**strophy syndrome: fat redistribution

Opportunistic Infection – Treatment

1. Neurology:
TB meningitis: as for pulmonary TB, but for 1-year duration
Cryptococcus: amphotericin + 5-flucytosine IV, fluconazole
Toxoplasma: pyrimethamine + sulphadiazine, or clindamycin
Lymphoma: dexamethasone and radiotherapy
CMV retinitis: ganciclovir IV (Ix: FBC, LFT), foscarnet IV (Ix: U&E)

2. Pneumonia:
TB: *R.I.P.E.* (p. 203) – N.B. Interaction with HAART; multi-drug resistance common
PCP: co-trimoxazole (trimethoprim + sulphamethoxazole) / dapsone + pentamidine

3. GIT:
Oesophagitis: Candida – fluconazole; CMV – ganciclovir; HSV – aciclovir
Cryptosporidium: paromomycin – decreases stool volume, but doesn't eradicate
Salmonella or Campylobacter: ciprofloxacin
MAI: azithromycin or clarithromycin

Opportunistic Infection – Prophylactic

1. PCP: cotrimoxazole or dapsone
2. Candida: amphotericin lozenges or oral fluconazole
3. TB: rifabutin

Other

1. Aphthous ulcers of mouth and oesophagus: corticosteroids, thalidomide
2. Weight loss: testosterone or anabolic steroids, growth hormone

Tuberculosis – Clinical

Epi

Inc: 1. Developed world: 5/100,000 p.a.; developing world: 500/100,000 p.a.
2. Most important disease in world: prevalence: 1/3 world population; 3 million die of TB p.a.
3. Increasing incidence, due to AIDS; drug resistance ↑; vaccination ↓

Age: Children and elderly most at risk, as cell-mediated immunity impaired

Geo: 1. Asian immigrants: come from endemic areas
2. Inner city vagrants: due to malnutrition, alcohol (CMI ↓); overcrowding; BCG uptake ↓
3. Blacks: genetic predisposition?

Aet: *Mycobacterium tuberculosis*: spread by aerosol or dust
M. bovis: spread by unpasteurized milk (mainly children) – GIT, bone, renal disease

Pre: any impairment of cell-mediated immunity – **5 Ds**:

Drugs: steroids, chemotherapy / BCG not given
Drug addicts, intravenous, esp. because of AIDS; alcoholics
Debility: dementia, diabetes, renal failure
Deficiency: malnutrition, esp. Vit D deficiency; malabsorption, e.g. post-gastrectomy
Dust: silicosis (metal or quarry workers); medical personnel

Path

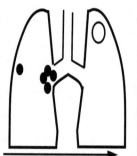

1° Infection

1. Ghon focus =
   midzone, subpleural,
   acute inflammatory lesion

2. Regional hilar lymph nodes
   → may cause obstruction and
   lobar collapse

PC

1. Asymptomatic or self-limiting:
   slight cough, fever, fatigue

2. Delayed type hypersensitivity
   (2–3 weeks postinfection):
   • Phylectenular conjunctivitis
   • Erythema nodosum
   • Lymphadenopathy

3. Lung invasion or milary spread
   occurs in only 5% at this stage

Reinfection or reactivation
due to:
• Genetic predisposition
• Virulent strain
• Cell-mediated immunity ↓
  e.g. steroid therapy

Post-1° Infection

1. Assmann's focus =
   apical, upper zone
   caseating granuloma

2. Granuloma may:
   • Fibrose and simply calcify, or
   • Cavitate (coalesces with others)
   • Invade lung

PC

1. Constitutional: due to cytokines:
   • Fatigue, malaise (IFN-γ)
   • Anorexia, weight loss (TNF-α)
   • Fever, night sweats (IL-1)

2. Lung invasion:
   • Due to granuloma invasion of
     bronchus or pulmonary artery,
     or lymphatics (→ SVC)
   • Presents as cough, esp. with
     green sputum or haemoptysis;
     chest pain

3. Miliary spread due to granuloma
   invasion of pulmonary vein

Epithelioid cells
(plump macrophages) or
Langhan's giant cells
(in centre of granuloma)

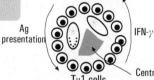

Ag
presentation

IFN-γ

T$_H$1 cells
(on periphery)

Central
necrosis

PC   *R.A.N.S.A.C.K.S. the whole body!*

Respiratory:

P.O.P.U.L.A.r presentations!
Pneumonia: lobar or bronchial
Obstruction, bronchial: • Lobar collapse (1° infection)
                     • Bronchiectasis (post 1°)
Pleurisy / **P**leural effusion / empyema
    if left for long, forms chest wall sinus ('empyema necessitans')
Upper respiratory tract: laryngitis, tonsillitis, otitis media
Lymphadenopathy, cervical:
Abscess, upper zone: • Cavitation ⇒ massive haemoptysis / mycetoma
                   • Fibrocalcification: tracheal deviation

Abdominal:
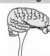
Acute peritonitis: diffuse, abdominal pain, due to disseminated miliary tubercules
Adenitis, mesenteric: right iliac fossa pain and mass (ileo-caecal lymph nodes)
Abscess, psoas: painful or painless groin swelling; femoral neuropathy
Ascites: high protein content; **A**dhesions: bowel obstruction
Addison's crisis: due to adrenal granulomas
Path: Colonization occurs via: • Swallowing sputum or milk (*M. bovis*)
                          • Blood or transcoelomic spread (i.e. from ovaries)

Neurological:

1. Basal meningitis–encephalitis:
       •Headaches, confusion, hydrocephalus, SIADH
       •Focal neurology (cranial neuropathy), tuberculoma, infarct
2. Fundus: choroiditis (miliary tubercles), papilloedema
3. Cord: spinal meningitis, block

Skin:

1. Lupus vulgaris: red–brown scaly plaques, scars
2. Erythema nodosum: tender
3. Erythema induratum (Bazin's dis.): deep purple, ulcerating nodules; assoc. chilblains
4. Papulo-necrotic tuberculides: firm, dusky, ulcerating papules on elbows, knees

Arthritis–osteomyelitis:
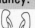
Path: Subchondral osteomyelitis ⟶ cartilage invasion: synovitis ⟶ may form sinus
Types: • Spine: discitis, vertebral collapse (kyphosis or 'gibbus') – esp. children
         • Knee, hip, ankle: esp. adults

Cardiac: Pericardial effusion, constrictive pericarditis; O/E: pulsus paradoxus; Kussmaul's Sx.; knock

Kidney:

1. Nephritis – cortex granulomas: PC: Painless haematuria, loin pain
2. Ureter blockage ⇒ hydro- or pyonephrosis; chronic renal failure
3. Cystitis

Sexual organs:
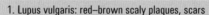
1. Salpingitis: PC: Fever, peritonitis, cervical excitation, amenorrhoea, infertility
               Complications: Endometriosis, oophoritis, vulvitis
2. Epididymo-orchitis: unilateral, hard painless testis swelling; 'string of beads' vas

Tuberculosis – Ix and Rx

Ix

Bloods: FBC: monocytosis
ESR: ↑↑

Urine: 3 x early-morning urines (EMUs) – see Microbiology

Microbiology:
Pulmonary:
1. Sputum, early morning: induce with hypertonic saline or gastric lavage, × 3
2. Bronchoscopy: bronchoalveolar lavage (BAL), transbronchial biopsy (TBB)
3. Pleural: aspirate, biopsy
4. Mediastinal lymph node biopsy, via mediastinoscopy or thoracotomy

Extrapulmonary:
1. Skin: lymph node, rash, sinus
2. Urine: early morning, × 3
3. Blood (special culture bottles); bone marrow biopsy

Laboratory methods:
1. Staining: alcohol + acid fast bacilli – Ziehl–Nielsen / auramine stain
2. Culture: Lowenstein–Jensen medium:
   • Slow growth: 1–8 weeks (each round of replication takes 24 hrs)
   • Cultures appear 'rough, tough + buff': dry, crumbly, not easily smeared
3. Serology (ELISA / haemagglutination): protein Ags 5, 6; plasma membrane Ag
4. PCR / RFLP: tracks different strains, e.g. outbreaks, multi-drug resistance

Radiology – CXR:

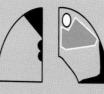

1° infection:
1. Mediastinal lymphadenopathy
2. Bronchial obstruction:
   • Lobar collapse
   • Bronchiectasis (long-standing)

Post-1° infection:
1. Fibrocalcification
2. Cavitate
3. Invasion: pneumonia

Pleural effusion

Skin test – Tuberculin:

1. Mantoux: needle injection
2. Heaf: circle of needles
Ingredient: **intradermal** injection of PPD
(purified protein derivative)
Dose: 1 unit if TB expected, or
10 units if high sensitivity required

48–72 hrs
i.e. time for
delayed-type
hypersensitivity
→

1. Mantoux:
disc diameter > 10 mm = +ve
(or > 15 mm if previous BCG)
*measure induration, not
erythema*
2. Heaf:
ring of induration = +ve
(or confluent disc if previous BCG)

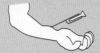

False -ve ('anergy'): miliary TB; co-existent HIV, measles, EBV
False +ve: previous BCG / infection; atypical mycobacteria
Side-effect: ulceration, abscess, lymphadenopathy

Rx

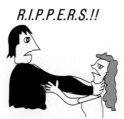

R.I.P.P.E.R.S.!!

Rifampicin: RNA polymerase inhibitor

Isoniazid: mycolic acid +metabolism inhibitor

+Pyridoxine (Vit B6): protects against isoniazid-induced neuropathy, esp. in alcoholics, diabetics

Pyrazinamide

Ethambutol

> Course
>> 6 months: R.I.P.E. for 2 months →   R.I. for further 4 months
>>   (as these 2 drugs are bacterio**cidal**)
>> 9 months: immunocompromised or multi-drug-resistant TB
>> 12 months: extrapulmonary or miliary TB
>> Compliance must be ensured: check urine is orange; use 'directly-observed therapy' (DOTS)
>
> ☠: All TB drugs can cause rash, N+V, and hepatitis, but the following side-effects are drug-specific:
>> Rifampicin: diarrhoea, stains bodily fluids orange, inc. contact lenses,
>>   liver inducer (e.g. reduces effectiveness of oral contraceptives, warfarin)
>> Isoniazid: fulminant liver failure, peripheral neuropathy, optic neuritis, SLE, ITP
>>   (N.B. if patient has slow-acetylator status then ↑ er efficacy, but ↑ er side-effects)
>> Pyrazinamide: vomiting prominent, gout (↓urate excretion), sideroblastic anaemia
>> Ethambutol: optic neuritis (colour vision must be checked at start and during follow-up), gout

Resistant TB ('multi-drug resistant' TB: MDR-TB):
   High-risk groups:
   - AIDS or IVDU; alcoholics; children
   - Travel from MDR-endemic area, e.g. Africa, Korea; or nosocomially acquired
   - Inadequate previous anti-TB Rx , esp. if prolonged
   Rx: R.I.P.E. +   Macrolide: azithromycin, clarithromycin
                      Aminoglycoside: capreomycin – ☠: Vertigo; renal, liver, WBC △
                      Cycloserine (+ pyridoxine) – ☠: Vertigo, fits, psychosis; megaloblastic anaemia
                      Ciprofloxacin

Streptomycin, thiacetazone; *para*-aminosalicylic acid – cheaper, but more side-effects (used in 3rd World)

Steroids: oral glucocorticoids used in TB meningitis or CNS tuberculoma; pericardial or pleural effusions

Surgery: e.g. for spinal disease–osteomyelitis / orchidectomy

Source isolate or face-mask – while still has +ve sputum smears (usually within 1 week of starting Rx)
     + contact-trace + notify CDC

Prophylaxis

1. BCG: • **Intramuscular** injection of live, attenuated *Mycobacterium bovis*
        • Given to 13-yr-olds; neonates at risk (e.g. Asian immigrants); health-care workers
2. Isoniazid in exposed children with +ve Heaf test

<u>Mycobacteria</u>

The following types of mycobacteria occur:

> *T.A.X.S.L.U.M.*
>
> *Mycobacterium* **T***uberculosis* (see p. 200)
> **A***vium intracellulare | cheloni*
> **X***enopi | kansasii*
> **S***crofulaceum*
> **L***eprae*: leprosy – see opposite
> **U***lcerans*: Buruli ulcer
> **M***arinum*: fish-tank granuloma

<u>Atypical Mycobacteria</u>

<u>*M. avium intracellulare* (MAI) | *M. cheloni*</u>

Epi: Immunocompromised: terminal phase of AIDS (CD4 count $< 50/mm^3$); elderly

> *M.A.I.*
>
> **M***egaly*: hepatosplenomegaly (Alk. Phos.↑), lymphadenopathy
> **A***naemia*: bone marrow infiltration
> **I***ntestine*: chronic diarrhoea, weight loss
> + Systemic: fever, night sweats

Ix: Cultures from urine, stool; blood; bone marrow; liver; lymph node

Rx:
> *Needs C.A.R.E.*
>
> **C**lofazimine, **C**iprofloxacin
> **A**zithromycin (or clarithromycin), **A**mikacin
> **R**ifampicin, **R**ifabutin (also used as prophylaxis in AIDS)
> **E**thambutol

<u>*M. xenopi | kansasii* | MAI</u>

Epi: Occurs in pre-existing lung lesions, e.g. bronchiectasis, fibrosis
PC: Lung cavities (but note that sputum cultures may be +ve in healthy people)

<u>*M. scrofulaceum* | MAI</u>

Epi: Children
PC: Lymphadenitis

<u>*M. ulcerans*</u>: 'Buruli ulcer'

Epi: Tropics
PC: Indurated, fluctuant nodule that breaks down to form painless ulcer with necrotic base
and extensive scarring

<u>*M. marinum*</u>: 'fish-tank granuloma'

Epi: Fish collectors, swimming pools
PC: Painless nodular ulcer

Leprosy

Epi   Inc: 10 million cases worldwide
Age: In endemic areas, acquired in childhood, but not manifest until teens–30s
Geo: Tropics, Mediterranean, Southern USA
Aet: *M. leprae*: spread by nasal aerosol from lepromatous leprosy patients;
         prolonged contact required, but bacteria may survive for < 7 days outside of body

PC   Incubation period: 2–15 years, as leprosy has slowest bacterial replication (12 days per cycle!)

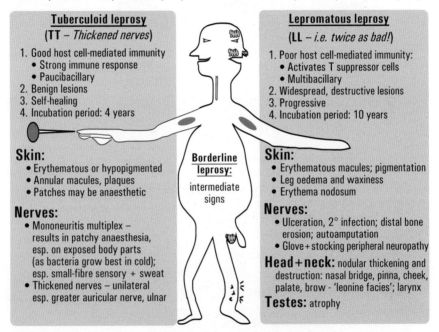

Tuberculoid leprosy
(TT – *Thickened nerves*)

1. Good host cell-mediated immunity
   • Strong immune response
   • Paucibacillary
2. Benign lesions
3. Self-healing
4. Incubation period: 4 years

Skin:
   • Erythematous or hypopigmented
   • Annular macules, plaques
   • Patches may be anaesthetic

Nerves:
   • Mononeuritis multiplex –
     results in patchy anaesthesia,
     esp. on exposed body parts
     (as bacteria grow best in cold);
     esp. small-fibre sensory + sweat
   • Thickened nerves – unilateral
     esp. greater auricular nerve, ulnar

Borderline leprosy:
intermediate signs

Lepromatous leprosy
(LL – *i.e. twice as bad!*)

1. Poor host cell-mediated immunity:
   • Activates T suppressor cells
   • Multibacillary
2. Widespread, destructive lesions
3. Progressive
4. Incubation period: 10 years

Skin:
   • Erythematous macules; pigmentation
   • Leg oedema and waxiness
   • Erythema nodosum

Nerves:
   • Ulceration, 2° infection; distal bone
     erosion; autoamputation
   • Glove + stocking peripheral neuropathy

Head + neck: nodular thickening and
   destruction: nasal bridge, pinna, cheek,
   palate, brow - 'leonine facies'; larynx

Testes: atrophy

Ix   **Bloods:**   IgM ↑ , ESR ↑; TPHA, Rh factor, ANA are often + ve
Lepromin test:

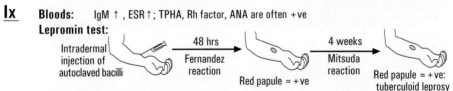

Intradermal injection of autoclaved bacilli — 48 hrs → Fernandez reaction — Red papule = + ve — 4 weeks → Mitsuda reaction — Red papule = + ve: tuberculoid leprosy

Biopsy: from skin scraping (either type); nerve biopsy (TT only); nasal septum scraping (LL only)
         Laboratory: a) Acid-fast bacilli smear for *M. leprae*
                  b) Inoculation: in armadillo or mouse foot pad (can't culture on artificial media!)

Rx   **Medical:** dapsone + clofazimine + rifampicin
   • Duration: 6 months (tuberculoid leprosy); 2 years or more (lepromatous leprosy)
   • ☠: Dapsone: neuropathy, erythema nodosum; N + V; Clofazimine: blue–black skin lesions, red urine
   • Steroids may be needed if lesions worsen acutely on starting Rx ('reversal reaction')
Surgery: amputation
Prophylaxis: BCG may protect, esp. in children

Syphilis

<u>**Bacterium**</u> *Treponema pallidum* subsp. *pallidum*

<u>**Epi**</u>   Transmitted sexually (horizontal) and transplacentally (vertical); rarely via blood products or fomites

<u>**PC**</u>

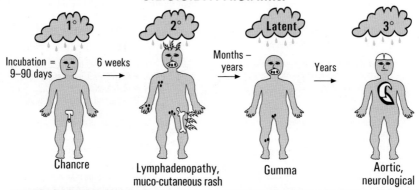

C.L.O.U.D.Y. A.G.A.I.N.

1°	2°	Latent	3°
Incubation = 9–90 days	6 weeks	Months – years	Years
Chancre	Lymphadenopathy, muco-cutaneous rash	Gumma	Aortic, neurological

Chancre: painless papule , breaks down to ulcer and erythematous ring on genitals, anus or mouth

Lymphadenopathy (generalized), fever, headache

Oral ulcers: 'snail-track'

Organomegaly: hepatomegaly, hepatitis

Uveitis

Urine: protein–nephrotic syndrome

Dermatological:
 1. Non-pruritic, maculopapular rash on palms, soles, trunk
 2. Scarring alopecia

Y: cond**Y**lomata lata =large pink–grey discs around vulva, anus or under breasts (highly infectious)

Arthralgia, nocturnal bone pain (periostitis), meningism

Gumma: granulomatous swellings in: skin (e.g. leg, foot, periorbital), oropharynx (tongue, palate)
   viscera (testis, liver, lung)

Aortic:
 1. Ascending aortic aneurysm
 2. Aortic regurgitation

Immune: paroxysmal cold haemoglobinuria

Neurological: classified according to onset of signs:
  2 months–2 years: • Meningitis (may occur during secondary stage)
           • Cranial nerve palsies, inc. deafness, vertigo, optic neuritis
  2 years–5 years: strokes (Heubner's endarteritis)
  5 years–15 years: general paresis of insane = dementia, psychosis, Argyll–Robertson pupils
  10 years +: tabes dorsalis = rombergism, Charcot joints, numbness and lightning pains

<u>**PC**</u> **Congenital syphilis**

my baby comes as something of a S.H.O.C.K.

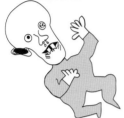

Sniffles (watery nasal discharge)

Saddle-shaped nose (also sunken maxillae and frontal bossing)

Hutchinson's incisors – notched, widely spaced;
  + Mulberry' molars – multiple cusps
  + Linear rhagades – scars around mouth

Optic atrophy, salt + pepper choroidoretinitis; keratitis – blindness

Otitic: sensorineural deafness

Clutton's joints (painless knee effusions); sabre shins

Cold haemoglobinuria, paroxysmal

Kills: 50% babies die pre- or perinatally!

<u>**Ix**</u>
1. Chancre swab with dark-ground microscopy: characteristic spiral-shaped bacterium
2. Serology: • Non-specific: anti-cardiolipin – e.g. VDRL (Venereal Diseases Research Lab) or
                                                              RPR (Rapid Plasma Reagin)

     • Advantage: becomes –ve with Rx
                   False +ves = infections (e.g. herpes, HIV, TB), SLE, pregnancy, elderly (10%)
                   False –ves: esp. in late syphilis, HIV
     • Specific: TPHA (Treponema pallidum Haemagglutination Assay) or
                   FTA (Fluorescent Treponemal Assay) or TPI (T.P. Immobilization)
                   Advantage: more specific, but remains +ve even when successfully treated
                   False +ves = non-venereal treponemes, leptospirosis, Lyme
     • CSF: Pleocytosis + Protein ↑ + Antibody Tests +ve

<u>**Rx**</u> 1. Procaine penicillin - IM 600 mg od x 10 days (2–3 weeks if tertiary disease)
     ☠: Jarisch–Herxheimer reaction = septic shock on initiating Rx, due to endotoxin release,
          which is most likely in 2° syphilis, but most dangerous in 3° syphilis. Risk can be reduced
          by administering steroids at same time.
     2. Contact-trace

<u>Non-Venereal Treponemes</u>

<u>**Def**</u>   These diseases are characterized by being:
          1. Non-venereal: transmitted skin-to-skin, esp. as children; shared kitchen utensils
          2. Endemic to Africa, S. and Central America

<u>**Types**</u>   • Yaws (*T. pallidum* subsp. *pertenue*) – West-Central Africa, S. America, SE Asia
          • Pinta (*T. carateum*) – S. and Central America
          • Endemic syphilis (*T. pallidum* subsp. *endemicum*) – Central Africa

<u>**PC**</u>   1°:   raspberry-like papules ('framboesia')
          2°:   lymphadenopathy; periostitis
          Latent: bone gummae – destroy facial bones

Borreliosis

Lyme Disease

Bacteria

Borrelia burgdorferi (USA, esp. New England (Lyme, Conneticut))
B. afzelii, or *B. garinii* (Middle Europe and Asia)

PC

S.N.A.C.K.

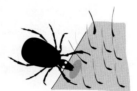

Vector:
deer tick
(*Ixodes scapularis*)

Skin: Erythema chronicum migrans: initial phase (days after infection)
- Annular erythema that expands from centre
- Accompanying fever / lymphadenopathy / headache
- Organism can be cultured from rash on Kelly medium

Neuro:
- Meningo-encephalitis
- Cranial neuropathy, esp. VII
- Peripheral neuropathy
- Lymphocytic meningo-radiculitis (Bannwarth's syndrome)

Arthritis: oligoarticular, esp. knees

Cardiac: heart block, inc. 3° (temporary – does not need pacing)

K: A**C**rodermatitis chronica atrophicans – only sign of *B. afzelii* / *B. garinii*

Ix
ELISA

Rx
Rash: tetracycline, doxycycline, amoxicillin
Systemic: benzylpenicillin, ceftriaxone

Relapsing fever

Louse-borne: *B. recurrentis* – Ethiopia (body lice occur with poor hygiene and overcrowding)
Tick-borne: *B. duTToni* – Sub-Saharan Africa (or *B. hermsii* – NW USA)
PC: Leptospirosis-like (see opposite):
- Flu-like symptoms with fluctuating high temperature (> 40°C), myalgia-arthralgia, headache
- Injected conjunctivae
- Respiratory (dry cough), neuro. (lymphocytic meningitis), gastro. (abdominal pain, vomiting)

Vincent's angina

B. vincenti: PC: acute gingivitis

Leptospirosis

Bacteria   *Leptospira interrogans* (serotype *icterohaemorrhagie* or *copenhageni* = 'Weil's disease')

Epi   Transmitted by contact of rats' urine with skin abrasions or mucous membranes, e.g. sewage workers.

PC   Types: 1. Anicteric (90%): flu-like, aseptic meningitis
2. Icteric   (10%): additional liver and renal failure, and DIC = 'Weil's disease'

M.O.U.R.N.S.

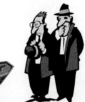

Anicteric: mortality rate < 1%
Weil's: mortality rate 10%

Myalgia: Severe calf, back, abdominal pain (flu-like with high fever)

Ophthalmic: • Injected conjunctivae
• Uveitis: iritis or retinochoroiditis – present several weeks – months later
• Deeply jaundiced due to hepatitis (Weil's disease)

Urine: • Proteinuria, red cells, white cells, granular, hyaline casts – invariable!
• Tubulointersitial nephritis; acute tubular necrosis (2nd week)

Respiratory: Cough, haemoptysis, chest pain

Neurology: • Aseptic meningitis – CSF: early neutrophilia, late lymphocytosis; high protein
• Encephalopathy

Skin: • Maculopapular rash
• Purpura, bruising due to vasculitis or DIC

Spleno- / hepatomegaly / lymphadenopathy

Ix   **B**loods : CK ↑
U&E: urea ↑, creatinine ↑ – in Weil's
LFT: bilirubin ↑, alkaline phosphatase ↑
FBC: neutrophilia, thrombocytopenia, haemolytic anaemia, deranged clotting, CK ↑
(N.B. viral hepatitis: ALT ↑ ↑, leucopenia and normal CK)

Urine: active urine sediment

Micro: 1. **1st week:** blood / CSF culture; **2nd–4th weeks:** urine culture (EMJH medium)
2. MAT = Microscopic Agglutination Test: rise in titre at 2nd week
3. Hanta virus serology – similar presentation with myalgia and meningism

ECG, **E**cho: associated myocarditis, pericarditis

Radio: CXR – lower-zone air-space shadowing

Rx   1. Antibiotics: Mild: doxycycline or amoxicillin
Severe: benzylpenillicin, ampicillin or erythromycin
☠: Jarisch–Herxheimer reaction (fever, myalgia)
2. Renal dialysis
3. Prophylaxis: Doxycycline 200 mg 1x/week, or vaccine – in exposed personnel

Rickettsia

Q.ua.R.T.I.L.E.S.

Q-Fever

Organism: *Coxiella burnetii*

Epi: Acquired from pregnant farm animals or pets, and rarely from other affected humans:

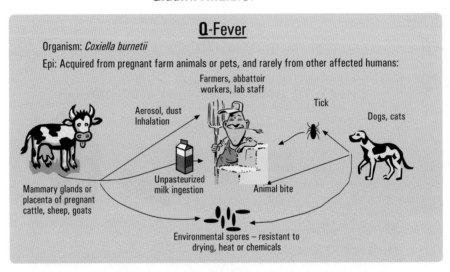

Farmers, abbattoir workers, lab staff

Aerosol, dust Inhalation

Tick

Dogs, cats

Unpasteurized milk ingestion

Animal bite

Mammary glands or placenta of pregnant cattle, sheep, goats

Environmental spores – resistant to drying, heat or chemicals

Typhus

Rocky mountain spotted fever
Organism: *Rickettsia rickettsii*
Vector: Rocky Mountain wood tick, American dog tick
Geog: South West USA, Mexico

TIck-borne typhus – other
Ehrlichiosis:
Organism: *Ehrlichia chaffeensis* (monocytes), *E. phagocytophilia* (granulocytes)
Vector: Deer tick
Geog: USA
Mediterranean spotted fever: Organism: *Rickettsia conorii*

Louse-borne:
Epidemic and Endemic typhus
Epidemic typhus:
Organism: *Rickettsia prowazekii*
Vector: Body lice (*Pediculus humanis*)
Geog: Poor hygiene, overcrowding, e.g. prisons, famine
Endemic typhus:
Organism: *Rickettsia typhi*
Vector: Flea; rats, cats, opossums act as reservoir
Geog: South USA

Scrub typhus
Organism: *Orientia tsutsugamushi*
Vector: Larval mite
Geog: SE Asia, Australia

Q-Fever

PC

F.R.I.C.T.I.O.N.

Flu-like symptoms – fever, myalgia
Respiratory – atypical pneumonia, i.e. mild, dry cough, but CXR shows consolidation or masses
Intestine (1) – D + V
Cardiac: acute phase – myocarditis, pericarditis; chronic – aortic valve endocarditis
Thrombosis – DVT, miscarriage; early platelets ↑ ⇒ later platelets ↓
Intestine (2) – granulomatous hepatitis
Organomegaly – hepatosplenomegaly
Neurological – headache common, meningoencephalitis, optic neuritis, parkinsonism

Ix

Serology: exists in 2 antigenic forms due to 'phase variation' of lipopolysaccharide:
Phase I Ag = chronic infection: highly infectious
Phase II Ag = acute   infection: avirulent

Rx

Tetracycline ± rifampicin, or ciprofloxacin

Typhus

PC

F.R.I.C.T.I.O.N.

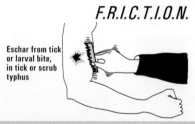

Eschar from tick
or larval bite,
in tick or scrub
typhus

Flu-like symptoms: fever, myalgia
Rash: 1. Eschar of original bite
            2. Vasculitic – maculopapular, purpura, haemorrhagic – esp. palms, soles (on 4th day)
Intestine (1): D + V, enterocolitis, GIT bleeding
Cardiac: arrhythmias
Thrombosis: DVT; limb gangrene: thrombocytopenia
Intestine (2): transaminitis
Oedema, peripheral and pulmonary: due to widepread increased vascular permeability,
            leads to sh**O**ck
Neurological: headache common, meningoencephalitis, ataxia, deafness

Ix

1. Serology: indirect IF (the 'Weil–Felix heterophile antibody test' is less sensitive and specific)
2. PCR, esp. *Rickettsia typhi*
3. Skin biopsy, esp. Rocky Mountain spotted fever

Rx

Tetracycline or chloramphenicol

Malaria

Plasmodium falciparum

Incubation period: 1–2 weeks (but may be up to 1 year)
Duration: 3 weeks, but mortality rate = 20%
Relapses do not occur – if successfully treated

F.A.L.C.I.P.A.R.U.M.S.

Flu-like:
  1. Fever: continuous, daily or paroxysmal (subtertian – every 36 hrs, or tertian – 48 hrly)
  2. Other: myalgia, lymphadenopathy

Anaemia: Intravascular haemolytic anaemia causes haemoglobinuria ('Blackwater fever')

Leucopenia / thrombocytopenia:
  1. Leucopenia: • Although B cells and IgM increased (inc. cryoglobulinaemia)
                • Imunodeficiency ⇒ herpes labialis, septicaemia, Burkitt's lymphoma (EBV)
  2. Thrombocytopenia (due to malaria or quinine) / DIC

Cerebral malaria (causes 80% deaths):
  1. Headache common
  2. Encephalopathy, cerebral oedema: drowsiness, seizures, pyramidal signs, psychosis
  3. Retinal haemorrhages, papilloedema, nystagmus

Intestine: diarrhoea + vomiting – common

Pulmonary oedema: due to ARDS, uraemia or injudicious rehydration

Acidosis, lactic: due to hypotension / parasite occlusion of tissue vessels

Renal: acute tubular necrosis 2° to shock ('algid'), or mesangiocapillary glomerulonephritis

Uraemia

Metabolic:
  1. Na ↓
  2. Glucose ↓: due to reduced hepatic gluconeogenesis, or quinine

Miscarriage

Splenomegaly / splenic rupture / hepatosplenomegaly: repeated infections over long time

Benign Malaria

Incubation period: *P. vivax* or *ovale*: 2–3 weeks
                   P. malariae: 3–6 weeks, although 10% present after 1 year
Duration: *P. vivax* or *ovale*: 1–2 months
                   P. malariae: 1–6 months, with recrudescences over 20 years

F.A.R.

Fever, paroxysmal:
  • *P. vivax / ovale* – tertian (i.e. every 3rd day); *P. malariae* – quartan (i.e. every 4th day)
  • Due to dormant hypnozoites in liver (*P. ovale / vivax*), or blood (*P. malariae*)
  • Fever regularity not seen in early infection

Anaemia, haemolytic: *P. vivax*

Renal – nephrosis: *P. malariae* (esp. in children)

Life-Cycle

Alternates between **spores** (products of asexual reproduction) and **gametes** (products of sexual reproduction)

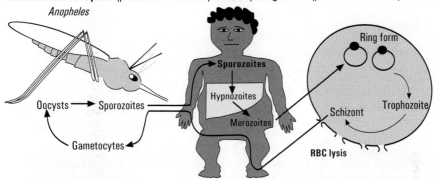

<u>Ix</u> **1. Thick and thin films x 3:**
- Parasitaemia > 2% = symptomatic; > 10% = exchange transfusion required
- May take several days to rise to true level after becoming symptomatic, so repeat films over 3 days
- Parasites may persist in blood for weeks–months after cure

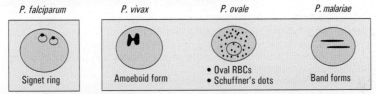

2. Bone marrow smear: may be needed in partially treated patients, with –ve blood smears.

<u>Rx</u>

P. falciparum

1. Quinine for 7 days (PO or IV)
   ☠ : Cinchonism: tinnitus, visual loss, abdominal pain, headache + thrombocytopenia; glucose ↓; renal failure
   Followed by further 7-day course of:
2. a) Fansidar (pyrimethamine + sulpadoxine), or
   b) Malarone (proguanil + atovaquone), or
   c) Tetracycline
3. Supportive:
   a) Tepid sponging / paracetamol
   b) Blood transfusion / exchange transfusion
   c) Phenobarbitone for cerebral malaria

Benign malaria

1. Chloroquine for 2 days
   Followed by further 2–3-week course of:
2. Primaquine: destroys liver phase hypnozoites in *P. ovale / vivax*, and therefore prevents relapse

   ☠ : • Haemolysis (if G6PD deficency)
   • Methaemoglobinaemia

Prophylaxis

1. Conservative: drain swamps; long sleeves; permethrin-impregnated nets; DEET lotion
2. Chemoprophylaxis: start 1–3 weeks pre-visit to endemic area → stop 4 weeks post-visit:
   a) Weekly chloroquine (☠ : Visual loss, fits, blood dyscrasia) + daily proguanil
   b) Weekly mefloquine (☠ : Acute psychosis, fits, arrhythmias)
   c) Daily doxycycline

Nematodes (roundworms)

Intestinal
S.N.A.K.E.

Strongyloides stercoralis
Inc: 1 month, and may last for decades due to autoinfection (*S.T.R.O.N.G.!*)
PC: worms penetrate skin from soil:

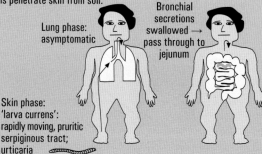

Lung phase: asymptomatic

Bronchial secretions swallowed → pass through to jejunum

GIT phase: epigastric pain (worsened by eating) diarrhoea; PR bleeding (colitis); malabsorption

Skin phase: 'larva currens': rapidly moving, pruritic serpiginous tract; urticaria

'Autoinfection':
1. Larvae invade jejenum (internal)
2. Perianal skin (external)

'Hyperinfection': severe autoinfection due to immunocompromise, e.g. steroids, that may occur after many years of asymptomatic infection, and become disseminated to CNS, myocarditis, and Gram –ve septicaemia

Necator americanus / *Ancylostoma duodenale* ('hookworm')
Inc: 1–3 months, and can last for several years (< 8 years for *A. duodenale*)
PC: 1. Skin phase: worm penetrates toe furrow: pruritus; serpiginous tract (cutaneous larva migrans)
    2. Lung phase: mild pneumonitis
    3. GIT phase: Fe-deficiency anaemia; hypoalbuminaemia

Ascaris lumbricoides ('human roundworm' – largest!)
Inc: 2 months, and lasts up to 1 year
Path: Eggs are ingested → larvae invade jejunal mucosa → enter portal vein and lymphatics → lung phase → swallowed to re-enter jejunum, where mature worm develops
PC: 1. Lung phase: dry cough, wheeze; CXR shows transient, round infiltrates (Löffler's pneumonitis)
     2. GIT phase: bowel, biliary, pancreas obstruction (esp. heavy infestation in children)

K : Anisa**K**iasis, capillariasis – raw fish; trichostrongyliasis – vegetation; abdominal angiostrongyliasis

Enterobius vermicularis ('pinworm' or 'threadworm')
Path: Larvae colonize appendix and caecum → worms migrate nocturnally to release eggs perianally
PC: Pruritus ani in children; abdominal pain, weight loss; vulvovaginitis; pelvic granulomas

Extra: rectal prolapse-causing – *Trichuria trichuris* ('whipworm')
Inc: 2–3 months, and may last for 5 years
Path: Eggs hatch in duodenum → larvae migrate and mature in caecum and colon
PC: Abdominal pain, PR bleeding (colitis); rectal prolapse – esp. in children

For all: Ix : 1. Stool samples for ova or larvae
                2. Eosinophilia (during migration phase of hookworm, *Ascaris*, *Strongyloides*)
                3. ELISA: *Strongyloides*
          Rx: Albendazole, mebendazole; thiabendazole (*Strongyloides*)

Tissue
F i.G.h.T.S.

Filariasis – lymphatic nematodes:
   Onchocerca volvulus – 'river blindness'
      Vector: *Simulium* blackfly
      PC: 1. Keratitis, choroidoretinitis, secondary optic atrophy
          2. Rash: generalized papular, pruritic
          3. 'Hanging groin' = inguinocrural lymph node blockage
      Ix: Skin snip – motile microfilariae
   Wuchereria bancrofti – 'elephantiasis'
      Vector: mosquitoes – *Aedes aegypti* or *Anopheles*
      PC: 1. Systemic: fever, myalgia, photophobia, diffuse lymphangitis, lymphadenopathy
          2. Local: leg lymphedema, hydrocoele, pleural effusion, ascites
      Ix: Blood film: parasites present
   Loa *loa*
      Vector: deerfly – *Chrysops*
      PC: 1. Calabar swellings of limbs (= evanescent angioedema)
          2. Subconjunctival worm
          3. Endomyocardial fibrosis
   Brugia *malayi*
      Vector: mosquitoes: *Mansoni* or *Anopheles*
      Rx for all : 1. Diethylcarbamazine (onchocerciasis: add suramin, ivermectin)
               2. Nodulectomy: prevents continued production of microfiariae

Guinea worm (*Dracunculus medinensis*)
   Path: Larvae swallowed in drinking water contaminated with vector *Cyclops* (freshwater crustacean)
      → invade stomach → migrate subcutaneously or to joints → female penetrates skin and release
      larvae into water
   PC: 1. Painful vesicle; subcutaneous nodule
       2. Arthritis

Toxocara canis / cati ('visceral larva migrans')
   Path: Eggs in soil contaminated by dog or cat faeces ingested by children →
      larvae migrate to liver and lungs → systemic spread
   PC: 1. Migration: asthma, fever, dermatitis
       2. Chronic: choroidoretinitis; hepatosplenomegaly
   Ix: Serology
   Rx: Diethylcarbamazine

Trichinella *spiralis*
   Path: Larvae swallowed in infected pork → invade small intestine, portal circulation → systemic spread
   PC: 1. Migration: periorbital oedema, fever, diarrhoea (+ eosinophilia)
       2. Muscles: myalgia, myopathy, myocarditis
       3. Other: meningo-encephalitis, gastroenteritis, pneumonia
   Ix: Muscle biopsy, serology
   Rx: Thiabendazole (intestinal phase) + steroids for systemic infection

Skin: 'cutaneous larva migrans'
   e.g. *Anclyostoma brasiliense*, A. *caninum*, *Uncinaria stenocephalia*, *Bunostomum phlebotomum*
   Path: Animal hookworms that cannot develop further in humans (human hookworms also cause initially)
   PC: Serpiginous, erythematous, pruritic, vesicular rash – esp. in children, and on feet; eosinophilia
   Ix: Skin biopsy

Cestodes (tapeworms)

There are 2 main types of disease, depending on which stage of the worm's life-cycle is ingested:
1. Larvae or proglottid segments: matures to produce adult tapeworm within the intestine
2. Eggs: penetrate intestine (as an 'oncosphere') and spread to brain, muscle, liver and lung

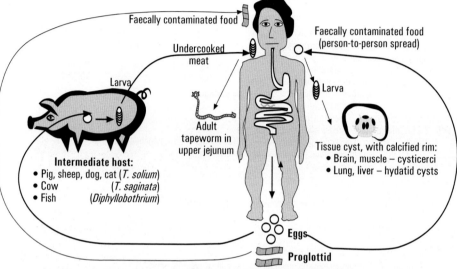

Faecally contaminated food

Faecally contaminated food
(person-to-person spread)

Undercooked
meat

Larva

Larva

Adult
tapeworm in
upper jejunum

Tissue cyst, with calcified rim:
• Brain, muscle – cysticerci
• Lung, liver – hydatid cysts

Intermediate host:
• Pig, sheep, dog, cat (*T. solium*)
• Cow   (*T. saginata*)
• Fish   (*Diphyllobothrium*)

Eggs

Proglottid

Survive in environment for months–years

Intestinal Tapeworms

P.h.D.

Pork tapeworm – *Taenia solium*

Epi: *T. solium* – pork : Africa, Latin America, SE Asia
    T. saginata – beef : Africa, Middle East
PC: 1. Perianal pain, inc. faecal passage of proglottids
    2. Epigastric pain, nausea, diarrhoea
    3. Appetite ↑, weight ↓
Ix: 1. Stool microscopy: eggs, proglottids
    2. Perianal swab with cellophane tape: detects eggs
    3. FBC: eosinophilia; IgE ↑
Rx: Praziquantel – single dose

Hymenolepis nana (dwarf tapeworm)

Epi: • Commonest cestode infection:
      endemic in temperate and tropical regions
    • Doesn't require intermediate host:
      auto-infection with eggs common
PC: Asymptomatic, or anorexia, abdominal pain, diarrhoea

Diphyllobothrium latum (fish tapeworm)

Epi: eggs are eaten in raw freshwater fish, e.g. Finland
PC: 1. Abdominal pain, diarrhoea, bowel obstruction
    2. Cholangitis, cholecystitis
    3. Vit B12 deficiency – due to consumption by worm

Tissue Tapeworms

P.E.T.S.

Pork tapeworm – *Taenia solium*

PC: Cysticerci form in brain, muscle, subcutaneous:
    1. Focal seizures, weakness
    2. Obstructive hydrocephalus, meningitis
    3. Subretinal: ocular parasite
Ix: 1. MRI brain: ring-enhancing cysts with scolex
    2. X-ray: 'cigar-shaped' calcifications in muscle
    3. ELISA of serum, CSF; tissue biopsy
Rx: Praziquantel / albendazole; prednisolone
    + anti-convulsants; CSF shunt

Echinococcus granulosus (dog tapeworm)

Epi: Dog-handlers, ingesting eggs in vegetables or water
PC: Hydatid cysts expand:
    1. Hepatic: RUQ pain, obstructive jaundice
    2. Lung: chest pain, haemoptysis
    3. Other organs: bone, brain, myocardium
Ix: Serum ELISA (fluid aspiration risks anaphylaxis!)
Rx: Cyst excision, with albendazole cover
Taenia solium (pork tapeworm) – see above

Sparganosis (spirometra tapeworm)

Epi: Water contains infected crustacean *Cyclops*
PC: Periorbital – orbital destruction

Trematodes (flukes)

S.C.O.F.F.s H.em P.

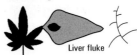
Liver fluke

Schistosomiasis (blood fluke = 'bilharzia')

Epi: Fluke (*Schistosoma* sp.) acquired from being bitten by freshwater snails e.g. in Lake Victoria, S. America

PC: Has acute and chronic manifestations, depending on which part of the life-cycle:

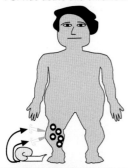 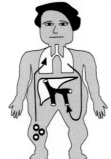 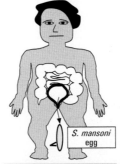 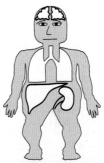

S. mansoni egg

Skin penetration	***Migration***	***Egg deposition***	***Systemic spread***
Freshwater snail eats fluke larvae ('miracidia') and releases cercariae ('freshwater bodies'). Cercariae attach to skin, lose tails, and penetrate to form 'schistosomulae'. PC: 'Swimmers' itch': dermatitis, papules generalized urticaria *Occurs on day 1, and may persist for fortnight*	Skin → lung → portal vein PC: 'Katayama Fever': • Lymphadenopathy • Hepatosplenomegaly • Cough, myalgia • Headache, diarrhoea • Encephalopathy, death *Occurs within first month; worst for S. japonicum* Outcome of migration:  1–2 cm	Schistosomulae settle in portal vein, and mature to form adult male and female pairs, which copulate for many years, and release eggs that are deposited in venules and incite local granulomatous reactions: PC: • Colon: *S. mansoni* – polyps, bleeding, protein-losing enteropathy; *S. japonicum* – colon carcinoma • Ileum: *S. japonicum* – colic, malabsorption • Bladder: *S. haematobium*- haematuria, squamous cell carcinoma	1. Liver: • Hepatosplenomegaly • Portal hypertension, due to periportal pipe-stem fibrosis 2. Lung: • Fibrosis • Cor pulmonale 3. CNS: • Brain (*S. japonicum*): focal seizures • Transverse myelitis / cauda equina syndrome (*S. mansoni/ haematobium*) 4. Renal: • glomerulonephritis

Clonorchis, Opisthorchis, Fasciola (liver flukes)

Epi: Raw fish in SE Asia (*Clonorchis, Opisthorchis*); raw liver or watercress in S. America (*Fasciola*)

PC: RUQ pain; cholangitis with secondary hepatitis or obstructive jaundice; cholangiocarcinoma

Fasciolopsis, Heterophyes (liver flukes)

Epi: Aquatic plants in SE Asia (*Fasciolopsis*); raw freshwater fish in Nile, China (*Heterophyes*)

PC: Abdominal pain, mucoid diarrhoea

Paragonimus westermani (lung fluke)

Epi: Crayfish, crab ingestion

PC: Lung – haemoptysis, bronchiectasis, bronchitis; brain – focal seizures, weakness

Rheumatology

Osteoarthritis – causes

Def   Common final pathological pathway of synovial joints, arising from variety of insults
(although commonly refers only to age-related '1° osteoarthritis', with no identifiable insult).

Causes

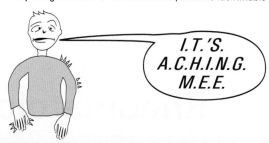

*I.T.'S.
A.C.H.I.N.G.
M.E.E.*

Idiopathic (1°) - i.e. age-related - *see opposite and p. 222*
Trauma – old fracture:
 due to abnormal joint loading after healing, ± articular surface damage
Softened bone: *see opposite*
 1. Developmental - congenital dislocation of hip, Perthes' disease, SUFE
 2. Osteochondritis
 3. Osteonecrosis (avascular necrosis)

 The remainder occur due to weakened cartilage:

Autoimmune
 - rheumatoid arthritis; seronegative arthropathies, SLE, polymyalgia rheumatica

Crystal: gout, pseudogout, hydroxyapatite, hypercholesterolaemia

Haemorrhage: haemophilia, previous AML
Infection:
 1. Septic arthritis, inc. viral, gonococcal, TB: Lyme; congenital syphilis (Clutton's joints)
 2. Reactive: endocarditis, rheumatic fever
 3. Foreign body arthropathy, e.g. rosethorn ⇒ symmetric polyarthritis

Neuropathic ('Charcot joints': gross changes of dislocation, disorganization and debris):
 1. Cord: syringomyelia (shoulders), syphilis, Vit B12 deficiency (hip, knee)
 2. Neuropathy: diabetes, leprosy, Charcot–Marie–Tooth disease (ankle, feet)
Genetic:
 • Osteogenesis imperfecta, Marfan's, homocystinuria, hyperlysinaemia
 • Immunodeficiency: Bruton's agammaglobulinaemia or common variable
Malignancy:
 1. Infiltration, inc. leukaemia, amyloid
 2. Paraneoplastic: giant-cell arteritis-like syndrome, HPOA (squamous cell carcinoma)
Endocrine–metabolic:
 O.W.T.C.H.A. – see opposite
Exogenous:
 1. Vitamin deficiency: D (rickets), C (scurvy)
 2. Kashin-Beck disease: fungal infestation of wheat in E. Europe

Idiopathic

Inc: 10% over-60s
Age: Linear increase with age (radiographic progression)
Sex: F > M (esp. knee, hand); M > F (elbow); M = F (hip)
Geo: White > Black
Aet: 1. Genetic: ∴ family history
     2. Cumulative repetitive movements: ∴ age
     3. Excess loading: ∴ obesity

Softened bone

1. Developmental:

  a) Congenital dislocation of hip = posterior hip dislocation due to acetabular flattening or joint laxity
       PC: • Neonate: failure to abduct flexed hips to 90°, and difficulty reducing head (Ortolani's test)
            • Child: waddling gait, hyperlordosis (bilateral), asymmetric skin crease (unilateral)
  b) Perthes' disease = avascular necrosis of femoral head secondary to minor trauma
       PC: Painful hip in 5–10 yr old, esp. boys
  c) Slipped upper femoral epiphysis = insufficiency fracture of physeal growth plate
       PC: Painful hip or knee at puberty, esp. obese, hypogonadal boys

2. Osteochondritis:

  a) Crushing: = necrosis of cuboidal bone in hand or feet, esp. during puberty
       Types: hand: lunate or capitulum; feet: metatarsal head or navicular
  b) Splitting (dissecans): = osteochondral fracture of convex joint, due to repeated minor trauma
       Types: medial femoral condyle, talus, capitulum (humeral part of elbow joint)
  c) Pulling (traction apophysitis): = bone that receives tendon insertion is pulled off during puberty
       Types: tibial tuberosity (Osgood–Schlatter), calcaneum (Sever's)

3. Osteonecrosis ('avascular necrosis')

F.I.N.A.L.I.T.Y.

Fractured: neck of femur, carpal (scaphoid, lunate), foot (talus, metatarsal head)
Infection: septic arthritis or osteomyelitis, TB, endocarditis
Nitrogen: following rapid decompression N_2 bubbles act as emboli, e.g. in deep-sea divers
Autoimmune: rheumatoid arthritis, SLE, vasculitis
Lipodystrophy: Gaucher's disease
Ischaemic: sickle cell anaemia, polycythaemia, diabetes, shock (e.g. acute pancreatitis)
Toxins: steroids (inc. pregnancy, Cushing's), alcohol
Young: Perthes' – as above

Endocrine–metabolic   *O.W.T.C.H.A.!*

Ochronosis (homogentisic acid oxidase deficiency – alkaptonuria); PC: Black cartilage
Wilson's disease
Thyroid: Graves' disease: acropachy, hypothyroidism
Calcium: Hyper- or hypoparathyroidism
Haemochromatosis
Acromegaly

Osteoarthritis – PC

PC   1° OA: 1. Distribution: localized (1–2 joints) or generalized (≥ 3 classes of joints)
              2. History: a) Pain ↑ed by movement; evening–night; stiffness ↑es after rest
                          b) Slow onset ⇒ flares every few months ⇒ deformity occurs late
              3. O/E: Crepitus felt on movement, due to osteophytes; locking; effusions

A. Foot / Hand

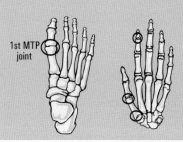

1st MTP joint

1. 1st MTP joint affected first

2. DIP and PIP joints (Heberden's and Bouchard's nodes):
   O/E: Binodular (cf. scleroderma – uninodular)
   • DIP only: Mild disease; post-menopausal; familial
   • PIP: 'Erosive OA' with synovitis
            Associated large-joint OA and cervical spondylosis

3. Thumb base: 1st MCP and CMC joints:
   O/E: Stiffness, subluxation and squaring of thumb base

   Familial 'persistent generalized osteoarthropathy' =
   • CMC + DIP + knee OA
   • Assoc. carpal tunnel syndrome, ulnar neuropathy

B. Hip

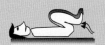

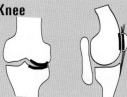

1. Pain inguinal; buttock; thigh, radiating to knee;
   limited passive internal rotation (normal: 50° external; 40° internal)

2. Fixed-flexion deformity: Thomas' test (see diagram):
   • Legs flat on bed: hyperlordosis apparent
   • Flex both hips to straighten back
   • Extend one hip, while holding pelvis straight ⇒
        fixed-flexion deformity apparent in hip

3. True shortening of leg:
   • Distance between ASIS and trochanter decreases
   • Telescoping may occur with severe instability

C. Knee

1. Medial compartment osteoarthritis
   • Varus and fixed flexion deformity
   • Gait disturbance:
       – bilateral: waddles
       – unilateral: Trendelenburg sign + ve: pelvis sags on diseased
                      side, on standing on one leg
2. Patello-femoral osteoarthritis
3. Baker's cyst

D. Spine

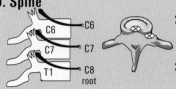

C6   C6
C7   C7
T1   C8
      root

1. Cervical spondylosis – facet joints: radiculopathy; myelopathy

2. Lumbar spondylosis – posterior disc and facet joints:
   radiculopathy; cauda equina syndrome, spinal stenosis,
   spondylolisthesis

3. Other: sacro-iliitis, skeletal hyperostosis (ligament ossification)

Other: Shoulder (glenohumeral, acromioclavicular, sternoclavicular), tibio-talar, temporomandibular

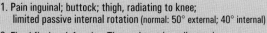

Osteoarthritis – Ix and Rx

<u>Ix</u>   X-ray

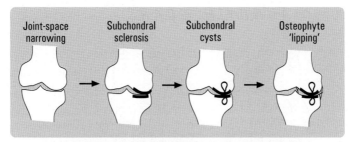

| Joint-space narrowing | Subchondral sclerosis | Subchondral cysts | Osteophyte 'lipping' |

☠:   Complications

1. Soft tissue swelling and effusion   ⇒ acute pain; locking
   – due to: a) Osteophyte separation
   b) Synovitis in 'erosive OA'
   c) Crystal deposition
2. Bone marrow vascular congestion   ⇒ chronic pain
3. Capsular fibrosis, bony ankylosis   ⇒ stiffness
4. Osteoporosis, 2° to immobility   ⇒ fracture

<u>Rx</u> Conservative

1. Physiotherapy:
   a) Exercise – pain ↓ , function ↑, power ↑
   b) Hydrotherapy – joint load ↓ , mobility ↑ ; heat or ice therapy – for acute flares
   c) Serial splintage – fixed flexion deformity (e.g. knee), stabilizes joints
2. Orthotics and occupational therapy:
   a) Stick, frame: joint load ↓ , mobility ↑ ; shoe-raiser for shortened leg
   b) Home appliances: stair + bath rail, firm chairs, high toilet-seat ('doughnut')

Medical

1. Effusion: Joint aspiration and injection of steroid (e.g. triamcinolone), hyaluronic acid, osmic acid
2. Analgesia:
   a) Mild: paracetamol, co-dydramol
   b) NSAIDs: ibuprofen, diclofenac, COX-2 inhibitors (if no arteriopathy) – for acute flares
      ☠: gastritis, peptic ulceration, ? enhances OA progression due to chondrocyte inhibition
   c) Other: capsaicin cream, TENS

Surgical

1. Arthroscopy: • Debride unstable cartilage and osteophytes (but recurrence common)
   • Drilling exposed bone causes cartilage remodelling
2. Osteotomy: a) Genu varum: • Realign tibial plateau by removing wedge from lateral tibia
   • Divide meduallary veins, which reduces pain
   b) 1st MTP joint: Keller's osteotomy – excision of proximal MTP and proximal phalanx
3. Arthroplasty: a) Hip, knee, elbow : replacement hemi or total
   b) 1st MTP joint: joint excision or insertion of Silastin sponge
4. Arthrodesis: fusion of joint removes pain and can improve resting position, but
   requires neighbouring joints to be normal to allow compensation

Rheumatoid Arthritis – PC

Def Multisystemic cell-mediated immune autoimmune disease, characterized by chronic synovitis

PC *A.N.N.O.Y.I.N.' S.C.A.R.S.*

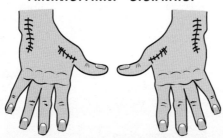

Arthritis:
- Small-joints, symmetric + generalized (≥3 joint areas)
- Pain + stiffness: ↑es with rest, e.g early morning stiffness
- Subacute onset ⇒ periodic + progressive; flare frequency ↓es , deformity ↑es ⇒ quiescence

Nodules (25%):
- Elbows, feet, ischial tuberosity; Achilles tendon; periosteal; visceral (e.g. lung, eye, bowel)
- EPI: - Elderly men; sero +ve; serositis, e.g. pleural effusions; may ulcerate and become infected

Nails and skin:
1. Longitudinal ridges, clubbing (if lung fibrosis), splinter haemorrhages (if vasculitis), palmar erythema
2. Vasculitis (10%), inc. dusky cyanotic digits, Raynaud's syndrome, cryoglobulinaemia livedo reticularis
3. Leg ulcers, inc. pyoderma gangrenosum; ankle oedema

Ophthalmology:
1. Keratoconjunctivitis sicca: 2° Sjögren's syndrome (40%) – associated lethargy + lymphoma
2. Episcleritis (also scleromalacia perforans); scleral nodules
3. Vasculitis: central retinal; anterior ciliary arteries (obliterative endarteritis)

Y: l**Y**mphadenopathy: proximal to affected joints; resembles giant follicular-cell lymphoma on histology

Immunocompromise: due to disease and immunosuppression; PC: pneumonia, infected leg ulcers

Neurology:
1. Peripheral - entrapment neuropathy, e.g. carpal tunnel syndrome; vasculitic mononuritis multiplex
2. CNS: ischaemic stroke due to medium-vessel vasculitis
3. Myositis: polymyositis or vasculitis (also hand wasting due to disuse atrophy)

Systemic: fatigue, low-grade fever, anorexia, weight loss, steroid side-effects (e.g. skin thinning)

Cardiac: pericarditis ± effusion, myo- or endocarditis, mitral regurgitation, coronary arteritis

Anaemia of chronic disease / **A**myloid AA (hepatosplenomegaly, malabsorption; renal failure)

Respiratory:
1. Pulmonary fibrosis: lower zone ± 2° pulmonary hypertension; adenocarcinoma
2. Pleurisy, pleural effusions, empyema
3. Rare: COAD, lung nodules, pneumonitis (esp. with methotrexate), bronchiolitis

Syndrome, Felty's (1%) = severe arthritis, splenomegaly, low platelets and neutrophils (leg spots, ulcers)

Still's disease ('juvenile chronic arthritis'): PC: evening rash coincident with fever

Arthritis

1. Upper Limb

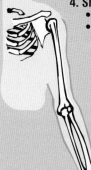

4. Shoulder / clavicle
- Shoulder: unable to abduct; rotator cuff tears, superior subluxation
- Acromioclavicular, sternoclavicular arthritis, subacromial bursitis

3. Elbow
- Unable to extend, olecranon bursitis

2. Wrist
- Extensor tenosynovitis and effusion: tender, hot, red, boggy swelling
- Volar subluxation of wrist joint, dorsal subluxation of distal radio-ulnar joint
- Prominent distal radius and ulnar: 'piano-key deformity' (radius), tendon rupture

1. PIP / MCP joints
- PIP: fusiform or sausage-shaped fingers. effusions, 2° osteoarthritis
- MCP: ulnar deviation of fingers, volar subluxation, Z-shaped thumb
- Deformities: swan-necking, bouttonière (tendon rupture), trigger finger

N.B.
joints numbered in
order of frequency with
which they occur

B. Lower Limb

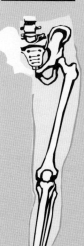

3. Hip
- Osteoporosis
- Avascular necrosis, inc. due to steroids
- Protrusio acetabuli
- Trochanteric bursitis: anterior thigh pain

2. Knee
- Genu valgus
- Baker's cyst = popliteal bursitis ruptures to cause acute pain and swelling in calf

1. Foot
- Toe clawing and hallux valgus
- Metatarsal callosities
- Volar subluxation of metatarsal heads: 'walking on pebbles'
- Talar, subtalar joint synovitis

C. Cervical Spine / Other Head–Neck

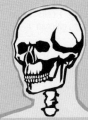

Uncommon:
1. Superior oblique tenosynovitis
2. TMJ – esp. young women
3. Crico-arytenoid – hoarseness

1. Atlanto-axial dislocation
Odontoid peg – atlas synovitis:
when separation ↑es to > 2 mm, on flexion:
- Cord compression (limb paraesthesia)
- Paroxysmal medullary dysfunction (e.g. vertigo, dysphagia, LOC) or vertebral artery TIA or stroke
- Head feels like falling forwards on flexing

2. Neurocentral joints of Luschka (C3–7) synovitis
Def: Synovial joints occur at upturned lateral lips of vertebral bodies
PC: Neck + head pain and stiffness, cord compression

Rheumatoid Arthritis – Epi, Ix and Rx

Epi

Inc: Prevalence 3% (women), 1% (men)
Age: Middle-aged
Sex: F:M = 3:1
Geo: Urban > rural in Blacks
Aet: Cell-mediated immunity: CD8$^+$ T cells
Pre: 1. Genetic: HLA-DR4 or -DR1 (relative risks of 6 and 2, respectively)
   2. Infection: commoner in Winter
   3. Estrogen: pregnancy + pill – protective; prolactin receptor mutation association

Ix

Bloods:

1. Rheu**M**atoid factor = Ig**M** (± IgG) directed against Fc of IgG, found in serum and synovial fluid
   • Tests involve agglutination of sheep red blood cells or latex (latter more sensitive)
   • High sensitivity (80%):   False –ves due to IgG rheumatoid factor
   • Low specificity: False +ves due to SLE, Sjögren's; infection (malaria, leprosy, rubella)
   Prognosis: titre (> 1/32) correlates with disease severity: erosions and systemic involvement
2. Other autoantibodies, or markers of inflammation:
   a) ANA +ve in 30%
   b) ESR, CRP   ↑ (correlates with severity)
   c) C3, C4, IgG ↑ or normal (unlike SLE)
3. Routine bloods:
   a) FBC: • Hb – normochromic, normocytic anaemia (ferritin ↓ if Fe-def.; ↑ if active inflammation)
        • WBC – eosinophilia, lymphocytosis in severe RA (except in Felty's syndrome – leucopenia)
        • Plt – thrombocytosis (except in Felty's syndrome – thrombocytopenia)
   b) LFT: Alk Phos. ↑, LDH ↑, albumin ↓

Microscopy – aspirate of synovial or serosal fluid:
   • Straw-coloured, turbid, low viscosity
   • Neutrophilia; CD8$^+$ T cells ↑
   • Complement Ig ↑, glucose ↓

Radiology – X-ray:

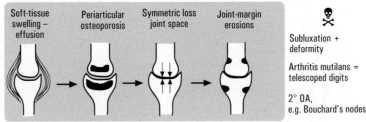

Soft-tissue swelling – effusion	Periarticular osteoporosis	Symmetric loss joint space	Joint-margin erosions	☠

Subluxation + deformity

Arthritis mutilans = telescoped digits

2° OA, e.g. Bouchard's nodes

Cervical X-ray: atlanto-axial distance should be < 2 mm on flexion
MRI: cervical cord compression by synovial hypertrophy
CXR: lower-zone fibrosis

Surgical – biopsy, e.g. of skin, nerve:
   Vasculitis: • Obliterative endarteritis e.g. retina, nailbeds
        • Necrotizing arteritis (large vessel), e.g. ischaemic colitis, CVA, PVD (limb)
        • Subacute arteritis (medium and small vessel), e.g. nerves (vasa nervorum), muscles

<u>Rx</u>

Conservative:
1. Rest: bedrest, splintage - for acute flare-up
2. Physiotherapy: stretching (decreases joint contractures); hydrotherapy; heat or ice therapy; orthotics, aids, inc. collar; neck protection during surgery
3. Diet: low-fat, high in omega–3 fatty-acids

Medical: *drug S.A.M.P.L.I.N.G.*

Steroids / NSAIDs

Ind: Steroids: • Acute flares: intra-articular; short oral course; IM or IV pulse
                • Maintenance (< 7.5 mg prednisolone od): decreases erosion and systemic disease
☠ 1. Steroids: add Na Bisphosphonate, omeprazole if given for > 3 months; check glucose, ABP
   2. NSAIDs: peptic ulcer, hypertension; fluid retention, renal failure, asthma
   3. COX-2 inhibitors (e.g. celecoxib): caution due to risk of stroke, ischaemic heart disease!

Disease-Modifying Anti-Rheumatoid Drugs (DMARDs)
1. Should always be used; 2. Takes several months to start working; 3. Efficacious for 1–2 yrs

Sulphasalazine:
☠: Oligospermia; headache, nausea, dizziness; rash

Antimalarials – chloroquine, hydroxychloroquine:
☠: Retinopathy (annual fundoscopy and visual fields); rash

Methotrexate (purine antagonist) – weekly PO or IM:
1st choice: as quicker onset of action: 1–2 months; and longest-lasting efficacy of approx. 6 yrs
☠: Liver failure; lung: fibrosis, acute pneumonitis; cytopenia; nausea

Penicillamine:
☠: Glomerulonephritis, obliterative bronchiolitis (acute SOB), cytopenia (esp. Hb, Plts.)
+myasthenia gravis; myositis; taste disturbance

Leflunomide (pyrimidine antagonist):
☠: Hypertension, diarrhoea, liver impairment, cytopenia

Infliximab or etanercept (TNF-α antagonists)
(etaneRCEPT = receptor antagonist; infliximAB = anti-TNF antibody):
☠: Opportunistic infections – TB, fungal, bacterial septicaemia; autoimmunity – SLE or MS

Nasty: azathioprine, mycophenolate, cyclophosphamide, cyclosporin A, chlorambucil:
☠: Immunosuppression; cytopenia; lymphoma and haemorrhagic cystitis (cyclophospamide)

Gold – IM or PO:
☠: Nephrosis, renal failure, cytopenia (or eosinophilia), diarrhoea (oral gold)

Surgical: arthroplasty (hip, knee, elbow); arthrodesis (wrist, atlanto-axial)
osteotomy (e.g. radial head, forefoot) + tendon transposition; synovectomy

Seronegative Arthropathies – 1

Def
1. Generalized arthropathy centred on axial skeleton, with systemic features
2. Negative rheumatoid factor
3. Familial component, esp. via association with HLA-B27

Types   *R.A.P.E.R.S.*

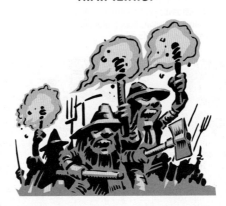

Reiter's syndrome:
      Assoc: STD or gastroenteritis
      PC: Arthritis, urethritis, conjunctivitis
Reactive arthritis:
      Assoc: STD, gastroenteritis, meningococcus
      PC: As for Reiter's, but only arthritis
Ankylosing spondylitis:
      Assoc: HLA-B27 – strongest association
      PC: Spondylosis, chest, arthritis, enthesopathy
Psoriasis:
      Assoc: Psoriasis, nail pitting
      PC: Arthritis
Enteropathic:
      Assoc: IBD, Whipple's or Behçet's syndrome
      PC: Arthritis
Rheumatic fever:
      Assoc: *Streptococcus pyogenes* (not HLA-B27)
      PC: Pancarditis, arthritis, subcutaneous nodules, Sydenham's chorea,
         erythema marginatum, streptococcal infection in past
Still's disease, adult-onset:
      PC: Arthritis, serositis, rash, organomegaly
Sarcoid
SAPHO:
      PC: **S**ynovitis, **A**cne, **P**ustulosis, **H**yper**O**stosis spine and costochondral joints

PC

S.C.A.R.E.D. S.L.O.U.C.H.E.R.S.

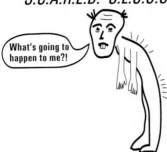

What's going to happen to me?!

Sacro-iliitis / **S**pondylosis:
   1. Sacro-iliitis:
      PC: Painful buttocks, hamstrings; thighs: ↑ in morning or with rest; difficult high-stepping
      O/E: Tender over SI joints – induced by pressure on sacrum centre and both iliac crests
   2. Spondylosis (fibrous bony ankylosis):
      PC: Stiff, painful back and neck
      O/E: Restricted lateral or anterior flexion; lumbar flattening or lordosis on forward flexion;
         thoracic kyphosis (wall–tragus distance ↑);
         Schober's Test: max. excursion of two points, 10 cm apart upwards from L5, is < 15 cm
   3. Complications: spinal fracture (inc. end-plate collapse); cauda equina syndrome, spinal fusion

Costochondritis:
      Sternocostal and costovertebral enthesitis, resulting in ankylosis; thoracic spondylosis
      O/E: Max. inspiratory excursion below breasts < 5 cm circumference increase

Arthritis: Asymmetrical, mono- or oligoarthritis, esp. women; knee, ankle, TMJ

Respiratory: 1. Chest wall ankylosis – restricted excursion and pain
              2. Apical fibrosis (*Aspergillus* may infect fibrotic lung)

Enthesopathy (painful inflammation of tendon and ligament insertions):
         pelvis (iliac crests, ischial tuberosity, greater trochanter), patella, Achilles,
         plantar fasciitis

Dactylitis

Systemic: fatigue, low-grade fever, anorexia – weight loss; ESR, CRP ↑
Liver and GIT:
      1. Fatty change, chronic active hepatitis, cirrhosis (Alk. Phos. ↑), sclerosing cholangitis
      2. Inflammatory bowel disease, inc. silent ileal ulcers

Ophthalmology: Iridocyclitis (anterior uveitis), phlyctenular conjunctivitis, episcleritis

Ulcers / Urethritis: Orogenital ulceration, inc. circinate balanitis

Cardiac: Aortic root fibrosis and regurgitation; myocarditis – arrhythmias

Haematology: Anaemia of chronic disease, DVT
              Sweet's syn. (purple plaques, fever, neutrophilia)

Extra: hepatosplenomegaly due to AA amyloid or adult-onset Still's disease (also lymphadenopathy)

Renal: IgA nephropathy, plasma IgA ↑

Skin: 1. Pyoderma gangrenosum (esp. UC): O/E: violaceous everted edge;
      2. Erythema nodosum or multiforme; 3. Vasculitis or Raynaud's syndrome; 4. Clubbing

Seronegative Arthropathies – Specific

Ankylosing Spondylitis

Epi **Inc:** Prevalence = 0.5% population
Age: Onset in teens – 30s
Geo: Native Americans, e.g. Pima (high HLA-B27 occurrence)
Sex: M:F = 3:1;   M – spondylosis, psoriasis; F – peripheral arthritis, Crohn's disease
Aet: Autoimmune attack against a cartilage glycoprotein, e.g. 'aggrecan'
Pre: 1. HLA-B27 in 95% (but B27 prevalence = 10%; so only 5% of people with HLA-B27 have ank. spond.)
2. MZ / DZ = 70:25; familial forms - milder severity
3. Infective: *Klebsiella pneumoniae, Campylobacter* (serology often +ve)

PC

S.C.A.R.E.D. S.L.O.U.C.H.ers

Sacro-iliitis / **S**pondylosis: back and buttock pain, stiffness
Costochondritis and thoracic ankylosis
Arthritis: mainly women sufferers: knees, ankles, shoulder
Respiratory: apical fibrosis; chest wall anylosis (restricted excursion and pain)
Enthesopathy: ligament insertion inflammation e.g. plantars, Achilles, knees
             (also responsible for spondylosis and sacro-iliitis)
Dactylitis

what's going to happen to me?!

Systemic: fatigue (esp. elderly); fever (low-grade); anorexia; weight loss
Liver / GIT: liver fatty change, alkaline phosphatase ↑, silent ileal ulcers
Ophthalmic: acute iridocyclitis (commonest complication) - poor prognosis
Urethritis
Cardiac: aortic regurgitation; heart block
Haematology: anaemia of chronic disease

Ix **B**loods: ESR, CRP ↑; IgA ↑; CK; alkaline phosphatase ↑
Radiology: X-ray

Sacro-iliac jts: 1. Blurred cortical margins
2. Erosions ('pseudowidening')
3. Sclerosis (esp. lower half)

Spine:

1. Initially upper lumbar spine

2. Calcification of annulus fibrosus ends = 'syndesmophytes'

1. Ossification of annulus and posterior longitudinal ligament ('bamboo spine')
2. Loss of joint space

1. Squared-off bodies
2. Sclerotic end-plate
3. Osteoporosis

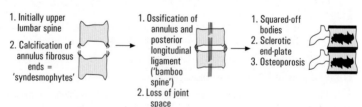

MRI – spinal arachnoid cysts

Rx **Conservative:** Physiotherapy; swimming; avoid contact sports
Medical: 1. NSAIDs: esp. indomethacin, phenylbutazone (most efficacious, but ☠ : cytopenias!)
2. Steroids: Pulsed methylprednisolone, CT-guided sacro-iliac injection, eye-drops for iritis
3. DMARDs: sulphasalazine, methotrexate (for peripheral arthritis), infliximab, thalidomide
Surgery: Total hip arthroplasty; spinal osteotomy – in severe cases only

Reiter's Syndrome

Def
1. Triad of *G.O.A.* – see below (if arthritis alone, then it is called 'reactive arthritis')
2. Systemic autoimmune reaction, secondary to cross-reactivity with Gram-negative bacteria:
    gastroenteritis (e.g. *Yersinia*, *Salmonella*, *E. coli*); STD (*Chlamydia*, Gonococcus)

Epi
Occurs in 1–2 % of those with associated infections, esp. in young, with equal sex distribution

PC
A real G.O.A.

Genital:
- Urethritis (discharge), prostatitis
- Pelvic inflammatory disease, cervicitis
- Orogenital ulcers, inc. circinate balanitis

Ophthalmic:
- Conjunctivitis, anterior uveitis

Arthritis:
- Lower limb, mono- or oligoarthritis
- Resolves within 6 months, although $1/3$ relapse
- Enthesopathy, inc. Achilles tendonitis, plantar fasciitis

+ Keratoderma blenorrhagica – pustular psoriasis on soles or palms
+ Diarrhoea

Ix
Micro:
- Microscopy and culture of blood; stool; urine; urethral, cervical + rectal swabs
- Serology: ligase chain reaction for *Chlamydia*, HIV, syphilis (if STD suspected)
- Joint aspirate: neutrophil or monocyte exudate, but sterile

Rx
Acute: rest initially, physio, later; aspirate effusions; NSAIDs ± steroids
Chronic: sulphasalazine, methotrexate or azathioprine (but must exclude HIV first!)

Psoriatic Arthropathy

Epi
2% population have psoriasis, of whom 7% develop arthropathy, esp. young men

PC

Arthritis	Skin
1. Small-joint, esp. DIP joints – commonest	1. Psoriasis: poor correlation with arthritis
2. Large-joint – symmetric or asymmetric	2. Nail pitting; onycholysis; horizontal ridging:
3. Sacro-iliitis; spondylitis	esp. on same digits with DIP arthritis
4. 'Arthritis mutilans' = telescoping of digits	**Iritis**

Distinction from rheumatoid arthritis
1. DIP joints   (rheumatoid: PIP joints)
2. Asymmetric, oligoarthritis   (rheumatoid: Symmetric, polyarthritis)
3. Sacro-iliitis, spondylitis   (rheumatoid: atlanto-axial disease)
4. Dactylitis – uniform-swelling (rheumatoid: spindle-shaped fingers)

Ix
X-ray : osteolysis of phalanx ends: 'Pencil-in-cup' deformity

Rx
1. NSAIDs: avoid steroids (worsen psoriasis on withdrawal)
2. DMARDs: Sulphasalazine, methotrexate, infliximab, etanercept (avoid antimalarials – worsen psoriasis)

Septic Arthritis

Predisposing

All the I's

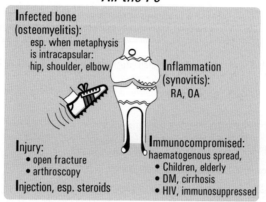

Infected bone
(osteomyelitis):
   esp. when metaphysis
   is intracapsular:
   hip, shoulder, elbow

Inflammation
(synovitis):
   RA, OA

Injury:
   • open fracture
   • arthroscopy
Injection, esp. steroids

Immunocompromised:
haematogenous spread,
   • Children, elderly
   • DM, cirrhosis
   • HIV, immunosuppressed

Organisms

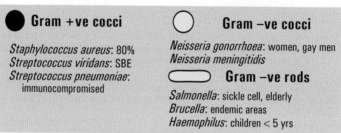

● Gram +ve cocci

Staphylococcus aureus: 80%
Streptococcus viridans: SBE
Streptococcus pneumoniae:
   immunocompromised

○ Gram –ve cocci

Neisseria gonorrhoea: women, gay men
Neisseria meningitidis

⬭ Gram –ve rods

Salmonella: sickle cell, elderly
Brucella: endemic areas
Haemophilus: children < 5 yrs

🪱 Atypical bacteria

Mycobacterium tuberculosis:
   • Children: discitis, vertebral body collapse. Adults: painful large-joint synovitis
   • Poncet's disease (reactive non-septic arthritis)

Mycobacterium bovis: carpal tunnel infection

Lyme disease: rash followed by recurrent large-joint arthritis

⬡ **Viruses**	**DNA**	**RNA**
	Parvovirus	Rubella
	EBV	Mumps
	Hep B	Enteroviruses: coxsackie, Hep A

The following cause a reactive, non-septic arthritis:
1. *Streptoccous pyogenes* ('rheumatic fever');
2. *Neisseria*, *Chlamydia*, or *Campylobacter* ('Reiter's syndrome')
3. HIV seroconversion

Patterns

1. Monoarthritis: pyogenic, TB
2. Polyarthritis: • Virus (rubella = rheumatoid-pattern in hands that lasts months)
   • Lyme
3. Migratory: Gonoccoccus: occurs several weeks after acute infection;
   moves between hand, wrist, and knee, before settling in 1 or 2 joints
4. Vertebral: TB (painless), staphylococal (painful)
   cause discitis, vertebral body collapse, psoas abscess, radiculopathy

PC ### Arthritis
   • Acute, severe pain; tender, hot effusion; muscle spasm (pseudoparesis)
   • Secondary osteomyelitis (tender along bone), sinus, abscess
   • Chronic immobility due to:
   Fibrous-bony ankylosis: begins within 24 hrs of infection!
   Secondary wasting and osteoporosis

Systemic
   • Fever, N+V
   • Associated: rash (virus, inc. parvovirus, gonococcus, Lyme), diarrhoea (parvovirus, enterovirus)
   • Risk groups: Black (sickle cell anaemia, pneumococcus), sexually active (gonorrhoea, HIV)

Ix ### Bloods
   1. FBC, ESR, CRP
   2. Uric acid, rheumatoid factor, ANA (acute gout and rheumatoid are differential diagnoses)

Urine: microscopic haematuria – SBE

Microbiology
   1. Blood cultures and serology: for suspected viral infections
   2. Synovial aspirate: urgent Gram stain

Radiology
   1. X-ray

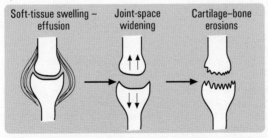

Soft-tissue swelling – effusion   Joint-space widening   Cartilage–bone erosions

1. Osteomyelitis:
   • Metaphyseal mottling
   • Perisoteal elevation
     (involucrum + sequestrum)
2. Fibrous or bony ankylosis
3. Dislocation:
   tense effusion

   2. Radio-isotope scan: reveals adjacent osteomyelitis, even in absence of X-ray changes

Rx 1. Antibiotics: • *S. aureus* – flucloxacillin, vancomycin, clindamycin (fusidic acid if osteomyelitis)
   • Coliforms – gentamicin (IV for first 2 weeks, PO for 6 weeks thereafter)
2. Surgery: Arthroscopy and drainage – indicates whether synovial damage and osteomyelitis
3. Supportive: • NSAIDs, e.g. indomethacin
   • Daily aspiration – relieves pain
   • Physio: 1st – splint or cast in appropriate position (hip: 30° flexion + adduction); rest
     2nd – gradual exercise from 1 week after acute stage

Gout

Def 1. Precipitations of NaHUrate (monosodium urate monohydrate) and uric acid crystals,
in synovial joints and soft tissue (cf. 'Pseudogout' = Calcium pyrophosphate crystals)
2. Occurs acutely and chronically against a background of hyperuricaemia, that is caused by:

Causes

G.O.U.T.Y.

Genetic: enzyme defects in purine metabolism:

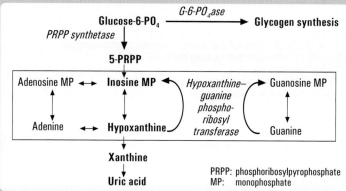

1. Lesch–Nyhan syndrome (X-linked) = HGPRT deficiency
   PC: Spasticity, mental retardation, self-mutilation
2. PRPP synthetase overactivity
3. Glycogen storage disease, type 1: glucose-6-phosphatase deficiency

Overproduction of uric acid:
1. Ingestion of purines: offal, oily fish
2. Increased cell turnover:
   - Myeloproliferative disease, leukaemia, myeloma, carcinomatosis – esp. with chemotherapy
   - Chronic haemolytic anaemia
   - Severe psoriasis
3. Hypoxia, e.g. cyanotic congenital heart disease, inc. Down's syndrome
   ATP production $\downarrow$ $\Rightarrow$ inosine $\Rightarrow$ xanthine production $\uparrow$

Underexcretion of uric acid:
1. 'Idiopathic' (95% cases) – often have positive family history
2. Chronic renal failure – due to decreased glomerular filtration rate, and hence urate clearance:
   - Esp. with hypertension
   - Tubular disease: uric acid may be lost excessively (hypouricaemia)
3. Acidosis: urate $\rightarrow$ uric acid $\rightarrow$ resorbed in renal tubules
   e.g. starvation, alcoholism (lactic acidosis)

Toxins:
1. Alcohol
2. Diuretics: thiazide, loop
3. TB Rx: pyrazinamide; ethambutol
4. Other: salicylates ($\therefore$ don't treat pain with aspirin!), cyclosporin, metformin

Y: h**Y**pothyroidism or h**Y**perparathyroidism

Epi   Inc: 5% hyperuricaemia → of which 15% have gout
Age: Middle-age or elderly - urate levels increase until 30 yrs (men) or menopause (women)
Sex: Men: 10–20 x ↑er
Geo: Urban, high social–classes
Pre: Wine-drinking, meat-eating, obese; hypertensive-IHD; type A personality

PC   **Acute:**

Triggers of A.T.T.A.C.K.

Arthritis
• Location:
small-joint monoarthritis
75% = 1st MTP ('podagra')
10% = > 1 joint
• Painful, red, shiny, desquamates
• Fever

Acute illness: infection, trauma, dehydration, exertion
Toxin-1: allopurinol, uricosuric
Toxin-2: diuretic, chemotherapy
Alcohol: esp. binge, withdrawal
Cold, **C**onsumption of high-protein meal
Ketoacidosis: DKA, starvation

Chronic: *A.R.T.*

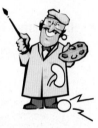

Arthritis: irregular nodules, recurrent flares;
tenosynovitis, olecranon bursitis
Renal: tubulointerstitial nephritis
Tophi: crystal deposition and calcification in skin (finger tips); pinna;
eyes; cartilage, bone, bursae, tendons

Ix   **B**lood: uric acid (< 480 μmol-males; < 390 μmol-females)
• But levels do not correlate with acute attack – an attack may be precipitated by a **reduction** in levels!
Urine: 24-hr uric acid, collected after a 70 g protein, purine-free diet
• Distinguishes 'overproducers' (high urinary uric acid) from 'underexcretors'
Micro: synovial aspirate microscopy:
• Polarized light: strongly negative birefringence (cf. pseudogout = weakly positive birefringence)
• Neutrophils contain crystals
• Blood-staining suggests pseudogout, or hydroxyapatite crystals (e.g. Milwaukee shoulder)
Radio: • Bone X-ray: subcutaneous calcification; 'moth-eaten' phalanges; 'punched-out' erosions
• Abdominal X-ray: Calculi - radiolucent, unless mixed with calcium

Rx   **Acute:**
1. NSAIDS, high-dose: e.g. indomethacin, diclofenac, azapropazone (but not asprin!)
2. Colchicine: microtubule assembly inhibitor; ☠: bloody diarrhoea, N+V, neuropathy
Chronic:
Strategy: wait > 1 month after acute attack; cover for 3 months with NSAID or colchicine;
continue indefinitely, inc. during attacks
1. Allopurinol (xanthine oxidase inhibitor): indicated in 'overproducers' or severe disease
☠: hypersensitivity reaction or rash - necessitates withdrawal; dyspepsia
2. Uricosuric (probenecid; NSAIDs, e.g. sulphinpyrazone, phenylbutazone) –
Indicated in 'underexcretors', mild disease, preserved renal function
☠: Renal stones (ensure high fluid intake, render urine alkali, e.g. K citrate)

Multisystemic Autoimmune Diseases

Classification

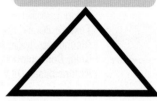

Rheumatoid Arthritis
Sjögren's Syndrome

Connective Tissue Diseases

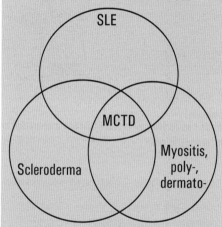

SLE

MCTD

Scleroderma

Myositis, poly-, dermato-

Associations
1. Anti-phospholipid syndrome
   (recurrent thromboses and miscarriages)
   – associated with SLE
2. Raynaud's disease / cryoglobulinaemia
3. Primary biliary cirrhosis
   – both 2. and 3. associated with connective tissue
   diseases, rheumatoid arthritis and Sjögren's

Vasculitides

Primary	With **g**ranuloma	Without granuloma
	⬤◯	◯ **p**-ANCA
Large	GCA, PMR Takayasu's	
Medium	Buer**G**er's	Kawasaki's **PAN**
Small	Chur**G**–Strauss We**G**ener's	Micro-**PAN** **HSP**
Special	Isolated CNS Co**G**an's	Behçet's Relapsing polychondritis

Autoimmune: connective tissue disease
Infection: ● HBV – PAN
● HCV – 'essential mixed cryoglobulinaemia'
● HIV, parvovirus B19, rickettsia
Neoplasia: lymphoma, carcinoma – paraneoplastic
Toxins

SLE, systemic lupus erythematosus
MCTD, mixed connective tissue disease

GCA, giant-cell arteritis
PMR, polymyalgia rheumatica
PAN, polyarteritis nodosa
HSP, Henoch–Schönlein purpura

Auto-Antibodies

RheuMatoid Factor

Def: Ig**M** directed against Fc portion of IgG
Positive: 1. Rheumatoid arthritis, Sjögren's, connective tissue disease (in 50%)
2. Malaria, leprosy, rubella
False −ve: Other Ab serotypes, e.g. IgG or IgA

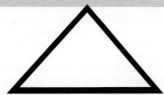

ANA (Anti-Nuclear Abs)

High sensitivity (SLE 95%), but poor specificity:
False +ve: rheumatoid arthritis, PBC, drugs, elderly
False −ve: complement deficiency, subacute cutaneous LE
Types: Classified according to:

Indirect immunofluoresence (HEP-2 cells)	ENA
Rim = **R**egular SLE	Double-stranded DNA Smith (Sm) antigen: • Small nuclear RNP
Diffuse = **D**rug-induced or regular SLE	Histone
Speckled = **S**ystemic • myositis • Raynaud's • cardiopulmonary	U₁ ribonucleprotein • MCTD Jo-1 (histidyl tRNA synthetase) • Myositis + pulmo. fibrosis
Speckled = **S**jögren's syndrome	SS-A (Ro); SS-B (La) • Sjögren's syndrome • Subacute cutaneous LE, or lupus nephritis (Ro) • Neonatal heart block
Nucleolar = scleroderma	Anti-Scl-70 • Diffuse cutaneous Anti-Centromere • Limited CREST

ANCA (Anti-Neutrophil Cytoplasmic Abs)

p-ANCA

Def: Abs against **p**erinuclear antigens: myeloperoxidase, cathepsin, elastase, lactoferrin, lysozyme

Diseases: *P.U.R.G.E.*

PAN, micro**P**AN (70% sensitivity) or Churg–Strauss syndrome
Ulcerative colitis, or:
• Chronic active hepatitis
• Primary biliary cirrhosis
• Primary sclerosing cholangitis
Rheumatoid arthritis with vasculitis
Glomerulonephritis, idiopathic crescentic
Endocarditis, HIV

c-ANCA

Def: Abs against **c**ytoplasmic antigens, esp. proteinase-3 (neutral serine protease)

Diseases:
1. Wegener's granulomatosis (90% sensitivity)
2. α₁-Anti-trypsin deficiency

N.B. ANCA titre indicates disease severity better than ESR or CRP

Anti-Cardiolipin IgG
Anti-phospholipid syndrome ± SLE

Anti-RBC, -platelet, or -lymphocyte Abs
Respective cytopenia ± SLE

Systemic Lupus Erythematosus (SLE)

<u>PC</u>

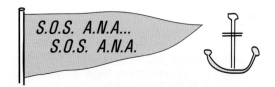

S.O.S. A.N.A...
S.O.S. A.N.A.

Skin 1. Photosensitivity due to IL-1 secretion from keratinocytes:
- Malar, 'butterfly', rash: erythematous maculopapular rash involving chin and ears
- Discoid LE: hyperkeratotic, follicular plugs; atrophic scars, raised erythematous rim
- Subacute cutaneous LE: extensive papules, annular, hypopigmented rash; fatigue
2. Alopecia: patchy or total
3. Vasculitis: purpura, cryoglobulinaemia, Raynaud's, nail fold infarcts, ulcers–nodules
4. Other: urticaria, bullae, erythema multiforme, lichen planus, panniculitis

Oral ulcers, or nasopharyngeal ulcers: aphthous – white base with red surround

Serositis: 1. Pleural effusions, pericarditis, peritonitis
2. Other respiratory: basal fibrosis, linear atelectasis, pulmonary hypertension
3. Other cardiac: 'Libman-Sacks endocarditis', myocarditis
4. Other GIT: abdominal pain, N + V + D

Arthritis:
1. Non-erosive arthritis of ± 2 joints: 'Jaccoud's arthropathy'
2. Joint effusions, contractures, avascular necrosis; tendonitis
3. Myalgia, myositis

Neurological:
1. Headaches – common
2. Seizures, psychosis, dementia, encephalopathy, cerebellar ataxia
3. Transverse myelitis, peripheral neuropathy

Anaemia and other haematological:
1. Haemolytic: direct Coombs' test +ve, warm agglutinins
2. Lymphopenia – immunosuppressed: miliary TB; toxoplasmosis; histoplasmosis, Candida
3. Thrombocytopenia

Splenomegaly, hepatomegaly (fatty change), lymphadenopathy

Ophthalmic: sicca, conjunctivitis, episcleritis, retinal vasculitis, cytoid bodies

Systemic: fever, fatigue, LOW

Acute **N**ephritis (or chronic): proteinuria (3+; > 0.5 g/24 hr) / cellular casts
Antibodies:
1. ANA +ve: inc. dsDNA, anti-Sm, false +ve VRDL (or LE cell prep. +ve)
2. Anti-cardiolipin (or lupus anticoagulant) ⇒ 'anti-phospholipid syndrome' =
arterial and venous thromboses (inc. recurrent miscarriages), thrombocytopenia,
liveo reticularis, nephritis, cerebral disease, endocarditis

Disease-defined by presence of any 4 of SOS, ANA and ANA

Epi   Inc: Prevalence = 1/ 10,000
Age: Onset 15–30 yrs
Sex: F:M = 9:1 (discoid LE = 2:1)
Geo: Black : White = 9:1; Blacks have higher anti-Smith Ag;
            SLE also highly prevalent in Chinese
Aet: 1. Inherited: C2, C4 deficiency (5%)
          2. Estrogen: OCP, pregnancy, menses worsen SLE
          3. Drug-induced:
             • Fast acetylators: Hydralazine
             • **SL**ow acetylators: *SL.I.P.P.E.D.*
                 Isoniazid
                 Phenytoin, **P**henothiazine (chlorpromazine)
                 Procainamide, **P**enicillin (or tetracycline)
                 Estrogen (oral contraceptive)
                 Diuretic (thiazide)
                 PC: Rash, serositis, pulmonary fibrosis (*NOT* neurological or nephritis)

Ix   1. ANA (anti-nuclear antibodies):

Indirect immunofluoresence (HEP-2 line)	Extractable nuclear Ag (antibodies to ENA)
Rim = **R**egular SLE	dsDNA: specific for SLE ssDNA: subacute cutaneous LE Smith (Sm) Ag: predicts nephritis
Diffuse = **D**rug-induced (or regular)	Histone
Speckled = A**SS**ortment (overlap)	U1-RNP: mixed connective tissue disease SS-A: predicts nephritis SS-B: protective against nephritis

2. Other auto-antibodies:
   a) Rheumatoid factor +ve in 40%
   b) Anti-cardiolipin ELISA IgG; or lupus anticoagulant assay (APTT ↑)
   c) Direct Coombs' test (warm agglutinins); anti-neutrophil, -lymphocyte, -platelet Abs

3. Other:
   a) ESR ↑ but CRP normal (unless superimposed infection or active serositis)
   b) Complement: C3, C4 ↓ (C3 normal in C1, C4 deficiency, or drug-induced SLE); CH50 ↓
   c) Biopsy, e.g. rash, renal, brain: fibrinoid necrosis; small–medium-vessel vasculitis

Rx   1. Symptomatic:
          a) NSAID, chloroquine – check vision annually
          b) Warfarin: antiphospholipid syndrome, if recurrent thrombotic episodes or miscarriages
         2. Immunosuppression:
          a) Steroids (flare-ups, chronically)
          b) Azathioprine, cyclophosphamide, IVIg
         3. Splenectomy, esp. if ITP

Scleroderma

Types

Scleroderma – Localized

1. Morphoea: plaque of thick, waxy skin
2. Linear scleroderma: en coup de sabre (linear alopecia), facial hemiatrophy
3. Eosinophilic fasciitis:
   - Acute inflammation, and cobblestone-like induration of all extremities, after exertion
   - Flexion contractures, carpal tunnel syndrome, myositis (CK normal)
   - Aplastic anaemia, myelodysplasia

Systemic Sclerosis - Limited

<u>PC</u>   *C.R.E.S.T.*

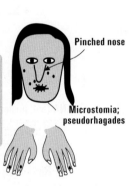

Pinched nose

Calcinosis, subcutaneous
Raynaud's phenomenon: may precede CREST by several years
Esophageal dysmotility: PC: Dysphagia (present in 50%)
Sclerodactyly: tight, tense, thick, tender, tanned skin
                  (oedema and fibrosis); ulcers; claw hand
Telangiectasia: no central arteriole, cf. liver disease

**Microstomia;
pseudorhagades**

N.B. Cutaneous disease is confined to forearms and face

Systemic Sclerosis – Diffuse

<u>Path</u>   Organ fibrosis

<u>PC</u>   *C.R.A.C.K.I.N.G*

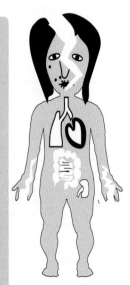

Cutaneous disease spreads to entire body
Respiratory:
     1. Pulmomary fibrosis
     2. Pulmonary hypertension
Arthritis:
     1. Non-erosive arthritis
     2. Tapered fingers; phalangeal tuft erosion and osteolysis
Cardiac:
     1. Restrictive cardiomyopathy
     2. Pericardial effusion
Kidney:
     1. Rapidly progressive renal failure, or chronic renal failure
        (Path: Intimal proliferation + medial fibrinoid necrosis)
     2. Malignant hypertension, flash pulmonary oedema
     3. Microangiopathic haemolytic anaemia (MAHA)
Intestine:
     1. Small bowel: dysmotility, bacterial overgrowth, malabsorption
     2. Large bowel: constipation, diverticulae,
                    pseudo-obstruction, pneumatosis coli
Neurological: polymyositis
Gastric: oesophageal dysmotility – peptic oesophagitis

Epi

Inc: Prevalence = 50 / 100,000
Age: 20–40s
Sex: F:M = 3:1 (esp. limited systemic sclerosis)
Geo: Choctaw Native Americans (Oklahoma) – highest incidence
Aet: Limited systemic sclerosis: small-vessel vasculitis
Diffuse systemic sclerosis: necrosis ⇒ overproduction of collagen and ground substance ⇒ fibrosis
Pre: 1. Industrial toxins: vinyl chloride, aromatics, epoxy resins – scleroderma-like disease
2. Iatrogenic – bleomycin; breast implants – localized scleroderma around silicon implants
3. Autoimmunity: Sjögren's, primary biliary cirrhosis, vitiligo

Ix

Bloods:
  1. Routine:
    Hb ↓ : • Normocytic, due to chronic inflammation or microangiopathic haemolytic anaemia
          • Macrocytic, due to Vit B12 deficiency (bacterial overgrowth)
    ESR ↑ ; urea and creatinine ↑
  2. Autoantibodies:
    • Limited systemic sclerosis: ANA: anti-centromere pattern
                            ENA: anti-centromere
    • Diffuse systemic sclerosis: ANA: anti-nucleolar pattern
                            ENA: anti-Scl-70 (topoisomerase)
    • Others: rheumatoid factor, cryoglobulins

Urine: RBC and WBC casts
ECG, Echo
Radio:
  1. CXR, high-resolution CT
  2. Barium swallow, meal + follow-through: abnormal in 90% systemic sclerosis
                                    dilated 2nd part of duodenum

Special:
  1. Oesophageal manometry
  2. Wide-angle microscopy (or ophthalmoscopy) of nail fold:
    • Limited systemic sclerosis: capillary enlargement
    • Diffuse systemic sclerosis: capillary enlargement and areas of capillary loss

Rx

Immunosuppressive:
  1. Penicillamine: also acts as an anti-fibrotic agent (inhibits collagen cross-linking):
    ☠: glomerulonephritis (nephrosis), cytopenias, myasthenia
  2. Other drugs: steroids, methotrexate, azathioprine, cyclophosphamide
  3. Autologous bone marrow transplant

Symptomatic:
cR.E.S.t 1. Raynaud's: nifedipine, IV prostacyclin
         2. OEsophageal dysmotility: metoclopramide, domperidone, proton-pump inhibitor
         3. Sclerodactyly: emollients (keep skin moist), subcutaneous relaxin (pregnancy hormone)

Diffuse 1. GIT: laxatives, cyclical antibiotics (bacterial overgrowth)
        2. Respiratory – pulmonary hypertension: IV prostacyclin
        3. Kidney: ACE inhibitors, beta-blockers

Sjögren's Syndrome

Def   Autoimmune destruction of exocrine glands that is either primary, or secondary to:
1. Rheumatoid arthritis (30% of RA pts); SLE, scleroderma, polymyositis; vasculitides
2. Organ-based autoimmunity: chronic active hepatitis, primary biliary cirrhosis, thyroiditis

Epi   **I**nc: Prevalence = 0.5–1% (primary SS)
Age: Onset commonest in 30s-40s
Sex: F:M = 9:1 (*same as SLE*)
Aet: Virus, e.g. EBV, causes cross-reactivity of CD4 cells with salivary gland antigen α-fodrin?
Pre: HLA-B8, -DR3 – associated with extraglandular involvement and auto-antibodies

PC

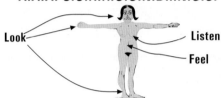

X.X.X. S.U.R.R.O.U.N.D.I.N.G.S.

Look   Listen   Feel

Xerophthalmia (dry eyes):
- Grittiness, soreness, photophobia, every day for > 3 months
- O/E: Keratitis, conjunctivitis, corneal ulcers (Rose Bengal stain)

Xerostomia (dry mouth):
- Dysphagia: need to take water to swallow ('cream cracker Sx'); awakes at night to drink water
- Bilateral parotid enlargement (uncommon in secondary Sjögren's; massive in HIV)
- Angular stomatitis, dental caries, fissured tongue; atrophic filiform papillae, oral candida

X: Ix: 2 out of 4 must be positive to establish diagnosis: see opposite

Skin: • Dry skin + dry hair
• Vasculitis, inc. Raynaud's syndrome, ulcers, urticaria, livedo reticularis

Ulcers: orogenital, corneal, leg ulcers (inc. pyoderma gangrenosum)

Rheum: reversible deformity, e.g. swan-necking PIP joints (Jaccoud's arthropathy)

Respiratory: • Dry respiratory passages: xerotrachea, bronchitis (dry cough), sinusitis
• Basal pulmonary fibrosis

Ophthalmic: xerophthalmia causes keratoconjunctivitis sicca and corneal ulcers

Urine: • Tubulointerstitial nephritis, renal tubular acidosis–nephrocalcinosis, osteomalacia
• Glomerulonephritis (vasculitis-associated)

Neurology: • Central nervous system vasculitis: seizures, multiple sclerosis-like syndrome
• Peripheral neuronopathy: sensory, painful, facial numbness, Rombergism

Deafness: sensorineural

Intestine: • Atrophic oesophagitis–gastritis (due to lack of mucosal barrier), achlorhydria
• Pancreatitis (subclinical)

Neoplasia: lymphoma or Waldenström's macroglobulinaemia (5% risk)

Genital: dyspareunia (dry secretions) – 30% pts (often presenting complaint)

Systemic: fatigue, anorexia, loss of weight, low-grade fever, lymphadenopathy

Differential Diagnosis

Causes of dry eyes and dry mouth

S.A.L.I.V.A.T.E.

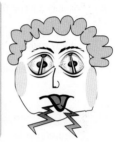

Sarcoidosis
Autoimune: Sjögren's (primary or secondary)
Lymphoma or Leukaemia (CLL) or graft-versus-host disease
Infection: TB
Virus: HIV 'sicca syndrome'
Amyloid
Toxin: anticholinergics, inc. tricyclic antidepressants
Endocrine: diabetes mellitus

*N.B. Glandular enlargement (Mikulicz's syndrome) is common
with these conditions*

Causes of dry, gritty eyes

1. Ocular: blepharitis, conjunctivitis, corneal ulcers, proptosis
2. Neurological: 5th or 7th cranial nerve palsies, myopathy
3. Vit A deficiency

Causes of bilateral parotid enlargement

1. Viral: mumps, EBV, influenza
2. Gastroenterological: cirrhosis, chronic pancreatitis, hyperlipoproteinaemia
3. Bulimia nervosa (painless)

Ix 1. Autoantibodies:
   • ENA: SS-A (Anti-Ro) , SS-B (Anti-La): associated with severe disease and extraglandular symptoms
   • ANA (immunofluorescent staining = speckled), rheumatoid factor, thyroid auto-antibodies
2. Schirmer's test < 5 mm in 5 min (usual > 15 mm)
3. Salivary function tests:
   salivary scintigraphy, parotid sialography, salivary flow test
4. Labial minor salivary gland histology:
   Clusters of CD4$^+$ lymphocytes around salivary acini (1 'focus' > 50 lymphocytes);
   + gland destruction; duct dilatation
      (cf. HIV: CD8$^+$ lymphocytes in glands; sarcoid: granulomas)

Rx 1. Symptomatic:
   • Sicca symptoms – artificial tears and saliva; oral pilocarpine; avoid anticholinergics or diuretics
   • Arthralgia: hydroxychloroquine

2. Immunosuppressants:
   steroids, IVIg or cyclophosphamide – used for extraglandular disease, e.g. vasculitis, respiratory

Autoimmune Myositis

Dermatomyositis

Epi   Inc: 1/100,000 p.a.
Age: Adults and **children**
Sex: F:M = 3:1
Aet: Primarily a **vasculitis** of muscle and skin capillaries ⇒ ischaemia + CD4 infiltration
Pre: **Malignancy:**
  • Present in 10%: Bronchial, Breast, Ovary, GIT, Lymphoma (Non-Hodgkin's)
  • May predate or postdate malignancy by 2 years

PC   Similar organ involvement as for diffuse systemic sclerosis:

C.R.A.C (k).I.N.G.

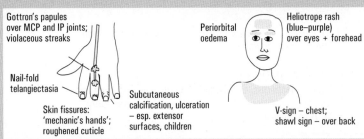

Cutaneous:

Gottron's papules over MCP and IP joints; violaceous streaks

Nail-fold telangiectasia

Skin fissures: 'mechanic's hands'; roughened cuticle

Subcutaneous calcification, ulceration – esp. extensor surfaces, children

Periorbital oedema

Heliotrope rash (blue–purple) over eyes + forehead

V-sign – chest; shawl sign – over back

Respiratory:
  • Pulmonary fibrosis: assoc. anti-Jo-1 (tRNA synthetase); anti-KL6 (mucin-like glycoprotein)
  • Respiratory muscle weakness

Arthritis: arthralgia; flexion contractures (children)

Cardiac: AV-conduction block, arrhythmias, myocarditis

Intestine: visceral myopathy – constipation, dysphagia

Neurological: • Proximal myopathy develops **acutely** over days–weeks
  • Bulbar and respiratory weakness

Gastro-oesophageal - dysphagia, due to involvement of striated muscle of oropharynx, upper oesophagus

Ix   **B**loods: • CK ↑↑
  • AutoAbs: anti-Jo1 (histidyl tRNA synthetase), anti-SRP (signal recognition particle)
EMG: Small-amplitude, polyphasic potentials; positive sharp-waves; fibrillations
Radio: • Plain X-rays – subcutaneous calcification
  • CT thorax–abdominal–pelvis, or PET scan – search for occult malignancy
Surgical: muscle biopsy (site can be guided by prior MRI)

Rx   1. Steroids: 80 mg od, taper over 10 weeks
2. Steroid-sparing drugs: methotrexate (acts faster), azathioprine, mycophenolate, IVIg

Polymyositis

Epi   Inc: 0.5/100,000 p.a.
Age: Adults **only**
Sex: F:M = 3:1
Aet: Primarily **myositis** ⇒ CD8 infiltration
Pre: 1. **Autoimmunity**: SLE, Sjögren's syndrome, RA
      2. **Infection**: HIV

PC   As for dermatomyositis, except:
      1. No cutaneous features
      2. Myopathy develops **sub-acutely** over weeks–months (cf. acutely for dermatomyositis)

Ix   As for dermatomyositis, except no need to hunt for neoplasia, but do HIV test

Rx   As for dermatomyositis

Inclusion Body Myositis

Epi   Inc: Commonest myopathy of > 50s
Age: **Elderly**
Sex: F:M = 1:3
Geo: Caucasians
Aet: **Myositis + degenerative** components:
      1. Myositis: similar to polymyositis
      2. Degenerative: vacuolated fibres, amyloid-positive inclusions, mitochondrial DNA deletions
Pre: 1. Autoimmunity
      2. Family history

PC   Myopathy:
   • **Distal** (foot extensors, wrist extensors, finger flexors), or quadriceps weaknesss
   • **Dysphagia** in 60%
   • **Sub-acute** onset over weeks–months
   • **Unresponsive to steroids**

Ix   **B**loods: CK – normal or slightly ↑

EMG: as for dermatomyositis

Surgical: muscle biopsy – distinguished from DM and PM due to rimmed vaculoes, amyloid-positive inclusions
      and abnormal mitochondria (ragged-red fibres and cytochrome-oxidase-negative fibres)

Rx   Immunosuppressants (steroids, azathioprine, IVIg) can be tried, but no or little response
is often found – in contrast to other inflammatory myopathies

Vasculitis

Types

P.A.I.N.T.

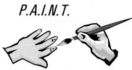

Primary

	With **G**ranuloma	Without granuloma **p-ANCA** +ve
Large	Giant-cell arteritis (polymyalgia rheumatica) Takayasu's arteritis	
Medium	Buer**G**er's disease (thromboangitis obliterans)	Kawasaki's disease Polyarteritis nodosa (PAN)
Small-vessel	Chur**G**–Strauss syndrome We**G**ener's **G**ranulomatosis	Micro-polyarteritis nodosa (PAN) Henoch–Schönlein purpura
Special	Isolated CNS vasculitis (granulomatous angiitis) Co**G**an's syn. (=vestibulocochlear Δ + keratitis)	Behçet's (venulitis; DVT) Relapsing polychondritis

Autoimmune: SLE, Sjögren's, rheumatoid arthritis, polymyositis, scleroderma

Infection: HBV – PAN; HCV – 'essential mixed cryoglobulinaemia';
VZV, CMV, syphilis – isolated CNS vasculitis; HIV; parvovirus B19;
Streptococcus (Behçet's, 'erythema elevatum diutium'); TB; rickettsia; histoplasmosis

Neoplasia: lymphoma, carcinoma (bronchus, ovary, renal cell)

Toxins: propylthiouracil, amphetamine, leflunomide (N.B. ANCA may be +ve)

Typical Presentations of Primary Vasculitides

GCA:
Epi: Elderly (> 60), women (2:1)
PC: Headache, proximal weakness, optic neuropathy
Takayasu's
Epi: Young, Asian women
PC: CVA, PVD, renal failure

Buerger's disease
Epi: Middle-aged, Mediterranean men;
smoking, HLA-B5 (B51)
PC: CVA, PVD, Raynaud's

Kawasaki's disease
Epi: Children
PC: Cervical lymph nodes, Conjunctivitis,
Cutaneous (rash), Coronary microaneurysms
Polyarteritis nodosa (PAN)
Epi: HBV-infection PC: see opposite

Churg–Strauss syndrome
Epi: Any age, M:F = 1.3:1
PC: Asthma, mononeuritis multiplex, eosinophilia
Wegener's granulomatosis
Epi: Whites, any age, M:F = 1:1
PC: ENT, pulmonary infiltration, renal failure

MicroPAN: As for PAN

Henoch–Schönlein purpura
Epi: Children (4–11), Boys, Post URTI; IgA ↑
PC: • Maculopapular rash on extensor surfaces
• Haematuria (IgA nephropathy)
• PR bleeding (ischaemic bowel, intussusception)

PC

Examine the S.U.R.R.O.U.N.D.I.N.G.S.

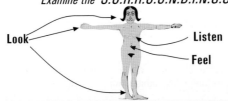

Look — Listen — Feel

Skin: PAN, WG: purpura, nodules, Raynaud's syndrome, infarcts, livedo reticularis

Ulcers: orogenital ulcers, esp. Behçet's

Rheumatology: arthralgia or myalgia (esp. PMR – morning stiffness); arthritis

Respiratory and Cardiac
    Respiratory: PAN, microPAN: pulmonary infarction, haemorrhage
                     Wegener's: haemoptysis; pulmonary infiltrates, atelectasis, nodules, cavitation
                     Churg–Strauss: asthma, fleeting eosinophilic infiltrates
    Cardiac: Takayasu's, PAN: MI, CCF, pericarditis, aortic regurgitation, aortic dissection, aneurysm

Ophthalmic: retinal infarcts ('cotton-wool spots'), uveitis, scleritis, conjunctivitis
                  Wegener's: orbital pseudotumour with proptosis

Urine: glomerulonephritis: proliferative or crescentic

Neurological: CNS: headache, stroke (both infarction and haemorrhage), fits, dementia, psychosis
                  PNS: neuropathy, mononeuritis multiplex (esp. CS, WG, PAN), myopathy (GCA)

Deaf (ENT)   Wegener's: deafness due to otitis media (conductive) or sensorineural
                  nasopharynx necrosis (epistaxis, sunken nasal bridge); sinusitis
                  subglottic stenosis (hoarseness, stridor); dacrocystitis

Intestine   PAN, HSP: mesenteric ischaemia (pain, perforation, PR bleeding, intussusception)
              PAN: cholecystitis; pancreatitis; hepatic infarction

Neoplasia: cyclophosphamide side-effect

Genito-urinary: PAN: ovarian, testicular–epididymal pain; Behçet's: ulcers

Systemic   1. Fever, weight-loss and anorexia, depression-fatigue
              2. Hypertension (suggests glomerulonephritis)
              3. Bloods: normocytic anaemia, CRP ↑, ESR ↑; polyclonal Ig ↑; complement normal

Ix

1. ANCA: • p-ANCA +ve in PAN, microPAN, HSP, Churg–Strauss
          • c-ANCA +ve in Wegener's granulomatosis (level indicates severity)
2. Angiogram (e.g. renal, cerebral, retinal): aneurysms, stenosis, beading, corkscrew collaterals
3. Biopsy: • Skin, renal, liver, nerve, muscle, brain: immunofluorescence for immune complexes, IgA
          • Superficial temporal artery (may be negative due to skip lesions)

Rx

1. Immunosuppression: steroids, cyclophosphamide, methotrexate, plasma exchange, IVIg
2. Anti-platelet / anti-coagulation: Kawasaki's, giant-cell arteritis if ischaemia, optic neuropathy
3. Surgery: angioplasty (Takayasu's), renal transplant (Wegener's, PAN)

Prog

1. Poor: PAN, microPAN, Churg–Strauss: 5-Yr SR = 50% treated; 10% untreated
2. Intermediate: Wegener's – 75% achieve remission, of whom 50% relapse: Takayasu's (variable)
3. Good: HSP (self-remitting usually), GCA (if steroids given promptly), Kawasaki's

Raynaud's Phenomenon

Def Episodic vasospasm of extremities (digits, pinnae, nose) in normal arterioles (idiopathic form)

PC 1. Pain
2. Characteristic pattern of colour change: white → blue → red
3. Chronic: ulcers and necrosis (not in idiopathic form)

Causes   P.A.I.N.T. P.O.T.

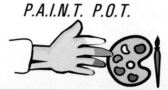

Primary ('Raynaud's disease') / **P**ulmonary hypertension:
  EPI: • Accounts for 50% of Raynaud's phenomenon
       • Women in 20–40s. Assoc: Primary pulmonary hypertension
  PC: Triggered by cold, emotion, smoking

Autoimmune: 1. Scleroderma (90% pts. have Raynaud's – due to digital vessel calcification)
                2. SLE, RA, poly- or dermatomyositis

Injury:
  1. Repetitive Injury: pneumatic drills, chainsaws, drums, piano
  2. Frostbite

Neurological: reflex sympathetic dystrophy, following trauma ('Volkmann's ischaemia')

Toxins:
  1.   Migraine Rx: beta-blockers (β_2-mediated), ergotamine; methysergide
  2.   Bromocriptine (ergot derivative)
  3.   ChemoRx: bleomycin, cisplastin
  4.   Heavy metals/vinyl chloride

Paraproteinaemia; polycythaemia; cold agglutinins – hyperviscosity
  1. Paraproteinaemia (myeloma, Waldenström's), esp. cryoglobulinaemia
  2. Cold agglutinins (e.g. mycoplasma, EBV, lymphoma), typhoid

Outlet obstruction, thoracic:
  1. Cervical rib; fascial band behind scalenus anterior; prominent transverse process C7
  2. Fractured 1st rib or clavicle; sleep-related
  O/E: • Symptoms ↑ and radial pulse ↓ with shoulder abduction to 90°, and external rotation
       • Supraclavicular fossa bruit

Thromboembolism:
  1. Atherosclerosis
  2. Buerger's disease (thromboangiitis obliterans)

Rx 1. Conservative: avoid cold; mittens and coats (cold induces generalized vasospasm); Stop Smoking.
2. PO meds: Ca antags (nifedipine), α_1-blockers (prazosin), losartan, fluoxetine (via platelet 5-HT effect)
3. IV prostacyclin
4. Sympathectomy

Cryoglobulinaemia

Def   Immunoglobulins that precipitate at 4°C

PC   *S.A.U.N.A.*

Skin: • Palpable purpura (leucocytoclastic vasculitis)
       • Raynaud's, with digital ulcers
       • Cold urticaria

Arthralgia: rheumatoid arthritis-like

Urine: mesangiocapillary glomerulonephritis

Neurology: mononeuritis multiplex, cranial nerve palsies

Additional: pericarditis, thyroiditis

The full syndrome is typical of mixed essential cryoglobulinaemia; other causes result predominantly in rash

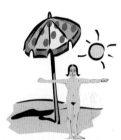

I prefer it hot

Causes   *P.A.I.N.*

Primary – 'mixed essential cryoglobulinaemia':
    most cases have chronic hepatitis C

Autoimmune
    1. SLE, RA, systemic sclerosis
    2. Primary biliary cirrhosis

Infection:
    1. Hepatitis C, B virus: 5% chronic hepatitis C patients develop cryoglobulinaemia
    2. Herpes (EBV, CMV)
    3. Bacteria: • Endocarditis
              • Streptococcus (esp. post-acute glomerulonephritis)
              • Leprosy, kala-azar, malaria (hyper-reactive form with splenomegaly)

Neoplasia
    1. Myeloma, Wegener's granulomatosis, amyloid
    2. CLL, Hodgkin's lymphoma

Ix   Type 1: monoclonal Ig – myeloma
       Type 2: polyclonal IgG (e.g. specific to hep C)   + **mono**clonal rheumatoid factor
       Type 3: polyclonal IgG (e.g. to herpes, bacteria) + **poly**clonal rheumatoid factor

Differential Diagnosis

1. Acrocyanosis
    PC: Cyanotic digits irrespective of ambient temperature
    Epi: Women in 20s
2. Erythromelalgia
    PC: Burning, erythematous extremities; feet > hands; worse in warmth and dependency; normal pulses
    Epi: Middle-aged men; myeloproliferative disease, nifedipine, bromocriptine. Rx: Aspirin

<u>Carpal Tunnel Syndrome</u>

P.O.M.E.G.R.A.N.A.T.E

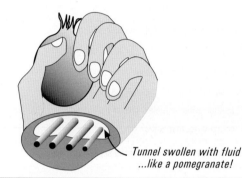

*Tunnel swollen with fluid
...like a pomegranate!*

Pregnancy

OCP (oral contraceptive pill)

Menopause, pre-menstrual

Endocrine:
   1. Acromegaly
   2. Hypothyroidism
   3. Diabetes mellitus

Gout

Renal:
   1. Nephrosis (fluid overload)
   2. Chronic renal failure or congestive cardiac failure (fluid overload)
      (and, as in CCF, symptoms worsen at night)
   3. Haemodialysis: accumulation of β_2- microglobulin
   4. AV – fistula: steals blood from median nerve vasa nervorum

Amyloid, multiple myeloma

Neuropathy: hereditary neuropathy with liability to pressure palsies
   (autosomal dominant)

Arthritis:
   1. Rheumatoid arthritis with associated wrist tenosynovitis
   2. Osteoarthritis, esp. familial 'persistent generalized osteoarthropathy'

Trauma: carpal fracture or anterior dislocation of lunate

Extra: TB, sarcoid

Path   Swelling of flexor synovial sheaths beneath flexor retinaculum, due to generalized fluid
accumulation, or synovitis.

PC   1. Pain and paraesthesia in hand – often more extensive than just lateral 3½ fingers!
    • Radiates up medial forearm and towards shoulder (thus mimicking a cervical root lesion)
    • Worse at night; relieved by shaking hand
  2. Clumsy hand or weak grip

O/E   1. Motor: wasting and weakness of hand muscles supplied by the median nerve:

L.O.A.F.

> **L**umbricals 1 + 2
> **O**pponens pollicis
> **A**bductor pollicis brevis (most sensitive)
> **F**lexor pollicis brevis

  2. Sensory: sensory loss over palmar aspect, and tips, of lateral 3½ fingers, and adjacent palm
(but not over thenar eminence, which is supplied by superficial palmar branch that
traverses **over** the transverse ligament!)

  3. Special: **T**inel's test   = **T**apping gently over carpal tunnel reproduces paraesthesia
              Phalen's test = **F**lexing wrist maximally for 1 min reproduces symptoms

Distinguish this pattern from diffuse wasting of hand muscles, whose causes are:
    • Upper motor–neuron: CVA, Parkinson's (disuse atrophy)
    • Cervical cord: syringomyelia
    • Anterior horns: motor neuron–disease, polio
    • Roots: cervical spondylosis
    • Brachial plexus. 'Klumpke's palsy'
    • Neuropathy:
              – Brachial neuritis (viral)
              – Mononeuritis multiplex (e.g. vasculitis)
              – Generalized neuropathy (CIDP, multifocal motor neuropathy)
    • Joints: e.g. rheumatoid arthritis
    • Constitutional: e.g. carcinoma, malnutrition

Ix   EMG: slowing of median nerve across wrist

Rx   *S.I.D.S.*

> **S**plint wrist
> **I**njection of hydrocortisone
> **D**iuretics
> **S**urgical decompression

Collagen and Elastic-Tissue Diseases

Defects in Collagen

Genetics: All are **autosomal dominant**, except severe forms of osteogenesis imperfecta and severe epidermolysis bullosa (autosomal recessive), and Alport's disease (X-linked)

Type I: Osteogenensis Imperfecta

<u>PC</u>   *O.S.T.E.OC. L.A.S.T.*

Osteopenia: frequent fractures; kyphoscoliosis;
              in utero fractures – short stature; perinatal death
Skin: thin, scarred
Teeth: dentinogenesis imperfecta
Eyes: blue sclera: also seen as familial trait, Ehlers–Danlos, Marfan's; PXE, pseudohypoPTHism
Otos**C**lerosis, and sensorineural deafness > 20 yrs
Ligament laxity: joint dislocations
Aortic regurgitation; mitral regurgitation
Systemic hyperthermia
Thyroid, hyper-

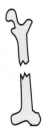

Type II: Achondroplasia

<u>PC</u>   *C.H.O.N.D.R.O.*

Craniofacial: frontal bossing, midface hypoplasia
Height: short – due to short thighs (rhizomelic), but normal trunk size
Orthopaedic: hip, pelvic abnormalities due to metaphyseal flaring
Neurological: spinal stenosis, cervicomedullary compression, hydrocephalus
Deafness: recurrent otitis media, partly due to cleft palate
Respiratory: restrictive defect; obstructive sleep apnoea, inc. central apnoea
Ophthalmic: cataracts, vitreal degeneration, retinal detachment

Type III: Ehlers–Danlos syndrome

<u>PC</u>   *E.L.A.S.T.I.c*

Eyes: keratoconus; ocular rupture (lysyl hydroxylase def. variant – AR)
Ligament laxity: hypermobile joints, osteoarthritis
Aortic regurgitation; **A**ortic dissection–aneurysm; mitral valve prolapse
Skin: Hyperextensible (cutis laxis), fragile (cigarette paper), purpura
Thoracic: kyphoscoliosis
Intestine: bowel or uterine perforation

Type IV: Alport's disease

<u>PC</u> Glomerular and interstitial nephritis (recurrent haematuria), sensorineural deafness, lenticonus

Type VII: Epidermolysis bullosa

<u>PC</u> Epithelial blisters and breaks following minor trauma
  • Mild: epidermal keratin
  • Severe: dermal collagen VII, or junctional laminin

<u>Defects in Elastic Tissue</u>

Fibrillin: Marfan's syndrome

<u>Path</u> 1. Fibrillin mutation - in epidermal growth factor-like regions of gene (chromosome 15)
2. Fibrillin is a constituent of **elastic** tissue and microfibrils, inc. suspensory ligaments of lens
3. Autosomal dominant (as opposed to phenotypically-similar homocystinuria: AR)

<u>PC</u>   *E.E.L.L.A.A.S.S.T.T.I.C.*

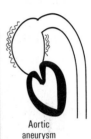

Aortic
aneurysm

Eyes: ectopia lentis (upward displacement, cf. homocytinuria - downwards)
Elevated (high-arch) palate
Limbs: • Long arms, fingers (arachnodactyly) and toes
              • Long trunk, i.e. upper:lower segment ratio increased
Ligament laxity: hypermobile joints (thumb sign, Walker–Murdoch wrist sign)
Aortic regurgitation; mitral regurgitation or mitral valve prolapse
Aortic: aneurysm–dissection (esp. ascending aorta)
Skin: striae
Skin: purpura on buttocks, shoulders
Thorax: pectus excavatum or carinatum, kyphoscoliosis; dural sac dilatation
Thorax: pneumothorax
Intestine: herniae
Circulation: varicose veins

Elastin (1): Pseudoxanthoma elasticum

<u>Path</u> 1. Calcium deposition in elastic fibres of skin; arteries and retina–choroid Bruch's membrane
2. Autosomal recessive / dominant, or as an effect of penicillamine; worsened by steroids!

<u>PC</u>   *E.L.A.S.T.I.C.*

Angioid streaks

Eyes: angioid streaks (also seen in Paget's, sickle cell disease, Ehlers-Danlos) - blindness
Ligament laxity: hypermobile joints; osteoarthritis
Aortic: regurgitation; mitral regurgitation
Skin: • 'Plucked-chicken' = coalesced yellow maculopapules; spares follicles
            • Hanging, lax skin folds: esp. neck, axillae, antecubital fossae
            • Purpura on buttocks, shoulders
Thorax: scoliosis, pneumothorax
Intestine: haematemesis
Circulation: hypertension, ischaemic heart disease, peripheral vascular disease; *and*
                   haemorrhage: subarachnoid, GIT, genito-urinary; haemoptysis

Elastin (2): Williams' syndrome

<u>Path</u> Sporadic large deletion on chromosome 7, incorporating elastin and actin-regulator *LIMK* genes

<u>PC</u>   *WI.L.LI.A.M.*

WIde mouth, short, upturned nose
Low growth. **L**ow **I**ntelligence but gregarious (opposite of autism)
Aortic stenosis – supravalvular; **M**etabolic – hypercalcaemia

Back Pain

<u>**Epi**</u>   1. Commonest cause of chronic disability in under-50s
2. 1% of general population are chronically disabled by back pain
3. 2nd most common primary care consultation (after viral URTIs)

<u>**Causes**</u>   *M.A.D.D.E.N.I.N.G. P.A.I.N.*

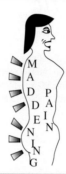

Mechanical: injury-related: ligament strain. Also fracture

Autoimmune:
  • Seronegative arthropathies – ankylosing spondylitis, enteropathic, etc.
  • Rheumatoid arthritis

Disc prolapse

Degenerative – other:
  • Adults: spondylosis, canal stensosis
  • Adolescents: kyphosis, spondylolisthesis, spondylolysis

Endocrine–metabolic:
  osteoporosis (microfractures, verterbral compression), osteomalacia, Paget's

Neoplasia – vertebral or cord

Infection: discitis, epidural spinal abscess, osteomyelitis – pyogenic, TB

Neurological: Guillain–Barré syndrome, meningoradiculitis
  haematomyelia (e.g. subarachnoid haemorrhage, AVM), spina bifida occulta

Gastroenterological or gynaecological or genito-urinary:
  • Gastroenterological: duodenal ulcer, pancreatitis
  • Gynaecological: endometriosis, pelvic inflammatory disease, ovarian cyst
  • Genito-urinary: prostatitis, pyelonephritis

Psychological

Aortic aneurysm or retroperitoneal haematoma

Ischaemic – sickle crisis

Neurofibromatosis

Mechanical

Cause: Minor injury, e.g. lifting heavy object or sudden deceleration in car accident
PC: Pain confined to lower back or neck, but no radiation to buttocks or legs
O/E: Paraspinal muscle spasm – if unilateral, causes scoliosis to that side

Autoimmune

Ankylosing spondylitis
PC: Lower back and buttock pain and stiffness, worse at night or morning; better with exercise
O/E: Loss of lumbar lordosis and exaggeration of thoracic kyphosis; reduced chest expansion

Rheumatoid arthritis
PC: Painful limitation of movement due to facet joint involvement

Disc Prolapse

Path:
- Disc prolapse most common at L4–5 or L5–S1, although may occur at any level
- Affected nerve root lies lower than affected disc space, e.g. L4-5 causes either L5 or S1 radiculopathy
- Lateral disc prolapse causes radicular pain; central disc prolapse causes cauda equina syndrome

PC:
- Lower back and leg pain, with variable sensory symptoms in leg; worsened by cough or sitting
- Bilateral leg pain, saddle anaesthesia, or sphincter–erectile dysfunction suggest cauda equina syndrome

O/E:
- Ipsilateral scoliosis; hip and knee kept in flexed position.
- Straight leg raising reduced (often to $< 30°$); Lasegue manoeuvre (pain on extending knee with hip flexed)
- Radicular signs: e.g. absent ankle jerk or numbness of 5th toe (both suggest S1 root lesion)

Degenerative – Other

Spondylosis
Path: Osteoarthritis-like changes in lumbar or cervical spine, e.g. flaval or facet joint hypertrophy
PC: Radiculopathy, myelopathy or headache (esp. cervical spondylosis)

Lumbar spinal stenosis (neurogenic claudication)
PC: Back, buttock or leg pain in elderly (rarely congenital); triggered by standing (unlike ischaemic claudication)
   or walking; relieved by sitting (unlike disc prolapse)
O/E: Radiculopathy may be present; normal peripheral pulses (to exclude ischaemic claudication)

Neoplasm

Vertebral: *B.O.N.E.1.M (Boney-M!)*

Breast, **B**ronchus, **O**varian, **N**ephro (renal, prostate, testes), **E**ndocrine (thyroid) – metastatic carcinoma
1° bone tumour – Ewing's, osteosarcoma
Myeloma / lymphoma

Cord:
1. Extradural: all causes of vertebral tumours (**BONE1M**)
2. Extramedullary: neurofibroma, meningioma, leptomeningeal metastases
3. Intramedullary: glioma, ependymoma, medulloblastoma 'drop' metastases

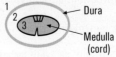

Bone Cysts

P.E.N.N.I.E.S.

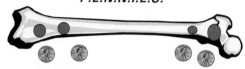

Primary   *S.A.F.E. (all benign)*

Simple bone cyst:
  Epi: Pre-pubertal
  PC: Pain or pathological fracture
  Rx: • Intracystic steroid injection
       • Curettage; pack with bone chips

• Central, metaphyseal
• Knee, proximal humerus,
   skull ('congenital cranial lacunae')

Aneurysmal cyst or AVM:
  Epi: Young adults

• Expanding, eccentric
• Blood-filled, trabeculated
• Long bone, spine, skull AVM

Fibrous cortical defect:
  Epi: Children

• Cystic centre, sclerosed edge
• Long bones

Enchondroma:
  Ollier's syndrome (multiple enchondroma)

• Tubular bones
• Specks of calcification

Endocrine: primary hyperparathyroidism

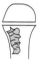

'Pepper-pot skull'

Neoplasia – primary – giant-cell tumour:
  Epi: 20–40 (epiphyses must have fused)
  Path: Multinucleate giant cells; stromal proliferation
  PC: Pain and swelling **near** joint; pathological fracture
  Prognosis: 1/3 benign; 1/3 local invasion; 1/3 metastasize

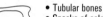

Soap-bubble /
ballooned cortex
in sub-articular site , e.g.
knee, distal radius,
proximal humerus

Neoplasia – secondaries: *B.O.N.E.1.M.*
  Breast, **B**ronchus
  Ovary, c**O**l**O**n
  Nephrology: renal, prostate
  Endocrine: tumour
  1°–primary
  Myeloma / Langerhans' cell histiocytosis

     also pseudotumour of haemophilia

Infection: osteomyelitis – 'Brodie's abscess'

• Metaphyseal
• Round, cystic centre
• Sclerosed edge

Electrolytes: gout

Sarcoid: dactylitis (enlarged phalanges)

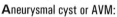
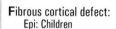

Sclerosis

P.E.N.N.I.E.s

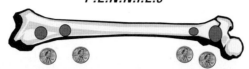

Paget's disease

Endocrine: secondary hyperparathyroidism – renal osteodystrophy

Neoplasia – primary – benign
  1. Osteoid osteoma: appears similar to Brodie's abscess
  2. Eccondroma; osteochondroma =cartilage-capped exostosis

Neoplasia – primary – malignant:

> **Osteosarcoma (50%):**
>   Epi: Bimodal 10–20%: and > 50% (Paget's); M:F = 2:1
>   PC: 1. Painful, swollen, warm limb; worse at night
>   2. Lung metastases – early
>   X-ray: 1. Mixed rarefaction and sclerosis
>   2. 'Codman's triangle' (periosteum lifts off shaft)
>   3. Sunray spicules: soft-tissue calcification
>
> Knee, proximal humerus
>
> **Chondrosarcoma** (derived from en- or ecchondroma) **(25%):**
>   Epi: Age > 40
>   PC: Enchondroma - indolent pain, swelling, pathological fracture
>   Ecchondroma - early swelling, except pelvic basin exostosis
>   X-ray: 1. ENC: medullary rarefaction, calcified specks
>   2. ECC: large exostosis, calcified specks in cartilage cap
>
> Girdles, metaphysis of long bones
>
> **Ewing's or reticular-cell sarcoma (15%):**
>   Epi: Age 10–20; associated with adrenal neuroblastoma
>   PC: 1. Pain, worsened by walking / limp
>   2. Swelling: warm, firm, rubbery, tender
>   3. PUO from liver, lung, bone metastases (like osteomyelitis)
>   X-ray: 1. Medullary rarefaction
>   2. Periosteal onion-skinning (reactive new layers)
>
> Diaphysis of long bones

Neoplasia – secondary:
  1. Metastatic carcinoma: breast, prostate, colorectal
  2. Myeloma (inc. POEMS syndrome); Hodgkin's lymphoma

Inflammation:
  1. Osteoarthritis
  2. Osteopetrosis

Exogenous:
  1. Lead ('pica'), radium, bismuth, phosphorus (match heads)
  2. Fluorosis, esp. Persian Gulf, India, China
  3. Vitamin A toxicity; X-ray – epiphyseal thickening; irregular opacification of lower ribs

Neurology

Headache – Acute

Causes

V.I.C.I.O.U.S.

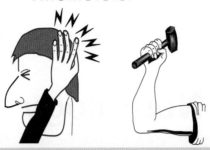

Vascular
1. Haemorrhage – subarachnoid; intracerebral haemorrhage
2. Infarction – esp. posterior circulation, arterial dissection
3. Venous sinus thrombosis

Infection / Inflammation
1. Meningitis:
   - Neutrophilic CSF: meningococal, pneumococcal, listeriosis, fungal; OR early viral or TB
   - Lymphocytic CSF: viral (enterovirus, HIV), TB, Lyme, syphilis; OR partially treated bacterial; autoimmune vasculitis, SLE, Behçet's syndrome; sarcoidosis
2. Encephalitis; ADEM
3. Brain abscess

Compression
1. Intraventricular or periventricular tumour, causing transient obstructive hydrocephalus, colloid cyst of 3rd ventricle, craniopharyngioma, pinealoma, brainstem tumour
   PC: Paroxysmal headaches, drop attacks, acute blindness
2. Posterior fossa lesion: tumour, AVM, Arnold–Chiari malformation, platybasia
   PC: Paroxysmal headaches, drop attacks, acute blindness
3. Pituitary enlargement:
   apoplexy, due to infarction of pituitary macroadenoma; post-partum hypophysitis

Intracranial pressure ↑ or ↓
1. Primary intracranial hypertension:
   PC: Headache worse on stooping or lying flat; visual disturbance (obscurations; 3rd cranial nerve palsy); tinnitus, triggered by weight gain
2. Spontaneous intracranial hypotension, due to CSF dural leak.
   PC: Headache worse on standing initially, but may become posture-independent later

Ophthalmic – acute glaucoma

Unknown (idiopathic)
1. 'Thunderclap headache' – variant of migraine (commoner in migraineurs):
   - Mimics subarachnoid haemorrhage
2. Situational: cough, exertion, coitus:
   - Mimics posterior fossa or ventricular lesion, sinusitis or dental abscess

Systemic
1. Hypertensive crisis: vasculitis, pre-eclampsia, phaeochromocytoma
2. Infection, e.g. sinusitis, tonsillitis, dental abscess, UTI, atypical pneumonia (e.g. mycoplasma):
   - May all cause meningism and encephalopathy, esp. in children and elderly
3. Toxins: carbon monoxide

Ix

Bloods

- WBC   – Neutrophils: bacterial meningitis, abscess, **LyMe** disease (**L**ymphocytes in **M**eninges)
             – Lymphocytes: **LiS**teria (**L**ymphocytes in **S**erum)
             – Monocytes: TB
- ESR, CRP   Meningitis

Urine

- MSU, glucose, protein

Microbiology

- Blood cultures
- Serology: bacterial meningitides, enterovirus, HIV, syphilis, cryptococcal (serum CRAG)
- CSF: do brain scan before performing lumbar puncture to exclude mass-lesion or manifest haemorrhage

Radiology

- CT head   1. Subarachnoid haemorrhage: blood in sulci, cisterns – sensitivity = 90% in first 24 hrs
             2. Mass lesions: intracerebral haemorrhage, abscess, tumour

- MRI   1. MRI: posterior fossa lesion, ADEM, CSF dural leak (brain and spine MRI with contrast)
             2. MRA: aneurysm, AVM, dissection, vasculitis; sensitivity for aneurysms > 5 mm = 90%
             3. MRV: cerebral venous thrombosis

- Angiogram: If aneurysm or AVM suspected, sensitivity = 90% (but risk of stroke due to procedure = 0.5%)

Special - CSF

- Opening   – Normal: 5–20 cmH$_2$O
  pressure   – Raised: subarachnoid haemorrhage, primary intracranial hypertension, meningitis
                – Depressed: spontaneous intracranial hypotension (avoid LP if history is suggestive!)

- Appearance   – Normal: clear
                – Xanthochromic (yellow): traumatic tap, subarachnoid haemorrhage, high protein
                – Bloody: traumatic tap, subarachnoid haemorrhage: ∴ if subarachnoid haemorrhage is a
                   possibility, send for immediate centrifugation and spectrophotometry on supernatant for
                   bilirubin (+ve between 12 hours and 2 weeks) and CSF ferritin (+ve in SAH)

- Microscopy,   – Normal: RBC count raised if traumatic tap, but should see decrease from bottles 1 to 3
  culture and   WBC count 0–4 (lymphocytes); deduct 1 WBC for every 700 RBCs
  sensitivity   – Neutrophilia: meningococal, pneumococcal, listeriosis, fungal; OR early viral or TB
                – Lymphocytosis: viral (enteroviruses, HIV), TB, Lyme, syphilis; OR partially treated bacterial
                   autoimmune vaculitis, SLE, Behçet's syndrome; sarcoidosis
                – Stains: Gram – bacteria, some fungal; Ziehl–Nielsen – TB; Indian Ink – Cryptococcus

- Chemistry   – Normal: Protein 0–0.45 g/l; deduct 0.01 g/l for every 1000 RBCs;
                   Glucose 2.8 - 4.2 mmol/l, or > 50% serum glucose
                – Protein > 1 g/l: bacterial, TB or fungal meningitis, or subarachnoid haemorrhage
                – Glucose < 40%: bacterial, TB, fungal or mumps meningitis

- Other   – Cryptococcal antigen (CSF CRAG), herpes class PCR, ACE, oligoclonal bands, cytology

Headache – Chronic

Causes

M.A.T.C.H.I.N.G. S.I.T.E.S.

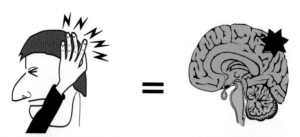

Migraine
Autonomic (trigeminal–autonomic cephalgias or TACs)
    1. Cluster headaches
    2. Paroxysmal hemicrania / SUNCT: briefer attacks relative to cluster headaches
    3. Hemicrania continua: continuous hemicranial pain with autonomic signs
Tension
Cervical disease / other surrounding structures: neck, eyes, ears, TMJ, teeth
Head injury / other triggers: cough, exercise, coitus, ice cream
Intracranial pressure ↑ or ↓
    1. ICP raised: • Tumour or meningeal infiltration; aneurysm or AVM
               • Primary intracranial hypertension: assoc. with cerebral venous thrombosis
    2. ICP low: • Spontaneous intracranial hypotension (due to CSF dural leak)
Neuralgia, trigeminal, paratrigeminal
Giant-cell, temporal arteritis

Systemic
    1. Organ failure: • Hypercapnia (e.g. obstructive sleep apnoea), hypoxia (e.g. mountain sickness)
                 • Uraemia, hepatic failure
    2. Anaemia; hyperviscosity
    3. Severe hypertension: accelerated-phase, pre-eclampsia, phaeochromocytoma
Inflammation
    1. Chronic infection, neoplasia
    2. Autoimmunity: SLE, vasculitides, Behçet's syndrome
    3. Sarcoid
Toxins
    1. Analgesics: excess opioids, caffeine, NSAIDs, paracetamol, triptans; or withdrawal from these
    2. Vasodilators: calcium antagonists, nitrates, monosodium glutamate (Chinese food)
    3. Others: anticonvulsants, sulphasalazine, steroids (corticosteroids, pill, HRT), alcohol
Endocrine
    1. Cortisol ↑ or ↓ (Cushing's or Addison's)
    2. Thyroxine ↑ or ↓
    3. APUDoma: phaeochromocytoma, carcinoid, mastocytosis – episodic headaches, with flushing
    4. Hypoglycaemia
Seizures – post-ictal
    Morning headaches if nocturnal fits

PC

Migraine

Temporal: Attack duration = 4–72 hrs;
may also develop background continuous headache ('transformed migraine')

Character: Throbbing, unilateral but may cross midline, severe; worse with movement; pt lies down

Assoc: N+V, photophobia, phonophobia, osmophobia:
- Premonitory symptoms in 50% (e.g. change in appetite, arousal, mood)
- Aura in 20% (preceding focal neurological sx, esp. visual)

Epi:
- Age: begins in childhood (as cyclical abdominal pain or motion sickness) or teens
- Sex: females > males; family history common
- Triggers: carbohydrates (cola, citrus, chocolate, alcohol); premenstrual; exertion; lying-in

Autonomic: trigeminal–autonomic cephalgias (TACs)

1. Cluster headaches

Temporal:
- Attack duration = 5 mins–3 hr
- Onset typically same time every night–day
- Cluster length = 2–12 weeks; remission length = 3 months–3 years

Character: non-throbbing; strictly unilateral peri- or retro-orbital pain; pt. paces room

Assoc: ipsilateral Horner's syndrome, lacrimation, nasal congestion or rhinorrhoea, sweating

2. Paroxysmal hemicrania / SUNCT

Paroxysmal hemicrania:
- Attack duration =5–45 mins
- Recur 5–30 x /day, usually chronic, may be episodic (i.e. in bouts)
- Respond well to indomethacin (also SUNCT and hemicrania continua)

SUNCT (short-lasting unilateral neuralgia with conjunctival injection and tearing):
- Attacks last 15–60 s, recur 5–30 x /hr

3. Hemicrania continua

Temporal: Continuous symptoms of cluster headache-like symptoms

Tension

Temporal: Attack duration = 30 min – continuous ('chronic daily headache' > 15 days / month)

Character: Tightness, pressure, heaviness, ice-pick pains, vertex-bitemporal; mild (pt works through)

Assoc: Mild photophobia, nausea, depression; dizziness (due to hyperventilation)

Epi: middle-aged men; triggered by alcohol

Cervical

Worse with head movements; TMJ – preauricular, temple pain; associated crepitus

Head injury

Assoc: Poor concentration, insomnia, irritable or depressed mood

Intracranial

Raised: worse with stooping; visual obscurations; obese women (primary intracranial hypertension)

Low: worsens on sitting or standing; associated with previous trauma, often minor

Neuralgia, trigeminal

Temporal: Attack duration = sudden, momentary pain, repeated in bursts:
- Triggered by touching trigger zone or action e.g. chewing, swallowing, talking

Character: Lancinating, in distribution of V2 or V3 dermatome typically

Giant-cell, temporal arteritis

Character: Unilateral temple pain and tenderness; worse at night; anorexia and weight loss; myalgia

Assoc: 'Law of 60' = > 60 years; ESR > 60; responds within days to prednisolone 60 mg od:
- Jaw claudication; anterior ischaemic optic neuropathy (blindness); ophthalmoplegia

Acute Confusional State

Def

1. Impairment in the **level** of consciousness (GCS), with a secondary global impairment in the **content** of consciousness (i.e. cognition) over hours, days or weeks (cf. dementia, which refers to primary impairment in cognition, with preserved alertness).
2. Specific terms refer to progressively deeper levels of unconsciousness:-
   a) Delirium: fluctuating consciousness with agitation, psychosis, etc.
   b) Encephalopathy: drowsy and disorientated
   c) Stupor: rousable only to pain

O/E

Glasgow Coma Scale: fluctuates – worse in evenings: ('sundowning')
Physical Examination: sympathetic overactivity: tachycardia, hypertension, diaphoresis
Mental State Examination
   Appearance: agitated, aggressive, but purposeless
   Affect: labile
   Thought: • Speech incoherent, rapid or slow
               • Delusions: paranoid, but poorly systematized and poorly sustained
               • Hallucinations: visual; illusions–distortions
   Cognition: • Globally impaired
   Insight: • Impaired

Causes

1. **Intracranial:** primary disturbance in structures subserving consciousness
2. **Extracranial:**
   a) Interruption of energy substrate delivery: glucose ↓, O_2 ↓, Hb ↓, blood supply ↓
   b) Alteration of neuronal membrane physiology: toxaemia, electrolyte disturbance

I.N.V.I.T.E. / P.A.S.S.   I.S.   F.R.E.E.

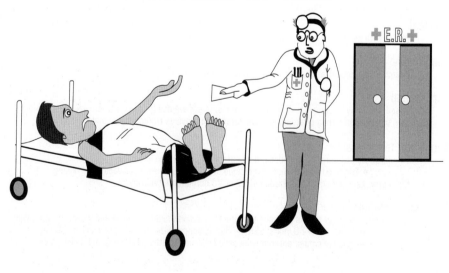

Acute Confusional State – Causes

I.N.V.I.T.E. / P.A.S.S. I.S. F.R.E.E.

Intracranial

Infection
- Meningitis: bacterial, TB, fungal, syphilis
- Encephalitis: HSV, VZV, Western Nile virus, Japanese encephalitis virus
- Other: abscess, HIV-dementia complex, malaria

Neoplasia
- Brain tumour: 1° or 2°
- Meningeal: carcinoma, melanoma, lymphoma
  - paraneoplastic syndrome

Vascular
- Infarction: non-dominant temporoparietal region; thalamic, upper brainstem
- Haemorrhage: subarachnoid haemorrhage
- Migraine: vertebrobasilar

Injury
- Trauma: diffuse brain injury; extradural or subdural haemorrhage

Toxins / nutritional
- 1. Prescribed: • β-blockers, anticholinergics, dopaminergics, steroids, NSAIDs
  - Overdose: anticonvulsants, paracetamol, aspirin, digoxin
- 2. Abused: • Alcohol: intoxication, withdrawal ('delirium tremens'), Wernicke's syndrome
  - Recreational: opioids, cannabis, amphetamines, LSD
- 3. Nutritional: Vit B12 deficiency

Epilepsy
- Postictal
- Non-convulsive status epilepticus: often complex partial seizures (temporal lobe)

Psychiatric
- Mania or catatonia

Autoimmune
- ADEM: postviral, vaccination; multiple sclerosis
- Cerebral vasculitis, SLE, antiphospholipid syndrome
- Anti-K^+ voltage-gated channel antibodies

Sarcoid

Special
- Degenerative dementia, esp. Lewy body; end-stage Alzheimer's; prion disease

Extracranial

Infection
- Pneumonia, esp. mycoplasma, legionella / endocarditis / tonsillitis
- Gastroenteritis, esp. campylobacter / leptospirosis / UTI / cellulitis / septic arthritis
  NB: infection presenting solely with confusion is most common in elderly or children

Systemic
- Haematological: anaemia, hyperviscosity, acute intermittent porphyria
- Autoimmune: SLE, vasculitis, Hashimoto's encephalopathy (anti-thyroid Abs)
- Hypothermia, hyperthermia

Failure, organ
- Respiratory / cardiac, due to ↓O_2 or ↑CO_2
- Renal / liver: due to toxins uraemia, plasma NH_4^+ ↑, CSF glutamine

Retention
- Acute urinary / faecal impaction

Electrolytes
- Na^+ or Ca^{2+}: ↓ or ↑; NH_4^+ ↑ (esp. valproate)

Endocrine
- Glucose: ↓ or ↑ (esp. HONK, insulinoma)
- Thyroxine: ↓ or ↑
- Steroid hormones: ↓ or ↑ (Addison's, hypopituitarism, Cushing's)

Coma – Causes

<u>**Def**</u> Persistent unconsciousness, i.e. inability to arouse the patient by painful stimuli.

<u>**Path**</u> Consciousness requires normal functioning of three 'systems':

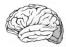

Cerebral cortex
An extensive area of cortex needs to be deranged before consciousness impaired i.e. diffuse process: e.g. encephalitis, trauma, epilepsy

Ascending Reticular Activation System (ARAS)
A limited set of areas need to be deranged for consciousness to be impaired: viz thalamus, upper brainstem: e.g. CVA, tumour, MS

Systemic
Metabolic factors may depress all brain regions, e.g. anoxia, toxins, septicaemia

<u>**Causes**</u>

I.N.V.I.T.E. / P.A.S.S. I.S. .F.R.E.E.

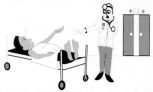

Intracranial

Infection: **Focal**: abscess. **Diffuse**: meningo-encephalitis, inc. AIDS, malaria, syphilis

Neoplasia: **Focal**: tumour. **Diffuse**: meningeal carcinoma or lymphoma
paraneoplastic limbic encephalitis

Vascular: **Focal**: large cerebral CVA, or basilar artery thrombosis
Diffuse: subarachnoid haemorrhage; cerebral venous thrombosis, cerebral anoxia

Injury: **Focal**: sub-, extradural, intracerebral bleed, contusion. **Diffuse**: axonal injury, oedema

Toxins: Opioids, alcohol (central pontine myelinolysis, Wernicke's syn.), sedative overdose

Epilepsy: Non-convulsive status epilepticus, post-ictal, anticonvulsant overdose

Psychiatric: Catatonia

Autoimmune: ADEM, vasculitis, antiphospholipid syndrome

Sarcoid

Special: Degenerative dementia, prion

Extracranial

Infection: Endocarditis, septicaemia

Systemic: SLE, vasculitis, Hashimoto's encephalopathy, hypo- or hyperthermia

Failure, respiratory / cardiac: ↑ CO_2, ↓ O_2

Renal / liver failure: toxin accumulation

Electrolytes: Na^+ ↑/↓, Ca^{2+} ↑/↓, NH_4^+ ↑

Endocrine: Glucose ↑/↓, thyroid ↑/↓, cortisol ↓

Coma – Management

B. Breathing

1. Oxygen: 60%
2. Ventilation if GCS < 9
3. Hyperventilation may be needed to treat raised ICP

1. ITU transfer, if ventilation required
2. Neurosurgeons if abscess, tumour, bleed or ICP bolt-monitor needed

C. Hydration

1. **Dextrose 50%, 50ml iv**
   - If hypoglycaemic

2. **Normal saline**
   Caution if
   - Severe hypertension
   - Pulmonary oedema
   - Alcoholic or hyponatraemia, as at risk of central pontine myelinolysis

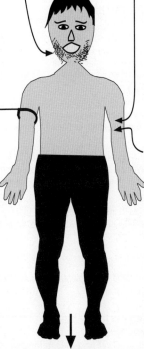

A. Assessment

1. **A.B.C.Disability**
   a) GCS:-
   - Eyes: *S.S.P.S.*
     Spontaneous, Spoken, Pain, Shut
   - Motor: *O.L.W.F.E.N.*
     Obeys, Localizes, Withdraws, Flex, Ext, None
   - Vocal: *O.C.I.I.N.*
     Orientated, Confused, Inappropriate, Incoherent, None
   b) Brainstem tests:
   - Pupils
   - Ocular movements
   - Corneal / gag
   - Respiration pattern

2. **C.O.A.T.**
   Cardiac monitor; O$_2$ sats; ABP, CVP line; TPR

3. **Investigations**
   Bloods:
   - Glucose
   - Arterial blood gases
   - FBC, U+E, LFT
   - Ca, PO$_4$, Mg, NH$_4$
   - Vit B12, drug levels, autoAbs, anti-neuronals, ACE
   Urine:
   - Toxicology / porphyrins
   Micro
   - Blood cultures; serology
   - CSU
   - LP (post-imaging)
   - Culture, spectrophotometry
   Monitor: GCS
   EEG, ECHO
   Radiology:
   - CT brain (urgent)
   - MRI, A, V

Nursing, bedsore avoidance, catheterize

Physio, flexion contracture avoidance

D. Drugs

1. **Vit B complex IV**
   (esp. thiamine – Vit B1)
2. **Antimicrobials:**
   - Cefotaxime IV
   - Aciclovir IV 10mg/kg tds
   - Also consider HIV / immunosuppressed: ? TB, fungal or toxoplasmosis
     – Foreign travel: ? malaria, W. Nile virus

   +

1. **Drug overdose:**
   - Naloxone 400 µg IV
   - Flumazenil 200 µg IV
2. **Anticonvulsants:**
   - Lorazepam, phenytoin,
   - Phenobarbitone IV
3. **Dexamethasone:**
   Indicated in
   – vasculitis
   – tumour

Dementia

Def Chronically impaired content of consciousness (i.e. cognition), with a normal level of consciousness.
that - affects multiple cognitive domains, e.g. memory, attention, language (cf. amnesia or aphasia)
- is acquired and progressive (cf. learning disability e.g. due to cerebral palsy)

Causes   *D.I.V.I.N.I.T.Y.*

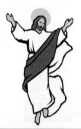

Degenerative / Developmental

Degenerative   Cortical   Subcortical
- Amyloidopathy   Alzheimer's disease   Prion disease
- Synucleinopathy Cortical Lewy Body disease   (MSA - dementia only late)
- Tauopathy   Frontotemporal dementia   PSP, CBD
- Other: Neurofilament dementia   Huntington's, Wilson's diseases

Developmental – *F.A.M.I.L.I.A.L.*
Fragile X, Aneuploidy (Down's), Mitochondrial, Ictal (myoclonic epilepsy syndrome)
Lipoidoses, Intermediary metabolism (glycogen storage disease)
Acidaemia, organic or Ammonaemia, or Ataxia spinocerebellar, Leucodystrophy

Infection
- Viruses: HSV; HIV, due to 'AIDS-dementia complex', PML (JC virus), TB, cryptococcus, toxoplasmosis
- Bacterial: syphilis (tertiary), Whipple's disease, TB (all cause low-grade, chronic meningitis)
- Other: fungal, prion: CJD (classical, new-variant)

Vascular
- Vascular dementia – cortical (multi-infarcts), subcortical (hypertensive arteriosclerosis, CADASIL)
- Subdural haematoma, chronic (also presents with fluctuating confusion, SIADH)
- Cerebral anoxia

Inflammation
- Sarcoidosis
- Vasculitis: inc. SLE, antiphospholipid syndrome, Behçet's syndrome
- Multiple sclerosis (late)

Neoplasia
- Brain tumour: e.g. frontal, callosal or temporal location
- Meningeal carcinoma, melanoma, lymphoma
- Paraneoplastic syndrome, esp. small-cell lung ca (anti-Hu limbic encephalitis), lymphoma (PML)

Injury / Epilepsy   Single or repetitive head trauma (dementia pugilistica); non-convulsive status

Toxin / Nutritional

Toxins   Alcohol; Anti-convulsants, long-term use, esp. phenytoin; lead; aluminium
Nutrition Vitamin B12, folate, or niacin deficiency; malabsorption syndrome e.g. coeliac

Y: hYpothyroidism, hYpercalcaemia, hYpoadrenalism (Addison's or hypopituitarism)
hYdrocephalus, normal-pressure – PC: dementia, gait apraxia and urinary incontinence
psYchiatric - depression ('pseudodementia')

Alzheimer's disease

Epi: 50%
Path: 1. Intracellular: neurofibrillary tangles (paired helical filaments)
      2. Extracellular: senile plaques; amyloid angiopathy (β-amyloid)
HPC 1. Memory loss, esp. spatial
      2. Language: empty speech, anomia
      3. Other cognitive: apraxia, attention, executive, mood (depression, aggression, psychosis)
      4. Other neurology: incontinence; primitive reflexes, myoclonus, epilepsy
Ix: MRI - medial temporal lobe atrophy occurs early
      EEG - loss of normal posterior alpha rhythm
Rx: Cholinesterase inhibitor: donepezil, rivastigmine

Cortical Lewy Body disease

Epi: 20%
Path: Lewy bodies (eosinophilic inclusion bodies, containing ubiquitin and neurofilament), predominantly
      within occipito-parietal cortex (cf. Parkinson's disease - occur predominantly within substantia nigra)
HPC: 1. Fluctuating cognitive dysfunction (esp. attention, visuospatial), and fluctuating consciousness
      2. Visual hallucinations, paranoid delusions
      3. Parkinsonism, inc. falls, sensitivity to neuroleptics, due to nigral Lewy Bodies
Ix: MRI, EEG - normal initially
Rx: Cholinesterase inhibitor

Frontotemporal dementia

Epi: < 5%
      Autosomal dominant cases linked with chromosome 17
Path: Pick bodies (argyrophilic tau cell-inclusions) + Pick Cells (swollen chromatolytic neurones)
HPC: 1. Behaviour
         • Overactive: disinhibition, distractibility, stereotypy, ritualism, predilection for sweet food
         • Underactive: apathy, withdrawal, emotion lack
      2. Primary progressive aphasia
         • Non-fluent (frontal)
         • Fluent (left anterior temporal) = 'semantic dementia'
      3. Other neurology: motor neuron disease (fasciculations deltoids); parkinsonism
Ix: MRI: frontal or temporal atrophy
Rx: none

Vascular dementia

Epi: 20%
Path: 1. Cortical:- Multiple and / or large infarcts – deficits determined by regions and size of infarcts
      2. Subcortical ('Lacunar'): Hypertensive arteriosclerosis (Binswanger's disease)
HPC 1. Pattern: abrupt onset, fluctuating course, stepwise deterioration, nocturnal confusion
      2. Patchy deficits; personality and insight preserved / Psychiatric: depression / emotional lability
      3. Pyramidal signs, 'marche à petit pas'
      4. PMH of hypertension, arteriopathy, atrial fibrillation, diabetes mellitus
Ix: MRI - extensive infarcts or small-vessel disease, with secondary atrophy
Rx: Treat predisposing factors - hypertension, diabetes; aspirin; statin

Parkinsonism

<u>**Def**</u> **Parkinsonism** refers to the constellation of signs listed opposite (tremor, rigidity, akinesia, etc.).
Parkinson's disease refers to the commonest cause of parkinsonism, viz primary neurodegeneration.

<u>**Causes**</u> *D.I.V.I.N.I.T.Y.*

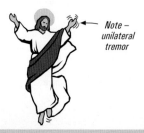

Note –
unilateral
tremor

Degenerative / Developmental
Degenerative
1. Idiopathic Parkinson's disease:
   Epi: Prevalence: 0.5% over 50 yrs old
   Path: • Degeneration of > 80% substantia nigra pars compacta dopaminergic neurons and other
         neuromodulatory systems of brainstem (e.g. locus coeruleus), and basal forebrain
       • Lewy bodies (eosinophilic inclusions) occur in areas of cell loss and in cerebral cortex
2. Parkinson's-plus (degeneration of basal ganglia plus another system):
   a) Multiple systems atrophy: parkinsonism–symmetric, poorly responsive to L-DOPA – and
         autonomic (postural hypotension, urinary frequency) and/or cerebellar and/or pyramidal signs
   b) Progressive supranuclear palsy *P.S.P.*
      Postural instability; **S**peech disturbance (+ dementia); **P**alsy, supranuclear down-gaze
   c) Corticobasal degeneration:
      • Cortical: aphasia, dysarthria, stimulus-sensitive myoclonus, apraxia (alien-hand), neglect
      • Basal-ganglia: Parkinsonism–asymmetric, intention or kinetic tremor
3. Dementia: Alzheimer's, frontotemporal dementia, cortical Lewy body disease
Developmental
1. Genetic: • Autosomal dominant: Huntington's disease - juvenile form
            • Autosomal recessive: Wilson's or Hallervorden–Spatz disease (*PANK-2* mutation), PKU
2. Perinatal: cerebral palsy (anoxia, kernicterus)

Infection
1. Streptococcus, group A: – post-infective encephalitis lethargicum (von Economo's disease)
2. Structural: syphilis, toxoplasmosis, cysticercosis, CJD

Vascular
1. Hypertensive arteriosclerosis PC: lower-body parkinsonism
2. Cerebral anoxia: opiate overdose, cardiac arrest, CO poisoning

Inflammation Vasculitis

Neoplasia Brain tumour affecting basal ganglia

Injury 'Dementia pujilistica': boxers

Toxin
1. Dopamine-receptor-2 antagonists: haloperidol, metoclopramide
   Dopamine depletors (presynaptic): tetrabenazine, methyldopa
2. Toxins: MPTP (heroin contaminant), manganese, cycad (endemic in Guam)

Y: hYdrocephalus, normal-pressure PC: lower-body parkinsonism

PC   *The Parkinson's patient is T.R.A.P.P.E.D.*

Tremor • Resting, 4–6 Hz, pill-rolling (less commonly, intention or postural 6–8 Hz tremor)
      • Initially unilateral
      • Worsened by stress, walking; reduced by relaxation, sleep

Rigidity • Lead-pipe, cog-wheeling (= rigidity + tremor)
      • May present subtly with pain or numbness in limb, or writer's cramp
      • When advanced, may cause foot dystonia, hand or swan-neck deformities, scoliosis

Akinesia (decreased frequency and decreased speed of movements):
      • Difficulty with repetitive movements, e.g. opposing finger + thumb
      • External cues and emotional input promote movement

Postural instability: stooped gait with festination and shuffling; retropulsion

Prose: monotone, quiet dysarthria, micrographia, drooling (due to reduced swallowing ↓)

Perseveration: when asked to clap 3 times, will clap more; palilalia;
              doesn't inhibit blinking with glabellar tap

Expression / **E**yes: mask-like face, stare (widening of palpebral fissures), blinking ↓ (5–10 / min)

Depression / **D**ementia: thought slowing / **D**epressed autonomics: constipation, detrusor instability

Rx   **Pro-dopaminergic**
    1. L-DOPA:
      • Given with dopa-decarboxylase inhibitor (carbidopa, benserazide) to minimize peripheral conversion
      • Side-effects: *D.O.P.A.M.I.N.E.*
        Dyskinesia, e.g. chorea – occurs after about 5 years of therapy with peak dose, or end of dose;
        On–**O**ff phenomenon; **P**sychosis, insomnia; **A**BP ↓ (postural hypotension); **M**ental addiction;
        Intestinal (diarrhoea); **N** + V; **E**xcretions – red urine

    2. Dopamine agonist
      • Oral: ergoline: (pergolide, cabergoline), non-ergoline (ropinirole, pramipexole)
      • Delays time to requirement of L-DOPA, but not as effective and causes confusion in elderly
      • Subcutaneous: apomorphine – indicated in pts with severe fluctuations due to L-DOPA

    3. MAO-B inhibitor (selegeline, rasagaline) – may increase time before L-DOPA needed
    4. COMT inhibitor (entacapone, tolcapone) – given with L-DOPA to increase its bioavailability

   Other
    1. Anticholinergics: benzhexol (trihexyphenidyl):
      • Good for tremor and drug-induced parkinsonism, but causes confusion in elderly
    2. Amantadine (indirect dopamine agonist + anticholinergic):
      • Good for dyskinesias, but causes livedo reticularis, ankle oedema and confusion
    3. Stereotactic surgery:
      • Thalamotomy, subthalamotomy, pallidotomy, subthalamic stimulators, fetal-cell grafts

Chorea

<u>Def</u>

C.H.O.R.E.A.

Continuous (brief jerks, e.g. forearm pronation–supination, tongue poking)
High-speed and brief
Odd or bizarre movements
Random (flit over body), irregular
Exacerbated by movement
Actions intruded upon by chorea, or chorea incorporated into normal activity e.g. lurching gait

<u>Causes</u>

H.I.T.T.I.N.G. M.E.

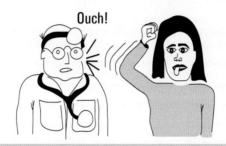

Ouch!

Hereditary

Dominant: 1. Huntington's disease:
  Epi: 35–50 yrs, onset inversely proportional to length of CAG trinucleotide repeat
  Path: Huntingtin (IT) gene: chromosome 4 (Huntingtin - Ͱ); caudate atrophy
  PC: Chorea or parkinsonism in young; apraxia; dementia, violence, depression
  2. Benign, hereditary chorea
Recessive: Wilson's disease
Complex: Acanthocytosis – 'neuroacanthocytosis' or McLeod's syn. (abnormal Kell blood group)

Infection / Inflammation
- *Streptococcus pyogenes*: Sydenham's chorea in childhood (cross-reactivity with basal ganglia)
- AIDS
- SLE, antiphospholipid syndrome

Toxins
- L-DOPA
- Neuroleptics (dopamine antagonists) – immediate or tardive, esp. orofacial or akathisia (legs)
- Phenytoin

Toxins Alcohol withdrawal or thiamine deficiency, pellagra

Ischaemic
- Cerebral palsy
- Small-vessel disease ('senile chorea' = vascular +degenerative damage to basal ganglia)
- Traumatic or anoxic brain injury; carbon monoxide poisoning

Neoplasia, in basal ganglia; or other mass-lesion – abscess, CVA, subdural haemorrhage:
  violent, flinging movements suggest hemiballismus due to subthalamic lesion

Gynaecological   chorea gravidarum (pregnancy) / oral contraceptive pill users

Myeloproliferative   Polycythaemia rubra vera
Endocrine   Thyroxine ↑ or ↓, glucose ↓ or ↑
Electrolytes Na^+ ↑ or ↓, Ca^{2+} ↓, Mg^{2+} ↓

Dystonia

Def

1. 'Abnormal tone': continuous co-contraction of agonist – antagonist pair with joint in unusual posture, e.g. flexed and pronated wrist with flexed digits, or inverted foot, or retrocollis with neck tremor
2. Types
   a) Idiopathic focal dystonia – this is the commonest form of dystonia:
      - Spasmodic torticollis
      - Hemifacial or blepharospasm
      - Oromandibular dystonia or spasmodic dysphonia
      - Writer's, musician's, or sportsman's cramp
   b) Secondary focal or generalized

Causes

H.I.T.T.I.N.G. M.E.

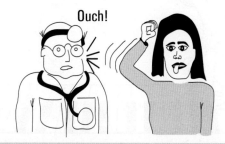

Ouch!

Hereditary
    Dominant: 1. Huntington's disease
                      2. DOPA-responsive dystonia (GTP cyclohydrolase mutation)
    Recessive: Wilson's disease
    Complex: Primary generalized dystonia (DYT 1 mutation)

Infection / Inflammation
- AIDS
- SLE, antiphospholipid syndrome

Toxins
- L-DOPA (or Parkinson's disease itself, esp. young onset)
- Neuroleptics (dopamine antagonists) – immediate or tardive
- Phenytoin, flunarizine (calcium antagonist)

Toxins Alcoholic liver disease; methanol

Ischaemic
- Cerebral palsy
- Small-vessel disease ('senile chorea' = vascular + degenerative damage to basal ganglia)
- Traumatic or anoxic brain injury; carbon monoxide poisoning

Neoplasia, in basal ganglia; or other mass-lesion – abscess, CVA, subdural haemorrhage; paraneoplastic

Groan! Depression / post-traumatic

Multiple sclerosis – with cord lesion

Electrolytes Ca^{2+} ↓ or idiopathic striatal calcification (Fahr's disease)

Tremor

Def   Regular, rhythmic oscillation, that needs to be distinguished from:
- Myoclonus: irregular, discontinuous jerks (however, asterixis = rhythmic myoclonus)
- Epilepsia partialis continua: abrupt onset, striking asymmetry

Types

R.A.P.I.D. TA.P.S.

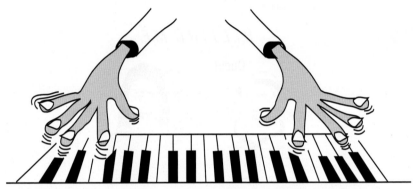

Resting
Cause: Parkinsonism
O/E: 4–6 Hz, 'pill-rolling' tremor of thumb–index finger; jaw tremor; ↑es with distraction;
postural or action tremor may also occur

Action / Postural
Cause: *see opposite*
O/E: 6–12 Hz (slows with age), worse with outstretched hand or movement, equally bad at
all stages of movement (i.e. 'kinetic tremor', as compared with intention tremor)

Intention
Cause: Cerebellar outflow: dentate nucleus, superior cerebellar peduncle, red nucleus
O/E: > 6 Hz, terminal tremor, past-pointing and ataxia on reaching or pointing;
severe, 'wing-flapping' tremor, inc. at rest and posture, suggests midbrain ('rubral tremor')

Dystonic
Cause: Mostly idiopathic, and as for dystonia
O/E: Varies depending on precise position of joint; associated cervical dystonia

TAsk-specific
Primary writing tremor

Psychogenic

Special
- Orthostatic – can be detected by palpating ankle dorsiflexor tendons or auscultating thighs
- Palatal tremor (previously called 'palatal myoclonus')

Causes

The following are causes of an **action or postural tremor**:

B.E.A.T.I.N.G.S.

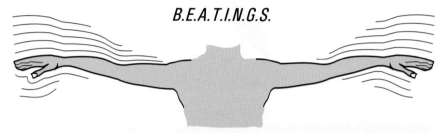

Benign essential tremor
- Epi: Autosomal dominant
- PC: Action > rest; arms, neck, voice tremor (discriminates from Parkinson's disease)

Endocrine
- Thyrotoxicosis, phaeochromocytoma, hypoglycaemia

Alcohol withdrawal ('delerium tremens')
- or caffeine, or opioid, withdrawal
- 'Delirium tremens'

Toxins
- Prescribed   – Lithium, tricyclic antidepressants
                – Salbutamol, theophylline
                – Phenytoin, valproate
- Drugs of abuse
- Lead, arsenic, mercury ('hatter's shakes')

Infection / Inflammation
- Infection: syphilis
- Inflammation: multiple sclerosis, SLE

Neuropathy, peripheral
- IgM paraproteinaemia, Charcot–Marie–Tooth disease (Roussy–Levy syn.)

Genetic
- Autosomal recessive – Wilson's disease

Sympathetic – enhanced physiological tremor
- Physiological tremor is present in everybody at 8–12 Hz, but is usually too small to be apparent. It may be enhanced by factors that increase sympathetic output: endocrine, toxins, fatigue, anxiety, hypothermia

Rx

1. Alcohol in moderation – improves essential tremor
2. Propranolol, primidone, topiramate
3. Botulinum toxin (Botox) injections
4. Surgery: ViM nucleus thalamus stimulation / lesion

Cerebellar Disease – Causes

D.I.V.I.N.I.T.Y.

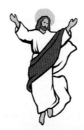

Developmental / **D**egenerative
Developmental
    1. Structural: Arnold–Chiari or Dandy–Walker malformations
    2. Spinocerebellar ataxias: • Autosomal recessive: Friederich's ataxia
                                   • Autosomal dominant: SCA 1-14
    3. Other genetic: ataxia telangiectasia, Refsum's disease, progressive myoclonic epilepsy
Degenerative
    1. Parkinson's-plus syndrome: multiple-systems atrophy (MSA)
    2. Prion: Gerstmann–Straussler–Schenker syndrome

Inflammation
    1. Multiple sclerosis
    2. Coeliac disease (or other malabsorption, e.g. Whipple's disease)

Vascular
    1. Infarction: PICA, AICA, superior cerebellar artery
    2. Haemorrhage

Infection
    1. Virus: VZV, EBV, HIV
    2. Bacteria: Mycoplasma, Legionella, abscess

Neoplasia:
    1. 1°: • Children: medulloblastoma (midline), haemangioblastoma (hemispheric), astrocytoma
            • Cerebellopontine-angle tumour: vestibular schwannoma, cholesteatoma, meningioma
    2. 2°: • Bronchus, breast, bowel
    3. Paraneoplastic syndrome, esp. small-cell lung cancer (anti-Purkinje cell = anti-Yo)

Injury
    Oxygen deprivation, carbon monoxide poisoning, heat stroke

Toxin / Nutritional
    1. **Alcohol (commonest cause):**
            • Causes anterior vermis degeneration or Wernicke's syndrome
    2. Anticonvulsants, in overdose or long-term use, esp. phenytoin
    3. Nutrition
            • Vit B12, folate or Vit E deficiency
            • Lead poisoning

Y: h**Y**pothyroidism

Cerebellar Disease – PC

D.A.N.I.S.H. PAST.R.Y.

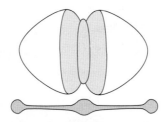

Dysdiadochokinesia
- Failure of rapidly alternating movements

Ataxia
- Limb, inc. gait
- Trunk, titubation (neck tremor)
- Gait: due to anterior vermis degeneration

Nystagmus
- Horizontal: ipsilateral hemisphere
- Downbeat: inferior cerebellum, e.g. Arnold–Chiari malformation, SCA

Intention tremor
- Tested by finger-to-nose, and heel-to-shin test
- Severe 'bat's wing' tremor suggests lesions of superior cerebellar peduncle or nuclei

Speech – Slurred, Staccato, and Scanning dysarthria
- Writing: enlarges

Hypotonia

PAST-pointing (hypermetria)
- Also seen with saccadic eye movements that overshoot and then correct themselves

Rebound: overcompensatory response to passive disturbance of position
- Reflexes: reduced (due to hypotonia) but pendular (due to overshoot)
- Riddoch's sign: hyperpronation and elevation of outstretched hand

Y: WIde-based gait
awRY head: head tilts to side of lesion, due to
imbalance of postural tone, dural irritation or 4th cranial nerve palsy

Additional Notes
1. **Ipsilesional** due to crossing of connections from motor to cerebellar cortex
2. Acute: nausea + severe vomiting; occipital headache
3. Chronic: signs may improve with time, due to compensatory mechanisms

Blackouts

Causes

C.R.A.S.H.

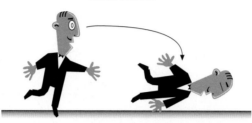

Head
1. Epileptic attacks
2. Non-epileptic attacks
3. Drop attacks

Reflexes
1. Vagal overactivity
   (venodilation + cardioinhibition)
   - Vasovagal syncope:
     constitutional or situational:
     cough, micturition, exercise, pain
   - P.O.T.S. = postural orthostatic
     tachycardia syndrome
   - Carotid sinus hypersensitivity;
     glossopharyngeal neuralgia
2. Sympathetic
   underactivity
   (postural hypotension)
   S.T.A.N.D. U.P.
   Salt deficiency: hypovolaemia,
            Addison's dis.
   Toxins:
   - Cardiac: diuretics, ACE
     inhibitors, a_1-antagonists,
     nitrates
   - Neuro: L-DOPA,
     antipsychotics, TCAs,
     benzodiazepines
   Autonomic **N**europathy:
      Guillain–Barré syndrome,
      diabetes (both peripheral);
      Parkinson's, MSA (central)
   Dialysis
   Unwell: chronic bedrest
   Pooling, venous: varicose veins,
      prolonged standing

Arterial
1. Vertebrobasilar
   insufficiency
   – Migraine
   – TIA or CVA, including
      subclavian steal
2. Shock
   See p. 30
3. Hypertension
   e.g. phaeochromocytoma

Systemic
1. Metabolic:
   hypoglycaemia or
   hypothyroidism
2. Respiratory:
   hypoxia or
   hypercapnia
3. Blood:
   anaemia or
   hypervicosity

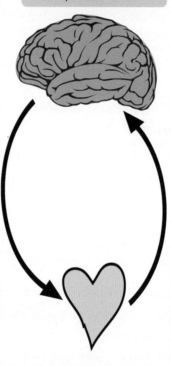

Cardiac
1. Bradycardia: heart block, sick sinus syndrome, tachy–brady syndrome
2. Tachycardia: SVT (atrial fibrillation, Wolff–Parkinson–White syndrome), VT
3. Structural: • Weak heart: LVF, pericardial tamponade
              • Blockage: aortic stenosis, HOCM, myxoma, pulmonary embolism, SVCO

Cardiac, reflex and arterial causes give rise to syncope, i.e. cerebral hypoperfusion

PC, Ix

Cardiogenic syncope
    Trigger: Exertion – esp. sinus bradycardia, SVT, outflow obstruction; drug
    Before: Palpitations, chest pain, dyspnoea or no warning
    During: As for vasovagal; brady- or tachycardic, ABP↓
              (*if prolonged* – cyanosed, apnoeic, brainstem signs or extensor plantars)
    After: Rapid recovery (*if prolonged* – confusion, focal neurological signs)
    Ix: ECG, 24-hr tape; ECHO; event recorder; intracardiac electrophysiological recording

Reflex – vasovagal
    Trigger: Prolonged standing, heat, fatigue, stress
    Before: • Gradual onset over minutes
              • Faint, nausea, anxiety, blurred or tunnel vision, visual spots or fading, tinnitus
    During: Pale grey, clammy, eyes closed; limp; bradycardic; ABP↓; quiet respiration
    After: Rapid recovery (may feel cold, nausea)
    Ix: Tilt-table testing – blood-pressure initially maintained $\Rightarrow$ HR↑ $\Rightarrow$ HR↓, ABP↓

Reflex – postural hypotension
    Trigger: Standing for short or long delay
    Before, During, After: As for vasovagal
    Ix: Tilt-table testing – blood-pressure drops immediately (esp. with autonomic failure)

Arterial
    Trigger: Arm elevation (subclavian steal)
    Before, During, After - as for vasovagal $\pm$ brainstem Sx (diplopia, nausea, dysarthria)
    Ix: MRA or duplex vertebrobasilar circulation

Systemic
    Before, During, After: As for vasovagal

Head – epileptic attacks
    Trigger: Flashing lights, fatigue, fasting
    Before: Complex partial seizure – 'strange feeling'; epigastric rising;
              olfactory hallucinations; déjà vu; automatism, grimacing
              frontal seizures – sudden onset; 'heralding cry'; occurs in frequent clusters
    During: Tongue-biting; urinary and faecal incontinence; stiffness (tonic phase); eyes open
              O/E: Sympathetic activation – pupillary dilation; tachycardic; ABP↑;
              cyanosed; reduced oxygen sats; pyrexia; brainstem signs
    After: Headache, sleeps, confused, Todd's paresis
    Ix: EEG; videotelemetry; serum prolactin at 10–20 min elevated

Head – non-epileptic attacks
    Trigger: Emotional stress; presence of other people; psychiatric history; sexual abuse
    During: Eyes closed firmly; head turns side-to-side; pelvic thrusts; flailing limbs;
              persists for > 10 min with no cyanosis and normal oxygen saturation

Dizziness – Causes

    1. **With impaired consciousness**
        Blackout causes: *C.R.A.S.H.*
    2. **Without impaired consciousness**
        Vertigo: spinning sensation – vestibular
        Imbalance - unsteady on feet: vestibular, cerebellar, extrapyramidal

Epilepsy

Causes   *D.I.V.I.N.I.T.Y.*

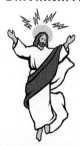

Degenerative / Developmental

Degenerative
Alzheimer's, prion disease

Developmental
Primary: • Generalized: generalized tonic–clonic seizures on awakening ± absences ± myoclonus
• Focal: benign rolandic, occipital
• Complex: Lennox–Gastaut syndrome
Secondary:
• Structural: mesial temporal sclerosis, cortical heterotopia, dysplasia
• Neurocutaneous: neurofibromatoses, tuberous sclerosis / PKU
• Progressive myoclonic epilepsy: *C.L.U.M.S.Y.*
(**C**eroid lipofuscinosis, **L**afora body, **U**nverricht-Lundborg; **M**itochondrial; **S**ialidosis; **Y**:DRPLA (Lu**Y**sian) or Huntington's)

Infection
• Viral encephalitis, esp. herpes simplex
• Bacterial abscess
• HIV, syphilis, Whipple's (or coeliac disease)

Vascular
• Large stroke, multi-infarcts, hyperviscosity syndrome, TTP
• Cortical venous thrombosis
• Cerebral AVM, angioma

Inflammation
• Rassmussen's encephalitis (anti-glutamate receptor)
• Multiple sclerosis
• SLE, antiphospholipid syndrome, vasculitis, sarcoidosis

Neoplasia
• Brain tumour: primitive neuroectodermal tumour (PNET), glioma
• Meningeal carcinoma, melanoma, lymphoma
• Paraneoplastic syndrome, esp. small cell lung cancer (anti-Hu limbic encephalitis)

Injury
• Head injury: early or late
• Cerebral anoxia

Toxins
• Withdrawal from alcohol; sedatives
• Drugs: penicillin, ciprofloxacin, opioids

Y: hYpoglycaemia, hYpocalcaemia (or Mg ? or Na?), hYperthermia

PC

Complex partial seizures   *A.A.A.A.A.*

> **A**ura: rising epigastric sensation; déjà vu; olfactory or auditory hallucinations
>
> **A**utonomic: change in skin colour, temperature, palpitations
>
> **A**bsence: motor arrest, motionless stare
>   last longer than typical absences of childhood
>
> **A**utomatism: lip-smacking, chewing, swallowing; fumbling, walking
>
> **A**mnesia: amnesia of entire attack usual

Cause: 1. Usually arise from mesial temporal lobe, esp. 'mesial temporal sclerosis'.
   2. Associated with febrile convulsions in childhood, but the complex partial
      seizures may not begin until middle-age.

Absences   *A.B.S.E.N.C.E.*

> **AB**rupt onset + offset
> **S**hort: usually < 10 seconds
> **E**yes: glazed, blank stare; slight blinking, eye-rolling
> **N**ormal: i.e. normal intelligence, examination, brain scan
> **C**lonus, or automatism: may occur, esp. as duration of attack increases
> **E**EG: 3 Hz spike-and-wave, with photosensitivity

Cause: 1. Typical absences (as described) are one of the 'primary generalized epilepsies',
      due to thalamic dysregulation
   2. Atypical absences (e.g. last longer; focal signs common) may form part of temporal
      or frontal-lobe seizures, or complexes e.g. Lennox–Gastaut syndrome

Ix

Bloods: prolactin 10 min after fit should be increased relative to baseline
Urine: e.g. toxicology
Micro: e.g. CSF PCR for HSV; HIV serology
EEG: resting or with provocation (hyperventilation, photosensitivity); sleep-deprived; telemetry
Radiology: MRI brain with fine temporal lobe cuts
Surgical: depth or subdural strip electrodes (pre-operative work-up)

Rx

Conservative: don't need to treat if one-off
Counsel: • can't drive for 1 year; careful in bath, ladders etc.
   • pregnancy (folate) and pill (interactions)
Drugs: • generalized: lamotrigine or valproate are 1st-line
   • partial: carbamazepine is 1st-line; levetiracetam is good adjunct
Surgical: e.g. temporal lobectomy; callosotomy; vagal nerve stimulator
Underlying cause: e.g. alcohol abuse counselling; antiviral for encephalitis

Stroke – Ischaemic

Causes   Based upon Virchow's Triad of thrombosis *(p. 474)*

1. Endothelial injury   Arterial ischaemia

A.D.V.I.S.E.

Atherosclerosis: hypertension, DM, cholesterol, smoking
Dissection: hypertension, Ehlers–Danlos, Marfan's; **D**ysplasia, fibromuscular
Vasculitis: autoimmune (PAN, giant-cell arteritis); infection (TB, syphilis)
Injury: trauma, catheterization (angioplasty), indwelling central line, radiation
Spasm: migraine
Embolism, cardiac: AF, endocarditis, myxoma

2. Stasis   Venous, ± arterial, ischaemia

O.R.

Occlusion: head–neck tumour   **R**aised SVC pressure: SVCO

3. Hypercoagulability   - Venous, ± arterial, ischaemia

H.E.P.A.R.I.N.I.S.E.

Hereditary: prothrombin, factor V Leiden genes, protein S, C deficiency, homocystinuria,
          mitochondrial (MELAS – stroke due to metabolic not vascular defect)
Endocrine: estrogens – pregnancy, OCP, HRT; androgens; diabetic HONK
Polycythaemia; **P**araproteinaemia; **P**NH
Autoimmune: antiphospholipid syndrome, SLE, Behçet's
Renal: nephrosis, dehydration
Injury
Neoplasia: adenocarcinoma, acute leukaemia
Infection: septicaemic; local – cellulitis; otitis media, sinusitis
Smoking; **S**enility (increasing age)
Exogenous: chemotherapy, steroids; COX-2 inhibitors

Ix

Bloods: FBC, U&E, cholesterol, ESR, CRP,
          autoAbs, thrombophilia screen
Urine: Glucose, blood; toxicology
Micro: VDRL, HIV serology, blood cultures
Monitor: ABP, Neuro. obs., glucose
ECG, **E**CHO
Radiology: • CXR
          • Brain: CT, MRI, MRA
          • Carotid Doppler USS

Rx   *R.A.M.P.S.*

Resuscitation + **R**egulation:
   O₂, nasogastric tube, fluids
   ABP, temperature, glucose, ICP
Acute stroke unit:
   SALT assesment – NGT, PEG?
   TED stockings, physiotherapy, OT
Medical:
   Antiplatelet, thrombolysis, statin
Prevention, secondary:
   Anticoagulant, antihypertensives
Surgery:
   Acute: decompression, shunt
   Elective: carotid endarterectomy or shunt

Stroke – Haemorrhagic

Causes

H.A.E.M.A.T.O.M.A.

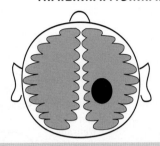

Hypertension
- Causes Charcot–Bouchard microaneurysm: putaminal / thalamic / brainstem bleed

Aneurysm
- Berry aneuysms occur at arterial bifurcations and usually cause subarachnoid haemorrhage
- Assoc. with hypertension, family history, APKD

Elderly
- Amyloid angiopathy causing lobar haemorrhages

Malformations
- AVM, cavernous angioma, moya-moya syn.

Autoimmune / infection
- Vasculitis, TB, endocarditis

Toxin
- Sympathomimetic: cocaine, amphetamines
- Warfarin (+ other causes of coagulopathy)

Occlusive venous or arterial disease
- Cerebral venous thrombosis
- Haemorrhagic transformation of infarct

Metastases / primary brain tumour
- Mets: bronchial, melanoma, choriocarcinoma (pregnancy, testes), thyroid, renal
- Glioma

Accident   Head injury

Ix

Bloods:	FBC, clotting, G&S, autoAbs
Urine:	Glucose (subarachnoid bleed); toxicology
Micro:	Blood cultures
Monitor:	ABP, neuro. obs., glucose
ECG:	Ischaemic changes in SAH
Radiology:	• CXR (pulmonary oedema in SAH)
	• Brain: CT, MRI, MRA
	• Cerebral angiogram
Special:	LP for xanthochromia if SAH suspected

Rx   *R.A.M.P.S.*

Resuscitation + **R**egulation:
O_2, nasogastric tube, fluids
ABP, temperature, glucose, ICP

Acute stroke unit / neuro-ITU:

Medical
Nimodipine, lactulose, opioid, phenytoin, recombinant factor VII

Prevention, secondary:
- Antihypertensives – give later, initially keep blood pressure high to avoid ischaemia

Surgery
- Aneurysm: – coil better than clipping
  – within 72 hrs
- AVM: embolization, gamma-knife

Acute Weakness

Cerebrum / Brainstem
1. Vascular: infarction, haemorrhage
2. Infection: encephalitis, abscess
3. Inflammation, e.g. ADEM

Cord
1. Vascular: anterior spinal artery infarction, AVM
2. Inflammation: transverse myelitis
3. Injury

Anterior horn cells
1. Infection: polio, West Nile virus
2. Paraneoplastic

Roots / Plexus
1. Proximal nerve inflammation: brachial neuritis
2. Plexitis: carcinoma, radiotherapy

Motor nerves (p. 292)
1. **Demyelinating**
   Inflammatory: GBS
   Toxin: diphtheria, buckthorn,
       seafood (ciguatoxin),
       suramin
   Systemic – uraemia
2. **Axonal**
   Porphyria, acute intermittent
   Autoimmune: vasculitis
   Infection: Lyme disease / ITU neuropathy
   Neoplastic: paraneoplastic, lymphoma

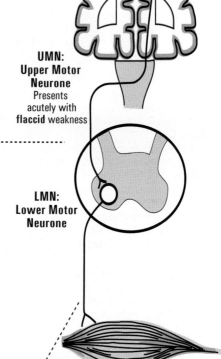

UMN:
Upper Motor
Neurone
Presents
acutely with
flaccid weakness

LMN:
Lower Motor
Neurone

NMJ: neuromuscular junction
esp. ocular and bulbar weakness
Muscle
esp. proximal weakness, myalgia

NMJ
1. Autoimmune: myasthenia gravis
2. Toxin: botulism
3. Neoplasia: Lambert–Eaton myasthenic syndrome

Muscle
Toxins: steroids, statins, ITU, cocaine, alcohol
Hereditary: periodic paralysis, malignant hyperthermia
Inflammation: myositis, trichinosis, HIV
Neoplastic: paraneoplastic
Electrolytes: $K^+\downarrow$, $PO_4\downarrow$
Rhabdomyolysis: due to any of above

Guillain–Barré Syndrome

Types

GBS =

AIDP: acute inflammatory **demyelinating** polyneuropathy   90%   – various antibodies
AMAN: acute motor (± sensory) **axonal** neuropathy   5%   – anti-GD1a antibodies
Miller–Fisher syndrome (ophthalmoplegia + ataxia + areflexia) 5% – anti-GQ1b antibodies
Acute sensory / autonomic neuropathy   1%

NB: AMAN constitutes 30–50% cases in China and South America

Causes

Cross-reacting antibodies to gangliosides (glycosphingolipids on myelin sheath or axolemma),
with clinical syndrome beginning 1–4 weeks, following exposure to:

1. Bacteria: *Campylobacter jejuni* (30%, esp. AMAN), *Mycoplasma*
2. Viruses: CMV, EBV, HIV, unidentified virus, e.g. flu (majority of cases)
3. Vaccines: esp. rabies

PC, Ix   *G.B.S. = A.I.D.P.*

Growing weakness
  • Typically, proximal weakness that ascends from legs to trunk, arms, head; nadir < 4 weeks
  • Variants include brachiocephalgic (bifacial palsies) or paraparesis (mimic cord lesion)
  • Areflexia very common; fasciculations may occur

Breathing and **B**ulbar problems / **B**ack pain
  • Respiratory support required in 25% due to bulbar and respiratory muscle weakness
  • Back pain common due to inflammation of proximal nerve roots

Sensory disturbance
  • Paraesthesia in extremities is often first symptom
  • Sensory ataxia common, esp. in Miller–Fisher syndrome

Autonomic neuropathy
  • Arrhythmias, labile blood pressure, urinary retention, constipation

Immune
  • Serology for anti-gangliosides; *Campylobacter*, HIV, etc.; stool sample

Demyelinating nerve conduction studies
  • Motor conduction velocities – slow; central motor conduction times (F-wave) – delayed

Protein in CSF
  • Protein usually > 1 g/l by second week
    white cells $< 4 \times 10^9/l$ (i.e. 'albuminocytological dissociation')
  • High CSF protein can cause papilloedema and optic neuropathies (check visual acuity)

Rx

1. Immunuosuppression: IVIg or plasma exchange – the earlier, the better
2. Supportive
   Airway / ventilation support: transfer to ITU if FVC < 1.0 l (15 ml/kg)
   Analgesia (NSAIDs, gabapentin, antidepressants)
   Autonomic: cardiac monitor; labetalol or noradrenaline etc.; laxatives; urinary catheter
   Antithrombotic: TED stockings, low-molecular-weight heparin
3. Physiotherapy: prevent flexion contractures

Prog

Death 5%; permanent disability 20%
Bad prognosis – rapid onset; *Campylobacter*-positive; Good prognosis – Miller–Fisher variant

Hand Wasting – Causes

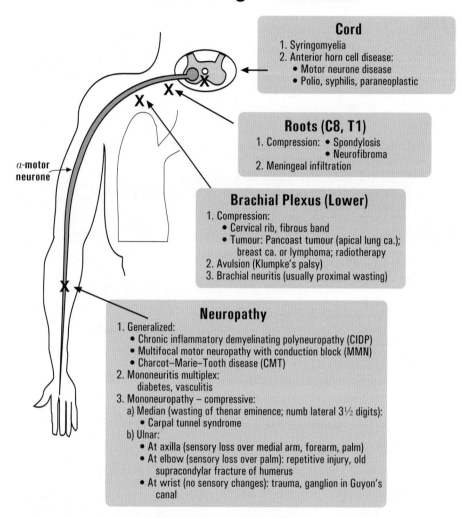

Cord
1. Syringomyelia
2. Anterior horn cell disease:
   - Motor neurone disease
   - Polio, syphilis, paraneoplastic

Roots (C8, T1)
1. Compression: • Spondylosis
   - Neurofibroma
2. Meningeal infiltration

Brachial Plexus (Lower)
1. Compression:
   - Cervical rib, fibrous band
   - Tumour: Pancoast tumour (apical lung ca.); breast ca. or lymphoma; radiotherapy
2. Avulsion (Klumpke's palsy)
3. Brachial neuritis (usually proximal wasting)

Neuropathy
1. Generalized:
   - Chronic inflammatory demyelinating polyneuropathy (CIDP)
   - Multifocal motor neuropathy with conduction block (MMN)
   - Charcot–Marie–Tooth disease (CMT)
2. Mononeuritis multiplex:
   diabetes, vasculitis
3. Mononeuropathy – compressive:
   a) Median (wasting of thenar eminence; numb lateral $3\frac{1}{2}$ digits):
      - Carpal tunnel syndrome
   b) Ulnar:
      - At axilla (sensory loss over medial arm, forearm, palm)
      - At elbow (sensory loss over palm): repetitive injury, old supracondylar fracture of humerus
      - At wrist (no sensory changes): trauma, ganglion in Guyon's canal

α-motor neurone

Distal Myopathy
Myotonic dystrophy

Other
1. Compartment syndrome – Volkmann's ischaemic contracture: fibrosis of wrist and finger flexors
2. Disuse atrophy:
   a) Rheumatoid arthritis (also causes carpal tunnel syn., ulnar neuropathy and mononeuritis)
   b) Long-standing neurodisability: Parkinson's, stroke, multiple sclerosis
3. Cachexia

Walking Disturbance – Causes

Apraxic (frontal lobes)
O/E: Wide-based, short steps,
out-turned toes,
+ dementia, incontinence,
primitive reflexes
1. Lacunar state: marche à petit pas
2. Normal-pressure hydrocephalus

UMN Bilateral
O/E: Spastic, scissoring
+ brisk jaw jerk,
pseudobulbar speech,
emotional incontinence,
sphincter dysfunction
1. Bihemispheric disease:
cerebral palsy, ALS
parasagittal meningioma
2. Cord lesion (myelopathy):
cervical spondylosis,
hereditary spastic paraparesis

UMN Unilateral
O/E: Circumducting, spastic gait
1. Cerebral hemisphere lesion:
CVA, MS, tumour
2. Hemicord (Brown–Séquard syn.):
MS, tumour

LMN Bilateral
O/E: Bilateral foot drop,
flaccid paraparesis, areflexia
1. Peripheral neuropathy:
CMT, Guillain-Barré syn., CIDP
2. Cauda equina:
lumbar disc prolapse
(also sphincter dysfunction,
saddle anaesthesia)

LMN Unilateral
O/E: Foot-drop: high-steppage gait
1. Radicular lesion, e.g. L5
2. Sciatic or lateral popliteal nerve:
trauma, diabetes, vasculitis

Mixed UMN + LMN
1. Conus medullaris lesion
2. Vit B12 deficiency
3. Motor neurone disease

Functional
O/E: Distractible, bizarre

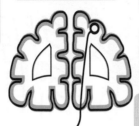

**UMN :
Upper Motor
neurone**

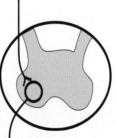

**LMN :
Lower Motor
Neurone**

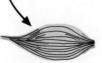

Myopathy Myasthenia
O/E: Waddling gait

Vestibular
O/E: Veering (ipsilateral),
Romberg's +ve, nystagmus,
drop attacks (paroxysmal)

Cerebellar
O/E: Wide-based, ataxic, nystagmus

Basal Ganglia
(Extrapyramidal)
1. Parkinsonism
O/E: Short-step, shuffling, flexed,
loss of arm swing, festinant
2. Choreiform
O/E: Lurching
3. Dystonia
O/E: Hand or foot held in
odd fixed position; torticollis
4. Myoclonus
O/E: Knees give way

Proprioceptive Loss
O/E: Romberg's +ve
1. Dorsal column disease:
• Vit B12 deficiency
• Syphilis, HIV
(mixed UMN + LMN disease)
2. Large-fibre peripheral neuropathy,
or dorsal-root ganglionopathy

Visual Loss

Other Medical
1. Vascular:
• Postural hypotension
• Intermittent claudication
2. Cardiac:
• Stokes-Adams attacks
3. Arthritis

Myelopathy

Cord Compression

Causes   *D.I.V.I.N.I.T.Y.*

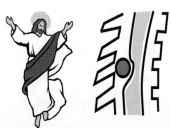

PC
1. Pain
2. Radicular symptoms

Degenerative / Developmental
Degenerative
- Cervical disc prolapse / cervical spondylosis
- Osteoporosis
- Paget's disease

Developmental
- Spina bifida (cauda equina syndrome / lipoma, haemangiomas)
- Klippel–Feil syndrome

Infection
- TB
- Pyogenic: – Epidural abscess
              – Infected intradural dermoid

Vascular
- Extradural haematoma

Inflammation
- Rheumatoid arthritis of atlanto-axial joint
- Ankylosing spondylitis: ↑ risk of vertebral fracture

Neoplasia
- Extradural: Vertebral – *B.O.N.E.1.M. (see p. 255)*
- Intradural, extramedullary:
  – Neurofibroma: 'dumb-bell'
  – Meningioma (esp. in thoracic cord, in middle-aged women)
  – Lipoma (assoc. with spina bifida)
  – Dermoid
- Arachnoid cyst

Injury
- Fracture
- Spondylolisthesis

Toxin / Nutritional
- Nutritional: rickets / osteomalacia

Y: kYphoscoliosis

Intrinsic Cord Disease

Causes   *D.I.V.I.N.I.T.Y.*

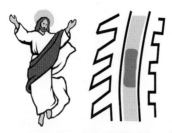

PC
1. Painless
2. Early sphincter /
   erectile dysfunction

Degenerative / **D**evelopmental
Degenerative
- Amyotrophic lateral sclerosis / primary lateral sclerosis

Developmental
- Friedreich's ataxia, and other spinocerebellar ataxias
- Hereditary spastic paraplegia

Infection
- Virus: HIV (selective dorsal column disease), HTLV-I, VZV
- Syphilis - 'tabes dorsalis' (selective dorsal column disease)

Vascular
- Infarction
  a) Thromboembolism, atheroma, diabetes mellitus
  b) Dissection of aorta
  c) Vasculitis, esp. polyarteritis nodosa
     (anterior spinal artery infarction causes spinothalamic loss)

Haemorrhage, intramedullary, inc. AVM (spinal haemangioma)

Inflammation
- Demyelination: – Multiple sclerosis, ADEM
                 – Postinfective transverse myelitis
                 – Devic's disease (transverse myelitis + optic neuritis)
- SLE, vasculitis
- Sarcoid

Neoplasia – intradural, intramedullary (rare)
- Glioma (esp. in cervical cord, in young adult)
- Ependymoma; haemangioblastoma (assoc. Von Hippel–Lindau syn.)

Injury
- Trauma: contusion, syrinx, myelomalacia secondary to compression
- Radiation myelitis

Toxin / Nutritional
- Toxin: lathyrism (chick-pea ingestion in India)
- Nutritional - Vit B12 deficiency (selective dorsal column disease)

Y: s**Y**ringomyelia

Anterior-Horn Cell Diseases

The following are causes of a pure lower motor neurone syndrome (wasting, fasciculations, weakness), with or without upper motor neurone signs.

A. S.K.I.N.N.Y. M.A.N.

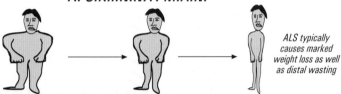

ALS typically causes marked weight loss as well as distal wasting

Amyotrophic lateral sclerosis (ALS) / other motor-neurone disease
Inc: 1/ 100 000 p.a.; prevalence - 5/100 000
Age: > 60 years
Sex: M:F = 1.5 : 1
Geo: Guam, West New Guinea, Japanese Kii Peninsula:
  • Associated with ALS–dementia–Parkinson's complex
Aet: • Neurotoxin: glutamate excess, e.g. higher in leather workers
  • Genetic: 10% are familial, of which 15% due to Cu-Zn SOD1 mutation
    (free-radical clearance enzyme)
Micro: • Degeneration of both LMN (anterior horns) and UMN (corticospinal tract)
  • Ubiquitin positive Bunina inclusion bodies are found within anterior horn cells

Spinal muscular atrophy (SMA)
Path: Autosomal recessive disorders linked to 5q
PC: • Infantile and childhood forms are severe and fatal within a few years
  • Adult-onset form causes mild proximal limb wasting

Kennedy's disease (bulbospinal muscular atrophy)
Path: Due to androgen receptor mutation, comprising CAG repeat on X chromosome
PC: • Head: facial fasciculations, bulbar palsy, dysarthria
  • Limbs: proximal wasting, postural tremor, sensory involvement
  • Endocrine: gynaecomastia, infertility, type 2 diabetes, prostate carcinoma

Infection
  • Acute: polio or West Nile virus; Lyme disease
  • Chronic: post-polio syndrome; syphilis (meningeal)

Neoplasia – 1
  • Direct motor nerve or meningeal infiltration

Neoplasia – 2
  • Paraneoplastic (esp. lymphoma) or radiotherapy to pelvis

Neoplasia – 3
  • Cervicomedullary tumour (or syringomyelia, or cervical spondylosis) may mimic ALS

Y: TaY–Sachs disease, adult-equivalent
  • GM2 gangliosidoses due to hexosaminidase deficiency

Monomelic Amyotrophy
  • Non-progressive wasting of one distal limb in young adult (i.e. 'benign')

Neuropathies, motor
  1. Multifocal motor neuropathy with conduction block: anti-GM1 anti-ganglioside
    • Important not to miss, as this can be treated successfully with IVIg!
  2. Toxins e.g. vincristine, lead

ALS / Motor Neurone Disease

Types / PC

A.P.P.L.E.S.

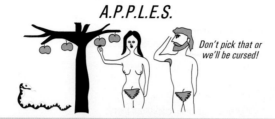

Don't pick that or we'll be cursed!

Amyotrophic lateral sclerosis (80%)
1. LMN: bulbar palsy, distal limb wasting, fasciculations, cramps
2. UMN: pseudobulbar palsy, spastic paraparesis, extensor plantars
3. Spares: • Ocular movements (III, IV, VI nuclei)
   • Bladder, anus control
   • Sensory signs (although symptoms may occur)

Progressive bulbar palsy (10%)
1. LMN: tongue atrophy and fasciculations, dysarthria, nasal regurgitation
2. UMN: pseudobulbar speech, brisk jaw jerk

Progressive muscular atrophy (10%)
LMN: • Fasciculations, distal limb wasting, claw hand
   • Respiratory: poor cough, tachypnoea

Lateral sclerosis, primary (1%)
UMN signs only

Extra features (1%)
Frontal dementia, parkinsonism – usually hereditary forms

SOD1 mutation, and other genetic forms of ALS
Younger onset, more severe course

Ix **Bloods**
1. CK: ↑ due to spasticity and cramps
2. Alternative diagnoses: anti-GM1 (anti-ganglioside Abs), VDRL, hexosaminidase

EMG
1. MND: fasciculations, fibrillation potentials; ↓ no. of spikes on maximum contraction
2. MMN: conduction block

Radiology
1. CXR
2. MRI brain and cervical cord

Special – CSF

VDRL, cytology

Rx

1. Riluzole: inhibits glutamate release – prolongs life by 3 months
2. Supportive: quinine (cramps); baclofen (spasticity); β-blockers (fasciculations); propantheline (drooling)
3. Other: nerve growth factors, IVIg, pyridostigmine (improves weakness in early MND)

Peripheral Neuropathy – Causes

Demyelination   *I.T.'S. T.H.I.N.*

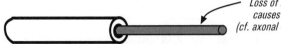

Loss of myelin sheath around axon
causes slowing of conduction
(cf. axonal – reduced action potential)

Acute
Inflammatory: Guillain–Barré syndrome
Toxin: diphtheria; arsenic, buckthorn berry
Syndrome: Refsum's disease; **S**ystemic: acute uraemic

Chronic
Toxins: amiodarone, suramin, industrial solvents
Hereditary:
  • Charcot–Marie–Tooth disease – type 1A (*PMP22* duplication); 1B (protein 0)
  • Hereditary neuropathy with liability to pressure palsies (*PMP22* deletion)
  • Metabolic: Refsum's disease, abetalipoproteinaemia, leucodystrophies
Inflammatory: chronic inflammatory demyelinating polyneuropathy, multifocal motor neuropathy
Neoplasia: myeloma, anti-myelin-associated glycoprotein IgM, POEMS syndrome

Axonal   *P.A.I.N. E.N.D.I.N.G.S. H.U.R.T.*

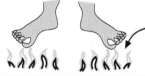

Predominantly sensory symptoms,
e.g. burning paraesthesia
(cf. demyelinating–motor symptoms)

Acute
Porphyria, acute intermittent: recurrent acute attacks, motor neuropathy
Autoimmune: vasculitis, cryoglobulinaemia, rheumatoid arthritis, Sjögren's syndrome, SLE
Infection: Lyme disease (painful lumbosacral polyradiculitis) / **I**TU or critical illness
Neoplasia: paraneoplastic (assoc. small cell lung carcinoma; anti-neuronal Abs), lymphoma

Chronic
Endocrine: diabetes, hypothyroidism, acromegaly (compression neuropathies, e.g. carpal tunnel)
Nutritional: Vit B12 deficiency (+myelopathy+dementia), thiamine deficiency (alcohol), coeliac
Drugs: chemotherapy (cisplatin, taxanes), antibiotics (isoniazid), nucleoside analogs (ddl)
Infection: HIV, leprosy
Neoplasia: infiltration (e.g. lymphoma, carcinoma), amyloidosis
Granulomatous: sarcoidosis
Systemic: amyloidosis

Hereditary: CMT disease type 2, HSAN, familial amyloid polyneuropathies, Fabry's disease
Uraemia / Respiratory failure (COAD): cirrhosis
Toxins: thallium (cockroach poison, causes hair loss, may be acute), lead (motor neuropathy)

Peripheral Neuropathy – Patterns

Mononeuropathy Multiplex *H.E.A.T.I.N.G. (some painful)*

Def Dysfunction of non-contiguous peripheral nerves, e.g. median ⇒ peroneal nerve

Causes
Hereditary neuropathy with liability to pressure palsies
Endocrine: diabetes, hypothyroidism, acromegaly
Autoimmune: vasculitis, cryoglobulinaemia
Toxin: lead (radial nerve, peroneal nerve palsies)
Infection: HIV, Lyme, leprosy / **I**nflammatory: CIDP variant (MADSAM, MMN)
Neoplastic: amyloid, direct infiltration with lymphoma or leukaemia
Granulomatous: sarcoid

Small-fibre Neuropathies *H.E.A.T.I.N.G. (most painful)*

Causes
Hereditary: HSAN, familial amyloid polyneuropathies
Endocrine: diabetes
Autoimmune: Sjögren's syndrome
Toxins: alcohol (large and small fibres, but painful)
Infection: HIV
Neoplastic: amyloid

Dorsal-Root Ganglionopathy *Sensory A.T.A.X.I.C.*

Causes
Acute: Guillain-Barré syndrome, esp. Miller–Fisher type
Toxins: cisplatin
Autoimmune: Sjögren's syndrome
Xs: excess Vit B6
Infectious, post
Carcinoma: paraneoplastic; also paraproteinaemia with anti-MAG

Palpable Nerves *L.A.R.G.E.*

Causes
Leprosy
Amyloidosis
Refsum's disease
Genetic, other: Charcot–Marie–Tooth types 1, 3; neurofibromatosis
Endocrine: acromegaly

Autonomic Involvement

Causes
Acute: Guillain–Barré syndrome, toxin (vincristine), paraneoplastic, porphyria
Chronic: diabetes, hereditary (HSAN, FAP), amyloid, HIV

Neuromuscular Junction Disease

<u>**Causes**</u>   *A.C.T.I.O.N.*

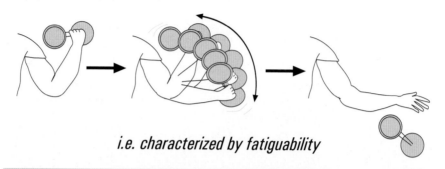

i.e. characterized by fatiguability

Autoimmune – myasthenia gravis
Path: Antibodies to skeletal muscle nicotinic-ACh receptors (nAchR), or muscle-specific kinase (MuSK)
     causing receptor endocytosis, receptor block and complement fixation
Types:
     Thymic hyperplasia (60%, esp. young women): high Ig level; good response to thymectomy
     Thymic atrophy   (20%, esp. old men):   low Ig level; poor response to thymectomy
     Thymoma   (10%, middle aged):   high Ig level; poor response to thymectomy
     Neonatal: due to placental transfer of IgG in 10% of myasthenic mothers (PC: arthrogryposis)
Assoc: HLA-B8, DR3; thyrotoxicosis, type 1 diabetes mellitus, rheumatoid arthritis, SLE

Congenital myasthenia
Path: Genetic defect in ACh receptor subunits, or presynaptic ACh synthesis or vesicle packaging

Toxins
Path: 1. Penicillamine: generates Ach-receptor Abs, and causes myasthenia gravis-like syndrome
      2. Other drugs may exacerbate primary causes of NMJ defects, e.g.
           Presynaptic: • Ca-channel antagonists: verapamil, magnesium, aminoglycosides
                        • Na-channel blockers: anti-arrhythmics (Ia, e.g. procainimide), β-blockers
                        • Black widow spider venom: depletes ACh from motor terminals
           Postsynaptic: anaesthetics: AChR blockers: atracurium, vecuronium, suxamethonium
           Pre- and Postsynaptic: ciprofloxacin

Infection – botulism
Path: 1. Clostridium botulinum toxin acquired from:-
           • Food-poisoning, esp. home-preserved food, cans
           • Food colonization, esp. infants, raw honey
           • Wound contamination, esp. intravenous drug users ('skin popping')
      2. Botulinum toxin (Botox) prevents docking of ACh vesicles with presynaptic cell membrane

Organophosphates, nerve gas
Path: Act as irreversible acetylcholinesterase inhibitors, causing cholinergic excess
      and depolarizing block

Neoplasia – Lambert–Eaton myasthenic syndrome
Path: Antibodies to presynaptic voltage-gated calcium channel
Types: 2/3 of cases are paraneoplastic (esp. small cell lung cancer); 1/3 are primary autoimmune

PC

Myasthenia gravis

Fluctuating weakness – fatiguable (worsens during day, with infection, drugs, dysthroidism)

> **Eyes:** • Ptosis, worse with sustained up-gaze; Cogan's lid twitch
> • Ophthalmoplegia, diplopia (if ptosis not complete)
>
> **Face:** weak, snarling-smile, jaw-droop
>
> **Bulbar:** nasal dysarthria; nasal regurgitation; aspiration
>
> **Neck:** marked weakness, head droop
>
> **Limbs:** proximal weakness, asymmetric, brisk reflexes
>
> **Ventilation:** ↓ FVC (worse on lying) – usually late

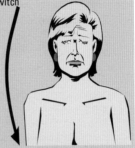

LEMS

As for myasthenia gravis, except: *L.E.M.S.*
Leg weakness early, Extra (areflexia, autonomic), Movement improves, Sensory symptoms

Botulism

As for myasthenia gravis, plus prominent **anticholinergic effects**:
• Ocular: iridoplegia, mydriasis, cycloplegia (blurred vision and diplopia are always early symptoms)
• Abdominal: nausea and vomiting (and vertigo); constipation; urinary retention
• Systemic: bradycardia, constipation

Ix

Bloods

1. AutoAbs: nAChR, MuSK, striated muscle (assoc. with thymoma), VG-Ca channel (LEMS)
2. TFT: dysthyroidism may precipitate myasthenic crisis
3. Associated autoimmunity: glucose, Vit B12, U + Es (Addison's), rheumatoid factor, ANA

EMG

1. Repetitive stimulation: ↓ in compound action potential in myasthenia (↑ with LEMS; botulinum toxin)
2. Single-fibre studies: jitter and block – represents delay between two fibres within one motor unit

'Tensilon' test

1. Patient injected with IV 'Tensilon' (edrophonium), which acts as short-acting cholinesterase inhibitor
2. Myasthenic crisis – resolution of weakness; cholinergic crisis – worsening weakness

Radiology

CT thorax: exclude thymoma

Rx

Myasthenia gravis

Anticholinesterases: pyridostigmine; ☠: N + V, colic, diarrhoea; bradycardia; cholinergic crisis (weakness)
Thymectomy (via mediastinectomy): success rate = 85% improve; 50% develop remission by 10 years
Immunosuppression: • Steroids (start at low dose to avoid initial 'steroid dip'), azathioprine (check TPMT level)
• IVIg, plasma exchange (myasthenic crises)

LEMS

3,4-Diaminopyridine, steroids, IVIg, plasma exchange

Botulism

Benzylpenicillin, intravenous: for active infection with *C. botulinum*
Antiserum, trivalent (anti A, B, E): within 24 hours

<u>Myopathy</u>

<u>Causes</u>

T.H.I.N.N.E.R.

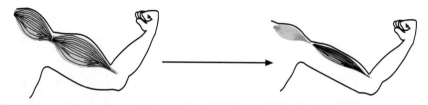

Toxins
Prescribed: **S**teroids, **S**tatins, **S**kin – etretinate
Immune – penicillamine, colchicine; **I**nfection – zidovudine, amphotericin; **I**TU (anaesthetics)
Chemotherapy: vincristine; **C**hloroquine, **C**arbimazole, **C**ardiology: amiodarone
K$^+$- losing diuretics: e.g. thiazides, carbenoloxone, liqourice
Drugs of abuse: alcohol, amphetamines, opioids, cocaine, barbiturates

Hereditary
Muscular dystrophy:
  XL: Duchenne, Becker, Emery–Dreifuss; AR: limb-girdle; AD: facioscapulohumeral, oculopharyngeal
Congenital myopathy
Myotonic dystrophy, myotonia congenita
Channelopathy: periodic paralysis (K$^+$), paramyotonia congenita, neuromyotonia
Metabolic: glycogen-storage, fatty-acid metabolism, mitochondrial disease

Inflammatory
Myositis: dermatomyositis; polymyositis; inclusion-body myositis (primarily a degenerative disease)
Infective: *Trichinella*, Cysticercosis, HIV
Sarcoidosis
(Polymyalgia rheumatica – causes proximal muscle pain, although power and CK usually normal)

Neoplasia
Carcinoma: advanced or paraneoplastic (inc. dermatomyositis)
Haematological: eosinophilia (e.g. tryptophan), amyloid, graft-versus-host disease

Nutritional
Ca^{2+} (or Mg^{2+}) $\updownarrow$: osteomalacia, due to poor intake, malabsorption, chronic renal failure
K$^+$ $\updownarrow$
Malnutrition, malabsorption: Vit E deficiency

Endocrine
Corticosteroids $\updownarrow$:
    • Cushing's syndrome: due to catabolic effects on muscle; acute or chronic
    • Hyperaldosteronism – due to ↓K$^+$, Hypoaldosteronism (Addison's) – mainly muscle fatigue
Thyroid $\updownarrow$
Other: acromegaly, diabetes – ischaemic infarction of thigh

Rhabdomyolysis
Toxins: Prescribed (e.g. statin + clofibrate, cyclosporin), neuroleptic malignant syndrome, drugs of abuse
Hereditary: Metabolic – McArdle's disease; CPT or acyl CoA deficiency; mitochondrial; malignant hyperthermia (ryanodine receptor gene)
Injury: Trauma, epilepsy

PC

Weak

Proximal pattern usually:
  a) Girdles, e.g. rising from chair, combing hair
  b) Ocular–lids, facial, bulbar, neck weakness (esp. myotonic dystrophy and myositis)
  c) Respiratory (nemaline, McArdle's myopathy, myositis)
Distal pattern: myotonic dystrophy, Emery–Dreifuss or FSH dystrophy, inclusion body myositis

Pain

Toxins (alcohol, heroin), **H**ereditary (McArdle's), **I**nflammatory (polymyositis), **N**eoplasia, **N**utrition ($Ca^{2+} \downarrow$)
Stiffness or cramps: better with movement – myotonia; worse with movement – paramyotonia

Associated

Arrhythmias: muscular dystrophy, myotonic dystrophy, mitochondrial myopathy
Infertility: myotonic dystrophy

O/E

Inspection:	wasting: proximal, symmetrical; ptosis; jaw droop; scapula winging; pseudohypertrophy calves
Tone:	normal; test for hand-grip release and percussion myotonia (thenar eminence, tongue) in myotonia
Reflexes:	relatively spared (except muscular dystrophy or myotonia, in which areflexia occurs)
Gait:	waddle
Other:	• Myotonia: frontal balding, cataracts, dilated cardiomyopathy
	• Mitochondrial myopathy: salt and pepper retinitis pigmentosa, deafness, dementia, ataxia
	• Myositis: periorbital oedema, rash, lower-zone pulmonary fibrosis

Ix

Blood:

  • CK ↑ , but normal in PMR, IBM, myotonia, mitochondrial myopathies, chronic steroids
  • AutoAbs – ANA, ENA, inc. anti Jo-1 (polymyositis), ESR ↑, AChR Abs (myasthenia mimics)
  • Genetics: dystrophin, FSH (facioscapulohumeral dystrophy); lactate ↑ in mitochondrial myopathy

Urine: myoglobin: rhabdomyolysis

Micro: ELISA

Monitor: FVC if dyspnoeic

ECG: muscular dystrophy, myotonic dystrophy, mitochondrial myopathy

EMG:

  • Small, brief, polyphasic potential (due to recruitment of ↑ed no. of weaker motor units)
  • Insertional activity, fibrillation potentials, positive sharp waves in polymyositis
  • Myotonia: waxing and waning amplitude and frequency: "dive-bomber / motor bike" revving sound

Radiology

  • CXR (polymyositis, sarcoid, carcinoma); MRI – directs muscle biopsy location

Surgical – biopsy

  • Lymphocytic infiltrate - myositis, sarcoidosis, dysferlinopathy
  • Mitochondrial myopathy - COX-staining, genetics and respiratory chain assay

Rx

Hereditary: myotonia – phenytoin, mexiletine (Na^+-channel blockers); dystrophy – myostatin inhibitors?
Inflammatory: steroids, IVIg
  • Distinction with steroid-induced myopathy can be made on basis of pain, CK, EMG, MRI and biopsy

Acute Visual Loss – Causes

Aqueous

Closed-angle glaucoma

Epi
Inc: 10% glaucoma
Age: Elderly
Sex: F:M = 3:1 (Whites)
Geo: Asians
Aet: 2 types:
    1: Apposition of back of iris to
       lens blocks aqueous flow
       ⇒ iris pushed forwards,
       blocking drainage
    2: Uveitis ⇒ iris adhesions
Pre: Hypermetropes (short eye)
Macro: Corneal oedema

PC:
1. Pain: eye, head; severe
   ↑ in evening (semidilated pupil)
   ↓ in sleep (pupil constricts)
2. N+V, photophobia
3. Vision: blurry, haloes

O/E:
1. Inspection: red eye, hazy cornea,
   pupil: fixed, semidilated
2. Palpation: tender, hard
3. Visual acuity ↓
4. Fundi: papilloedema
Late: anterior synechiae,
   grey atrophy of iris, lens flecks

Ix: Intraocular pressure > 21 mmHg
   (often 40–80 mmHg)

Rx: 1. Acetazolamide (top / IV)
    2. Mannitol (IV)
    3. Urgent iridotomy: laser /
       surgical

Vitreous

Vitreal haemorrhage

Epi:
    1. Diabetes mellitus
    2. High myope
PC:
    1. Floaters
    2. Blurred vision

O/E:
    1. Visual acuity ↓
    2. Red reflex ↓

Retinal detachment / tear

PC:
    1. Floaters
    2. Flashing lights
       (retinal traction)

Retina

Central retinal artery or vein (or branch) occlusion

Epi:
    Artery: thromboembolism,
      e.g. diabetes, AF, aortic stenosis
    Vein: hypertension, diabetes,
      hyperviscosity
PC:
    Visual loss:
    • Sudden onset ± offset
    • Curtain descending ± rising
O/E:
    1. Altitudinal scotoma
    2. Fundoscopy:
       Arterial: pale retina,
       embolus at bifurcation,
       macular cherry-red spot
       Vein: flame haemorrhages,
       papilloedema (sausage-strings
       – hyperviscosity)
    3. Late: rubeosis iridis, glaucoma

Macular degeneration

Epi:
    1. Disciform type > 60 yrs old
    2. Central serous
chorioretinopathy
    = leakage of fluid into subretinal
      space: side-effect of steroids
PC:
    1. Metamorphosia, micropsia,
    2. Positive central scotoma
    3. Photo-stress test +ve

Examination

1. Characteristic
   eye or retinal
   appearance
2. Usually unilateral

Trabecular
meshwork +
canal of   Ciliary
Schlemm   body

Flow of aqueous humor shown

Optic nerve
V.I.S.I.O.N. & O.P.T.I.C.

Vascular: anterior ischaemic optic neuropathy (AION)
1. Thromboembolic
2. Vasculitis: giant-cell arteritis, SLE, antiphospholipid syn.

Inflammatory – 'optic neuritis'
1. Multiple sclerosis
2. Devic's disease
3. ADEM

Sarcoid / other granulomatous CRION (chronic relapsing inflammatory optic neuropathy)

Infection:
1. Virus, e.g. VZV
2. TB, syphilis
3. Sinus infection (contiguous)

Other: GBS

Neoplasia: lymphoma, leukaemia

Ocular

Papillitis / papilloedema

Toxin: sildenafil, methanol, tobacco/alcohol

Inherited: Leber's hereditary optic atrophy (mitochondrial disease)

Compression: tumour, trauma, carotid aneurysm

CSF / Chiasm
Intracranial pressure ↑

Epi:
1. Mass lesion, e.g. tumour
2. Cerebral venous thrombosis
3. Primary intracranial hypertension

PC: Visual obscurations

O/E: Papilloedema

Obstructive hydrocephalus

Pituitary apoplexy

Cortical
Vascular

Epi: causes of vertebrobasilar insufficiency:
1. Thromboembolic, inc. AF, cardiac catheterization, hyperviscosity
2. Hypoperfusion, inc. vasovagal, arrhythmia, post-cardiac arrest
3. Migraine usually hemifield loss
4. Trauma

Occipital epilepsy

Functional
O/E:
1. Optokinetic nystagmus present with rolling striped drum
2. Tunnel vision that does not widen with distance

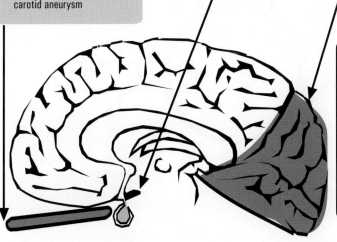

Examination
1. Optic disc abnormal (optic neuritis, AION, papilloedema) or normal (retrobulbar neuritis; cortical)
2. Unilateral (optic nerve), sequential (optic nerve or chiasm), bilateral (cortex or chiasm)

Optic Atrophy – Causes

= O.P.T.I.C.

Papillitis / Papilloedema

Papillitis or retrobulbar neuritis = inflammation of optic nerve head or behind nerve head

V.I.S.I.O.N.

Vascular: 'AION' or 'PION' (anterior or posterior ischaemic optic neuropathy)
1. Thromboembolic
2. Vasculitis: giant-cell arteritis, SLE, antiphospholipid syn.

Inflammatory: 'optic neuritis':
1. Multiple sclerosis
2. Devic's disease
3. ADEM

Sarcoid / other granulomatous: CRION (chronic relapsing inflammatory optic neuropathy)

Infection:
1. Virus
2. TB, syphilis
3. Sinus infection – contiguous

Other: GBS, vaccination

Neoplasia: lymphoma, leukaemia

Chronic papilloedema may also cause optic atrophy, e.g. due to primary intracranial hypertension

Toxins / Nutritional

Toxins
1. Chloroquine
2. Isoniazid, ethambutol
3. Lead, thallium

Nutritional
1. Vit B12 deficiency
2. Vit B1 deficiency – 'tobacco/alcohol amblyopia'
   • Due to combination of cyanide in tobacco and thiamine (Vit B1) deficiency
   • Strachan's syndrome is association of this with peripheral neuropathy, ataxia and dermatitis

Inherited

1. Leber's hereditary optic atrophy (LHOA):
   Epi:
   • Mitochondrial disease
   • Men are more symptomatic
   • Onset in 20–30s
   PC:
   • Attacks of acute visual loss, sequentially in each eye
   • Ataxia, cardiac defects
   O/E: initially papilloedema, circumpapillary telangiectasia

2. Neuropathy-associated
   • Charcot–Marie–Tooth disease
   • Refsum's disease

3. Ataxia-associated:
   • Friedreich's ataxia
   • Leukodystrophies

4. D.I.D.M.O.A.D.
   = **D**iabetes insipidus, **D**iabetes mellitus, **O**ptic **A**trophy, **D**eafness (autosomal recessive)

NB: Hereditary causes are often associated with **retinitis pigmentosa**, which presents as nyctalopia (night-blindness)

Ocular

1. Glaucoma
   chronic open-angle: presents with visual loss due to arcuate scotomas and tunnel vision
2. Graves' disease
3. High myopia

Compression

1. Neoplasia:
   • Optic nerve tumour: glioma, sheath meningioma
   • Pituitary tumour
   • Meningeal ca., leukaemia
2. Carotid aneurysm
3. Paget's disease

Papilloedema – Causes

ICP ↑

D.I.V.I.N.I.T.Y.

Developmental: hydrocephalus – esp. obstructive
Infection: meningo-encephalitis
Vascular: • Large cerebral infarct or bleed with oedema
  • Subarachnoid haemorrhage
Inflammation: vasculitis, sarcoid
Neoplasia: • Brain tumour, or spinal cord tumour (high CSF protein)
  • Meningeal
Injury: trauma
Toxin/Nutritional
  • drug overdose, alcohol, lead poisoning;
    estrogens (OCP, pregnancy), Vit A excess
  • Vit B12 deficiency
Y: • h**Y**pertension, idiopathic intracranial (assoc. obesity)
  • h**Y**ponatraemia (esp. rapid), h**Y**pocalcaemia (esp. hereditary)

Pseudopapilloedema

1. Hypermetropes
2. Drusen on disc
3. Medullated nerve fibres

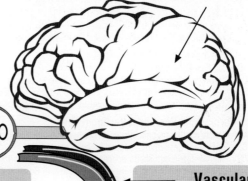

Papillitis

V.I.S.I.O.N.

Vascular – 'AION'
  (anterior ischaemic optic
  neuropathy):
  • Thromboembolic
  • Vasculitis: giant-cell arteritis
Inflammatory: 'optic neuritis':
  multiple sclerosis / ADEM
Sarcoid / CRION
Infection:
  • Virus, TB, syphilis
  • Sinus infection – contiguous
Other: Guillain–Barré syndrome,
  due to high CSF protein
Neoplasia: lymphoma, leukaemia

Vascular

Arterial flow ↑
  1. Malignant hypertension
  2. CO_2 retention
  3. Haematological:
    • Chronic anemia (high-output state)
    • Polycythaemia
    • Coagulopathy, e.g. DIC
Venous flow ↓
  1. Venous occlusion
    • Central retinal vein occlusion
    • Cavernous sinus thrombosis,
      carotico-cavernous fistula
    • SVCO
  2. Compression of optic nerve:
    • Optic glioma / meningioma
    • Orbital cellulitis
    • Thyroid eye disease

Vertigo

Def   Illusory sensation of movement, esp. rotation

Causes

Physiological   e.g. post-rotation, caloric testing
Visual / Somatosensory   e.g. refractive error, extraocular muscle palsy, peripheral neuropathy
Vestibular

I.M.B.A.L.A.N.C.E.

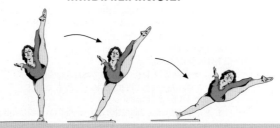

Peripheral

Infection / **I**schaemia / **I**njury – labyrinthitis
Path: Virus (associated with URTI), ischaemia (internal auditory artery), head injury
PC: Severe vertigo, N+V for days–weeks; deafness may also occur if cochlea involved

Ménière's disease
Path: Endolymphatic oedema
PC: 1. Paroxysmal vertigo for 20 min – 3 hrs, severe; associated N+V, aural fullness
        – may also present as paroxysmal drop attacks or ataxia with past-pointing
     2. Low-frequency deafness and tinnitus: initially paroxysmal, later continuous

Benign Paroxysmal Positional Vertigo (BPPV)
Path: Utricle sheds otoconia into posterior semicircular canal; often follows labyrinthitis
PC: Vertigo for secs–mins, induced by head rotation
O/E: Hallpike manouvre elicits upbeat–torsional nystagmus that exhibits:
        a) Latency; b) Adaptation; c) Fatiguability; d) Position-changing with return of position

Aminoglycosides (e.g. gentamicin) / furosemide

Lymph, peri-, fistula
Path: Trauma, congenital deformity, or superior-canal dehiscence
PC: Paroxysmal vertigo, high-frequency deafness, esp. when lying on ear
O/E: Nystagmus evoked by loud sound (Tullio's phenomenon) or pressure in external meatus

Arterial
1. Migraine, vertebrobasilar:
   PC: Headache, N+V may accompany, or occur at other times; focal numbness; dysarthria
2. TIA / stroke (e.g.in arteriopath, atrial fibrillation) PC: Attacks usually shorter than migraine

Nerve, vestibulocochlear lesion
Path: acoustic neuroma, meningitis, sarcoidosis, base of skull fracture

Central

Central lesions / **C**ervico-medullary lesion / **C**hannelopathy (episodic ataxia)
Path: Brainstem demyelination (multiple sclerosis, ADEM), tumour, VZV

Epilepsy, complex partial / **E**xtra: psychogenic

<u>Deafness</u>

<u>Causes</u>

<u>Conductive</u>

W.I.D.E.N.I.N.G.

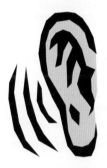

Wax in external auditory meatus

Infection – otitis media
Path: • Acute: *Streptococcus pyogenes, Haemophilus influenzae*
      • Chronic ('glue ear'): assoc. large adenoids, cleft palate, Down's syn., TB
O/E: Effusion on otoscopy

Drum perforation: noise injury; barotrauma (e.g. pilots, divers)

Extra: ossicle discontinuity – otosclerosis, trauma (note: normal otoscopy)

Neoplasia: glomus jugulare, carcinoma

INjury

Granulomatous: Wegener's / sarcoid

<u>Sensorineural</u>

D.I.V.I.N.I.T.Y.

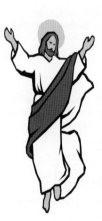

Developmental / **D**egenerative
  Developmental:
    1. Genetic: connexin mutation, Refsum's disease, Waardenburg's syndrome
    2. Congenital: TORCH infections, esp. syphilis (late-onset), rubella
    3. Perinatal: anoxia (cerebral palsy)
  Degenerative: Presbyacusis: high-tone deafness

Infection
    1. VZV (O/E: Vesicles on eardrum!), measles, mumps, influenza
    2. Meningitis: *Haemophilus influenzae*

Vascular
    1. Ischaemia: internal auditory artery 'AICA' – sudden hearing loss and vertigo
    2. Haemorrhage: superficial siderosis (slow haemorrhage following old brain op.)

Inflammation:
  Vasculitis, sarcoid

Neoplasia
    1. Cerebellopontine angle tumour, e.g. acoustic neuroma
    – commonest cause of unilateral sensorineural deafness
    2. Meningeal carcinoma, leukaemia, melanoma

Injury
    1. Noise: 4 kHz notch in audiogram, later high-frequency
    2. Trauma: including trivial head injury

Toxins
  Gentamicin, furosemide, quinine, aspirin

Y: l**Y**mph
    1. Endol**Y**mph h**Y**drops = Ménière's disease: low-tone deafness
    2. Peril**Y**mph fistula (ruptured oval or round window)

Facial Nerve Palsy

Anatomy

- The facial nerve (cranial nerve VII) has a long course, with branches at different points
- The location of the lesion can be ascertained by testing the several functions that it serves, as well as by testing functions of adjacent structures

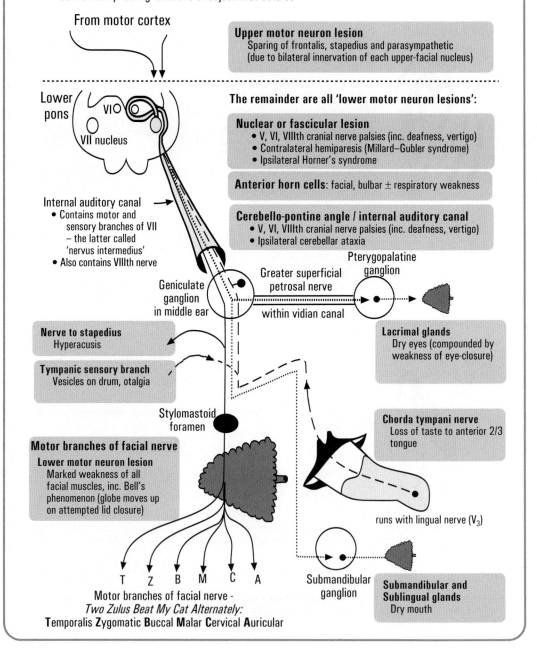

From motor cortex

Upper motor neuron lesion
Sparing of frontalis, stapedius and parasympathetic
(due to bilateral innervation of each upper-facial nucleus)

Lower pons
VI○
VII nucleus

The remainder are all 'lower motor neuron lesions':

Nuclear or fascicular lesion
- V, VI, VIIth cranial nerve palsies (inc. deafness, vertigo)
- Contralateral hemiparesis (Millard–Gubler syndrome)
- Ipsilateral Horner's syndrome

Anterior horn cells: facial, bulbar ± respiratory weakness

Internal auditory canal
- Contains motor and sensory branches of VII – the latter called 'nervus intermedius'
- Also contains VIIIth nerve

Cerebello-pontine angle / internal auditory canal
- V, VI, VIIIth cranial nerve palsies (inc. deafness, vertigo)
- Ipsilateral cerebellar ataxia

Geniculate ganglion in middle ear

Greater superficial petrosal nerve

within vidian canal

Pterygopalatine ganglion

Nerve to stapedius
Hyperacusis

Tympanic sensory branch
Vesicles on drum, otalgia

Lacrimal glands
Dry eyes (compounded by weakness of eye-closure)

Stylomastoid foramen

Chorda tympani nerve
Loss of taste to anterior 2/3 tongue

Motor branches of facial nerve

Lower motor neuron lesion
Marked weakness of all facial muscles, inc. Bell's phenomenon (globe moves up on attempted lid closure)

runs with lingual nerve (V₃)

T Z B M C A

Submandibular ganglion

Submandibular and Sublingual glands
Dry mouth

Motor branches of facial nerve -
Two Zulus Beat My Cat Alternately:
Temporalis **Z**ygomatic **B**uccal **M**alar **C**ervical **A**uricular

Causes

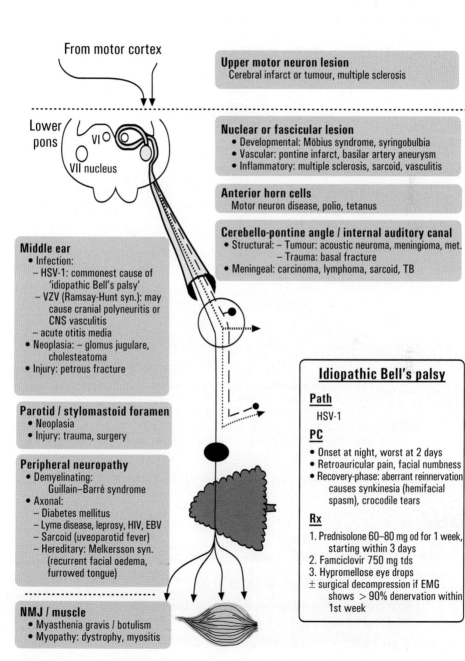

From motor cortex

Upper motor neuron lesion
Cerebral infarct or tumour, multiple sclerosis

Lower pons

VI

VII nucleus

Nuclear or fascicular lesion
- Developmental: Möbius syndrome, syringobulbia
- Vascular: pontine infarct, basilar artery aneurysm
- Inflammatory: multiple sclerosis, sarcoid, vasculitis

Anterior horn cells
Motor neuron disease, polio, tetanus

Cerebello-pontine angle / internal auditory canal
- Structural: – Tumour: acoustic neuroma, meningioma, met.
             – Trauma: basal fracture
- Meningeal: carcinoma, lymphoma, sarcoid, TB

Middle ear
- Infection:
  – HSV-1: commonest cause of 'idiopathic Bell's palsy'
  – VZV (Ramsay-Hunt syn.): may cause cranial polyneuritis or CNS vasculitis
  – acute otitis media
- Neoplasia: – glomus jugulare, cholesteatoma
- Injury: petrous fracture

Parotid / stylomastoid foramen
- Neoplasia
- Injury: trauma, surgery

Peripheral neuropathy
- Demyelinating:
  Guillain–Barré syndrome
- Axonal:
  – Diabetes mellitus
  – Lyme disease, leprosy, HIV, EBV
  – Sarcoid (uveoparotid fever)
  – Hereditary: Melkersson syn. (recurrent facial oedema, furrowed tongue)

NMJ / muscle
- Myasthenia gravis / botulism
- Myopathy: dystrophy, myositis

Idiopathic Bell's palsy

Path
HSV-1

PC
- Onset at night, worst at 2 days
- Retroauricular pain, facial numbness
- Recovery-phase: aberrant reinnervation causes synkinesia (hemifacial spasm), crocodile tears

Rx
1. Prednisolone 60–80 mg od for 1 week, starting within 3 days
2. Famciclovir 750 mg tds
3. Hypromellose eye drops
± surgical decompression if EMG shows > 90% denervation within 1st week

Neurofibromatosis

Type 1

<u>Epi</u>   Prevalence = 1 / 3000 (**30%** sporadic mutations)

<u>Gene</u>
1. Chromosome 17
2. Autosomal dominant tumour suppressor gene (as for all neurocutaneous syndromes)
3. Neurofibromin gene normally inhibits Ras-GTPase mitogenic signalling

<u>PC</u>

C.A.F.E. N.O.I.R.

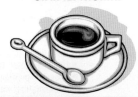

Café-au-lait spots: > 5 spots of > 1.5 cm diameter (or > 5 mm, prepuberty)

Axillary freckling, also inguinal

Fibromas, neuro-
   1. Subcutaneous: soft, firm, lobulated, mobile at right-angles to nerve only
   2. Plexiform: overgrowth of nerve trunk and overlying tissues, esp. temporal scalp
      PC: a) Cutaneous masses
         b) Compression:
            • spine / nerve roots: myelopathy, radicular pain, muscle atrophy
            • cranial nerves: trigeminal neuralgia, cerebellopontine angle tumour
            • GIT: bowel obstruction, bleeding
        c) Sarcomatous transformation in 10%

Eye 1. Lisch nodules (iris hamartomas); 2. Retinal astrocytoma; 3. Optic nerve glioma

Neoplasia
      1. CNS: meningioma, ependymoma, astrocytoma; complicating obstructive hydrocephalus
      2. Chronic or acute myeloid leukaemia
      3. MEN2b syndrome = medullary carcinoma, thyroid, phaeochromocytoma, marfanoid

Orthopaedic
      1. Spine - canal stenosis, spina bifida, kyphoscoliosis, short stature; 2. Sphenoid dysplasia

IQ ↓ / epilepsy

Renal: Wilms' tumour, renal artery stenosis / **R**espiratory: pulmonary fibrosis, pneumothorax

Type 2

<u>Epi</u>   Prevalence = 1 / 50,000

<u>Gene</u> Chromosome **22** (**MERLIN** gene = cytoskeletal proteins: Moesin, Ezrin, Radizin)

<u>PC</u>   *Think of diseases in 2s:*

Bilateral acoustic neuromas; also meningiomas, ependymomas
Bilateral posterior subcapsular cataracts
    (café-au-lait spots and peripheral neurofibromas occur rarely)

Neurocutaneous Diseases – Other

S.O.N.S. of neurofibromatosis

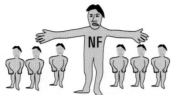

Tuberous Sclerosis

<u>Gene</u>   Chromosome 11 (80% sporadic mutations); autosomal dominant

<u>PC</u>

Skin
- Adenoma sebaceum (angiofibromata): papular rash around nose, worsens after puberty
- Shagreen patch (lumpy plaque), ashleaf macule (depigmentation seen with Wood's lamp)
- Periungual or intraoral fibromas

Ocular
- Retinal phakomas (50%; appear yellow), retinal pigmentation, optic disc drusen

Neurology
- Epilepsy (75%); IQ ↓ (50%)
- Brain tumours: subependymal tubers (hamartomas), lateral ventricle gliomas

Systemic
- Renal: adult polycystic kidney disease, angiomyolipomata (66%; cause loin pain, haematuria)
- Respiratory: pulmonary cysts, pneumothorax, pulmonary fibrosis
- Cardiac: rhabdomyosarcomas that cause arrhythmias and CCF

Sturge–Weber Syndrome

<u>PC</u>

Skin
- Port-wine stain (capillary haemangioma) on face
  - although most port-wine stains are not associated with the syndrome
- Associated with ipsilateral intracranial calcified haemangioma whose location depends on dermatome involved by stain: Vi – occipital; Vii – frontal or parietal

Ocular
- Strabismus, congenital glaucoma (appears as buphthalmos or 'ox-eye'), optic atrophy

Neurology
- Epilepsy (due to 'tramline' calcification of cortical vessels); IQ ↓
- Infantile hemiplegia–hemiatrophy

Von Hippel–Lindau Disease

<u>Gene</u>   Chromosome 3 (*VHL*)

<u>PC</u>

Skin   • Polycythaemia, secondary to renal cysts or cerebellar haemangioblastoma

Ocular   • Retinal angioma

Neurology • Cerebellar or spinal cord haemangioma (-blastoma)

Systemic • Polycystic kidney disease, renal cell carcinoma
- Adrenal phaeochromocytoma
- Other: epididymis, liver, pancreas cysts

Endocrinology

Diabetes Mellitus – Causes

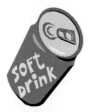

P.E.P.S.I. & C.O.K.E -
make sure it's diet!

Primary
　　Type 1: autoimmune destruction of β-cells of pancreatic islets of Langerhans: always causes IDDM.
　　　　Epi: Inc: Prevalence = 1–2% population, and rising
　　　　　　Age: Children – 30 yrs
　　　　　　Aet: a) Genetic: DR3, 4 ↑es risk, but MZ Concordance = 50 %
　　　　　　　　　b) Infection: CMV, EBV, coxsackie, congenital rubella (seasonal onset of diabetes)
　　　　　　　　　c) Cows' milk in babies: bovine serum antigen cross-reacts with β-cell protein p69
　　　　　　Path: anti-islet-cell Abs (esp. glutamic acid dehydrogenase) &/or anti-insulin Abs
　　Type 2: peripheral insulin resistance ± insulin ↓ ± hepatic glucose efflux ↑: causes IDDM or NIDDM.
　　　　Epi: Inc: Prevalence = 5%
　　　　　　Age: Increases with age, but inherited types occur in children
　　　　　　Geo: Indian, African
　　　　　　Aet: a) Genetic: MZ concordance = 90%
　　　　　　　　　b) Syndrome X = DM + central obesity + ↑ABP + ↑ lipids, due to ↑ liver fat synthesis
　　　　　　　　　c) Amylin deposition in islets (= hypoglycaemic hormone secreted by islet cells)
　　Hereditary: 1. Insulin hyposecretion: MODY (Maturity Onset Diabetes of Young) – like type 2 DM
　　　　　　　　　　　Aet: glucokinase or hepatocyte nuclear transcription factor Δ (autosomal dominant)
　　　　　　　　2. Insulin resistance: leprechaunism; lipodystrophy

Endocrine
　　1. Stress Hormone Excess: *in temporal order of release:*
　　　　　Adrenaline　→　Glucagon　　→　Glucocorticoid　→ Growth Hormone　→　　T4
　　　　　(Phaeochromo-　(Glucagonoma)　(Cushing's)　　(Acromegaly)　　(Thyrotoxicosis)
　　　　　cytoma)
　　2. Stress Response: sepsis, surgery, trauma → hypercortisolaemia → insulin resistance
　　　　　　　　　　　　　sub-arachnoid haemorrhage
　　3. Estrogen: gestational diabetes; polycystic ovaries syn.; oral contraceptive pill

Pancreatic disease: chronic pancreatitis, (alcohol, cystic fibrosis, malnutrition);
　　　　　haemochromatosis; pancreas ca.(late)

Steroids

Inherited:
　　1. Neurological: myotonic dystrophy; Friedreich's ataxia; ataxia telangiectasia; Huntington's chorea
　　2. Glycogen storage disease
　　3. Other - Lawrence-Moon-Biedl syn; DIDMOAD (Diabetes Insipidus, DM, Optic Atrophy, Deafness) syn.

Chromosomal: Down's, Turner's, Kleinfelter's syndrome

Organ failure: liver / congestive cardiac failure

Kidney failure: due to insulin resistance; insulin hyposecretion; peritoneal dialysis (glucose in dialysate)

Exogenous: diuretics (thiazides, loop), adrenergic stimulants (salbutamol, amphetamines),
　　　　　pancreatic toxins (pentamidine), chemo Rx (e.g. alloxan)

Insulin – Physiology

The causes, complications and treatment of diabetes are most easily understood by appreciating the normal regulation and actions of insulin:

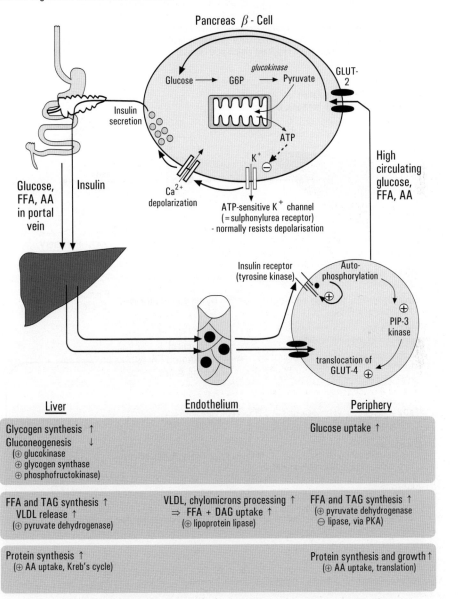

Pancreas β - Cell

Liver	Endothelium	Periphery

Glycogen synthesis ↑
 Gluconeogenesis ↓
   (⊕ glucokinase
   ⊕ glycogen synthase
   ⊕ phosphofructokinase)
		Glucose uptake ↑

FFA and TAG synthesis ↑
   VLDL release ↑
   (⊕ pyruvate dehydrogenase)
	VLDL, chylomicrons processing ↑
	   ⇒ FFA + DAG uptake ↑
	   (⊕ lipoprotein lipase)
		FFA and TAG synthesis ↑
		   (⊕ pyruvate dehydrogenase
		   ⊖ lipase, via PKA)

Protein synthesis ↑
   (⊕ AA uptake, Kreb's cycle)
		Protein synthesis and growth ↑
		   (⊕ AA uptake, translation)

Key: ⊕ insulin activates; ⊖ insulin inhibits; FFA free fatty acids; TAG triacylglyceride; DAG diacylglyceride; PKA protein kinase A; AA amino acids; GLUT glucose transporter; PIP phosphatidylinositol phosphate

Diabetic Ketoacidosis

Path Combination of **insulin deficiency** (e.g. first presentation, forgot insulin, inadequate dosage) and
sympathetic stimulation (e.g sepsis, MI, volume depleted, cocaine), results in:-
1. Glucose uptake ↓ and glucose release ↑   ⇒ hyperglycaemia
2. Osmotic diuresis → hypovolaemia → tissue ischaemia and renal failure ⇒ lactic acidosis
3. Compensation for lack of intracellular glucose by lipolysis (with resultant ketosis)
    and proteolysis (with resultant amino-acid release)   ⇒ metabolic acidosis

Insulin   ↓
Sympathetic stimulation   ↑
Glucagon, growth hormone, cortisol ↑

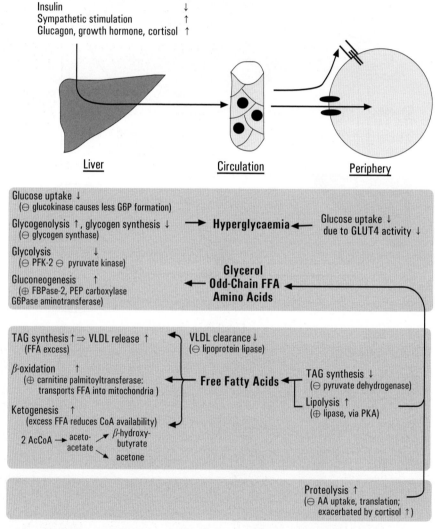

Liver   Circulation   Periphery

Glucose uptake ↓
 (⊖ glucokinase causes less G6P formation)

Glycogenolysis ↑, glycogen synthesis ↓   **→ Hyperglycaemia ←**   Glucose uptake ↓
 (⊖ glycogen synthase)   due to GLUT4 activity ↓

Glycolysis   ↓
 (⊖ PFK-2 ⊖ pyruvate kinase)   **Glycerol**
                                              ← Odd-Chain FFA ←
Gluconeogenesis   ↑   **Amino Acids**
 (⊕ FBPase-2, PEP carboxylase
 G6Pase aminotransferase)

TAG synthesis ↑ ⇒ VLDL release ↑   VLDL clearance ↓
 (FFA excess)   (⊖ lipoprotein lipase)

β-oxidation   ↑   TAG synthesis ↓
 (⊕ carnitine palmitoyltransferase: **Free Fatty Acids ←**   (⊖ pyruvate dehydrogenase)
 transports FFA into mitochondria)
                                                                Lipolysis ↑
Ketogenesis   ↑   (⊕ lipase, via PKA)
 (excess FFA reduces CoA availability)

  2 AcCoA → aceto- ↗ β-hydroxy-
            acetate   butyrate
                    ↘ acetone

                                                               Proteolysis ↑
                                                                (⊖ AA uptake, translation;
                                                                 exacerbated by cortisol ↑)

Key: ⊕ activation; ⊖ inhibition; FFA free fatty acids; TAG triacylglyceride; PKA protein kinase A;
AA amino acids; GLUT glucose transporter; FBPase fructose-1,2-biphosphatase; PEP phosphoenolpyruvate;
PFK phosphofructokinase; G6P glucose-6-phosphate; AcCoA acetyl coenzyme A; VLDL very-low density lipoprotein

PC   *D.K.A.*

Diuresis, osmotic / **D**ehydration
PC: polyuria, polydipsia, blurred vision (refractive error due to hyperglycaemic osmotic shift)
O/E: fast, thready pulse; hypotensive; collapsed veins; dry skin, tongue; skin turgor ↓; temp. ↓
Complications: cerebral oedema (confusion, coma); acute renal failure; deep-vein thrombosis

Kussmaul's breathing (deep sighs; also air hunger) / **K**etotic breath
K$^+$: initially hyperkalaemic, but becomes hypokalaemic with insulin Rx; risk of cardiac arrest

Abdominal
• Abdominal pain ('acute abdomen') - consider acute pancreatitis due to hyperlipidaemia
• N+V - consider acute gastric dilatation, but appetite ↑ (due to hypothalamic uptake ↓)

Ix Bloods
• U&E: urea: ↑↑ due to dehydration, proteolysis; creatinine ↑ (inc. false +ve due to ketone-bodies)
  Na$^+$: ↓ (peripheral osmotic activity, and hyperlipidaemia causing pseudohyponatraemia)
  K$^+$: initially ↑ ⇒ ↓ with insulin Rx; HCO$_3^-$↓ (weakness; SOB), and Cl$^-$↑: both occur on Rx
  anion gap (Na+K)-(Cl+HCO3-) > 18mmol/l, due to ketone bodies, lactate
• Arterial-blood gas: metabolic acidosis: PO$_4$ < 24 mmol/l, base excess > 2 mmol/l
• Glucose: typically 15 - 33 mmol/l; triglycerides ↑ (VLDL or chylomicrons)
• Ketone bodies; ratio of β-hydroxybutyrate: acetoacetate ↑es with hypoxia, due to shock
• FBC: neutrophilia (leukaemoid reaction); AST ↑ due to shock

Urine • glucose + + +
       • ketones +, but may be falsely negative if shocked or hypoxic, due to high BHB:AcAc ratio.
Microbiology   MSU, blood cultures
Monitor   2-hourly blood glucose, K$^+$
ECG   myocardial infarction (cause or effect); effects of hyper- or hypokalaemia
Radiology   CXR - infection; PAXR - gastric dilatation; ground-glass appearance

Rx   ITU:
                                 • NaHCO$_3$: If pH < 7.1, and SBP < 90mmHg
                                 • Dexamethasone: If cerebral oedema

B. Ventilatory support
1. O$_2$
2. Ventilation, if persistent
   acidosis

C. Hydration
1. Type:
   • Colloid 500 ml: If SBP < 90 mmHg
   • N. saline: 2l in 2° ⇒ 2l in 4° ⇒ 4l in 24°
   • 5% dextrose when glucose < 15 mmol/l
   • 10% dextrose if persisting acidosis and ketosis
2. KCL
   • Add 20 mmol to each litre after 1st litre
   • Titrate: [K$^+$] of 3 mmol/l = 300 mmol deficit
   • Caution if oliguric
3. Phosphate: IV or po as K$^+$ or Na$^+$ acid salt

A. Assessment
C.O.A.T.I.N'
Cardiac monitor
O$_2$
ABP
TPR ⇒ space blanket?
Input + output chart
(inc. nasogastric tube,
   urine catheter)
Neurological observations

D. Medication
1. IV Soluble Insulin (50 units in 50 ml N. saline)
   • 10 units stat ⇒ 6 - 10 units / hr
   • Sliding scale (e.g. 3 units / hr, while BM > 15)
2. Treat precipitant: e.g. antibiotics, thrombolysis
3. LMW heparin

Diabetes – HONK

Def   Hyperosmolar non-ketoacidosis

Path   1. Sustained, **partial** insulin deficiency, leads to hyperglycaemia (via ↓ glucose uptake and ↑ glucose release), but **not** β-oxidation of lipids or ketogenesis. Consequently, **acidosis does not occur initially**, and the condition presents later than DKA with very high glucose levels and extreme dehydration.
2. Predisposing: type 2 (NIDDM) or type 1 (IDDM) with inadequate insulin dose, plus supervening stress, e.g. sepsis, myocardial infarction, stroke, or initiation of diabetogenic drug (e.g. steroid, thiazide).

PC   HONK presents similarly to DKA, except for the following features:

H.O.N.K.

Hyperosmolar / **H**ypernatraemia / **H**yperglycaemia
All are more extreme than in diabetic ketoacidosis
PC: • Polyuria, polydipsia
• Fatigue
• Blurred vision (refractive error due to hyperglycaemic osmotic shift)
O/E: Fast, thready pulse; hypotensive; collapsed veins; dry skin, tongue; skin turgor ↓; temp. ↓
Complications: Cerebral oedema (confusion, coma); acute renal failure; deep-vein thrombosis
Ix: Typical values:
    Osmolality, serum   > 350 mosm/kg
    Na$^+$ > 150 mmol/l
    Glucose   > 35 mmol/l

O: n**O** ketosis / n**O** acidosis / n**O** vomiting or hyperventilation
• Ketosis may occur if patient fails to eat
• Acidosis may occur later, if pre-renal renal failure develops

Neurological
1. Lethargy, confusion, coma
2. Focal – seizures (e.g. Jacksonian); cranial nerve palsies
3. Strokes – due to intravascular depletion, and resultant hyperviscosity

Negative: Gram –ve septicaemia + other infections, e.g. pneumococcal pneumonia

K: Coagulation complications: DVT, CVA, DIC, acute pancreatitis

K$^+$: total body K$^+$ is lower than in DKA, and so is more unstable with Rx

Rx   HONK is treated similarly to DKA, except for:-

H.o.N.K.

Half-**N**ormal saline (0.45%) is used for rehydration, unless systolic blood pressure < 90 mmHg (use normal saline), or when glucose < 15 mmol/l (use 5% dextrose)

Half-**N**ormal insulin rate: 3 units / hour

K: Coagulation prophylaxis: subcutaneous LMW heparin

K$^+$: monitor more frequently at 30 min after insulin Rx, and 2-hourly thereafter

Diabetes – Lactic Acidosis

Path
Lactic acidosis is more likely to occur in diabetics, due to:
1. Inhibition of gluconeogenesis • Metformin therapy (type 2 DM (NIDDM))
                                   • Liver or renal failure
2. Hypoxia secondary to pneumonia or CCF
3. Shock, e.g. pancreatitis

PC
1. Hyperventilation
2. Fatigue, confusion, coma

Ix
Bloods
Lactate > 5 mmol/l (also apparent as a wide anion gap,
            where anion gap = $(Na^+ + K^+) - (Cl^- + HCO_3^-) > 18$ mmol/l)
ABGs: metabolic acidosis
Renal: may demonstrate renal impairment as a cause of lactic acidosis
Glucose: normal – slightly

Urine
Ketone –ve

Microbiology
Blood, urine, CSF cultures

ECG

Radiology
CXR – pneumonia

Rx
1. Underlying cause
2. O_2 (± ventilation)
3. IV $NaHCO_3$ – ☠ = paradoxical intracellular acidosis!
4. Haemodialysis, to clear lactic acid, and to clear sodium when $NaHCO_3$ given

Prog
Poor, when due to underlying organ failure

Diabetes Mellitus – Chronic Complications

PC *C.A.N.N.O.N.I.C.A.L.*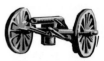

Macrovascular

Cardiology – ischaemic heart disease
Epi: Premenopausal women relatively most affected due to loss of protective effect of estrogen
PC: 1. Myocardial infarction / acute coronary syndromes:
- Classically 'silent' due to coexisting autonomic neuropathy
- More often complicated by cardiac failure and shock
- Rx involves intensive insulin regime, usually with IV 'sliding scale'
2. Cardiomyopathy = left-ventricular failure in presence of normal CXR and angiogram

Arterial insufficiency – peripheral vascular disease
PC: 1. Intermittent claudication ⇒ rest pain, due to tibial or iliofemoral artery insufficiency
2. Ulcer, gangrene *(see opposite)*

Neurological – large-vessel or lacunar stroke / TIA

Microvascular

Neurological – peripheral and autonomic neuropathy
1. Peripheral • 'Glove and stocking' sensory neuropathy; amyotrophy (painful, wasted
quadriceps); cranial neuropathies
- Mononeuritis multiplex
- Entrapment (carpal tunnel or ulnar neuropathies); ulcers *(see opposite)*
2. Autonomic: impotence, frequency, gustatory sweating, gastroparesis, postural hypotension

Ophthalmopathy
Lens / glaucoma / retinopathy *(see opposite)*

Nephropathy, inc. **N**ephrotic syndrome
1. Microalbuminuria (albumin excretion rate: 30–300 mg/day) ⇒ nephrotic syn. (> 3g/day)
2. Chronic renal failure
3. Renal tubular acidosis type 4: hyporeninaemic hypoaldosteronism (long-standing type 1 DM)

Immunocompromise
1. Bacteria: boils, UTI, pneumonia, osteomyelitis
2. Other: Candida (pruritus vulvae, balanitis), mucormycosis (proptosis), TB

Cutaneous
1. Pigmentation: acanthosis nigricans, diabetic dermopathy (pigmented scars on shins)
2. Necrobiosisis lipoidica diabeticorum (erythematous plaque, sunken, yellow atrophic skin)
3. Other: vitiligo (association with type 1 DM), scleroderma-like skin, granuloma annulare

Arthritis
1. Cheirarthropathy = limited joint mobility and contractures; 'prayer sign': can't appose palms
2. Pseudogout
3. Charcot's joints (neuropathic)

Lethargy / **L**oss of weight

Foot Ulcers

May be due either to arterial insufficiency or to neuropathy

Ischaemic ulcer	Neuropathic ulcer

Ischaemic ulcer

PC:
  Painful ulcer (sensation preserved)
  Colour: white on lying → red on standing

O/E:
  Site: foot margin
  Edge: ragged
  Skin: • Pale, cold, thin, hairless
         • Absent-weak pulses; bruits

Associations
  Infection: pus, crepitus, foul odour
  (also with neuropathic ulcer)

Neuropathic ulcer

PC:
  Painless and numb
    – pt ignores repetitive trauma

O/E:
  Site: metatarsal heads, calcaneum
  Edges: cleanly punched-out ulcer
  Skin: • Surrounding callus
         • Dry, fissured skin (sweat loss)
         • Warm, erythema, oedema,
           distended veins (sympathetic loss)

Associations
  • Pes cavus, claw toes, Charcot joints,
  • Lisfranc deformity: neuropathic subluxation
    of tarsal and metatarsals → convex sole

Ophthalmopathy   (50%)

1. Lens: • Acute blurred vision, due to osmotic-induced swelling of the lens (DKA)
           • Cataracts: senile or juvenile 'snowflake'
2. Glaucoma – open-angle, or closed-angle due to rubeosis iridis
3. Retinopathy:

Background	Preproliferative	Proliferative
1. Fluorescein angiogram: leakiness ↑ 2. Haemorrhages: a) Dot = microaneurysm b) Blot = deep retina c) Flame = superficial 3. Hard exudates: lipoprotein precipitates	1. Cotton-wool spots: retinal infarction 2. Venule dilatation; looping; beading 3. Intraretinal microvascular abnormalities (IRMA) 4. Avascular; featureless periphery	1. New vessels leashes and fronds on disc or vein bifurcations 2. Haemorrhages vitreous; preretinal 3. Rubeosis iridis: anterior extension of angiogenesis 4. Advanced: retinal fibrosis and tear

± Maculopathy: may occur at any stage, due to hard exudates; oedema; ischaemia involving fovea
± Other: retinal vein or artery thrombosis; ischaemic papillitis; lipaemia retinalis (if chylomicrons ↑)

Diabetes Mellitus – Diagnosis

Urinalysis

Method: Glucose oxidase or reducing-substance reagent
Sensitivity = 30%
　　　　False –ve: elderly, due to higher renal threshold;
　　　　(normal threshold for glycosuria > 7–13 mmol/l blood glucose)
Specificity = 99%
　　　　False +ve:
　　　　1. Glomerular filtration ↑ed, e.g. pregnancy
　　　　2. Tubular resorption ↓ed, e.g. renal tubular acidosis
　　　　3. Reducing substances (only, if using reducing-substance reagent), e.g.:
　　　　　　● Drugs, inc. salicylates, isoniazid, L-DOPA, tetracycline, Vit C
　　　　　　● Galactosaemia, fructosaemia, homogentisic acid (alkaptonuria)

Plasma Glucose

Method: 1. Capillary ('BM'), or venous sample (use fluoride oxalate tube – inhibits RBC glycolysis)
　　　　2. Two samples, on different occasions required (unless plainly symptomatic)
　　　　3. Postprandial glucose should not be taken < 2 hrs, due to normal high variability

Fasting (8-hr)		Postprandial (2-hr post 75 g glucose load)	
Normal	< 6 mmol/l	Normal	< 7.8 mmol/l
Impaired fasting glycaemia	6–7 mmol/l	Impaired glucose tolerance	7.8–11 mmol/l
Diabetes mellitus	> 7 mmol/l	Diabetes mellitus	> 11 mmol/l

Guidelines from American Diabetes Association 1997;
WHO guidelines suggest diabetes mellitus if fasting glucose > 7.8 mmol/l

Oral Glucose Tolerance Test (OGTT)

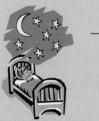 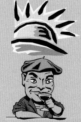 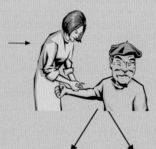

1. Normal diet for 3 days
　prior to test
2. Fast overnight
　(allowed water)
3. No smoking or exercise
　allowed during test

75 g glucose drink

Fasting
glucose

1- and 2-hour
glucose
(postprandial)

Interpret results as shown
for plasma glucose above

Diabetes Mellitus – Monitoring

The 4 C's

Control, glycaemic
1. Record of acute complications: DKA, hypoglycaemic episodes
2. Self-monitoring
   a) Urine dipstick
      Indications:
         a) children during infection (ketone sticks), or unwilling to prick finger
         b) elderly or type 2 DM: tight glycaemic control unnecessary (but higher renal threshold)
      ☠ Can't detect hypoglycaemia, and reflects mean glycaemia since bladder last emptied
   b) Capillary-blood glucose ('BM stick')
      Mechanism:
         glucose oxidase reagent + glucose → hydrogen peroxide → redox potential change
      Target: aim for 4.4–6.7 mmol/l (fasting) or 4.4–9 mmol/l (2-hour postprandial)

	Fasting (8-hr)		Postprandial (2-hr post 75g glucose load)
Desirable	4.5–7.0 mmol/l	Desirable	4.5–9.0 mmol/l
Acceptable	< 7.8 mmol/l	Acceptable	< 10.0 mmol/l

   Adjust insulin dose only after several days of abnormal pattern;
   do not adjust with every measurement (i.e. the 'sliding-scale approach')

3. Glycated Haemoglobin (HbA1c)
   Mechanism:
      a) HbA-valine + glucose → irreversible non-enzymatic glycation → HbA1
      b) electrophoresis separates HbA1 into more stable component HbA1c
   Indication: Reflects total glucose exposure over previous 6–8 weeks (RBC half-life):
      a) detects poor compliance with Rx
      b) prognostic indicator for retinopathy
   Target:

Normal:	5–8 % HbA1/HbA
Acceptable:	8–9.5 % HbA1/HbA

   False –ve: haemolysis: ↑ RBC turnover; false +ve: abnormally migrating Hb variants

Complications
1. Peripheral pulses, ABP, cardiac and carotid auscultation
2. Fundoscopy, sensory testing; feet inspection (inc. nails)
3. Urine albumin:creatinine ratio; U+Es

Competency with insulin administration, 'BM' monitoring; check insulin injection sites

Career / contraception, etc: psychosocial, domestic, occupation

Diabetes – Conservative Rx

D.E.L.A.Y.S. complications!

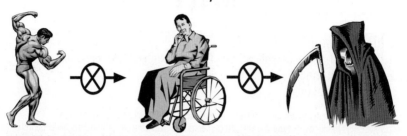

Diet
1. High-Carbohydrate (should be $> 60\%$ of calorie intake)
   - Select food with low glycaemic index (defined as plasma glucose at 3 hours after 50 g carbohydrate, relative to that of white bread)
   - Examples: complex carbohydrates, not mono- or disaccharides
   - Aspartame sweetener
2. Low-Fat (should be $< 20\%$ of calorie intake)
   - High polyunsaturates, e.g. vegetable oil; low eggs; milk-cheese; fried food
   - Drugs: orlistat (gut lipase inhibition), sibutramine (SNRI)
   - Surgery: gastric banding, gastric bypass (roux-en-Y) –
     $\downarrow$ es mortality in type 2 patients with body mass index $> 40\text{kg/m}^2$
3. Low-Protein (should be $< 15\%$ of calorie intake): Select fish; pulses
4. High-Fibre: high-soluble fibre $\downarrow$ es glucose absorption from gut $\Rightarrow$ overcomes requirement for phase 1 insulin release in type 2 diabetes

Exercise improves glycaemic control; $\downarrow$ CVS complications, $\downarrow$ weight

Lipids:
1. Monitor LDL:HDL cholesterol ratio and fasting triglycerides
2. Have a lower threshold for starting a statin

ABP $\uparrow$ (hypertension):
1. Reduce salt intake, alcohol
2. Drugs:
   - ACE inhibitors or A-II antagonists are best due to their reno-protective effects
   - β-blockers discouraged as they mask hypoglycaemia
   - Thiazides: cause hyperglycaemia

Yearly check-up
1. Ophthalmological assessment: Snellen chart, dilated fundoscopy
2. Renal function: albumin: creatinine ratio or 24-hour urine albumin

Smoking, Spirits and Sex
Smoking: increases risk of all complications
Spirits (alcohol): avoid alcohol binges (hypoglycaemia)
     or heavy consumption (hidden calories, hypertension)
Sex: • Contraception: use progestogen-only pill, as estrogen $\uparrow$ es glucose
     • Pregnancy: will need more intensive monitoring

<u>Diabetes – Rx of Complications</u>

Underlying causes
1. Hyperglycaemia:
    - Intensive insulin regimen: fasting glucose < 7 mmol/l; postprandial glucose < 9 mmol/l
    - Continuous sc insulin infusion: improves neuropathy, but may temporarily worsen retinopathy
    - Tolrestat: inhibits aldose reductase, which catalyses glucose + NADPH $\Rightarrow$ sorbitol (but ineffective!)
2. Hypertension and hyperlipidaemia control

Macrovascular
Relationship with glycaemia occurs at *low* HbA1c ($\therefore$ difficult to reduce risk with glucose control)

Cardiac: ischaemic heart disease – aspirin, anti-anginals, angioplasty, CABG

Arteriopathy: peripheral vascular disease – aspirin, angioplasty, bypass

Neurological: carotid disease – aspirin, endarterectomy

Microvascular
Relationship with glycaemia occurs at *high* HbA1c ($\therefore$ glycaemic control improves outcome)

Neurological:
1. Peripheral neuropathy:
    a) Intensive insulin or continuous insulin infusion
    b) Amitriptyline or gabapentin for neuropathic pain
    c) Prosthetics, e.g. foot calipers
2. Autonomic, e.g. impotence: sildenafil; intracavernosal or intra-urethral alprostadil (PGE1); vacuum
    postural hypotension hypotension: increase salt and water intake: fludrocortisone

Ophthalmopathy:
1. Cataract replacement: ☠ = worsening maculopathy ($\therefore$ perform laser Rx beforehand)
2. Argon laser photocoagulation:
    Indication: Early proliferative changes; perimaculopathy – laser applied in 'macular grid'
    Mechanism: • Focal Rx: ↓ es haemorrhage
    • Panretinal (1000–8000 burns): ↓ es release of vascular endothelial growth factor
    $\Rightarrow$ decreases blindness by 60% – ☠ = visual field loss
3. Vitrectomy:
    Indication: persistent vitreal haemorrhage, retinal detachment, severe proliferation

Nephropathy:
1. ACE inhibitors or A-II antagonists:
    Indication: Microalbuminuria
    Mechanism: Delays progression of nephropathy and treats hypertension
    ☠ = acute renal failure (if renal artery stenosis);
    hyperkalaemia (if hyporeninaemic hypoaldosteronism)
2. Protein restriction (< 50 g / day for 70 kg man) – reserved for established nephropathy

Feet
1. Hygiene: wash, dry and use moisturising cream daily; correctly fitting shoes; avoid ingrowing nails;
    avoid bare feet; meticulously inspect, and refer early for corns, calluses, etc.
2. Ulcer care: remove callus; swab; dressing; cast for pressure relief;
    antibiotics (e.g. co-amoxiclav, clindamycin)
3. Surgical: debridement + lavage; osteotomy for neuropathy or osteomyelitis; arterial bypass;
    amputation

Diabetes Mellitus – Insulin

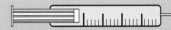

Types

Origin
1. Porcine or bovine insulin has problem of antigenicity ⇒ allergy, resistance
2. Recombinant human form has higher risk of hypoglycaemia, due to faster absorption and shorter effect

Preparation
1. Soluble: • IV: Peak 5–10 min; duration 30 min – used in DKA, HONK, perioperative
              • SC: Peak 2 hrs; duration 6 hrs – used as maintenance therapy
2. Suspension (S/C): complex of insulin with zinc crystals (Lente) or protamine (Isophane)
              • Onset 1-2 hrs; peak: 4-12 hrs; duration: < 24 hrs
3. Biphasic: soluble + suspension, e.g. Mixtard 30 = 30% soluble + 70% Isophane
              • Pens allow easy delivery of combination
4. Recombinant insulin analogue, e.g. insulin glargine or insulin detemir
              • Allows once-daily delivery

Regimens

Initiation:
Type 1 DM: start at presentation, e.g. DKA; but may need to ↓ dose or stop over weeks–months, due to
              'honeymoon period' = temporary partial islet-cell recovery
Type 2 DM: used if poor control in spite of oral hypoglycaemics; give metformin at same time (to ↓ weight)
              Benefits: Microvascular complications ↓ by 25%; post-MI mortality ↓ by 50% at 1-year
Maintenance:
1. 'Split-mixed' program:
              morning + evening biphasic insulin doses, given half-hour before breakfast + supper
2. 'Basal-bolus' program:
              bedtime long-acting + short-acting half-hour before every meal (adjust dose according to meal size)
Temporary adjustments:
1. Illness: vomiting, perioperative, pregnancy:
              • Dose must ↑ to counter sympathetic activation even if not eating, but check BMs 2–4-hourly
              • Continuous infusion (SC or IV) may be required; tolerate BM 8–10 if IHD or pre-CABG
2. Exercise   • Decrease dose before and 24 hrs post-exercise; as blood flow ↑ and glucose utilization ↓
              • Avoid injecting exercised limb: ↑ absorption; carry chocolate bar

Side-Effects ☠   G.L.A.R.G.I.N.E.

Glucose - low (hypoglycaemia): risk factors =
   • Elderly (can tolerate higher BM's because of less concern of chronic complications)
   • β-blockers (mask symptoms), alcohol binge

Local
   • Lipohypertrophy (due to lipogenic and growth effect) – Rx: rotate sites; lipoatrophy (allergy); bruising
   • Inadvertent IM injection, or limb injection (→ more rapid + unpredictable effect) – Rx: if IM then pinch skin

Atherogenesis – in high concentrations

Resistance, insulin > 200 units / day:
   • Associations: animal insulin (Ab formation), acanthosis nigracans, congenital receptor deficiency

Gain of weight in type 2 DM ∴ give with metformin

INstability – 'dawn phenomenon' or 'Somogyi effect':
   Insulin given too early in evening ⇒ hypoglycaemia through night ⇒ rebound hyperglycaemia by morning
   due to sympathetic activation, and growth hormone, cortisol release

Electrolyte – hypokalaemia: in DKA Rx

Diabetes Mellitus – Oral Hypoglycaemics

Acarbose

Mechanism:

Inhibits intestinal α-glucosidase, thereby decreasing starch and sucrose hydrolysis, and so decreasing absorption of glucose

☠ : Diarrhoea, flatulence, abnormal LFTs

Guar Gum

Inhibits glucose–Na+ co-transporter

GIT-acting drugs

Sulphonylureas: glibenclamide, gliclazide

Mechanism:

1. Inhibits ATP-dep. K$^+$ channel in islet β-cell $\Rightarrow$ ↑es basal secretion of insulin and ↑es phase 1, glucose-mediated stored-insulin secretion
2. Tissue sensitivity to insulin ↑

Types: Metabolism:

1. Long-acting   (48-hr): chlo**R**propamide   **R**enal
2. Intermediate (24-hr): glibenclamide, glimepride   Renal
                      (12-hr): gliquazone; gliclazide; glipizide   Liver
3. Short-acting   To**L**butamide   Liver

☠ : appetite ↑, weight gain; hypoglycaemia (if long-acting or organ failure); resistance (β-cell dysfunction, receptor downregulation)

Meglitinide analogues: repaglinide, netaglinide

Mechanism: Similar to sulphonylureas, but shorter acting (∴ take with meals), and have lesser risk of hypoglycaemia

Insulin secretagogues

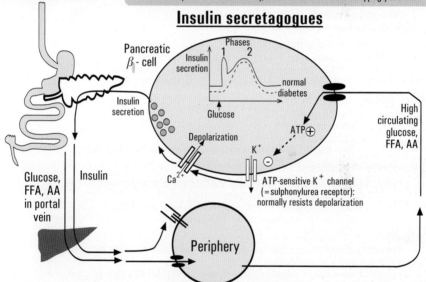

Insulin Sensitizers

Biguanides: metformin

Mechanism:

1. ↑ glucose uptake in presence of background insulin, and BM < 14 mmol/l
2. ↓ gluconeogenesis in liver, from lactic acid
3. LDL + VLDL ↓ and do *not* increase appetite:
   ∴ used in **Big** people

☠ 1. GIT Sx e.g. diarrhoea, dyspepsia, anorexia
   2. Lactic acidosis: esp. if organ failure
   3. Megaloblastic anaemia: Vit B12 absorption ↓

Thiazolinediones: rosiglitazone, pioglitazone

Mechanism:

↑ nuclear PPr receptor γ-subunit $\Rightarrow$ ↑ tissue responsiveness to insulin

☠ : Troglitazone withdrawn due to fatal liver failure, but others appear safe

Hypoglycaemia

Causes   Divided into: 1. Reactive (occurs after drug or 2–5 hrs postprandially)
                                    2. Fasting (occurs > 5 hrs postprandially)

I.A.T.R.O.G.E.N.I.C.

Insulin (i.e. in diabetics)
- Insulin excess: distinguished from endogenous insulin by plasma C-peptide absence
- Sulphonylureas, esp. chlorpropamide, glibenclamide, esp. in elderly and renal impairment
- β-blockers: $\beta2 \Rightarrow$ gluconeogenesis $\downarrow$, glucagon secretion $\downarrow$; $\beta1 \Rightarrow$ masks sympathetic response
  (although sweating may still occur, being mediated via muscarinic receptor M3)

Alcohol
- Acute: alcohol dehydrogenase $\Rightarrow$ NADH $\uparrow$ $\Rightarrow$ hepatic gluconeogenesis $\downarrow$
- Chronic: ACTH deficiency, malnutrition

Toxins
- Aspirin overdose (esp. in children), paracetamol overdose (hepatic necrosis)
- Quinine, pentamidine
- Ackee (hypoglycine) – Jamaican vomiting sickness

Reactive – 'postprandial hypoglycaemia'
- Idiopathic: symptoms occur 1–2 hrs after heavy carbohydrate meal
- Secondary: mild NIDDM, post-gastrectomy (= 'dumping syndrome')
                        TPN (following sudden cessation of IV hypertonic dextrose)

Organ failure – renal / liver
  Causes: a) Gluconeogenesis $\downarrow$
            b) Insulin metabolism $\downarrow$
            c) Glycogen reserve $\downarrow$: liver failure only
            d) Renal dialysis: glucose-rich dialysate causes reactive hypoglycaemia

Glycogen storage disease / **G**alactosaemia
- Glycogen storage disease 1 (von Gierke's): glucose-6-phosphatase or translocase deficiency
  PC: Stunted growth, hepatomegaly, hepatic adenoma
  Ix: G.L.U.T.: Glucose $\downarrow$, Lactic acidosis, Uric acid, Triglycerides $\uparrow$
- Galactosaemia and Fructose Intolerance – both cause reactive hypoglycaemia in infants

Endocrine
- Hypoadrenalism: Addison's, due to hypocortisolism (adrenaline deficiency does **not** cause)
- Hypothyroidism: esp. myxoedema coma
- Hypopituitarism (due to TSH and ACTH deficiency; isolated GH deficiency does **not** cause)

Neoplasia
- Insulin-secreting (commonest cause of fasting hypoglycaemia):
  a) Insulinoma: 70% solitary adenoma, 10% multiple (MEN-1), 10% ectopic, 10% malignant
      – commonest in women in 50s
  b) Nesidioblastosis – esp. children
  c) Carcinoid
- Insulin-like growth factors / insulin-receptor autoantibodies:
  a) Adrenal or hepatocellular carcinoma
  b) Mesothelioma, large retroperitoneal fibrosarcoma; haemangiopericytoma
  c) Hodgkin's lymphoma (insulin receptor autoAbs – may also occur without neoplasia)

Infection: malaria

Catabolic states: starvation, esp. neonates, due to $\downarrow$ glycogen reserve, sepsis, maternal diabetes

PC

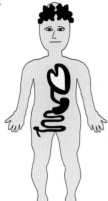

F.A.S.T.i.N.G.

Fatigue / **F**ierce (aggressive) / **F**unny turn / **F**ocal neurological signs
i.e. 'neuroglycopenic symptoms'
- Worse in morning, preprandially, or post-exercise; relieved by meal
- Also headache
- Focal neurological signs: transient hemiplegia, diplopia, dysarthria, ataxia, perioral paraesthesia

Appetite ↑
Sympathetic – pallor ($\alpha 1$ receptor) / **S**weating (M3 receptor)
Tachycardia, palpitations ($\beta 1$ receptor) / **T**remor ($\beta 2$ receptor)
Neurological: • Seizures, confused, coma
          • Chronic: amnesia, dementia, psychosis
(may also occur 2° to frequent diabetic asymptomatic 'hypo's')

Gain, weight: chronic hypoglycaemia, esp. with insulinoma

(Whipple's Triad of Insulinoma: wt gain + hypoglycaemia sx + blood glucose ↓)

Ix

Blood: 1. Capillary blood glucose < 2.5 mmol/l (normal = 3.5–5.5 mmol/l)
- *Hyper*glycaemia: may occur – if taken postprandially in Insulinoma (due to poor insulin release)
- Rapid drop in glucose level in hyperglycaemic pt may precipitate hypoglycaemic symptoms
2. Insulin + C-peptide high, in presence of glucose < 2.5 mmol/l (⇒ endogenous production);
proinsulin (> 20% insulin ⇒ insulinoma);
insulin antibodies (present ⇒ exogenous insulin)
3. Hydroxybutyrate (low due to insulin suppression of FFA oxidation)

Urine: sulphonylurea assay (also from blood sample)

Radiology: MRI abdomen

Special:
1. Hypoglycaemic Suppression Test:
    • Overnight, or 48-hr, or post-exercise   Measure 6-hrly:
    • Insulin (e.g. 3 u/hr IVI)   i) Glucose
    • Glucagon, tolbutamide or leucine (all IVI)   ii) Insulin: > 0.5 x basal level ⇒ insulinoma
                                        iii) C-peptide (longer $t_{1/2}$), but must be kept in fridge
2. Pancreatic vein sampling: intraoperative

Rx

Acute: 1. 20 g glucose po, or 50 ml dextrose 50% w/v iv ± dextrose infusion drip:
            use large vein, and leave needle in vein for a while, to reduce risk of thrombophlebitis
2. Glucagon (1 mg im): onset = 15 min; offset = 30 min
            contraindicated in liver failure or insulinoma
3. Dexamethasone (IV) 5 mg qds, or mannitol – treats cerebral oedema, once normoglycaemic

Chronic: 1. Dumping syndrome: • Frequent small snacks of complex carbohydrates
                              • Dietary fibre, guar gum, acarbose
2. Diabetics: review medication / education regarding eating, exercise / MedicAlert bracelet

Insulinoma: 1. Diazoxide or thiazide: inhibits insulin release (used preoperatively)
2. Streptozotocin: inhibits β-cell growth (used in malignant disease)
3. Adenoma resection, subtotal pancreatectomy

Hypopituitarism – Causes

Anatomy

Acidophilic *P.G. Tips tea – acid-like*
Prolactin
Growth hormone

Basophilic *F.L.A.T. – base*
FSH
LH
ACTH
TSH

Anterior pituitary ← → Posterior pituitary

ADH
Oxytocin

Causes

D.I.V.I.N.I.T.Y.

Developmental
    1. Hypothalamic: Kallman's syndrome – gonadotrophin deficiency and anosmia
    2. Pituitary: genetic panhypopituitarism (*Pit1* or *Prop1* mutations), isolated GHRH deficiency
    3. 'Empty sella syndrome':
        – congenital: usually a rim of pituitary tissue exists to allow normal pituitary function
        – acquired: pituitary mass may silently infarct with CSF replacement

Infection
    TB, toxoplasmosis, fungi (PCP, histoplasmosis)

Vascular
    1. Infarct: diabetes, vasculitis, Sheehan's syn. (postpartum haemorrhage – delayed presentation)
    2. Haemorrhage or compression by internal carotid aneurysm

Inflammation / **I**nfiltrative
    1. Autoimmune: lymphocytic hypophysitis
    2. Sarcoidosis, granulomatous hypophysitis
    3. Haemochromatosis, histiocytosis X

Neoplasia
    1. **Pituitary: Macroadenoma (commonest):**
        Gonadotrope: silent or non-functioning, i.e. no secretion or secretion of uncombined
    in order of α (constant) or β subunits
    frequency   Acidophils: prolactinoma (hyperprolactinaemia), growth hormone (acromegaly)
        Basophils: ACTH (Cushing's – usually microadenoma), TSH (hyperthyroidism – rare)
    2. Hypothalamic: craniopharyngioma (Rathke's pouch); pineal germinoma, chordoma
    3. Other: brain metastasis, glioma, meningioma, arachnoid cyst

Injury: surgery, trauma, birth injury (2nd commonest)

Toxin: radiotherapy – for brain tumour

Y: ps**Y**chosocial deprivation: GHRH deficiency

Hypopituitarism – PC

Endocrine Dysfunction

1. If the cause of hypopituitarism is a functioning pituitary macroadenoma, the clinical syndrome will be dominated by the effects of excess secreted hormone:
   - prolactin (infertility, galactorrhoea)
   - GH (acromegaly)
   - uncommon- ACTH (Cushing's); TSH (thyrotoxicosis)
2. Hypopituitarism due to any cause results in the following order of endocrine deficiencies:

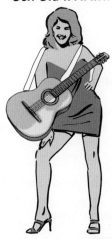

Sex G.u I.T.A.R.

Sex hormone-releasers - gonadotrophins: FSH, LH
1. Menopause-like symptoms
   amenorrhoea, infertility, hot-flushes loss of pubic / axillary hair, dyspareunia, breast atrophy
2. Loss of libido; impotence; infertility (azoospermia); regression of secondary sex characteristics (soft testicles, fine facial wrinkles)
3. Adolescent: delayed puberty
4. Anaemia: normochromic, normocytic

Growth hormone
1. Children: failure to grow
2. Weakness, muscle atrophy, fatigue, depression
3. Abdominal obesity, cholesterol↑, HDL↓ ⇒ atherosclerosis

Increased prolactin (due to loss of tonic dopamine inhibition)
   Galactorrheoa, amenorrhea or impotence, infertility

TSH: hypothyroidism

ACTH: hypocortisolism ⇒ hypomineralocorticoidism
   (teleogically, most important function of pituitary gland!)

Renal (ADH): Diabetes insipidus

Tumour Growth

Cerebral
- Personality change
- Focal epilepsy or hemiparesis – either direct compression or via carotid artery occlusion in cavernous sinus
- Obstructive hydrocephalus

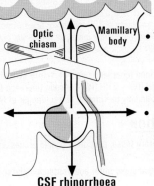

Ophthalmological
- Visual-field deficit (70%): superior-outer quadrantanopia or bitemporal hemianopia
- Bilateral central visual acuity or red-vision loss (esp. pituitary apoplexy)
- Cranial nerve palsies III, IV, Va, VI via cavernous sinus occlusion

Optic chiasm

Mamillary body

Hypothalamic
- Temperature, sleep, appetite dysregulation

Dura stretching
- Chronic headache in 40% – also due to endocrine effects
- Acute headache: pituitary apoplexy – also meningism, drowsiness, bilateral central visual field loss – due to haemorrhagic infarction of pituitary tumour

CSF rhinorrhoea

Hypopituitarism – Ix

Pituitary Function Tests

In order of hormone deficiency:

Sex G.u I.T.A.R.

Sex hormone-releasers – gonadotrophins: FSH, LH
 Bloods: 1. Testosterone ↓ (men) or estradiol ↓ (women)
   2. FSH and LH ↓
   3. Anaemia: normochromic, normocytic
 Dynamic: LHRH challenge: basal LH normally ↑ x2

Growth hormone
 Bloods: 1. IGF-1↓ or ↑ if GH-macroadenoma is cause of hypopituitarism
   2. Cholesterol ↑
 Dynamic: 1. Insulin tolerance test: GH normally ↑ to > 20 IU/l
    (glucose must ↓ to < 2.2 mmol/l)
   2. GHRH challenge (or L-arginine or L-DOPA): GH should ↑ to > 20 IU/l

Increased prolactin
 Bloods: Prolactin > 3600 mIU/l: prolactinoma (commonest functioning macroadenoma)
    500–3600 mIU/l: infundibular disconnection, e.g. other type pituitary tumour

TSH
 Bloods: TSH↓; fT4↓
 Dynamic: TRH challenge: TSH normally ↑ to 5–20 IU/l at 20 min;
    < 5 IU/l : hypopituitarism; > 20 IU/l : hypothalamic disease (supersensitivity)

ACTH
 Bloods: 1. Early-morning cortisol ↓ (often normal in early adrenal insufficiency)
   2. ACTH ↓
   3. Other: Na^+↓, K^+↑; glucose↓; eosinophils ↑, lymphocytes ↑
 Dynamic: 1. Synacthen test: should be normal in pituitary insufficiency
   2. Insulin tolerance test: cortisol normally > 600 mmol/l, or ↑ x2 from baseline
   3. CRH challenge: basal ACTH ↑es 2–4-fold
 Cushing's (rarely): 24-hour urine free cortisol; overnight dexamethasone suppression test

Renal (ADH): Diabetes insipidus
 Bloods: Serum osmolality and Na^+ ↓
 Urine: Urine osmolality ↑
 Dynamic: Water-deprivation test (for 8 hrs) – diabetes insipidus is diagnosed if:
    body weight ↓ > 3% /h
    serum osmolality > 300 mosm/kg; urine osmolality < 300 mosm/kg
   • Since cortisol deficiency may give false –ve, give dexamethasone before test
   • Correctable by prior administration of intranasal desmopressin ('cranial diabetes')

Dynamic tests are performed together as part of **'triple stimulation test'**, i.e.
LHRH (IV) + TRH (IV) + insulin tolerance test
Insulin tolerance test is seldomly performed, due to danger of hypoglycaemia in adrenal deficiency

Anatomical Localization

1. Skull X-ray: enlarged pituitary fossa, erosion of clinoid processes (historical test)
2. MRI / CT brain
3. Goldman perimetry: bilateral upper outer quadrantanopia; later, bitemporal hemianopia

Hypopituitarism – Rx

Tumour

1. Medical
a) Prolactinoma: dopamine agonists (bromocriptine, quinagolide, cabergoline):
  - Shrink prolactinomas
  - Shrink 10% of other pituitary macroadenomas, inc. non-functioning

b) Acromegaly: somatostatin analogues (octreotide, lanreotide):
  - Inhibit secretion of GH-secreting adenomas, but only cause shrinkage in 10%

2. Trans-sphenoidal / trans-frontal hypophysectomy
Ind: first-line Rx in non-functioning adenomas; acromegaly; Cushing's
  - Improves visual acuity / field in 70% pts
  - ☠: Recurrence in 20% (reduced by radiotherapy)

3. Radiotherapy (external / yttrium implant)
Ind: Used as an adjuvant to surgery, or where surgery inappropriate

Hormone Replacement

Sex hormone-releasers - gonadotrophins: FSH, LH
  - ♀: EthinylE2 or conjugated E2 for 1st–3rd weeks +
      medroxyprogesterone in 3rd week (if uterus)
      ⇒ withdrawal bleed on 4th week
  - ♂: Testosterone for low libido
      Testosterone enanthate (im every 2 weeks) / decanoate (PO) /
      transdermal or implant
  - Fertility:
    a) Human menopausal gonadotrophins
    b) Human chorionic gonadotrophins (LH analogue)
    c) Recombinant GnRH: – simulates normal pulsatile release of GnRH via pump
                         – less risk of ovarian hyperstimulation and multiple gestation

Growth hormone
    a) Human recombinant, subcutaneous GH
    b) GHRH – experimental: simulates normal pulsatile release of GH

Increased prolactin: only need to treat if prolactinoma – see under Tumour (above)

TSH
      T4 : 75–150 µg / day
      ☠ • AF, angina, osteoporosis
         • Addisonian crisis: must replace cortisol first, if deficiency exists

ACTH
      a) Hydrocortisone: 10 mg mane + 5 mg noon + 5 mg evening
      b) MedicAlert bracelet – Need to ↑ in event of illness or operation, e.g. 20 mg tds–qds
          NB Fludrocortisone unnecessary, as ACTH is not a significant releaser of aldosterone

Renal (ADH)
      Desmopressin : DDAVP (PO / intranasal)

Hyperprolactinaemia

Causes

Higher Brain Centres

Stress: pain (inc. venepuncture), infection, organ failure, esp. renal

Sleep: pre-awakening

Seizures: 10–20 min postictal or syncope

Sex: orgasm

Hypothalamus

Dopamine ⊖ ⊕ TRH Estrogen

Loss of Dopamine Inhibition

1. Hypothalamo–Infundibular disconnection:
   a) Pituitary tumour (any type) or craniopharyngioma
   b) Pituitary surgery (with damage to stalk)
   c) Pituitary radiotherapy
   d) Sarcoid, TB, histiocytosis X

2. Dopamine antagonists:
   a) Neuroleptics, TCAs, SSRIs or opioids
   b) Metoclopramide
   c) Verapamil

Endocrine Stimulation

1. Hypothyroidism:
   T4 ↓ ⇒ TRH ↑ ⇒ PRL ↑

2. Estrogen:
   a) Pregnancy
      • ↑ es size of pre-existing prolactinoma
      • < 12 weeks postpartum
   b) Polycystic ovaries
   c) Pill (OCP)

Autonomous Secretion

1. Pituitary tumour: commonest (40%)
   a) Prolactinoma
      • Microadenoma: women – present early
      • Macroadenoma: men – present later!
   b) Acromegaly
2. Ectopic prolactin secretion:
   small-cell lung, renal cell carcinoma

Prolactin

Sensory afferents to hypothalamus

Chest Wall Stimulation

1. Breast-feeding; self-examination
2. Trauma
3. VZV of thoracic dermatome

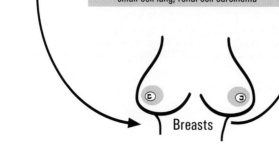

Breasts

PC   **1. Galactorrhoea**: women (rare in men)

       2. Hypogonadotrophic hypogonadism (GnRH ↓, gonadotrophins ↓, sex steroids ↓)
          a) ♀: Amenorrhoea, infertility
          b) ♂: Loss of libido, impotence, infertility (azoospermia)
          c) Osteoporosis

       3. Panhypopituitarism (if due to prolactinoma)
          a) Endocrine deficiencies *(Sex G.ul.T.A.R. – p. 327)*
          b) Mass effect: headache, hemianopia

Ix   **1. Prolactin** (daytime levels)

mIU/l	Cause
< 500	Normal
500–3600	Any cause, except prolactin macroadenoma ∴ *if MRI shows pituitary macroadenoma, then cause* *is infundibular disconnection and the treatment is surgery*
> 3600	Prolactin macroadenoma or pregnancy ∴ *if MRI shows pituitary macroadenoma, treat with* *dopamine agonist*

       2. Dynamic tests
          a) Prolactin: give domperidone or metoclopramide
          b) Hypopituitarism: triple stimulation test – LHRH, TRH, insulin tolerance test

       3. MRI Pituitary ± visual fields

Rx   **1. Dopamine agonists:** Bromocriptine, quinagolide, cabergoline (less side-effects)
          Ind: a) Secreting prolactinomas: first-line therapy
                  90% respond: – within hours, prolactin level normalizes
                               – within days–weeks, tumour shrinks
                               – can attempt withdrawal after 2 years, as tumour fibroses
                b) Non-secreting prolactinoma + pregnancy:
                    – give prophylactically for 6 months pre-conception to ↓ risk of tumour expansion
                    – bromocriptine also used for symptomatic expansion during pregnancy
          ☠: N + V, postural hypotension, Raynaud's syn., nasal stuffiness, constipation

       2. Trans-sphenoidal microadenectomy
          Ind: a) Intolerant or resisant to dopamine agonists
                b) Non-secreting tumour / disconnection:
                    90% cure, but may relapse

       3. Radiotherapy
          Ind: Adjunct to surgery

Acromegaly

Growth Hormone – Normal Physiology

Growth hormone is required for both **growth** and the **catabolic response** in stressful situations

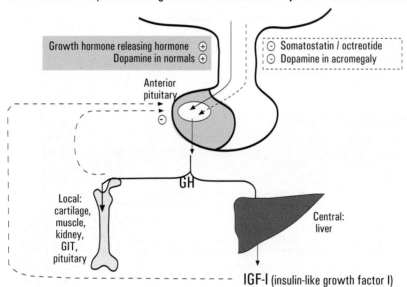

| Growth hormone releasing hormone ⊕ | ⊖ Somatostatin / octreotide |
| Dopamine in normals ⊕ | ⊖ Dopamine in acromegaly |

Anterior pituitary

Local: cartilage, muscle, kidney, GIT, pituitary

GH

Central: liver

IGF-I (insulin-like growth factor I)

Linear growth   Stress response → catabolism

Causes

Pituitary

Epi: Prevalence 5 / 100 000; age 30–50 years (uncommonly children)

Types:

1. Adenoma (90%):
   a) G-Protein Gsα activating mutation → autonomous growth hormone ± prolactin secretion
   b) **A**cidophilic adenomas → **A**cromegaly
2. Genetic syndrome with pituitary adenoma (9%):
   a) Multiple Endocrine Neoplasia 1 (MEN-1):
      Pituitary adenoma, **P**arathyroidism, hyper-, **P**ancreatic insulinoma or gastrinoma
   b) McCune–Albright syndrome = polyostotic fibrous dysplasia + pigmented patches,
      due to Gsα activating mutation in mosaic of tissues
   c) Carney complex: spotty pigmentation + myxomas + endocrine tumours
   d) Familial acromegaly and gigantism: loss of heterozygosity in tumour cells
3. Carcinoma (1%)

Extrapituitary

Types:

1. GHRH secretion:
   APUDoma (e.g. bronchial carcinoid), small-cell carcinoma, hypothalamic hamartoma
2. GH secretion:
   pancreatic islet cell

PC — *G.I.A.N.T. C.O.N.K.*

Growth: *'acromegaly'* = extremity enlargement
  Nose: broad; enlarged sinuses; supraorbital ridge prominence
  Mouth: prognathism; teeth parting; loss; deep voice; macroglossia
  Skull: frontal bossing; hat size ↑
  Hands: spade-like (e.g. ring size ↑); hyperhidrosis
  Feet: shoe size ↑; heel pad thickening (on X-ray)
  Gigantism: if onset occurs before epiphyseal fusion (children)

Insulin resistance or diabetes mellitus (25%)
  Diabetes mellitus; acanthosis nigricans; skin tags
  Hypertriglyceridaemia (due to ↓ lipoprotein lipase activity)

Arthritis
  Hips, knees; spine (kyphosis, spinal stensosis, cauda equina syn.)

Neurology
  Headache; carpal or tarsal tunnel syndromes; proximal myopathy

Tumour effects
  Homonymous hemianopia
  Panhypopituitarism, inc. hypogonadism
  Hyperprolactinoma: galactorrhoea, hirsutism, amenorrhoea

Cardiac
  Hypertension
  Ischaemic heart disease; CVA: mortality rate = 2x ↑
  Dilated cardiomyopathy; cardiac failure

Obstructive sleep apnoea in 60%, due to macroglossia

Neoplasia: colonic polyps, adenocarcinoma

Kidney stones / hypercalciuria
  Normocalcaemic, but PO_4 ↑ and Vit D ↑

Ix   1. Insulin-like growth factor I (IGF-I):   does not fluctuate over course of day (unlike GH)
        2. Oral-glucose tolerance test (OGTT): GH normally become undetectable following glucose challenge

Rx   Surgery (trans-sphenoidal or transfrontal hypophysectomy):
        • Curative for 90% microadenomas (i.e. < 1 cm); less successful for macroadenomas
        • ☠: Panhypopituitarism in 10%; meningitis; haemorrhage
      Medical:
        1. Somatostatin analogue: octreotide or lanreotide (inhibits GH and PRL secretion):
            • Rapid relief of headache, perspiration, obstructive sleep apnoea and carpal tunnel in > 90% pts
        2. Dopamine agonists: bromocriptine, cabergoline:
            • Effective in only 10%, but have additive effect with octreotide
        3. GH-receptor antagonists: pegrisomant
      Radiotherapy:
        GH levels decrease slowly over 10 years

Hypothyroidism – Causes

H.A.T.R.E.D.

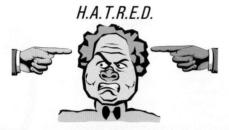

Hashimoto's thyroiditis

Epi: Middle-aged women; assoc. with other organ-based autoimmune disease, e.g. DM
Path: Lymphocytic and macrophage infiltrate with lymphoid follicles
Course: T4↓ ⇒ euthyroidism in 40% ; a few pts begin / become temporarily hyperthyroid
Ix: Anti-thyroglobulin (TG) and anti-myeloperoxidase (MPO)

Atrophic / Autoimmune, other / Amyloid and other infiltrative

1. Atrophic thyroiditis:
   Path: Fibrosis (limited to capsule) and deposition of hydrophilic glycosaminoglycans
   Course: May represent end-stage Hashimoto's or carbimazole-treated Graves'
   Ix: Anti-TSH receptor-blocking Abs (cf. Graves' = anti-TSH receptor-stimulatory Abs)
2. Autoimmune, other:
   • Graves' disease: late, or following radio-iodine therapy or surgery
   • Riedel's thyroiditis (part of multifocal fibrosclerosis: e.g. alveolitis, mediastinitis)
   • Scleroderma
3. Amyloidosis, sarcoidosis, haemochromatosis

Toxins / nutritional

1. Anti-thyroid treatment: carbimazole, radio-iodine (^{131}I), surgery
2. Other toxin:
   • Lithium, tolbutamide, aminosalicylic acid
   • Cassava excess: thiocyanate inhibits iodide uptake in thyroid ('trapping')
3. Nutritional: iodine excess or deficiency:
   • Excess: amiodarone (blocks iodination and coupling reactions), or nuclear fallout: (^{131}I)
   • Deficiency: endemic cretinism in Andes, Himalayas, New Guinea (> 10% population)
     Epi: associated with high $CaCO_3$ in water; pregnancy (high demand)
     PC: Massive goitre; often euthyroid due to compensation

Resistance to thyroid hormone

• Autosomal dominant condition, resulting from thyroid receptor β mutation
• Cases are often clinically euthyroid, but have abnormal TFTs – ↑TSH, ↑fT4 and ↑fT3
    PC: Learning disability, delayed skeletal maturation, goitre; occasionally thyrotoxic!

Endocrine

1. Hypopituitarism, e.g. pituitary tumour; order of endorine deficiency =
   (*Sex G.ul.T.A.R.* = sex hormones⇒ GH ⇒TSH⇒ ACTH ⇒ADH: *p. 326*)
2. Addison's disease: due to cortisol ↓ or polyglandular autoimmunity (PGAS-2)
   Ix = Anti-adrenal, anti-MPO

Developmental

1. Thyroid aplasia; ectopic thyroid (e.g. lingual, trachea) – commonest congenital cause
2. Dyshormonogenesis: peroxidase or iodine transferase deficiency
   PC: Deaf mutism, learning disability = Pendred's syndrome
   Ix: Perchlorate discharge test: KClO4 leaches out unincorporated ^{131}I
3. Down's or Turner's syndromes

Hypothyroidism - PC

S.H.O.W.I.N.G. O.F.F.
(their signs)

Skin
1. 'Myxoedema'
   = non-pitting, doughy oedema due to impaired hyaluronidase,
     leading to mucopolysaccharide accumulation
   - Facies: puffy, toad-like, apathetic; malar flush;
     peaches and cream (β-caroteinaemia)
   - Tongue: macroglossia, glossitis (pernicious anaemia)
   - Voice: hoarse, gruffy (myxoedmatous larynx)
2. Other: erythema ab igne, pruritus
3. Hair: alopecia; loss of outer 1/3 eyebrow

HypOmetabolism / Heart disease
1. Cold intolerance; hypothermic (myxoedema coma)
2. Cardiac:
   - Bradycardia (worsened with digoxin!)
   - Dilated cardiomyopathy (glycosaminoglycan infiltration)
   - Ischaemic heart disease: direct effect and via hypercholesterolaemia

HypOglycaemia / HypERcholesterol and -triglyceridaemia
Ophthalmic
1. Xanthelasma (and tendinous xanthoma): due to hypercholesterolaemia
2. Bitemporal hemianopia
      due to pituitary enlargement from thyrotroph hyperplasia
3. Grave's ophthalmopathy
      suggests Graves' disease that is 'burnt-out' or overtreated

Weight gain, anorexia
Intestinal: constipation, abdominal distension (inc. ascites)
Neuropsychiatric
1. Dementia (esp. amnesia) / depression (and paradoxical mania)
   - Congenital T4 ↓: mental retardatation – 'cretinism'; assoc. posterior fontanelle enlargement
   - Juvenile-onset T4 ↓: mental-slowing only
2. Cerebellar ataxia, dizziness, drop-attacks
3. Muscle: proximal myopathy (CK, AST, LDH ↑), slowly relaxing reflexes, myotonia
4. Carpal tunnel syndrome
5. Deafness (otitis media or Pendred's syndrome)

Goitre
Firm, irregular: Hashimoto's thyroiditis
Firm, regular: Graves' disease ('burnt-out' or treated)
Woody, hard: Riedel's thyroiditis
No goitre: atrophic thyroiditis

Oedema / effusions: pericardial, pleural, ascites, joint
Females: menorrhagia or amenorrhoea
Fertility: infertility delayed or premature puberty; galactorrhoea
               – all due to secondary hyperprolactinaemia

Hypothyroidism – Ix and Rx

Ix Bloods

TFT

TSH ↑ : most sensitive test

> False −ve: secondary hypothyroidism due to hypopituitarism (TSH ↓)
> False +ve: • 'Sick euthyroid': e.g. recovery phase of severe systemic illness
> • Generalized thyroid resistance (patients will have high T4 and T3)

fT4 ↓ : False −ve: subclinical hypothyroidism (still requires Rx due to higher risk of
> ischaemic heart disease; clinical symptoms occur with TSH
> > 5 x upper-limit normal)
> False +ve: 'sick euthyroid', due to T4 degradation ↑ and rT3 formation ↑

fT3 ↓ : False −ve: common, because ↓ TSH causes preferential release of T3
> rather than T4
> False +ve: 'sick euthyroid':
> • Reduced free T3 is the commonest consequence of severe
> illness; extremity of age (elderly, infants), and drugs
> (amiodarone, dexamethasone, propranolol)
> • Due to ↓ peripheral conversion of T4 ⇒ T3, and increased
> conversion of T4 ⇒ rT3 (reverse T3)

NB: **Free** T4 and **free** T3 are better than total amounts, as they are not influenced by
changes in thyroxine-binding globulin (TBG), which may decrease in severe illness, and
increase with states such as hepatitis, pregnancy or taking the contraceptive pill

AutoAbs
- Anti-myeloperoxidase (MPO) or anti-thyroglobulin (TG): Graves'; Hashimoto's
- Anti TSH-R blocking Abs: atrophic thyroiditis, athyrotic cretinism

Other
Biochem: Na^+ ↓; cholesterol, triglycerides ↑; CK, AST, LDH ↑ (sarcolemma damage)
FBC: Macrocytic anaemia; megaloblastosis suggests coexistent pernicious anaemia
Cause: ESR ↑↑ – Riedel's thyroiditis; Synacthen test – Addison's; FSH, LH – pituitary failure

Radiology / Surgical

Hashimoto's thyroiditis may present with asymmetric goitre, which can be confused with
multinodular goitre or carcinoma. In these cases, USS and FNA help to distinguish.

Rx Thyroxine, lifelong:

Dose 25–200 μg/day
☠: 1. Angina or myocardial infarction in elderly, so:
    • Introduce dose gradually (by 25 μg every 3 months)
    • Cover with β-blocker
2. Addison's – due to unmasking of hypoadrenalism or hypopituitarism:
    • Prior Synacthen test if hypoadrenal features; or, if in doubt
    • Cover with hydrocortisone
3. Acute psychosis
Ix: Maintain TSH < 5 mU/L

KI: if deficient

Hypothyroidism Rx – Complications

Myxoedematous Coma

Precipitants

1. Sedatives
2. MI, CVA
3. Infection

B. Ventilatory support

Ventilate: pts often develop
type 2 respiratory failure

A. Assessment

1. *A.B.C.D.*
2. *C.O.A.T.*
   Cardiac monitor:
      bradycardia,
      heart block,
      long QT interval
   O_2
   ABP
   TPR: hypothermic
3. Warming

C. Hydration

1. **CVP line**
2. **IV fluids**
   - Often hypertensive due to
     compensatory catecholamines,
     but hypovolaemic
   - Hypotension is a poor prognostic sign
   - Give 5–50% dextrose, as often
     hypoglycaemic
   - Inotropes are ineffective

D. Medication

1. **Hydrocortisone:** pretreat
2. **Thyroxine**
   a) Liothyronine (IV T3):
      - 5–20 µg od for 3 days
      - Rapid onset and offset
      - Overcomes need to convert
        peripherally, which is suppressed
        in coma and infection
      ☠: – labile concentrations
         – angina (give prophylaxis GTN)
   b) T4 PO or nasogastric, 25-50 µg od
3. **Antibiotics, broad-spectrum**

Complications

Hypoglycaemia: 50% dextrose, 50 ml
Seizures (25%): anticonvulsants
Psychosis: antipsychotics
ICP ↑: ITU, hyperventilation, inotropes

Hyperthyroidism – Causes

G.A.I.N. of F.U.N.C.T.ioN.

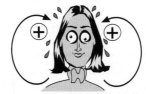

Hyperstimulation

Graves' disease
Epi: Prevalence: 1–2%; F:M = 10:1, esp. postpartum; age: 20–40
Path: Lymphocytic infiltrate with follicles; follicle cell hyperplasia, columnar metaplasia;
  scalloping of colloid adjacent to follicle cells due to active endocytosis
Course: 1. T4 ↑ ⇒ 40% euthyroidism ⇒ 20 % T4 ↓ (may present as hypoT4ism)
  2. Neonatal thyrotoxicosis due to maternal LATS (IgG) crossing placenta in
    3rd trimester
Ix: Anti-TSH receptor stimulatory Abs ('long-acting thyroid stimulator')

Follicle Destruction

Autoimmune, other
1. Hashimoto's thyroiditis: early
2. Postpartum lymphocytic thyroiditis
   PC: Painless goitre
   Course: Temporary T4 ↑ or ↓ ⇒ 10% develop permanent hypoT4ism
   Ix: Anti-TSH receptor blocking Abs

Infection: de Quervain's thyroiditis (viral, granulomatous)
Epi: Women, 20–40 yrs, assoc. with HLA-B35
Path: Coxsackie, influenza or EBV
PC: Subacute; painful goitre or dysphagia; fever
Course: Transient ↑T4 ⇒ mild ↓T4 (exhaustion) ⇒ recovery over 2–4 months

Autonomous Secretion

Nodular goitre (toxic multinodular goitre or Plummer's disease)
Epi: Age > 50
Cause: Long-standing non-toxic goitre, or iodine deficiency

Follicular adenoma (> 2.5cm) / Follicular thyroid carcinoma (esp. metastatic)

U: McCUne–Albright syndrome: GTP activating mutation

Neoplasia: ovarian teratoma (benign struma ovarii): T4 secretion

Choriocarcinoma: hydatidiform mole; TSH-related peptide secretion

Toxins
1. Iodide, inc. amiodarone (Jod–Basedow disease)
2. Thyroid tissue ingestion: e.g. hamburgers; epidemic (T4-toxicosis, with normal T3)
3. T4 over-replacement

Neoplasia: pituitary adenoma – TSH-secreting (rare)

Hyperthyroidism – PC

S.H.O.W.I.N.G. O.F.F.
(their signs)

Skin
1. Sweaty, erythematous palms; smooth, salmon-pink face
2. Graves' disease-associated
   a) Pretibial myxoedema:
      - Thickened skin over legs, feet; clearly demarcated; erythema; pruritic
      - Accentuated hair follicles (peau d'orange)
   b) Acropachyderma:
      - Clubbing; onycholysis, thick skin, hypertrophic periosteum
3. Autoimmune-associated: vitiligo, alopecia

Hypermetabolism / **H**yperdynamic circulation
1. Fever, esp. with thyrotoxic storm, or viral infection
2. Hyperdynamic circulation:
   - Rapid, bounding pulse or atrial fibrillation
   - Hypertension
   - High-output cardiac failure, dilated cardiomyopathy

Hyperglycaemia

Ophthalmic
1. Upper lid retraction (sympathetic stimulation of levator palpebrae superioris)
   O/E: Staring; infrequent blinking; lid lag, on rapid descent
2. Graves' disease ophthalmopathy:
   Path: due to deposition of hydrophilic glycosaminoglycans in
         retro-orbital fat pad; lymphocyte infiltrate; muscular fibrosis
   O/E: a) Exophthalmos: superior limbic keratitis (grittiness),
            chemosis (discomfort, worse in morning)
        b) Ophthalmoplegia, esp. upward and outward
        c) Retro-orbital compression: optic nerve atrophy ($\downarrow$ visual acuity), papilloedema, glaucoma

Weight loss, hyperphagia

Intestinal
1. Diarrhoea, malabsorption, abdominal pain, N + V (severe in 'thyrotoxic storm')
2. Cholestasis (periportal fibrosis)
3. Hyposplenism

Neuropsychiatric
1. Emotionally labile, psychosis, depression, anxiety, fatigue
2. Tremor (fine, positional), chorea
3. Proximal myopathy (rarely ptosis), or hypokalaemic periodic paralysis (esp. in oriental men)

Goitre
PC: Dysphagia, stridor, dysphonia (due to recurrent laryngeal nerve palsy (esp. if carcinoma)
O/E: Palpation: • Diffuse and smooth – Graves'; diffuse and multinodular – toxic multinodular or Hashimoto's
             • Focal and mobile – cyst or adenoma; focal and immobile – carcinoma or lymphoma
             • Tender – viral thyroiditis
     Auscultation: bruit in Graves', carcinoma
     SVCO: esp. on raising arms (Pemberton's sign)
     Lymphadenopathy: Graves', carcinoma, lymphoma

Osteoporosis / hypercalcaemia

Females: oligomenorrhoea (less commonly menorrhagia, due to $\uparrow$ PRL), gynaecomastia

Fertility: infertility

Hyperthyroidism – Ix and Rx

Ix Bloods

TFT
- Free T3 ↑: most sensitive test, as free T4 will be normal in T3-thyrotoxicosis
- TSH ↓: but will be ↑ in TSH-secreting tumours, e.g. choriocarcinoma, pituitary adenoma

AutoAbs
- Anti-TSH receptors: 100% specific; 90% sensitive for Graves'
  Only clinical use is in 3rd trimester to detect babies at risk of thyrotoxicosis
- Anti-myeloperoxidase (MPO), anti-thyroglobulin (TG): Graves', Hashimoto's, viral, postpartum

Other
Biochem: Ca ↑, Mg ↓, Bilirubin ↑, ALP ↑, Glucose ↑, Ferritin ↑
FBC: Normochromic Normocytic anaemia, Lymphocytosis
Cause: ESR ↑ (viral thyroiditis), β-hCG ↑ (choriocarcinoma)

Radiology: ^{99m}Tc – pertechnate scan

Diffuse uptake	No uptake	Nodular uptake	Cold nodule = less activity than normal
Graves'	1. Viral thyroiditis 2. Postpartum thyroiditis 3. Ingestion of iodine or thyroxine	1. Toxic multinodular goitre 2. Follicular adenoma 3. Ectopic thyroid	1. Benign 2. Malignant (20% of cold nodules)
		↓ **USS:** cystic vs solid cystic less likely to be cancer **FNA or surgical excision**	NB: neoplastic nodules may also be 'hot'

Rx *be S.T.R.I.C.T. with them!*

Symptomatic: atenolol (anxiety, palpitations); digoxin, warfarin (atrial fibrillation)

Thiourea: Carbimazole or propylthiouracil (PTU)
Mechanism: ↓ thyroid peroxidase, ↓ oxidative coupling, ↓ T4→T3, immunomodulation
Indication: Graves' or toxic multinodular goitre: Rx for 18 months → 50% relapse
☠: Hypersensitivity (rash, arthralgia, hepatitis – within 6 weeks), agranulocytosis

Radio-Iodine ($^{131}I_2$)
Mechanism: Iodine is only taken up by 'hot' nodules: the rest of the gland is atrophic
Indication: Toxic multinodular goitre or adenoma in over-40s
☠: • HypoT4ism (esp. in Graves'), malignancy, teratogenic (avoid in women), hypoPTHism
    • Flare-up: thyrotoxic storm (add thiourea before), ophthalmopathy (add steroids)

Cause-specific:
Viral – aspirin, steroids; gynae – surgery; iodide ingestion – Na perchlorate

Thyroidectomy, partial
Indication: Treatment-resistant Graves'; large goitre or adenoma
Method: Pretreat with thioureas for 3 months (avoids thyrotoxic storm), KI for 1 week
☠: Recurrent laryngeal nerve palsy (ENT exam before), hypoPTHism (usually transient)

Hyperthyroidism Rx – Complications

Thyrotoxic storm

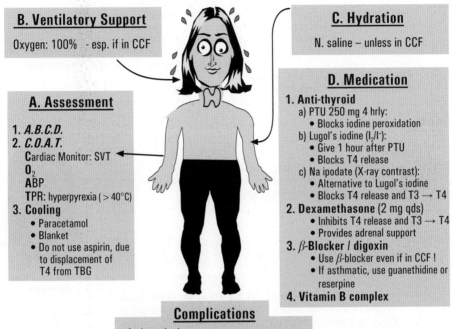

B. Ventilatory Support

Oxygen: 100% - esp. if in CCF

C. Hydration

N. saline – unless in CCF

A. Assessment

1. *A.B.C.D.*
2. *C.O.A.T.*
   Cardiac Monitor: SVT
   O_2
   ABP
   TPR: hyperpyrexia (> 40°C)
3. Cooling
   - Paracetamol
   - Blanket
   - Do not use aspirin, due
     to displacement of
     T4 from TBG

D. Medication

1. **Anti-thyroid**
   a) PTU 250 mg 4 hrly:
      - Blocks iodine peroxidation
   b) Lugol's iodine (I_2/I^-):
      - Give 1 hour after PTU
      - Blocks T4 release
   c) Na ipodate (X-ray contrast):
      - Alternative to Lugol's iodine
      - Blocks T4 release and T3 → T4
2. **Dexamethasone (2 mg qds)**
   - Inhibits T4 release and T3 → T4
   - Provides adrenal support
3. **β-Blocker / digoxin**
   - Use β-blocker even if in CCF !
   - If asthmatic, use guanethidine or
     reserpine
4. **Vitamin B complex**

Complications

- Anti-psychotics
- Anti-arrhythmics / heart failure treatment
- Anti-diarrhoeals / analgesics for abdominal pain

Graves' ophthalmopathy

Rx
1. Conservative: sleep propped up, lubricant eye drops, guanethidine (adrenaline release ↓)
2. Medical: diuretics, steroids (e.g. prednisolone 60 mg od)
3. Radiotherapy
4. Surgery: lateral tarsorraphy, medial orbital wall decompression

Neonatal thyrotoxicosis

Path
1. Transplacental transfer of maternal TSH receptor Abs (LATS) to neonate
2. Check neonatal TFTs at birth and 1 week – maternal antithyroid drugs may initially mask

Rx
1. Pregnancy:
   - Symptomatic: allows sparing or avoidance of thiourea, esp. at 3rd trimester
   - Thiourea (low-dose, as Graves' goes into partial remission, and risk of causing neonatal
     hypothyroidism and goitre, with stridor)
2. Neonate: β-blockers and carbimazole
3. Breast-feeding mother: propylthiouracil

Goitre

PC 1. 'Lump in the neck'; 2. Dysphagia; 3. Stridor; dyspnoea

O/E **Inspection:** Signs of Graves' or myxoedema; scar; lingual thyroid (look at back of tongue)
Palpation: Method: palpate from behind; get patient to swallow:
- Diffuse (smooth or irregular) vs nodular
- Other masses: – Thyroglossal cyst (elevates on tongue protrusion)
  – Cervical lymphadenopathy (Graves', papillary carcinoma)
  – Delphian node: midline above isthmus (papillary carcinoma)
Auscultation: Bruit in Graves' or carcinoma
Manoeuvres:
- Transillumination: cystic vs solid nodules
- Pemberton's sign: arm elevation causes SVCO with retrosternal goitre

Causes

Euthyroid
1. Simple goitre: assoc. women, smoking
2. Nodules: non-toxic (i.e. euthyroid): assoc. ionizing radiation
3. Iodine deficiency, compensated

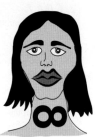

**8% population
have palpable
goitres!**
(4x more common
in women)

T4 ↑ *G.A.I.N. of F.U.N.C.T.I.O.N.*
Graves' disease: diffuse enlargement
Autoimmune, other: postpartum thyroiditis
Infection: de Quervain's thyroiditis (painful, fever, systemic upset)
Nodular: toxic multinodular goitre – multiple nodules (irregular)
Follicular adenoma: single nodule
Neoplastic: metastatic follicular carcinoma
Toxin: amiodarone

T4 ↓ *H.A.T.R.E.D.*
Hashimoto's: firm and irregular (may be mistaken for neoplasm)
Autoimmune, other: Riedel's – woody hard
Toxin / Nutritional: iodine deficiency:
a) Endemic mountainous regions – often massive goitre !
b) Pregnancy – increased demand
Resistance to thyroid hormone (hereditary, often euthyroid)
Developmental: ectopic thyroid may be observed, e.g. back of
tongue, above thyroid cartilage

Ix 1. Bloods:
a) TFTs (and associated bloods, e.g. glucose, if autoimmune disease suspected)
b) Thyroglobulin ↑ in most thyroid diseases and benign adenomas, but especially high in neoplasia
c) AutoAbs : anti-TSH R; anti-myeloperoxidase (MPO) or anti-thyroglobulin (TG)

2. Radiology:
a) Neck X-ray: calcification: papillary ca. (stippled – psammoma bodies); medullary ca. (dense calcification)
b) Pertechnetate scan ⇒ if single nodule ⇒ USS ± FNA (as for thyrotoxicosis – see p. 340)

Thyroid Tumours

PC

1. Thyroid nodule

Epi: a) 50% population have nodules *of any size*
    b) 5% population have nodules that are *palpable*:
       • 10% of those palpable nodules removed surgically are neoplastic
       • 5% of multinodular goitres are neoplastic

2. Local infiltration

1. Dysphagia (oesophagus)
2. Haemoptysis (trachea); hoarseness, dysphonia (recurrent laryngeal nerve)
3. Neck pain: radiates to jaw and ear

3. Endocrine (rare)

1. Follicular Carcinoma (metastatic): thyrotoxicosis
2. Medullary Carcinoma • Cushing's (ACTH)
                  • MEN-2a (associated phaeochromocytoma, hyperPTHism)

Types

Papa's. F.A.M.i L.y

PAPillary (80%) – young adults (20–30s), esp. females
    Aet: Radiation, iodine deficiency (TSH overstimulation), *ptc* oncogene
    Path: Psammoma bodies: stippled calcification (radio-opaque on CXR)
    PC: Fixed multifocal neck mass + lateral cervical lymphadenopathy + lung invasion
    Rx: T4 – decreases TSH stimulation; surgery or ^{131}I in elderly
    Prog: good: 5-yr survival: 95% (best prognosis young, women); but 10% relapse after 10 yrs

Follicular (15%) – middle-aged
    PC: • Metastasizes early (lung - snowstorm appearance on CXR; bone)
           • Thyrotoxicosis
    Prog: 5-yr survival: 50% (poor prognosis: Hurthle-cell variety)

Anaplastic (2%) – elderly, esp. females
    Path: spindle and giant cells
    Prog: 5-yr survival: 10%

Medullary (2%) – young
    Path: • Parafollicular C cells (APUDoma derived from neural crest cells)
          • Secrete calcitonin: forms amyloid and raises plasma calcitonin
    PC: • Cervical lymphadenopathy
          • Diarrhoea (secretion of prostaglandin, 5-HT, polypeptide)
          • Endocrine: MEN-2a or 2b (assoc. phaeochromocytoma, hyperPTHism), ACTH
    Ix: • Basal calcitonin; ^{131}I-MIBG scan

Lymphoma: 1% – elderly
    Aet: Assoc. Hashimoto's thyroiditis, chronic lymphocytic thyroiditis
    Path: Immunoblastic (large-cell histiocytic)

Adrenal Insufficiency

Causes   A.D.D.I.S.O.N.'S.

1° Hypoadrenalism ('Addison's disease')
PC: Pigmentation. Ix: ACTH↑

Autoimmune (90%)
F:M = 3:1
Assoc: PGAS-1; 2
Ix: • Anti-adrenal Abs (in 50%; may be transient)
     • Steroid-receptor-blocking Abs

Deficiency, enzyme – 1
Congenital adrenal hyperplasia: 21-hydroxylase deficiency (defect in 90%)
PC: masculinization of female; male infertility (not all become Addisonian)

Deficiency, enzyme – 2
Adrenoleucodystrophy (X-linked, usually)
PC: Epilepsy, mental retardation, spasticity

Infection
1. TB
2. AIDS-related: CMV, histoplasmosis
3. Meningococcaemia (Waterhouse–Friedrichsen syn.) – adrenal haemorrhagic infarction

Sarcoidosis

Other infiltrative disease
1. Amyloidosis
2. Haemochromatosis

Neoplasia
1. Metastases: esp. from breast
2. Adrenal vein thrombosis: e.g. from renal cell carcinoma

Surgery: bilateral adrenalectomy for Cushing's disease

2° Hypoadrenalism
PC: No pigmentation. Ix: ACTH↓

Secondary: late complication of hypopituitarism

Steroid therapy, during:
1. Withdrawal, after several months of treatment
2. Intercurrent infection or trauma, when demand exceeds supply

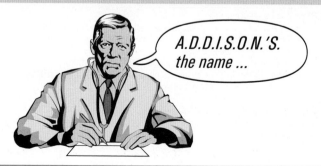

A.D.D.I.S.O.N.'S. the name ...

<u>**PC**</u>   *W.A.S.H.E.D. O.U.T.*

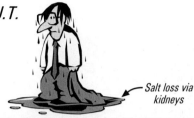

Salt loss via kidneys

Weakness / **W**eight loss and anorexia

Abdo pain ↓ ('acute abdomen'):
       crisis often triggered by infection, trauma or surgery (i.e. high steroid-demand)

Skin   1. Hyperpigmentation of skin creases and buccal mucosa (1° hypoadrenalism)
            – due to high ACTH or melanocyte-stimulating hormone
          2. Hair loss: bodily hair, esp.females
          3. Vitiligo

Hypotension, postural / shock

Eosinophilia: wheeze, asthma attack

Diarrhoea + vomiting / constipation

O: hyp**O**glycaemia

U&Es: Urea ↑, Na ↓, K ↑, Ca ↑ (thiazide-like ↓ Na resorption from distal convoluted tubule)

Thyroid: hypothyroidism, responsive to steroids

<u>**Ix**</u>   1. Plasma cortisol < 200 nmol/l
      2. Short Synacthen test (SST)
          Method: Synacthen 250μg (IV or IM ACTH analogue) → measure cortisol at 0, 30, 60 min
                  (ensure patient switched to dexamethasone or prednisolone first – not hydrocortisone)
          Result: Cortisol > 550 nmol/l: normal;
                   Cortisol < 550 nmol/l: adrenocortical insufficiency (1°, 2°)
      3. Differentiation of 1° vs 2° hypoadrenalism
          a) ACTH - high in 1°, but not 2° hypoadrenalism
          b) Aldosterone at 30 min into SST: rise in 2° but not 1° hypoadrenalism
          c) Depot Synacthen Test: give Synacthen 1 mg IM → measure cortisol at 0, 6 and 24 hrs
             • No cortisol rise: 1° hypoadrenalism
             • Cortisol peaks at 24 hrs: 2° hypoadrenalism
             • Cortisol peaks at 6 hrs (to 900 mmol): normal

<u>**Rx**</u>   1. Acute
          a) Normal saline infusion; 50% dextrose if hypoglycaemic
          b) Hydrocortisone 100 mg 4 hrly
      2. Chronic
          a) Hydrocortisone 20 mg mane + 10 mg evening
          b) Fludrocortisone 0.1 mg od (not required if on high-dose hydrocortisone, or if 2° hypoadrenalism)
      3. Education
          MedicAlert bracelet; double hydrocortisone dose if intercurrent illness or enzyme-inducer

Cushing's Syndrome

PC　Glucocorticoids enhance breakdown of glycogen and protein to glucose and amino-acids, respectively:-

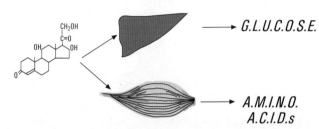

$\longrightarrow$ G.L.U.C.O.S.E.

$\longrightarrow$ A.M.I.N.O.
A.C.I.D.s

Glucose ↑　　• Diabetes mellitus; hyperphagia

Lipids
- Fat redistributed centripetally: buffalo hump; moon facies; supraclavicular fat pad
- Hyperlipidaemia

Ulcers, gastic • Esp. if taking NSAIDs

Children　　• Growth suppression

Osteo-
- Osteoporosis: esp. vertebral bodies; rib fractures with prominent callus formation
- Osteonecrosis: avascular necrosis of bone, esp. femoral head (vasoconstriction)

Skin
- Thinning, purple striae (> 1cm wide), bruises, telangiectasia, plethoric cheeks
- Acne; hirsutism, due to increased androgen secretion from adrenals
- Hyperpigmentation - due to ACTH excess
- Poor wound healing

Electrolytes • K^+ ↓; alkalosis – esp. when due to ectopic ACTH

ABP ↑　　　• Diastolic hypertension, due to fluid retention and oedema

Myopathy　• Proximal weakness, wasting, hoarseness (inhaled steroids - vocal fold myopathy)

Immunocompromise / Infections
- TB reactivation; *Aspergillus*
- Viruses - extensive disease: measles; VZV; HSV (corneal dendritic ulcer - topical)
- Candidiasis, esp. oral with inhaled steroids

Neuropsychiatric
- Fatigue, depression
- Depression; psychosis; mania; emotional lability
- Primary intracranial hypertension

Ocular
- Cataracts
- Glaucoma usually only from local steroid action (eye drops or nebulizer)

Abdomen　　• Acute pancreatitis

Coagulopathy • Hypercoagulability, e.g. DVT

Infertility　　• Amenorrhoea or impotence (pregnancy $\Rightarrow$ fetal adrenal hypoplasia)

Dependence, steroid
- Relative hypoadrenalism occurs during infection or trauma, necessitating an increase in steroid dose

Causes

Plasma cortisol suppressible by high-dose dexamethasone
   Pituitary: 'Cushing's disease'   (60%)
      Pituitary Microadenoma (< 1cm) = 95% Cushing's disease
      Epi: young females (age = 25-35; F:M = 3:1)

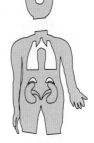

Plasma cortisol insuppressible by high-dose dexamethasone
   Adrenal adenoma / carcinoma / nodular hyperplasia (30%)
   Ectopic ACTH or CRH   (10%)
      e.g. bronchial (small cell carcinoma or adenoma); ovarian ca.; APUDomas
      Epi: elderly males

   Steroid therapy (commonest overall cause)
   'PseudoCushing's': alcoholism; depression; obesity; anorexia nervosa

Ix

Bloods   1. Morning cortisol (normal < 700 nmol/l) - screens for Cushing's syndrome
   2. ACTH ↑: ectopic ACTH ≫ pituitary > adrenal cause
   3. Na⁺ ↑; K⁺ ↓; alkalosis – may be only abnormality in ectopic ACTH secretion
   4. FBC: neutrophilia, lymphopenia

Urine: 1. 24-hour free cortisol: (normal < 140nmol /day)
   2. 17-Hydroxycorticosteroid: ↑ in pituitary; ectopic ACTH
      17-Ketosteroid: ↑ in adrenal carcinoma, ectopic ACTH

Radio: 1. Pituitary MRI - detects 60% microadenomas
   2. CXR / Chest CT
   3. Abdominal CT – Bilateral adrenal hyperplasia
               – Adrenal nodules: small = adenoma; large, necrotic = carcinoma

Special: 1. Low-dose dexamethasone (DXM) test
      • Method: 0.5mg qds for 2 days (or 1 mg nocte) ⇒ measure plasma cortisol next morning
      • Result: morning cortisol > 140nmol/l: Cushing's syndrome (not 'PseudoCushings')
   2. High-dose dexamethasone (DXM) test
      • Method: 2mg qds for 2 days ⇒ measure plasma cortisol next morning
      • Result: – plasma cortisol ↓ to 50% baseline: pituitary (but not macroadenomas)
               – plasma cortisol does not suppress: ectopic ACTH; adrenal; steroid Rx
   3. Inferior-petrosal sinus sampling: IV CRH ⇒ 60 mins sample of sinus and plasma
            ACTH and cortisol: ↑ in pituitary cause (bilateral sampling enables localization)

Rx   **Pituitary**
   1. Trans-sphenoidal microadenectomy - 80% cure rate; ☠ panhypopituitarism
   2. Chemical adrenalectomy - mitotane or 11-hydroxylase inhibition with metyrapone or ketoconazole
   3. Surgical adrenalectomy - ☠ Addison's syn; Nelson's syn: pigmentation due to pituitary disinhibition

Adrenal
   1. Adenoma: resection: ☠ Addison's due to previous contralateral adrenocortical atrophy
   2. Carcinoma: resection; mitotane; radiotherapy for bone mets. (overall 5 year SR = 20%)

Ectopic ACTH
   Primary tumour - resection / chemotherapy; Advanced - adrenalectomy as for Cushing's disease

Hypermineralocorticoidism

1° Hyper-Aldosteronism

Adenoma, adrenal (Conn's) - 75% of primary hyperaldosteronism; esp. women in 30-50s

Bilateral nodular hyperplasia

Carcinoma, adrenal - rare

Defective gene: glucocorticoid remediable aldosteronism (GRA) - chimeric gene of aldosterone synthase with 11β-Hydroxylase-1 promoter, resulting in ACTH-sensitive secretion of aldosterone in zona fasciculata

PC Diastolic hypertension (but no oedema, due to 'aldosterone escape'); weakness, due to K$^+$ $\downarrow$

Ix Bloods
1. K$^+$ $\downarrow$, Mg^{2+} $\downarrow$, metabolic alkalosis (Na$^+$ $\uparrow$ - uncommon)
2. Aldosterone $\uparrow$ $\uparrow$; renin $\downarrow$; ratio of aldosterone (pg/ml) : plasma-renin-activity > 400
   - Stop diuretics for 2 weeks; correct K$^+$
   - Prior salt-loading (NaCl 1.2g od) increases sensitivity, but avoid if SBP > 115mmHg
   - Effect of standing on aldosterone: Conn's - paradoxical $\downarrow$; Normal or BNH - $\uparrow$
3. Synacthen: Conn's - aldosterone slight $\uparrow$; BNH - no effect; GRA - aldosterone $\uparrow$ $\uparrow$

Radiology
1. High-resolution CT: adenomas > 1cm; BNH - bilateral adrenal cortex enlargement
2. Selective adrenal vein catheterization: compare aldosterone:cortisol ratio from each side
3. Radiolabelled cholesterol + dexamethasone (inhibits normal steroidogenesis): uni- vs bilateral

Rx Adenoma or ca.- surgery ; BNH - spironolactone, amiloride; GRA - dexamethasone ($\downarrow$ es ACTH)

2° Hyper-Aldosteronism

Reninism, primary: renin-secreting renal or ovarian tumour

Renovascular disease: renal artery stenosis; malignant hypertension

Gitelman's syndrome: $\downarrow$ NaCl resorption in distal convoluted tubule defect $\Rightarrow$ thiazide-like diuresis

Bartter's syndrome: $\downarrow$ NaCl resorption in ascending Loop of Henle $\Rightarrow$ frusemide-like diuresis

Hypovolaemia: congestive cardiac failure, hypoalbuminaemia, profuse sweating

PC Renovascular: hypertension, weakness due to K$^+$ $\downarrow$
     G.B.H: hypotension, weakness due to K$^+$ $\downarrow$, Mg^{2+} $\downarrow$

Ix Bloods: Na$^+$, Cl$^-$, K$^+$, Mg^{2+} – all $\downarrow$; renin $\uparrow$
    Urine Ca^{2+} - Gitelman's – $\downarrow$ Bartter's – $\uparrow$ (also, prostaglandins $\uparrow$)

Rx Bartter's – amiloride, ACE inhibitor, indomethacin (reverses juxtaglomerular hypertrophy)

Hypo-Aldosteronism ('Apparent Hypermineralocorticoidism')

Adrenal hyperplasia, congenital -11β-hydroxylase or 17α-hydroxylase deficiency (autosomal recessive)

B: 11 β-hydroxysteroid dehydrogenase deficiency (autosomal recessive), or excess liquorice

Cushing's syndrome

DOComa: 11-deoxycorticosterone-secreting adrenal tumour

Excess Na$^+$ resorption from distal-convoluted tubule: Liddle's syn (autosomal dom. mutation of Na$^+$ channel)

PC virilization of females - 11β-hydroxylase def.; hypogonadism -17α-hydroxylase deficiency

Ix Bloods: 11-deoxycorticosterone $\uparrow$ in congenital adrenal hyperplasia and DOComas
    Urine: ratio of urine cortisol:cortisone $\uparrow$ in 11BHSD deficiency

Rx congenital adrenal hyperplasia, 11BHSD deficiency - dexamethasone

Steroid Synthesis

The three main steroid types - mineralocorticoids (aldosterone); glucocorticoids (cortisol), and sex steroids are synthesized in the outer, middle and inner layers of the adrenal cortex, respectively:

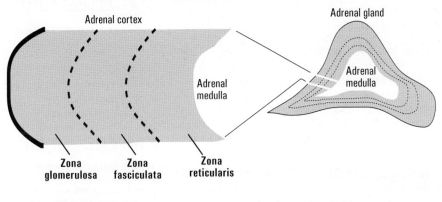

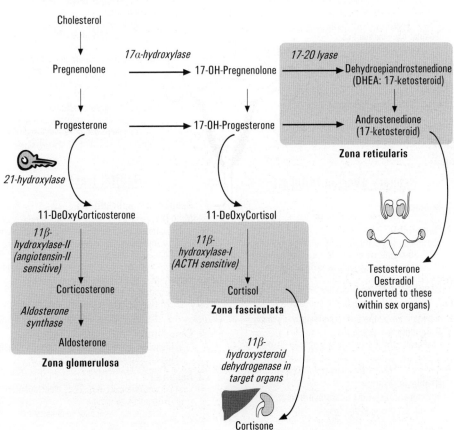

Amenorrhoea – Causes

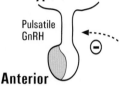

Hypothalamus

Pulsatile
GnRH

⊖

**Anterior
Pituitary**

Gonadotrophins
(FSH, LH)   Estrogen

Ovary

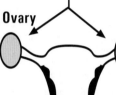

Hypothalamus – Pituitary

1. Constitutional
   a) delayed puberty (inherited)
   b) anorexia, anxiety, exercise, severe illness

2. Hypothalamus - Pituitary
   D.I.V.I.N.I.T.Y.
   Developmental: Kallman's syn: = failure of migration of GnRH cells from olfactory epithelium
   Infection: TB, meningitis
   Vascular: infarction
   Inflammation: hypophysitis
   Neoplasia:
      – craniopharyngioma, pinealoma
      – pituitary adenoma
   Injury: surgery, radiotherapy
   Toxins: e.g. neuroleptics
   Y: h**Y**drocephalus

3. Endocrine
   a) prolactin ↑
   b) T4: ↑ or ↓
   c) cortisol: ↑ or ↓, diabetes

Estrogen excess

Mechanism:
 • Excess, acyclical estrogen switches off pituitary gonadotrophs
 • Breakthrough bleeding may occur

1. Pregnancy; 'Pill'; post-pill

2. Ovarian tumour, estrogen-secreting
   a) Granulosa-theca cell
   b) Mucinous
   c) Brenner

3. Hyperandrogenism
   Mechanism:
      androgens are aromatized to estrogen in adipose tissue
   Causes:
   a) Polycystic ovaries syndrome –
      Epi: 10% of women, esp. obese
      Path: exaggerated adrenarche (adrenal androgens at puberty)
      Ix: estrone ↑,
         androstendione ↑,
         LH ↑, FSH ↓
   b) Cushing's syndrome
   c) Carcinoma: adrenal, ovarian
   d) Female pseudohermaphroditism

Primary ovarian failure

1. Menopause

2. Congenital
   a) Turner's syn (XO or mosaic with XX or XY)
   b) 17,20-desmolase or 17α-hydroxylase deficiency
   c) Galactosaemia - galactose toxic to ovaries

3. Acquired < 40 years (premature ovarian failure)
   T.A.I.N.T.
   Toxins - chemotherapy, radiotherapy, smoking
   Autoimmune - oophoritis
      Schmidt's syn. = oophoritis + thyroiditis + Addison's
   Infection - mumps, chlamydia, gonorrhoea
         (pelvic inflammatory disease)
   Neoplasia, ovarian
   Temporary resistant ovary syndrome:
      normal estrogen and follicles, but ovaries become FSH insensitive

Genital tract

1. Pseudohermaphroditism
   Male (XY, female ext. genitalia, no uterus)
   a) Testicular feminization - androgen resistance
   b) 5α reductase deficiency = 'Penis-at-12'
   c) Congenital adrenal hyperplasia:
         3β-hydroxysteroid dehydrogenase deficient
   Female (XX, virilized genitalia, no uterus)
      Congenital adrenal hyperplasia:
      21-Hydroxylase deficiency: Addison's
      11-Hydroxylase deficiency: hypertension

2. Congenital
   a) Mullerian agenesis: vaginal or uterine atresia
   b) Imperforate hymen or vaginal septae

3. Acquired
   a) Cervical stenosis, e.g. 2° to electrocautery
   b) Asherman's syndrome:
         intrauterine synechiae secondary to curettage
   c) TB, trauma (inc. hysterectomy!)

Amenorrhoea – PC

<u>**Types**</u>
- Primary amenorrhoea: no menses by 15 years old
- Secondary amenorrhoea: failure of previously normal menses
  - most causes of amenorrhoea may present in either way, including congenital causes that may present as secondary amenorrhoea

PC *The cause may be suggested by the patient's S.H.A.P.E.*

Syndrome, congenital
1. Turner's syndrome (XO)
   - Short stature, shield chest, wide-carrying angle
   - Coarctation of aorta, ASD, mild learning disability, acalculia
2. Enzyme defect: tall stature (failure of epiphyseal closure by estrogen)
3. Kallman's syndrome (X-linked)
   - Puberty delay; anosmia, sensorineural deafness, colour blind; renal agenesis, short metacarpals, bimanual synkinesia

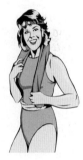

Hair
1. *Hairy and obese:* PCOS (Stein-Leventhal syndrome)
   - Acne, hirsutism on upper lip; subumbilical; thighs
   - Associated acanthosis nigricans, diabetic retinopathy etc.
2. *Hairy and medium:* other causes of virilization and hirsutism
   - Congenital adrenal hyperplasia (21- or 11β-hydroxylase deficiency)
   - Adrenal carcinoma
3. *Hairy and thin:* anorexia nervosa: lanugo
4. *Hairless* (pubic hair absence)
   - Testicular feminization (normal breasts)
   - Delayed puberty (small breasts)

ABP
1. Hypertension: 17α- or 11β-hydroxylase deficiency
2. Hypotension: 21-hydroxylase deficiency; Addison's

Private parts
1. Vagina
   - Haematocolpos: imperforate hymen / vaginal septae - cyclical pain
   - Blind-ending: Mullerian agenesis or testicular feminization
   - Vulval atrophy: ovarian failure
2. Cliteromegaly / labial enlargement or fusion
   - Polycystic ovaries syndrome
   - Congenital adrenal hyperplasia (21- or 11β-hydroxylase deficiency)
   - Adrenal carcinoma
3. Breasts
   - Enlargement: estrogen-secreting tumour
   - Atrophy: ovarian failure

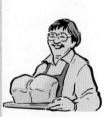

Endocrine
1. Menopause (ovarian or hypothal-pit. failure)
   hot flushes, night sweats, headaches, osteoporosis
2. Puberty
   precocious or delayed
3. Addison's:
   21-hydroxylase deficiency or Schmidt's syndrome (autoimmune)
   - latter also assoc. with hypothyroidism

Amenorrhoea – Ix

Hypothalamus – Pituitary

1. Pituitary hormones

FSH:
Low:
- Pituitary failure
- Polycystic ovaries (FSH:LH ratio < 1:3)
- Genital tract defect (normal estrogen levels)

High:
- Ovarian failure (as no −ve feedback)

Prolactin:
- Cause of amenorrhoea
- Also raised in PCOS

TSH, T4:
- Cause of amenorrhoea
- Also low in hypopituitarism

2. Gonadorelin test
Inject GnRH (IV or SC) ⇒
FSH+LH ↑↑ in Kallman's syn.
FSH+LH ↓ in hypopituitarism

3. MRI head
- Pituitary tumour, esp. prolactinoma,
- Craniopharyngioma

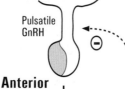

Hypothalamus

Pulsatile GnRH

⊖

Anterior pituitary

Gonadotrophins (FSH, LH)

Estrogen

Ovary

Estrogen Excess

1. Androgens
a) Serum testosterone ↑:
- DHEA ↑
- Androstenedione ↑ (principal circulating androgen)

b) Sex-hormone-binding globulin ↓ (binds testosterone preferently)

c) Urine 17-ketosteroids ↑↑
- PCOS
- Congenital adrenal hyperplasia
- Adrenal or ovarian carcinoma (dexamethasone suppresses 17-KS in PCOS and CAH, but not carcinoma)

2. Other bloods
a) β-HCG: pregnant?!
b) Glucose ↑: PCOS

3. Pelvic–abdominal USS
a) PCOS
- Bilateral, multiple, small follicular cysts in 'necklace' around edge; stromal, endometrial hyperplasia
b) Adrenal or ovarian carcinoma

Ovaries

1. Estrogen and Progesterone
Low:
- Ovarian failure
- Pituitary failure
- Testicular feminisation

Variable: • PCOS

Cyclical:
- Distinguishes vaginal obstruction (cyclical) from testicular feminization (acyclical)

2. Sex chromosome analysis:
Turner's syndrome (+ PCR of sex-determining region of Y)

3. Autoimmune cause:
a) AutoAbs: anti-ovarian; thyroid; adrenal Abs
b) Glucose: diabetes mellitus occurs as part of Schmidt's syndrome

Genital Tract

1. Cervical mucus analysis
- Stretchiness – spinnbarkeit
- Ferning on microscopy

2. Progestagen withdrawal bleed
Method:
- Exclude pregnancy
- Give medroxyprogesterone for 5 days; then stop
- If no bleed then give oral conjugated estrogen for 14 days prior (to prime uterus)

Results:
- Bleed: PCOS or other excess estrogen
- Bleed after estrogen
- Pituitary or ovarian failure
- No bleed: genital tract damage

3. Hysterosalpingogram or hysteroscopy
- Cervical stenosis / Asherman's syndrome

<u>Amenorrhoea – Rx</u>

<u>Hypothalamus – Pituitary</u>

1. Gonadotrophins / GnRH
   a) Human menopausal
      gonadotrophins (or purified
      FSH) + mid-cycle β-HCG
      (simulates LH)
   b) Pulsatile GnRH in portable infusion
      pump:
      • Improves efficacy of
        gonadotrophins

2. Clomiphene
   • Estrogen partial agonist: FSH ↑
   • Ovary stimulant

3. Prolactinoma treatment
   • Dopamine agonists
     Rx prior to pregnancy due to
     risk of expansion!

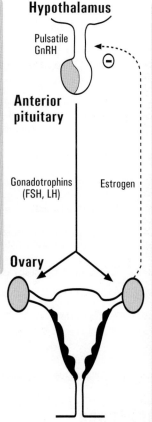

Hypothalamus

Pulsatile
GnRH

⊖

**Anterior
pituitary**

Gonadotrophins   Estrogen
(FSH, LH)

Ovary

<u>PCOS</u>

1. Hormonal
   a) Gonadotrophins / GnRH /
      clomiphene: ↑es fertility by
      ↑ing FSH
   b) Buserelin: ↓es LH
   c) OCP: ↓es ovarian and adrenal
      androgen production

2. Obesity
   a) Diet
   b) Insulin sensitizers:
      metformin or roglitazone:
      • ↓es ovarian androgen
        production by ↓ing insulin
        secretion, as insulin has
        direct ovarian effect
      • ↑es fertility, but stop drug
        in pregnancy

3. Hirsutism
   a) Topical: epilation, electrolysis,
      cover-up, H_2O_2 bleach
   b) 'Dianette' = cyproterone acetate
      (anti-androgen) + ethinylE2
      (contraceptive, as cyproterone
      is teratogenic)
   c) Spironolactone

4. Electrocautery of cysts
   Wedge resection of large cysts
   • ↓es ovarian androgen
     production and ovarian
     adhesions

<u>Primary Ovarian Failure</u>

If fertility desired:
   1. Low-dose prednisolone: induces ovulation
   2. Ovum donation + cyclical gonadotrophins

If fertility not desired:
   1. Combined OCP:
      • Regularizes periods
      • ↓es ovarian androgen production
   2. HRT (conjugated estrogens + progestagen):
      • Used in ovarian or pituitary failure as
        prophylaxis against osteoporosis

Turner's XY mosaic
   Gonadectomy, as at risk of dysgerminoma

<u>Genital Tract</u>

Surgery
   Cervical stenosis / Asherman's syndrome:
   dilatation

Male Sexual Problems

Gynaecomastia

Causes

P.E.C.T.O.R.A.L.I.s

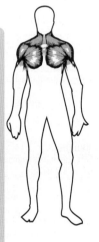

Physiological
Neonatal, puberty (often unilateral; resolves within 1 year), elderly

Endocrine
1. Hypogonadism:
   - Hypogonadotrophic: Kallman's syn., hypopituitarism, hyperprolactinaemia
   - Hypergonadotrophic, e.g. Klinefelter's, mumps orchitis, orchidectomy
2. Other: thyrotoxicosis, Cushing's (both ↑aromatase activity), diabetes

Carcinoma
1. Testis tumour: Leydig cell ⇒ estrogen; choriocarcinoma ⇒ β-HCG
2. Adrenal tumour
3. Ectopic: bronchial, liver, renal

Toxins – C.U.P.S.
Cardiac: spironolactone, digoxin, amiodarone, calcium antagonists
Ulcer: cimetidine, proton-pump inhibitors
Psychiatric: anti-dopaminergics, TCAs, opiates, cannabis, amphetamines
Steroids: goserelin, flutamide, ketoconazole, metronidazole, anabolic steroids

Organ failure
1. Cirrhosis: sex-hormone-binding globulin ↑, testis atrophy, alcohol ↑es estrogen
2. Chronic renal failure: prolactin ↑; testicular failure

Refeeding syndrome: post-fast

Adrenal: congenital adrenal hyperplasia (excess testosterone)

Local stimulation (via hyperprolactinaemia): breast cancer, VZV, thoractomy

Infection: TB, HIV

Rx   1. Medical: testosterone, danazol, tamoxifen. 2. Surgical: reduction mammoplasty + liposuction

Impotence

Causes

P.A.T.E.N.T.S.

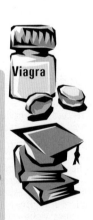

Psychological: anxiety, depression
Arterial:
  - Aorto-iliac thrombosis (Leriche's syndrome)
  - Sickle-cell anaemia
Toxins-1:
  - Alcohol or drug abuse
Endocrine:
  - Diabetes mellitus (autonomic neuropathy, arteriopathy)
  - Hypogonadism; hyperprolactinaemia; dysthyroidism
Neurological:
  - Autonomic neuropathy; cord disease, esp. MS; cauda equina lesion
Toxins: as for gynaecomastia (C.U.P.S.)
  e.g. spironolactone, digoxin, β-blockers, α_1-antagonists
Systemic: liver, renal failure, carcinoma

Rx   1. Oral: sildenafil. 2. Intra-urethral or intracavernosal alprostadil. 3. Prosthesis or vacuum. 4. Psychotherapy

Male Infertility

Hypothalamus – Pituitary

1. **Constitutional**
   Anorexia: anxiety, severe illness,
   e.g. organ failure, carcinoma
2. **Hypothalamus – Pituitary**
   D.I.V.I.N.I.T.Y.
   Developmental:
   - Kallman's syndrome
   - Prader–Willi syndrome
   - Spinocerebellar ataxia
   Infection: TB, meningitis
   Vascular: infarction
   Inflammation: sarcoid
   Neoplasia:
   - Craniopharyngioma
   - Pituitary adenoma
   Injury: surgery, radiotherapy
   Toxins: e.g. neuroleptics
   Y: h**Y**drocephalus
3. **Endocrine**
   a) GH ↑ or ↓
   b) Prolactin ↑
   c) T4 ↑ or ↓

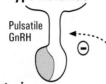

Hypothalamus

Pulsatile
GnRH

⊖

**Anterior
pituitary**

Gonadotrophins
(FSH, LH)   Testosterone

Testes

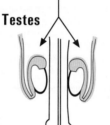

Estrogen excess

1. Congenital adrenal hyperplasia
2. Cushing's syndrome
   (and Addison's disease)
3. Anabolic steroids

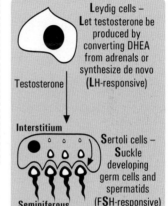

Leydig cells –
Let testosterone be
produced by
converting DHEA
from adrenals or
synthesize de novo
(**L**H-responsive)

Testosterone

Interstitium

Sertoli cells –
Suckle
developing
germ cells and
spermatids
(F**S**H-responsive)

Seminiferous
tubule

Primary Testicular Failure

1. **Congenital**
   a) Klinefelter's syndrome (XXY):
      - Small, firm testes, but potent
      - Gynaecomastia, breast carcinoma
      - Eunuchoid: gigantism, short spine, long limbs,
        high voice, learning disability, unemotional
   b) Androgen resistance:
      - 5α-reductase deficiency ('penis-at-12')
      - Myotonic dystrophy
      - Spinobulbar muscular atrophy

2. **Acquired**
   T.A.I.N.T.
   Toxins:
   - Chemo-, radiotherapy, smoking, alcohol
   - Digoxin, spironolactone
   - Sulphasalazine, phenytoin, nitrofurantoin
   Autoimmune: polyarteritis nodosa orchitis
   Infection: mumps, mycoplasma, TB,
            STD (gonococcus, chlamydia)
   Neoplasia, testis
   Temperature ↑: crytorchidism, varicocoele
   Torsion / Trauma: inc. hernia repair

Spermatazoa defects

1. **Genetic** – *60% cases of male infertility!*
   a) Microdeletions Yq xsome, inc.
      - AZoospermia Factor (AZF),
      - Deleted in Azoospermia (DAZ)
   b) Germinal- or Leydig-cell aplasia

2. **Autoimmune**
   Membrane-bound anti Ig-A
   (inc. vasectomy, infection, familial)

3. **Immotility**
   a) Cystic fibrosis
   b) Kartagener's syndrome: associated
      dextrocardia, bronchiectasis, sinusitis

Precocious Puberty

__Def__   Development of secondary sexual characteristics < 8 years (in girls) or < 9 years (boys)

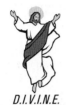

D.I.V.I.N.E.

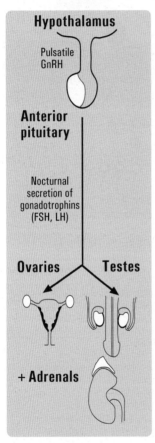

Hypothalamus

Pulsatile
GnRH

**Anterior
pituitary**

Nocturnal
secretion of
gonadotrophins
(FSH, LH)

Ovaries   **Testes**

+ Adrenals

True

Def: Premature activation of hypothalamo–pituitary–gonadal axis

Causes: *D.I.V.I.N.E.*

> **D**evelopmental – idiopathic: accounts for 2/3 of cases;
>   girls > boys; often familial
> **I**nfection: meningo-encephalitis, congenital infections
> **V**ascular: perinatal anoxia
> **I**njury, head / hydrocephalus
> **N**eoplasia – hypothalamic:
>   craniopharyngioma, hamartoma, neurofibroma
> **E**pilepsy, idiopathic
> **E**ndocrine: hypothyroidism ⇒ FSH↑

PC: 1. Boys: spermatogenesis   + virilization
        Girls: periods   + feminization
           i.e. appropriate sexual characteristics – isosexual
    2. Growth spurt;
       eventual short stature (premature epiphyseal fusion)

Ix: FSH↑, LH↑; Gonadorelin challenge ⇒ LH↑ > FSH↑

Rx: Long-acting gonadorelin analogue (goserelin): ↓ es gonadotrophins

Pseudo

Def: Excess sex steroids or activation of steroid receptors,
      independent of HPA axis

Causes: *G.A.M.E.S.*

> **G**onadal tumour:
>   • Testis (teratoma, Leydig cell) ⇒ testosterone, estrogen
>   • Ovarian tumour (granulosa cell) or ovarian cysts
> **A**drenal:
>   • Congenital adrenal hyperplasia
>   • Adrenal tumour (suggested by > 6 cm mass in adrenals)
> **M**cCune–Albright syndrome:
>   Path: autonomous LH receptor activity, via mutated Gsα
>   PC: Polyostotic fibrous dysplasia; café-au-lait spots
> **E**xogenous sex steroids / Ectopic gonadotrophins:
>   hepatoblastoma; pineal dysgerminoma ⇒ β-HCG, AFP
> **S**yndrome – testotoxicosis:
>   LH receptor mutation on Leydig cells, in boys only

PC: 1. Secondary sexual characteristics only (gonad, adrenal causes)
    2. Heterosexual precocity, i.e. boys ⇒ breasts; girls ⇒ virilized

Ix: 1. FSH↓, LH↓; Gonadorelin challenge ⇒ no response
    2. Urine 17-ketosteroids ↑: gonadal or adrenal cause;
       dexamethasone ⇒ 17-KS↓ in congenital adrenal hyperplasia
    3. MRI or CT adrenals; USS testes or pelvis

Rx: 1. Medroxyprogesterone acetate, ketoconazole
    2. Anti-androgens: cyproterone acetate, spironolactone

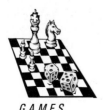

G.A.M.E.S.

Delayed Puberty

Def   No development of secondary sexual characteristics by 14 years

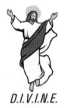

D.I.V.I.N.E.

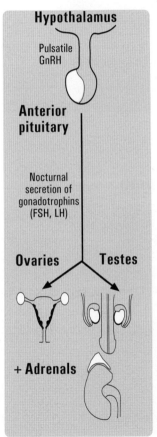

Hypothalamic – Pituitary Failure

Causes: *D.I.V.I.N.E.*

Developmental:
1. Idiopathic: commonest cause in boys; often familial
2. Kallman's syndrome:
   - Anosmia, due to failure of GnRH cells to migrate from olfactory mucosa (also deaf occasionally)
   - Cryptorchidism, microphallus, renal agenesis
3. Other syndromes:
   - Prader–Willi (hyperphagia, hypersomnolence, diabetes)
   - Lawrence–Moon–Biedl (retinitis pigmentosa, polydactyly, cardiac defects)

Infection: meningo-encephalitis, TB
Very ill: inc. anorexia, anxiety, strenuous exercise
Inflammation: sarcoid, SLE
Neoplasia: hypothalamic craniopharyngioma, hamartoma
Endocrine:
1. Hypopituitarism, or 'isolated gonadotrophin deficiency'
2. Hyperprolactinaemia
3. Thyroid or cortisol abnormalities (high or low); diabetes

Ix: FSH↓, LH↓
Rx: Pulsatile gonadorelin or gonadotrophins

Gonadal Failure

Causes:

Congenital:
1. Turner's syndrome (XO or mosaic with XX or XY):
   Commonest cause in girls
   PC: Webbed neck, wide-carrying angle, coarctation
2. Enzyme defect – e.g. 17α-hydroxylase deficiency
3. Klinefelter's syndrome (XXY):
   - Small, firm testes, azoospermia (but not impotent)
   - Gynaecomastia, breast carcinoma
   - Eunuchoidal: gigantism (short spine, long limbs), high-voice, learning disability, aggressive

Acquired: *T.A.I.N.T.*
Toxins: chemotherapy, radiotherapy, surgery, smoking
Autoimmune, inc. Schmidt's syndrome
Infection: mumps, chlamydia (PID) oophoritis
Neoplasia: testis or ovarian
Trauma: testis torsion

Ix: 1. FSH↑, LH↑
       2. Karyotype / buccal smear for Barr body (sex chromatin)
Rx: Anabolic steroids; ethinylestradiol + progestagen

Neuroendocrine Tumours

Neuroendocrine tumours are mostly derived from neural-crest cells, and secrete amines or peptides. They are also known as APUDomas as they all exhibit **A**mine **P**recursor **U**ptake and **D**ecarboxylation.

 C.A.P.I.T.A.L.S.

Carcinoid tumours / syndrome – *see p. 360.*
Adrenal phaeochromocytoma
Pancreatic endocrine tumours, including:
Islet-cell tumours
Thyroid medullary carcinoma
Additional – CNS glanglioblastoma, neuroblastoma, paragangliomas
Lung – small-cell carcinoma
Skin – melanoma

Ix: Most can be detected with an ^{131}I-MIBG scan

Adrenal Phaeochromocytoma

Epi
10% Familial MEN-2a,b syndromes, neurofibromatosis 1, von Hippel–Lindau syn.
10% Bilateral (50% of familial are bilateral)
10% Malignant
10% Extra-adrenal, e.g.
- Organ of Zuckerkandl (sympathetic ganglia below inferior mesenteric artery)
- Bladder wall: symptoms triggered by micturition!

PC
Paroxysmal hypertension: weakness, anxiety, tremor, sweat, headache, N+V, for 15 min
Postural hypotension (due to decreased plasma volume)
Palpitations, ischaemic heart disease, cardiomyopathy
Pallor (not flushing)
Pain (chest, epigastric, abdominal due to constipation)

Ix
Bloods: 1. Chromogranin A ↑ ; 2. Glucose ↑
Urine: 24-hour acid urine collection: VMA, HMMA, metadrenaline, free catecholamines ↑
Radiology: 1. CT, MRI Abdo; 2. ^{131}I-MIBG scan
Special: Pentolinium suppression test

Rx
1. Crisis: IV phentolamine or labetalol
2. Surgery: requires preoperative phenoxybenzamine + β-blocker for 3 weeks
3. Metastases: ^{131}I-MIBG

Pancreatic Endocrine Tumours (PETs)

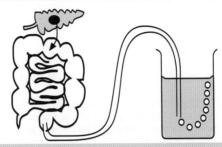

G.I.V.E.S.
G.A.S.

Glucagonoma (α-cells)
PC: 1. Diarrhoea, loss of weight
2. Diabetes mellitus
3. Necrolytic migratory erythema, glossitis–stomatitis, nail dystrophy
4. Deep-vein thrombosis
Ix: Failure of glucose suppression following arginine stimulation

Insulinoma (β-cells) – *Most common*
PC: Fasting hypoglycaemia (*see p. 324*)
Ix: Proinsulin:insulin ratio increased, C-peptide raised

VIPoma = 'Werner–Morrison syn.' (δ1-cells: vasoactive intestinal peptide)
PC: **W**atery **D**iarrhoea (> 1 l/day) with **H**ypokalaemia and **A**chlorhydria ('W.D.H.A.')

Ectopic endocrine secretions
GHRH – acromegaly; ACTH – Cushing's; ADH – SIADH; PTH – hyperPTHsim

Extra diarrhoea-causing secretions
PPoma (pancreatic polypeptide), neurotensinoma, calcitoninoma

Somatostatinoma (δ-cells)
PC: 1. Diarrhoea, loss of weight, steatorrhoea
2. Gallstones (relaxes gallbladder)
3. Diabetes mellitus, hypertension

GAStrinoma = 'Zollinger–Ellison syndrome' – *2nd most common*
Epi: 30% MEN-I syndrome; 10% multiple
Site: Islet cells; duodenum or adjacent to (G-cells); ectopic (parathyroid, ovary)
PC: 1. Peptic ulcers – multiple
2. Diarrhoea, malabsorption, steatorrhoea, Vit B12 deficiency
Ix: 1. Fasting serum gastrin (stop PPI / H2-antagonists for 1/52)
2. Secretin test (IV): paradoxical ↑ in gastrin (normally gastrin suppressed)
3. CT abdomen, selective angiography of pancreas

Rx 1. Somatostatin analogue (octreotide or lanreotide): improves diarrhoea in all
2. Specific: • Glucagonoma: zinc, high-protein diet, aspirin (not warfarin)
• Insulinoma: diazoxide, streptozocin
• Gastrinoma: high-dose omeprazole

Prognosis
About 2/3 of all islet-cell tumours metastasize (except insulinoma 10%; gastrinoma 30%)

Carcinoid Tumours

Def

Carcinoid tumours are one of the APUDomas, characterized by silver staining and the presence of cell markers chromogranin A, neuron-specific enolase and synaptophysin (on immunofluorescence), and somatostatin receptors.

Carcinoid syndrome occurs when a carcinoid tumour secretes biologically active peptides that reach the systemic circulation. The main secreted products are 5-hydroxytryptamine (5-HT or serotonin), tachykinins (substance P) and prostaglandins.

PC

Carcinoid tumours – local

GIT
- Abdominal pain, GI bleeding, obstruction
- Peritoneal fibrosis (esp. midgut or ovarian carcinoid)

Bronchial
- Cough, haemoptysis, incidental finding on CXR

Carcinoid syndrome – systemic

F.I.V.E. - H.T. - A.M.I.N.E

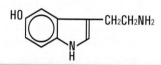

Flushing / Facial oedema
- Acute paroxysms of flushing, wheals, pruritus, lacrimation, salivation, hypotension that last 5 min – days
- Triggered by alcohol, cheese, straining, salbutamol
- Causes of flushing: *M.A.M.A.*
    Menopause, Alcohol, Mastocytosis, APUDoma, Autonomic neuropathy

Intestinal – diarrhoea, weight loss

Valve fibrosis – right-sided lesions (e.g. pulmonary stenosis), except bronchial carcinoid (left side)

E: WhEEze (esp. foregut tumours)

Hypoglycaemia

Telangiectasia, facial cyanosis – due to repeated attacks of flushing

Arthritis

Metastases – liver (hepatosplenomegaly), bone (pain)

Nicotinamide deficiency ('pellagra') – dermatitis of sun-exposed areas

Endocrine – Multiple endocrine neoplasia (MEN-1):
- Acromegaly (GHRH secreted by bronchial carcinoid)
- Cushing's syndrome (thymic carcinoid)
- HyperPTHism

Epi

The proportion of **carcinoid tumours** is:

	GIT 65%		Lung 30%		Other 5%
					Breast, thymus, ovary, testes
	Mets	Carcinoid syndrome	Mets	Carcinoid syndrome	Ovary and testes: 50% get carcinoid syndrome
Small bowel	60%	10%	Bronchial 5%	10%	
Rectum	5%	0%			

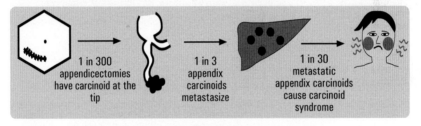

1 in 300 appendicectomies have carcinoid at the tip	1 in 3 appendix carcinoids metastasize	1 in 30 metastatic appendix carcinoids cause carcinoid syndrome

Ix

Blood: 5-HT, 5-hydroxytryptophan (5-HTP), histamine, chromogranin A ↑

Urine: 5-hydroxyindoleacetic-acid (5-HIAA) ↑ – levels act as prognostic marker
- False +ve: walnuts, bananas, paracetamol, aspirin, levodopa
- False –ve: atypical foregut carcinoids (urine 5-HT or 5-HTP ↑ instead)

Radio: 1. CT / MRI
2. Selective angiography
3. Octreotide scintigraphy: ligand for type 2 somatostatin receptors on tumour

Special: Provocative flushing with pentagastrin or adrenaline

Rx   1. Symptomatic:
- Flushing: somatostatin analogue (octreotide), diphenhydramine, ranitidine
- Diarrhoea: ketanserin, ondansetron
- Wheeze: aminophylline, steroids (avoid salbutamol!)

2. Curative:
- Resection: localized tumour or limited hepatic metastases
- Hepatic artery embolization
- Chemotherapy / radiotherapy: streptozocin, doxorubicin, interferon-α, ^{131}I-MIBG

Prognosis

5-year survival rate: local - 95%; lymph nodes - 65%; hepatic 20%
Tumours < 1 cm – curable; > 2 cm – frequently metastasize

Multiple Endocrine Neoplasia

All are autosomal dominant; all are caused by inactivating mutations of tumour suppressor genes

Type 1

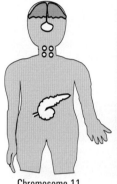

Chromosome 11
(gene = *menin*)

Midline 'P' organs

Pituitary: hyperplasia, adenoma

Parathyroid gland: hyperplasia, adenoma

Pancreas islet cell: hyperplasia, adenoma
    a) Gastrinoma: peptic ulcers (Zollinger–Ellinson syn.)
    b) Insulinoma: hypoglycaemia
    c) VIPoma: watery diarrhoea, K^+ ↓ (Werner–Morrison syn.)

Type 2

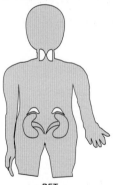

RET
('REarranged during
Transfection') =
tyrosine kinase

Paired (i.e. 2) organs

Thyroid: medullary carcinoma

Adrenals: phaeochromocytoma

Type 2A	Type 2B
PArAthyroid adenoma	**Big**: Marfanoid habitus
Anus: Hirschsprung's disease	**Big** tumours:
Amyloid:	mucosal, GIT neuromas
cutaneous lichen planus	

Other

Carney complex: 1. Adrenal, testicular, pituitary adenomas
                         2. Myxomas
                         3. Spotty pigmentation

von Hippel–Lindau syndrome:
                         1. Phaeochromocytoma, pancreatic islet-cell neoplasms
                         2. Renal tumours
                         3. CNS tumours, esp. cerebellar haemangioblastoma

Polyglandular Autoimmune Syndromes

Two main types exist: type 1 – childhood-onset and type 2 – adult-onset

Type 1 PGAS

Inc: Rare
Age: Childhood
Sex: M = F
Aet: • *APECED* gene = Autoimmune PolyEndocrinopathy, Candidiasis, Ectodermal Dystrophy
    • Autosomal recessive; chromosome 21

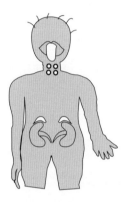

P.G.A.S.

Parathyroidism, hypo-
GIT:
    • Mucocutaneous candidiasis (esp. oral)
    • Malabsorption
    • Pernicious anaemia
    • Chronic active hepatitis
Addison's disease
Skin:
    • Dystrophy of teeth (enamel), nails, hair (alopecia)
    • Vitiligo
    • Otosclerosis

Type 2 PGAS (Schmidt's Syndrome)

Inc: Common
Age: Adulthood
Sex: F > M
Aet: • Polygenic: HLA-DR3 and -DR4-associated
    • Autosomal dominant with incomplete penetrance

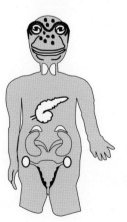

T.O.A.D. – P.G.A.S.

Thyroidism, dys-: Grave's or Hashimoto's disease
Oophoritis / **O**rchitis: infertility
Addison's disease
Diabetes, type 1

Pituitary: lymphocytic hypophysitis
GIT:
    • Coeliac disease
    • Pernicious anaemia
Additional: myasthenia gravis
Skin: vitiligo

Clinical Chemistry

Acid–Base Balance

Acidosis has two types of 1° cause, each being compensated by the other system:

- **Respiratory:** $PaCO_2$ ↑, due to ventilation ↓
  ⇒ renal compensation, via HCO_3^- resorption, and acid and NH_4^+ excretion
- **Metabolic:** HCO_3^- ↓ due to acid gain (high anion gap) or bicarbonate loss (low anion gap)
  ⇒ respiratory compensation, by $PaCO_2$ ↓

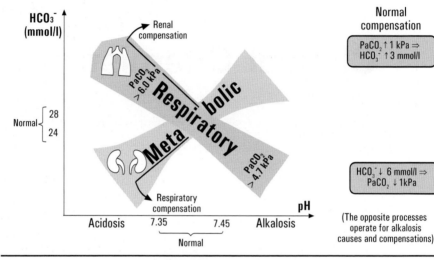

Normal compensation

$PaCO_2$ ↑1 kPa ⇒ HCO_3^- ↑3 mmol/l

HCO_3^- ↓ 6 mmol/l ⇒ $PaCO_2$ ↓1kPa

(The opposite processes operate for alkalosis causes and compensations)

HCO₃⁻ (mmol/l)

Renal compensation

$PaCO_2 > 6.0$ kPa

Respiratory

Metabolic

28
Normal
24

$PaCO_2 > 4.7$ kPa

Respiratory compensation

Acidosis   7.35   7.45   Alkalosis   pH

Normal

Respiratory

Acidosis: failure of CO_2 excretion via lungs

Ventilatory failure:

Obstructive	Restrictive
Small airways: COAD	Pulmonary fibrosis
Intrathoracic: cancer, lymph node	Neuromuscular: sedation, polio
Foreign body	Skeletal: spondylosis

Diffusion failure: Late pneumonia; ARDS

Alkalosis: hyperventilation due to stimulation of lung irritant receptors or medulla

Lung: 1. Fluid: pulmonary oedema; early pneumonia
2. Pulmonary embolism; atelectasis
3. Pneumothorax; flail chest

CNS: *I.N.V.I.T.E. I.S. F.R.E.E.:*
1. Intracranial: **I**nfection (meningitis), **N**eoplasia, **V**ascular, **I**njury, **T**oxin (aspirin, adrenaline)
Extra - pain, anxiety
2. Extracranial: **I**nfection – septicaemia; **S**ystemic – anaemia, hypotension, high altitude
Failure: cardiac, liver; **R**ecovery from metabolic acidosis;
Endocrine-1 – thyrotoxicosis; **E**ndocrine-2 – pregnancy, progesterone

Iatrogenic: mechanical ventilation, respiratory stimulants (e.g. doxapram)

Metabolic

Acidosis: classifed by size of anion gap $= (Na^+ + K^+) - (Cl^- + HCO_3^-)$: Normal: 8–18 mmol/l

K.I.L.L.E.R. T.R.I.G.G.E.R.

High Anion Gap: Organic acid gain

Ketoacidosis: DM, alcoholism (due to binge drinking, starvation)

Intake of organic acid: aspirin overdose, methanol, ethylene glycol
  High osmolar gap: Osmolality $- (2 \times Na^+ + glucose + urea) > 15$ mmol/l

Lactic acidosis, type A: tissue hypoxia:
  • Shock, hypoxia, poisoning: carbon monoxide, cyanide, TCA overdose

Lactic acidosis, type B: metabolic abnormality:
  • Gluconeogenesis $\downarrow$: liver failure; paracetamol overdose; metformin
  • Formation $\uparrow$: neoplasia (e.g. leukaemia), infection (e.g. malaria, epilepsy)

Enzyme mutation:
  • Glycogen storage disease (G6Pase deficiency), mitochondrial disease,
    methylmalonic aciduria

Renal failure (GFR < 20 ml/min): uraemic toxins, lactic acid

Low Anion Gap: bicarbonate loss, failure of acid excretion, hyperchloraemia

Toxins:
  • Cardiac: ACE inhibitors, A-II receptor blockers, K^+-sparing diuretics, acetazolamide
  • Other: statins, trimethoprim, pentamidine, cyclosporin, cation-exchange resin

Renal tubular acidosis
  • $K^+ \downarrow$: RTA-1 = failure of acid excretion (severe – most tubulointerstitial nephropathies)
       RTA-2 = bicarbonate loss (isolated or part of Fanconi's syndrome)
  • $K^+ \uparrow$: RTA-4 (hypoaldosteronism)

Intake of ammonium: hyperalimentation (TPN), NH4Cl

Gastrointestinal: diarrhoea, esp. VIPoma

Gastrointestinal: ureterosigmoidostomy, ileostomy, fistulae (pancreatic, biliary)

'Expansion acidosis' = rapid IV NaCl infusion

Renal failure (GFR: 20–50 ml/min): failure of acid excretion

NB: • *Bicarbonate loss $\Rightarrow$ high urine NH₄⁺*
   • *Failure of acid excretion $\Rightarrow$ absent urine NH₄⁺*
     – where urine NH₄⁺ can be estimated from Urine Cation Gap = $(Cl^- + HCO_3^-) - (Na^+$

Alkal O sis: Mostly causes of hyp**O**kalaemia *(p. 375)*

C.a.R.D.I.ac

Corticosteroid excess:
  • 1° Hyperaldosteronism: adrenal adenoma, BNH or carcinoma; GRA
  • 2° Hyperaldosteronism: renin-secreting tumour, renal artery stenosis, Gitelman's syn.
  • Hypoaldosteronism: Liddle's syn., 'apparent mineralocorticoid excess' syn.

Renal: osmotic diuresis

Drugs: diuretics (e.g.thiazide, furosemide), penicillin, salbutamol

Intake of K^+ or Mg^{2+} $\downarrow$ (i.e. hypoMgaemia)

Intestinal loss: vomiting, villous adenoma of rectum

Hyponatraemia

Causes

Other solute	Excess water	Sodium loss
'PseudoHyponatraemia'		

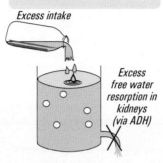

Excess intake

Excess free water resorption in kidneys (via ADH)

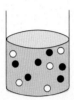

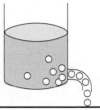

HOG (High Osmolar Gap)

Def:
Osmolar gap = actual - estimated
Estimated osmolality =
$2 \times (Na^+ + K^+) + Urea + Glucose$
High osmolar gap > 10 mmol/l

Causes:
1. Hyperosmolality
   – hyperglycaemia,
     e.g. diabetes, TPN
   – mannitol iv
2. Normal osmolality
   – hyperlipidaemia, e.g:
     diabetes, nephrosis
   – hyperproteinaemia, e.g.
     paraproteinaemia
   – NG-feed

LAG (Low Anion Gap)

Def:
Anion Gap =
$(Na^+ + K^+) - (Cl^- + HCO_3^-)$
Low Anion Gap: < 8 mmol/l

Mech: positive protein charge ⇒
   – displaces Na^+ from plasma
     to interstitium
   – compensatory ↑Cl^-

Causes:
   – Hypoalbuminaemia,
     e.g. nephrosis
   – Paraproteinaemia

Polydipsia (> 1.2l / hr)

Causes: *P.I.N.T.*
Psychogenic polydipsia;
   beer potomania
   = alcohol excess with
     inadequate solute in diet
Iatrogenic: post-operative IVI
Neuro: thalamus VMN lesion
TURP (bladder instillation)

Chronic hypovolaemia
(appropriate ADH excess)

Causes:
Oedematous states
(secondary hyperaldosteronism)
   – CCF, nephrosis, cirrhosis
   – pregnancy
Mech:
   – hypovolaemia ↑es ADH release
   – GFR↓ impairs distal tubular
     diluting capacity
   – "sick cell" syndrome =
     ↓Na^+K^+ATPase;
     ↓ intracellular protein
   – hypothal. osmoreceptor resets

SIADH
(inappropriate ADH excess)

Causes:
   P.I.N.T.S. – see opposite

Mech: ADH causes free water
   resorption from distal
   convoluted tubule and
   medullary collecting duct

Renal

Causes:
   – Diuretics (thiazide / loop)
   – TubuloInterstitial Nephritis
   – Hypoaldosteronism
     (RTA type IV)
     : e.g. Addison's; DM

Extra-renal

GIT, esp. villous adenoma,
   fistula, stoma

Skin
Blood

*N.B. Hyponatraemia never due
to inadequate salt intake!*

SIADH - Causes

P.I.N.T.S.

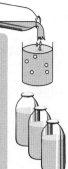

Pulmonary
  Infection esp. Legionella, TB (and rifampicin), abscess
  COAD; asthma; bronchial carcinoma
  CPAP or ventilation

Infection AIDS, pneumonia

Neurological
  CNS – meningo-encephalitis (esp. children)
      – stroke, traumatic brain injury, tumour, dementia
      – also causes "cerebral salt-wasting syndrome"
  PNS – autonomic neuropathy: acute intermittent porphyria, GBS
  Pain (and NSAIDs)

Toxins
  CNS – drugs of abuse: opiates, ecstasy, smoking
      – neuropsychiatric: carbamazepine, chlorpromazine; TCA, SSRI
      – anaesthetics, inhalational
  Chemotherapy: vincristine, cisplatin, cyclophosphamide
  Clofibrate; **C**hlorpropamide

SLE

Systemic
  Thyroid   – hypothyroidism
  Neoplasm – carcinoma of prostate, bladder, pancreas; carcinoid; lymphoma
  Malnutrition

PC Chronic
          – asymptomatic, or lethargy
      Acute (or late chronic)
          – headache / N+V
          – cerebral oedema: confusion, fits, coma, death
          – weight gain: due to intracellular swelling; **but no oedema or hypertension**
            (hypovolaemia with cerebral salt-wasting sydrome)

Ix **B**loods: Na$^+$ < 135
              Urea ↓; Uric acid ↓
              ADH ↑

      Urine: Urine Osmolality > 300 mosm/kg
              Urine Na$^+$ > 20 mmol/l: due to hypervolaemia, inhibition of RAAS, and ↑release of ANP

      Special: Water Load Test: Ensure Na$^+$ > 125. Drink 1.5 l
              ⇒ Normal: > 80% water excreted in 5 hrs; and urine osmolality < 100

Rx 1. Underlying cause
      2. Fluid restrict: 500–1000 ml/day
      3. Demeclocycline 900–1200 mg/day
      4. 3-5% hypertonic saline iv, if CNS symptoms occur.
          ☠: Central pontine myelinolysis, if too rapid correction in chronic hyponatraemia (e.g. alcoholic)
          Path: Pontine, basal ganglia, cerebral demyelination
          PC: quadraparesis; pseudobulbar palsy or mutism; fits, 1–2 days after Na$^+$ correction

Polyuria – Polydipsia

Def   Polyuria = urine volume > 3 litres / 24 hours

Causes

Concentrated urine (urine osmolality > 300 mosm/kg)

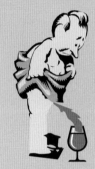

1. Osmotic diuresis
- Diabetes mellitus (glycosuria)
- TPN (urea)
- Mannitol

2. Tubulointerstitial disease
- Resolving acute tubular necrosis, or post-obstructive uropathy
- Medullary cystic disease
- $K^+\downarrow$, $Ca^{2+}\uparrow$

Dilute urine (urine osmolality < 250 mosm/kg)

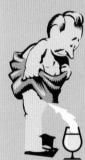

1. Diabetes insipidus
- Cranial
- Nephrogenic

2. Primary polydipsia
- Psychiatric: primary, anxiety, psychosis
- Neurological: head injury, MS, sarcoid
- Toxins: antipsychotics, tricyclics, lithium, carbamazepine

Ix   **B**lood:
- Glucose
- $K^+\downarrow$, $Ca^{2+}\uparrow$ (nephrogenic diabetes insipidus)
- Osmolality

Urine
- Osmolality

Special
- Water-deprivation test
- ADH-osmolality plots, during water deprivation test or hypertonic saline challenges *(p. 373)*

<u>Hypernatraemia</u>

<u>**Causes**</u>   *D.R.I.E.D. out*

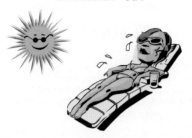

Deficiency – water restriction
- Debilitated, dementia, dysphagia, upper GI obstruction
- Hypothalamic disease may cause reduced thirst repsonse (adipsic hypernatraemia)

Renal – water loss via osmotic diuresis
- Diabetes mellitus; TPN or NG feeding (high urea); IV mannitol

Intestinal or other water loss
- GIT: infantile gastroenteritis, large solute load (e.g. NG feed)
- Skin: acclimatization to high temperature
- Lung: hyperventilation (esp. in dry air), COAD

Excess salt
- Excess salt intake, e.g. seawater; excess IV normal saline
- Excess salt resorption, i.e. hypermineralocorticoidism

Diabetes Insipidus *with* water deprivation
- Cranial: insufficient ADH release to hypernatraemia
- Nephrogenic: insufficient ADH sensitivity to hypernatraemia

Diabetes Insipidus

Causes

Cranial   Path: Hypothalamus, infundibulum or posterior pituitary lesion

D.I.V.I.N.I.T.Y.

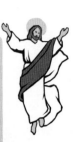

Developmental / inherited
- Autosomal dominant: AVP-neurophysin II gene
- Autosomal recessive: Wolfram's or DIDMOAD syndrome
  (**DI**, **D**iabetes **M**ellitus, **O**ptic atrophy, **D**eafness + bladder atony)
- Congenital: midline malformation (adipsia)

Infection
- Basilar meningitis, e.g. TB

Vascular
- Infarction: Sheehan's syndrome, sickle cell anaemia
- Anterior communicating artery aneurysm

Inflammation
- Lymphocytic infiltration of stalk – resolves in 3 yrs
- Sarcoid (also causes nephrogenic DI)
- SLE, Wegener's (midline granulomatas)

Neoplasia
- 1°: pituitary adenoma **with** suprasellar extension; craniopharyngioma
- 2°: metastases to pituitary or hypothalamus

Injury: trauma or craniotomy – lasts 1 day to 3 weeks

Toxin: alcohol

Y: pregnanc**Y**: placental vasopressinase (remits post-partum)

Nephrogenic   Path: Collecting duct or tubulointerstitial disease

T.U.B.U.L.A.R. p.H.

Toxins: lithium, amphotericin B, rifampicin, meflurane

Ureteric: vesicoureteric reflux, obstruction

Blood vessel disease: sickle cell, vasculitis, acute tubular necrosis

Uric acid ↑, calcium (plasma or urine) ↑, potassium ↓

Lymphoma, myeloma, amyloid

Autoimmune: SLE, Sjögren's syndrome

Radiation

Papillary necrosis: sickle cell, diabetes mellitus

Hereditary:
- X-linked recessive: *VR2* gene; results in cAMP ↓ ; presents in infancy
- Autosomal recessive: *aquaporin 2* gene

PC 1. Polyuria and polydispia
2. Fatigue: due to nocturia, and volume depletion that only occurs if deprived of water
3. Symptoms may be masked by concomitant adrenal insufficiency due to equimolar Na$^+$ loss, and unmasked by steroid Rx

Ix **B**loods: • Na$^+$: normal, or ↑ if patient is denied access to free water (↓ = primary polydipsia)
• Osmolality > 300 mosm / kg
Urine: • Osmolality < 300 mosm / kg; i.e. unable to concentrate urine

Special:
1. Water-deprivation test

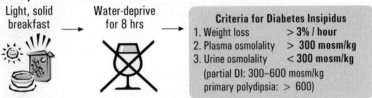

Light, solid breakfast → Water-deprive for 8 hrs →

Criteria for Diabetes Insipidus	
1. Weight loss	> 3% / hour
2. Plasma osmolality	> 300 mosm/kg
3. Urine osmolality	< 300 mosm/kg
(partial DI: 300–600 mosm/kg	
primary polydipsia: > 600)	

N.B. 1: Co-existent hypocortisolism: give pretest dexamethasone if cortisol deficiency possible
N.B. 2: Cranial vs nephrogenic DI: give nasal desmopressin and allow free access to water:
Cranial DI: urine gets concentrated: ↓ urine volume + ↑ urine osmolality
Nephrogenic DI: urine can't be concentrated: ↑ urine volume + ↓ urine osmolality

2. ADH radioimmunoassay, plus hypertonic saline IV challenge
Right-sided shift patterns:

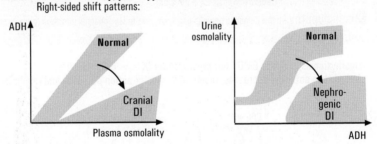

Rx

Cranial
1. Desmopressin (intranasal DDAVP): has advantage over AVP in having less pressor activity
2. **C**arbamazepine, **C**hlorpropamide, **C**lofibrate – are all causes of SIADH

Nephrogenic
1. Adequate water supply but Na$^+$-restrict: causes physiological ↓ urine output
2. Thiazide, e.g. chlothalidone: causes physiological ↓ urine output
3. Indomethacin
4. High-dose intranasal desmopressin in partial nephrogenic diabetes insipidus

Hyperkalaemia

Causes   *C.A.R.D.I.A.C.!*   plasma conc.
> 5mmol/l

Corticosteroid deficiency
- Addison's disease
- Hyporeninaemic hypoaldosteronism (RTA–type 4): e.g. diabetic nephropathy
- Aldosterone resistance: e.g. post-obstruction nephropathy

Acidosis, metabolic
- Poisoning with aspirin, ethylene glycol, methanol poisoning
- Diabetic ketoacidosis (not lactic acidosis due to free movement of anions into cells)

Renal failure – acute or chronic

Drugs
- Cardiac – ACE inhibitors, angiotensin-II receptor antagonists
  – diuretics: spironolactone, amiloride, acetazolamide
  – digoxin, beta-blockers (overdose)
- Nephrotoxic (tubulo-interstitial):
  – cyclosporin, tacrolimus
  – NSAIDs, trimethoprim

Intake ↑ : citrus foods; IV fluids (iatrogenic)

Intestinal, gastro- : haemorrhage

Artefactual
- Haemolysis, or blood clots, esp. prothrombotic states - Ix: PO_4↓, Ca^{2+}↓, glucose ↓
- Hereditary stomatocytosis (autosomal dominant) - red-cells leak K^+ at room temperature

Cell-lysis:
- Catabolic states: anorexia nervosa, trauma, chemotherapy
- Massive blood transfusion, esp. > 7 days old

Channelopathy - hyperkalaemic periodic paralysis, due to Na^+-channel mutation (autosomal dominant)

PC   Dysrhythmias, e.g. VT, EMD - but presents late (K^+ > 6.5 mmol/l) !
(membrane potential decreases, resulting in shorter action potential and repolarization)

ECG

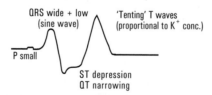

QRS wide + low
(sine wave)

'Tenting' T waves
(proportional to K^+ conc.)

P small

ST depression
QT narrowing

Rx 1. Cardioprotection: calcium chloride IV 10ml 10%
2. Acute • Insulin (IV soluble - 'Actrapid') + glucose (IV 50g of 50% glucose),
               followed with sliding scale of soluble insulin and dextrose
          • Salbutamol
          • $NaHCO_3$ with dialysis to remove Na^+
3. Chronic • Renal - loop diuretic; dialysis
          • GIT   - K^+ restrict; Na^+ or Ca^{2+} polystyrene sulphonate exchange resin (PO, PR)

<u>Hypokalaemia</u>

<u>Causes</u>   *C.A.R.D.I.A.C.!*   plasma conc.
                                                          < 3.5mmol/l

Corticosteroid excess – hypermineralocorticoidism
  • 1° Hyperaldosteronism: – adrenal adenoma, BNH or carcinoma
                          – glucocorticoid remediable aldosteronism
  • 2° Hyperaldosteronism: – renin-secreting tumour, renal artery stenosis
                          – Gitelman's, Bartter's syndromes, hypovolaemia
  • Hypoaldosteronism: Liddle's syn, 'apparent mineralocorticoid excess' syn.

Acidosis, renal-tubular, types 1 and 2

Renal – over-diuresis
  • Recovery phase of acute-tubular necrosis
  • Osmotic diuresis e.g. diabetes mellitus, TPN feeding

Drugs
  • Cardiac: diuretics (thiazide, loop, osmotic)
  • Nephrotoxic (tubulo-interstitial): penicillins, amphotericin B
  • β-2 agonists: salbutamol, aminophylline ($\uparrow$ es Na^+-K^+-ATPase)
  • Insulin: conjoint glucose-K^+ cell influx

Intake $\downarrow$ or Mg^{2+} deficiency, e.g. alcoholism, malabsorption, diuretics

Intestinal
  • Vomiting, naso-gastric tube suctioning
  • Diarrhoea, esp. villous adenoma of rectum; purgative abuse
  • Surgery: fistula, ureterosigmoidostomy

Artefactual: sample taken downstream from IV drip

Cell-proliferation: anabolic states, e.g. convalesence from trauma, surgery, TPN feeding

Channelopathy: hypokalaemic periodic paralysis, due to dihydropyridine Ca^{2+}-channel mutation
                 (autosomal dominant)

<u>PC</u>   1. Neurological: weakness: skeletal muscle (hypotonia); smooth muscle (constipation / ileus)
                          fatigue, confusion, depression
       2. Nephrogenic diabetes insipidus
       3. Dysrhythmias: bradycardia, heart block, SVT, VT, digoxin toxicity potentiation

<u>ECG</u>

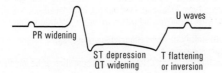

PR widening

ST depression   T flattening
QT widening   or inversion

U waves

<u>Rx</u>   1. K^+ replacement: PO or IV
            • Max conc. = 40 mmol / litre; max rate < 30 - 40 mmol / hr
            • Estimate total deficit, e.g. K^+ = 3 mmol/l $\Rightarrow$ 300 mmol deficit
            • Measure K^+ every few hours / ECG monitor
       2. Mg^{2+} replacement (if VT): IV $MgSO_4$ 8 ml 50%

Hypocalcaemia

Causes Two-step process:

1. Correct for albumin:
for every 4 g/l of albumin below 40 g/l allow 0.1 mmol/l from lower limit of Ca (2.2)

2. Measure PTH (parathyroid hormone), **ALP** (alkaline phosphatase) and **vitamin D**

PTH ↓　　　　　　　*I. A.M.*

Injury to parathyroid gland (commonest):
- Thyroidectomy, laryngeal carcinoma
- Parathyroidectomy (for ↑ Ca): 'Hungry bone syndrome' = rapid uptake of Ca + Mg + PO_4

Autoimmune – parathyroid inflammation
- Includes polyglandular autoimmune syndrome type 1 = PGAS:
  PTH, thyroid ↓; GIT (pernicious anaemia); Addison's; Skin (teeth, nail dystrophy, alopecia, candida)

Aplasia: isolated or DiGeorge syndrome = 3rd + 4th pharyngeal pouch aplasia =
'CATCH 22' syn. = Cardiac; Arterial; Thymus defects (immunodeficiency)
Craniofacial Δ; Hypocalcaemia; 22 = chromosome affected

Malignancy (carcinoma, lymphoma) / **M**etabolic (haemochromatosis, Wilson's)

Magnesium deficiency: • Alcoholism, chronic diarrhoea, coeliac
　　　　　　　　　　　• Drugs: cycloporin, amphotericin, cisplatin, furosemide

---

PTH ↑　　　　　*V.I.B.R.A.T.I.N.'*

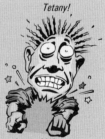

Tetany!

Vitamin D deficiency / impaired activation
= rickets (children) or osteomalacia (adults) *(p. 380)*
- Deficiency: diet, malabsorption, e.g. coeliac
- Activation: cirrhosis; chronic renal failure

Inherited: pseudohypoPTHism ('Albright's osteodystrophy')
Path: PTH-receptor insensitivity in proximal convoluted tubule
⇒ failure of Ca resorption and PO_4 excretion
- Type 1: renal adenylate cyclase, G protein sα subunit deficiency ⇒ ↓ urinary cAMP
- Type 2: post-adenylate cyclase transduction abnormality ⇒ normal urinary cAMP
PC: Type 1 (autosomal dominant):
  1. Short: height, 4th + 5th metacarpal and metatarsal length, IQ
  2. Oculocutaneous: subcutaneous calcification, cataracts, blue sclera
  3. Endocrinopathy: type 2 diabetes (and obese), hypogonadism, hypothyroidism
     (the presence of this phenotype, but normal calcium = 'pseudopseudohypoPTHism'!)

Burns, and other causes of cell lysis (infarction; haemolysis; sepsis; tumour lysis)
- Due to hyperphosphataemia
- Also caused artefactually by delayed serum separation or haemolysis

Rhabdomyolysis: releases phosphate

Acute pancreatitis (saponification)

Toxins: • Citrate, e.g. blood transfusion, heparin, protamine, glucagon, fusidic acid
　　　　• Bisphosphonate

Infection: *Legionella pneumophila* pneumonia

Neoplasia: prostate carcinoma

PC

General
- Neurological:
  - Sensory: numbness, perioral paraesthesia
  - Motor: hyperexcitability – cramps, hyper-reflexia, tetany, stridor
    - Chvostek's Sx (tap facial nerve → twitching) / Trousseau's Sx (carpopedal spasm)
  - CNS: seizures, depression, dementia, parkinsonism (basal ganglia calcification)
- Oculocutaneous:
  - Photophobia, papilloedema, subcapsular cataracts due to ectopic calcification
  - Subcutaneous calcification (if PO_4 ↑)
- Cardiac: ventricular tachycardia (due to prolongation of QT), electromechanical dissociation

Specific for cause
- Low PTH:
  1. Polyglandular autoimmune syndrome: *P.G.A.S.*
  2. DiGeorge syndrome = *C.A.T.C.H.22.*
- High PTH:
  1. Osteomalacia, rickets *(p. 380)*: bone pain and fractures; proximal myopathy; TB susceptibility
  2. PseudohypoPTHism *(see opposite)*: short; oculocutaneous, endocrinopathy

Ix

Bloods: 1. Calcium: corrected total calcium < 2.2 mmol/l
2. PTH: if normal, consider causes of hyperPTH-related hypocalcaemia (osteomalacia, etc.)
3. ALP ↑: osteomalacia; rickets; ALP normal: hypoPTHism or pseudohypoPTHism
4. Vit. D: 25-HCC ↓ 1,25-DHCC ↓ – poor intake; liver failure
           25-HCC ↑ 1,25-DHCC ↓ – chronic renal failure
           25-HCC ↑ 1,25-DHCC ↑ – vitamin D resistance
5. • PO_4 ↑ - hypoPTHism, pseudohypoPTHism or chronic renal failure
  • PO_4 ↓ – osteomalacia; rickets (except that due to CRF)

Urine: 1. PO_4 ↓: hypoPTHism or pseudoPTHism
2. cAMP, post-intravenous PTH: classifies pseudohypoPTHism

Micro: Throat / vaginal swab for candida

ECG: Hyp**O**calcaemia Pr**O**l**O**ngs QT interval

Radiology: X-rays

PseudohypoPTHism

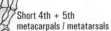

Short 4th + 5th
metacarpals / metatarsals

Osteomalacia

Looser's zones

Cortical thinning

Rx

Calcium supplements
1. Calcium gluconate (IV): use cardiac monitor
2. Calcium carbonate (PO)

Vitamin D
1. Ergocalciferol (D2): non-hydroxylated
   ☠: hypercalcaemia due to long half-life (must monitor for first few weeks)
2. Alfacalcidol (1α-HCC) or calcitriol (D3) – hypercalcaemia less likely

Hypercalcaemia

<u>**Causes**</u> Two-step process:

1. Correct for albumin, since physiologically inert, bound calcium increases with serum protein.
Hence total calcium increases with hypergammaglobulinaemia, or dehydration (urea ↑).

2. Measure PTH (parathyroid hormone) and **ALP** (alkaline phosphatase)

PTH ↑ (ALP normal)   *P.T.H.*

Primary hyperPTHism – **commonest**
  Epi: Prevalence = 1% population; typically women in 30–50s
  Aet: Hyperplasia (15%), adenoma (80%), carcinoma (5%)
  Pre: • Hereditary, esp. when bilateral tumours present
    • MEN syndromes: I (pituitary, pancreatic islet-cell tumour) or IIA (thyroid ca., phaeochromocytoma)
  PC: Usually asymptomatic, unless additional cause occurs, e.g. carcinoma

Tertiary hyperPTHism: following renal transplant in a patient with prior 2° hyperPTHism,
  Vit D and Ca rise, but parathyroid gland continues secreting autonomously

Hypocalciuric hypercalcaemia, familial (autosomal dominant, numerous mutations):
  Path: Incorrectly set Ca sensor on parathyroid and renal tubules causes ↑PTH secretion
    and ↑ Ca resorption in distal-convoluted tubule
  PC: Hypercalcaemic from birth (cf. primary PTH) – usually benign

---

PTH ↓   *S.T.O.N.E.S.*

Sarcoidosis; and TB (ALP ↑) due to 1α-hydroxylase activity in granulomas

Toxins (ALP normal)
  • Vit D or A, or antacids ('milk-alkali syndrome')
  • Thiazide diuretics (also diuretic phase of acute tubular necrosis)
  • Lithium: *PTH is actually ↑*!

Osteoblast and **O**steoclast turnover increased (ALP ↑)
  • Fracture, esp. with Paget's, puberty or immobility

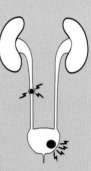

Neoplasia
  ALP ↑
    • Bony metastases, e.g. breast, bronchial – **2nd commonest**
      (due to prostaglandin release causing osteoclast activation)
    • Lymphoma, leukaemia: due to 1α-hydroxylase activity
  ALP normal
    • Myeloma
    • Carcinoma (PTH-related peptide): squamous cell bronchial, renal, liver, pancreas

Endocrine
  ALP ↑   thyrotoxicosis
  ALP normal   Addison's, acromegaly, androgen excess

Syndromes (ALP normal)
    • Jansen's syndrome: autonomous PTH-receptor activity
      PC: Severe hyperPTHism-like bone disease in children, premature death
    • William's syndrome:
      PC: **WI**de mouth, **L**ow growth, **L**ow **IQ**, **A**ortic stenosis, **M**etabolic (Ca ↑)

PC

'Bones'   • Bone pain, due to subperiosteal resorption
          • Arthralgia (pseudogout; chondrocalcinosis)

'Stones' • Renal stones
          • Tubular dysfunction: diabetes insipidus (polyuria, polydipsia), acidosis

Abdominal 'groans'
          • Abdominal pain (inc. peptic ulcers, acute pancreatitis)
          • N + V
          • Constipation

Psychological 'moans'
          • Fatigue, depression, psychosis, dementia

Ix

Bloods: • Essential:
              1. Calcium: corrected total calcium > 2.6 mmol/l
              2. PTH: if normal, consider causes of hyperPTHism
              3. ALP
            • Auxillary:
              1. $PO_4\downarrow$ – hyperPTHism; lymphoma; $PO_4\uparrow$: carcinoma
              2. $Cl\uparrow$, $HCO_3\downarrow$: HyperPTHism
              3. Other: albumin ↓ – neoplasia; ESR ↑ – hyperPTHism or neoplasia; ACE ↑ – sarcoid

Urine: 1. Ca: • Hypercalciuric (< 99% tubular resorption) – all causes, except:
                      • Hypocalciuric (> 99% tubular resorption) – familial hypocalciuric hypercalcaemia
             2. Bence-Jones proteinuria: myeloma

Micro: Consider TB (CXR, Mantoux, etc.)

ECG: Short QT interval (hyp**O**calcemia pr**OlO**ngs the QT)

Radiology: 1. X-rays

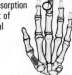
Subperiosteal resorption
of radial aspect of
middle–proximal
phalanges

Brown tumour

○ Tufting of distal phalanges

             2. Radioisotopes: • Parathyroid (pertechnetate – thallium or MIBI, to subtract out thyroid)
                                • Technetium bone scan: bone metastases

Special: selective neck venous catheterization for hyperPTHism

Rx

General   1. High fluid intake (normal saline infusion) + furosemide (↑ es Ca excretion)
          2. Bisphosphonates: pamidronate IV, clodronate
          3. Cytotoxins (IV mithramycin, gallium); calcitonin (IV or IM); cellulose phosphate resin
          4. Dietary restrict, e.g. for hereditary causes

Specific 1. Prednisolone is indicated for:
               a) Sarcoid or TB; b) Myeloma or lymphoma; c) Addison's; d) Vit D or A excess
          2. HRT (estrogen + progesterone): may obviate surgery in postmenopausal hyperPTHism
          3. Surgery: for primary hyperPTHism, where Ca > 3.0 mmol/l
                       – neck exploration with adenoma resection or partial PTHectomy

Osteomalacia and Rickets

Def   Defective mineralization of osteoid, that leads to reductions in global skeletal mass and density.
(Osteoid = composite of collagen type 1, glycosysaminoglycans and proteoglycan, secreted by osteoblasts.)

Osteomalacia: defect occurs **after** epiphyseal fusion in adults

Path

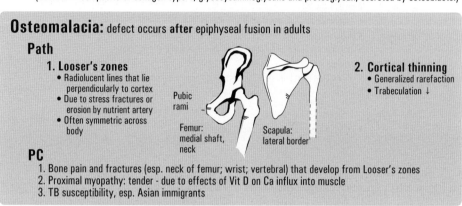

1. Looser's zones
- Radiolucent lines that lie perpendicularly to cortex
- Due to stress fractures or erosion by nutrient artery
- Often symmetric across body

Pubic rami

Femur: medial shaft, neck

Scapula: lateral border

2. Cortical thinning
- Generalized rarefaction
- Trabeculation ↓

PC
1. Bone pain and fractures (esp. neck of femur; wrist; vertebral) that develop from Looser's zones
2. Proximal myopathy: tender - due to effects of Vit D on Ca influx into muscle
3. TB susceptibility, esp. Asian immigrants

Rickets: defect occurs **before** epiphyseal fusion in children

Path

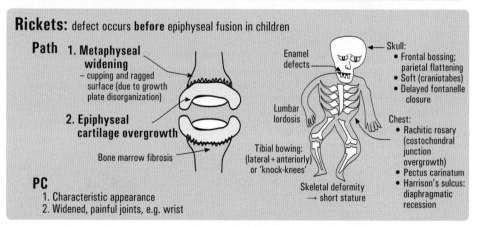

1. Metaphyseal widening
  – cupping and ragged surface (due to growth plate disorganization)

2. Epiphyseal cartilage overgrowth

Bone marrow fibrosis

Enamel defects

Lumbar lordosis

Tibial bowing: (lateral + anteriorly) or 'knock-knees'

Skeletal deformity → short stature

Skull:
- Frontal bossing; parietal flattening
- Soft (craniotabes)
- Delayed fontanelle closure

Chest:
- Rachitic rosary (costochondral junction overgrowth)
- Pectus carinatum
- Harrison's sulcus: diaphragmatic recession

PC
1. Characteristic appearance
2. Widened, painful joints, e.g. wrist

Vit D physiology

Vitamin D is actually a hormone, because:-
1. Endogenously produced: with adequate sunlight, no dietary fortification is required
2. Homeostatic control • Activated by ↓ Ca and ↓ PO$_4$
   • Its action is to increase Ca and PO$_4$ via GIT (absorption) + bone (resorption)

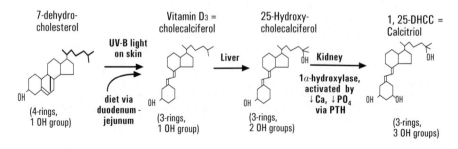

7-dehydro-cholesterol

UV-B light on skin

diet via duodenum - jejunum

(4-rings, 1 OH group)

Vitamin D3 = cholecalciferol

Liver

(3-rings, 1 OH group)

25-Hydroxy-cholecalciferol

Kidney

1α-hydroxylase, activated by ↓ Ca, ↓ PO$_4$ via PTH

(3-rings, 2 OH groups)

1, 25-DHCC = Calcitriol

(3-rings, 3 OH groups)

Causes 1. Due to either **Vitamin D** or **Phosphate** deficiency (but not calcium deficiency!).
2. Vitamin D deficiency causes
- Decrease in GIT absorption of Ca and PO_4
- Secondary HyperPTHism with consequent increased Ca renal resorption and PO_4 renal loss

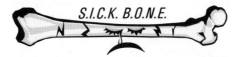

S.I.C.K. B.O.N.E.

↓ Vitamin D

Supply
a) Sunlight: housebound, debilitated, elderly
b) Diet: Asian chapatis / Vegans
c) Fat malabsorption (Vit D = fat-soluble): e.g. coeliac; chronic pancreatitis

Inherited
a) Renal 1α-hydroxylase deficiency
 ('Vit D-dependent rickets type 1'; auto. recessive)
b) Resistance to vitamin D
 ('Vit D-dependent rickets type 2'; auto. recessive)

Cirrhosis esp. primary biliary cirrhosis, due to -
 – 25-hydroxylase activity ↓
 – Vit D plasma-binding protein synthesis ↓
 – Bile salt synthesis and circulation ↓

Kidney failure
a) 1α-hydroxylase deficiency
b) Nephrosis: Vit D plasma-binding protein loss

Babies (pregnancy) / Breast feeding
 – Due to increased demand (also trauma)

ONcogenic rickets

Endocrine: HypoPTHism or pseudohypoPTHism

Enzyme inducers, e.g. phenytoin

↓ PO4

Supply
a) Diet (eggs)
b) Malabsorption e.g. coeliac, vomiting
c) Antacids: containing Mg or Al

Inherited
'X-linked dominant hypophosphataemic rickets'
 = Vitamin D resistance in GIT and
 proximal convoluted tubule
 (Ix: normal Calcium levels!)

Cirrhosis esp. alcohol bingers or post-glucose
 – Acetate displaces muscular PO_4
 – Poor absorption of PO_4 from PCT

Kidney: renal tubular acidosis
 • Distal (type 1)
 • Proximal (Fanconi's syndrome)
 e.g. 2° to myeloma, Wilson's

Binge alcohol drinking

ONcogenic rickets
 esp. neurofibromatosis, cavernous haemangioma,
 and giant-cell tumour of bone

Endocrine: hyperaldosteronsim

Ix
1. Ca : Normal (initially, due to 2ndary HyperPTHism) ⇒ ↓ (severe hypovitaminosis D) (except in renal failure when ↑) PO_4 ↓
2. Alkaline phosphatase ↑
3. PTH ↑
4. Vit D: 25-HCC ↓; 1,25-DHCC ↑ – supply ↓; demand ↑; cirrhosis (1,25-DHCC ↑ due to 2ndary ↑ PTH)
  25-HCC ↑; 1,25-DHCC ↓ – chronic renal failure (1,25-DHCC ↓ in nephrosis)
  25-HCC ↑; 1,25-DHCC ↑ – Vit. D Resistance

5. Urine: Renal Tubular Acidosis: pH > 5.5, aminoacids, glucose:

Rx Depends on cause:
Supply: Vit D2 (ergocalciferol); Vit D3 (cholecalciferol) + UVB light
Malabsorption or Resistance: High-dose or intramuscular vitamin D + calcium
Liver / Renal Disease: Calcitriol or 1-AlphaCalcidol (in renal failure) ☠: HyperCalcaemia
HypoPO4aemia, e.g. RTA: Oral PO4, but must correct Ca and Vit D first (or will worsen!)

Osteoporosis

Def 1. Bone mineral density < 2.5 standard deviations (-2.5 T) from normal young adult,
adjusted for race and gender; in presence of normal bone composition.
2. Due to imbalance between osteoblast synthesis vs osteoclast resorption.
3. Localized (due to trauma, disuse, reflex sympathetic dystrophy) vs generalized (see below).

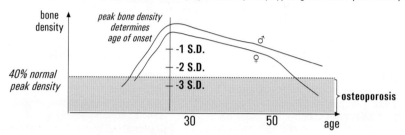

Causes *P.E.N.S.I.O.N.E.R.S.*

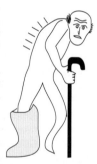

Primary
Epi: 5% of population have, of which 10% get fractures every year
Predisposing: *White and Light* (i.e. Caucasian, low body mass index),
genes, e.g. vitamin D receptor gene,
inactivity esp. in youth
Types: 1: Post-menopausal women (50-70 yrs)
Site: vertebral body; radius - trabecular bone
Ix: low PTH
2: Elderly (70 + yrs)
Site: femur neck, humerus, tibia - cortical bone
Ix: high PTH

Endocrine: steroid-related
1. Cushing's
2. Hypogonadism, inc: Turner's or Klinefelter's syn.
3. Addison's disease

Neoplasia: myeloma, lymphoma, carcinoma (PTH-related peptide)

Steroids / **S**moking, alcohol / other toxins
1. Heparin, warfarin;
2. Anti-convulsants (also cause vit D deficiency)
3. Lithium, buserelin, cyclosporin, thyroxine
N.B. must have annual DEXA scan if on steroids for > 3 months

Intestine / nutrition
1. Malnutrition, anorexia nervosa,
2. Malabsorption (of Ca, Vit D, Vit C), TPN

Organ failure: cirrhosis, esp. primary biliary cirrhosis; haemochromatosis

Neurological: dementia, MS, epilepsy

Endocrine: T4 ↑, PTH ↑, PRL ↑, acromegaly, type 1 DM (IDDM), pregnancy

Rheumatological - rheumatoid arthritis; ankylosing spondylitis; TB arthritis

Syndromes: osteogenesis imperfecta; Marfan's; homocystinuria; Ehlers-Danlos

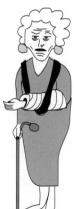

<u>PC</u> Often asymptomatic and picked up by routine DEXA scanning

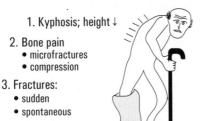

  1. Kyphosis; height ↓
  2. Bone pain
     • microfractures
     • compression
  3. Fractures:
     • sudden
     • spontaneous

<u>Ix</u> **B**lood: 1. Ca: normal, except for certain secondary causes:
                ↑ in malignancy; hyperPTHism; ↓ in malnutrition; malabsorption; osteomalacia
                PO_4: normal
             2. Alkaline phosphatase – normal: or ↑ if fracture

   Urine: Bone resorption markers ↑
             • Hydroxyproline / creatinine ratio (also ↑ by gelatin, gravy)
             • Pyridinium cross-links, e.g. total free deoxypyridinoline (unaffected by diet)

   Radio: 1. X-rays • generalized osteopenia: thin cortex and trabeculae
                        • fractures, esp. biconcave vertebral compression
             2. DEXA (Dual-Energy X-ray Absorptiometry)
                • Lumbar spine and femur neck 2-D mineralization area ⇒ estimates bone density
                  ☠: can't account for differences in bone depth as 2-D only; spondylosis falsley elevates
                     density
                • T-scores relate individual result to normal young adult population: (T < -2.0 to −2.5
                     ⇒ treat)
                • Z-scores relate individual result to normal age-matched population
             3. Quantitative CT: advantage in estimating 3-D mineralization density

<u>Rx</u> **A**void: smoking, alcohol, steroids; **A**ctivity: exercise in youth ↑ es peak bone density
   Bisphosphonates: etidronate, alendronate
        Mech: pyrophosphate analogue gets adsorbed onto hydroxyapatite crystals, before being
              phagocytosed and then inhibiting osteoclast ATP metabolism or protein prenylation
              ⇒ 50% ↓ in fracture risk (treatment and prophylaxis)
        ☠: poor absorption (take before breakfast); oesophagitis (stay upright for 30 mins); ↓ Ca

   Calcium (taken with bisphosphonates or calcitonin) / Mg / Strontium
   D, vitamin
   Estrogens
        Mech: ↑ osteoblast and ↓ osteoclast activity
        a) HRT: estrogen ± progestagen (for protection against uterine ca.)
           50% ↓ in fracture risk; ☠: breast carcinoma
        b) SERMs (Selective Estrogen Receptor Modulators): raloxifene, tamoxifen
           • 40% ↓ in fracture risk; ☠: uterine carcinoma (tamoxifen only)
           • Protective against breast ca., esp. estrogen-dependent types

   Fluoride - osteoprogenitor stimulator
   Growth hormone / anabolic steroids
   Hormones: calcitonin (nasal): ↓ es osteoclast activity, ↓ es Ca
                 PTH (sc, 'teriparatide'): ↑ es osteoblast activity, ↑ es Ca

Paget's Disease

Def 1. Bone mineral density increased + disordered bone architecture + brittleness
2. Excessive osteoclastic activity, and overcompensatory osteoblastic remodelling and sclerosis

Epi **I**nc: 4% of over-40s (although majority are asymptomatic)
Age: 50+: ↑ing incidence thereon
Sex: M > F
Geo: White Anglo-Saxons (W. Europe, Australia)
Aet: Paramyxovirus, e.g. canine distemper virus (found in osteoclasts)
Micro: cycles of osteolysis and sclerosis occur in different parts of the same bone simultaneously:

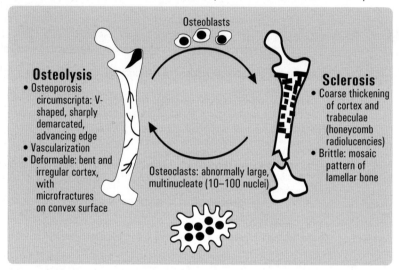

Osteoblasts

Osteolysis
- Osteoporosis circumscripta: V-shaped, sharply demarcated, advancing edge
- Vascularization
- Deformable: bent and irregular cortex, with microfractures on convex surface

Osteoclasts: abnormally large, multinucleate (10–100 nuclei)

Sclerosis
- Coarse thickening of cortex and trabeculae (honeycomb radiolucencies)
- Brittle: mosaic pattern of lamellar bone

Sites

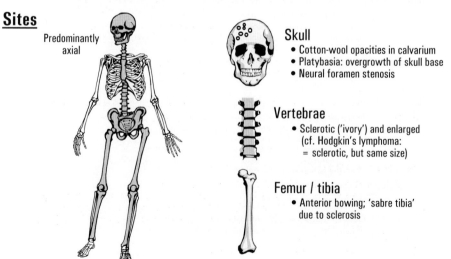

Predominantly axial

Skull
- Cotton-wool opacities in calvarium
- Platybasia: overgrowth of skull base
- Neural foramen stenosis

Vertebrae
- Sclerotic ('ivory') and enlarged (cf. Hodgkin's lymphoma: = sclerotic, but same size)

Femur / tibia
- Anterior bowing; 'sabre tibia' due to sclerosis

PC

Often asymptomatic, but picked up by X-rays + Alk. Phos. ↑ ↑

P.V.C. B.O.N.E.S.

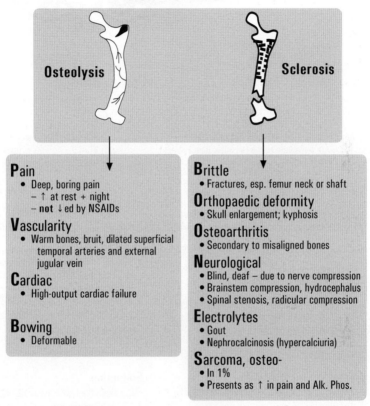

Osteolysis

Sclerosis

Pain
- Deep, boring pain
  - ↑ at rest + night
  - **not** ↓ed by NSAIDs

Vascularity
- Warm bones, bruit, dilated superficial temporal arteries and external jugular vein

Cardiac
- High-output cardiac failure

Bowing
- Deformable

Brittle
- Fractures, esp. femur neck or shaft

Orthopaedic deformity
- Skull enlargement; kyphosis

Osteoarthritis
- Secondary to misaligned bones

Neurological
- Blind, deaf – due to nerve compression
- Brainstem compression, hydrocephalus
- Spinal stenosis, radicular compression

Electrolytes
- Gout
- Nephrocalcinosis (hypercalciuria)

Sarcoma, osteo-
- In 1%
- Presents as ↑ in pain and Alk. Phos.

Ix

Blood: 1. Ca normal (but ↑ in immobility or fracture); PO_4 normal
2. Alk Phos. markedly ↑ ↑ ↑

Urine: 1. Ca ↑
2. Bone resorption markers: hydroxyproline:creatinine ratio or pyridinium crosslinks

Radio: 1. X-rays: sclerosis and osteolysis *(see opposite)*; used for Rx monitoring
2. ^{99}Tc bone scan: identifies 'hot-spots' of osteoblastic activity

Rx

Analgesics: NSAIDs only good for arthritis or fractures

Bisphosphonates: alendronate, clodronate, pamidronate IV
Mech: Pyrophosphate analogue is adsorbed onto hydroxyapatite crystals, before being phagocytosed and then inhibiting osteoclast ATP metabolism or protein prenylation
☠: Poor absorption (take before breakfast), oesophagitis (stay upright for 30 min), ↓ Ca

Calcitonin, nasal : ☠: ↓ Ca

Deformity: osteotomy for bowed tibia; joint replacements for osteoathritis

Hyperlipidaemia

Causes

P.E.A.R.L.S.
(xanthomata are pearl-like papules)

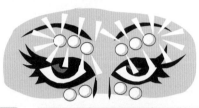

Cholesterol ↑

Primary (familial)
1. Familial hypercholesterolaemia
   Prev: a) Heterozygote: 1/500
         b) Homozygote: 1/250,000
   Aet: LDL-receptor or ApoB100 mutations
        or polygenic forms (all auto. dom.)
   PC: Premature ischaemic heart disease:
       a) Heterozygous: by 40 (cholesterol 7-13 mmol/l)
       b) Homozygous: by 20 (cholesterol > 13 mmol/l)
       c) Polygenic: by 40 (cholesterol 6-9 mmol/l)
   Ix: LDL ↑ = type IIa
   Rx: • Statins ineffective
       • Plasmapharesis: homozygous disease
2. Familial combined hyperlipidaemia
   Aet: ApoB overproduction in liver (auto. dom.)
   Ix: LDL+VLDL ↑ (cholesterol + triglycerides ↑)
3. Cerebrotendinous xanthomatosis
   Aet: bile acid synthesis defect (auto. rec.)
   PC: progressive learning disability and ataxia
   Ix: cholestanol ↑, but choleterol normal
4. Familial causes of HDL ↓
   LCAT deficiency (corneal opacity)
   Tangier disease (orange tonsils; neuropathy)

Endocrine
1. Cushing's (cholesterol + triglycerides ↑)
2. Hypothyroidism

Anorexia nervosa / **A**cute intermittent porphyria

Renal: nephrosis

Liver
1. Cholestasis, e.g. primary biliary cirrhosis
2. Hepatoma

Steroids / other toxins
1. Glucocorticoids, Progestagen
2. Cylosporin
3. Thiazide: (cholesterol + triglycerides ↑)

Smoking: HDL ↓

Triglycerides ↑

Primary (familial)
1. Familial hypertriglyceridaemia
   Prev: 1/600
   Aet: • Lipoprotein lipase mutation (auto. rec.)
        • Apo-CII mutation (LPL activator)
   Ix: a) VLDL ↑   = type IV (auto. dom.)
       b) Chylmicrons ↑ = type I (auto. rec.)
                          esp. Children

       c) VLDL ↑ +   ⎫
          Chylmicrons ↑⎬ = type V (auto. rec.)
                          ⎭
   Triglyceride levels very high in types I and V
2. Familial dysbetalipoproteinaemia
   Prev: 1/10,000
   Aet: • Accumulation of remnant lipoprotein due
          to impaired ApoE recognition by liver
        • Apo E2/E2 homozygotes (1% popultn.)
          plus obesity, diabetes, or menopause
   Ix: IDL ↑ (broad − β) = type III
3. Glycogen storage disease
4. Lipodystrophy

Endocrine
1. Diabetes type 2 - also HDL ↓
2. Acromegaly

Alcoholism - but HDL ↑ /
   Obesity - also HDL ↓

Renal: chronic renal failure

Liver: acute hepatitis

Steroids / other toxins:
1. Glucocorticoids,
   Estrogen (OCP, HRT, Pregnancy) - but LDL ↓
2. Beta-Blockers; furosemide
3. Chlorpromazine; etretinate; protease inhibitors

Stress / **S**epsis / **S**urgery (ileal bypass)

PC

O.X.- C.H.O.P.S.

Ophthalmic
   Cholesterol ↑ - xanthelasma palpebrum; corneal arcus (normal > 50 yrs); corneal opacity when HDL ↓
   Triglycerides ↑ - lipaemia retinalis (white optic disc and vessels, when TG > 10mmol/l)
Xanthomata
   Cholesterol ↑   a) Tendinous (normal skin colour as lie deep; Achilles, MCP, elbow)
                 b) Cutaneous: Homozygous FH only
   Triglycerides ↑   a) Eruptive (pruritic, skin-colour papules, pustules; buttocks / elbows)
                 b) Striate palmar (orange-yellow papules on creases) – *Type III hyperlipidaemia*
                 c) Tuberous (large, pink-red nodules on bony prominences) – *Type III hyperlipidaemia*
Cardiac: cholesterol ↑ or type III triglycerides ↑ or diabetes - atherosclerosis (esp. coronary); aortic stenosis
Haematology: cholesterol ↑ (esp. cholestasis or LCAT deficiency) - target cells
Organomegaly (hepatosplenomegaly): triglycerides ↑
Pancreatitis, acute: triglycerides ↑, when TG > 10mmol/l
Special: arthritis – Cholesterol ↑ (homozygous FH)

Ix

1. **Cholesterol:**   Total > 5.2 mmol/l: LDL > 4.0; HDL < 1.0; HDL / total cholesterol < 0.25
2. **Fasting triglyceride:** Total > 2.0 mmol/l (if > 11, consider ↑ chylomicrons)
3. **Plasma appearance** (after overnight storage at 4° C) - allows phenotype classification:-

clear	turbid - milky	creamy supernatant	turbid + creamy supernatant	
LDL ↑ only **Type IIa**	VLDL ↑ **Type IIb or IV**	Chylomicrons ↑ **Type I**	VLDL ↑ + Chylomicrons ↑ **(Type V)**	IDL (broad-*β*) ↑ **(Type III)**

Rx

Conservative: 1. Diet - cholesterol ↓ by < 10%; 2. Exercise - HDL ↑; 3. Alcohol, smoking, diabetes

Cholesterol ↑   *S.E.A.P.*

Statins: simva-, prava-, atorvastatin
   • HMG CoA reductase inhibitors cause upregulation of
     LDL receptors on liver
   • Triglycerides ↓: Atorvastatin only
   • ☠: GIT Sx.; Myositis; LFT △
Ezetimibe - GIT cholesterol absorption ↓
Anion-exchange resin – cholestyramine
   • Binds bile acids in small bowel, and so prevents hepatic
     conversion of cholesterol to bile acids
Probucol
   • Cholesterol synthesis ↓ + LDL atherogenicity ↓

Triglycerides / cholesterol ↑

1. **Fibrates:** clo-, bezafibrate, gemfibrozil
   • TG ↓ by 30%; Chol ↓ by 15%; HDL ↑
   • ☠: as for statins, esp. rhabdomyolysis
2. **Nicotinic acid**
   • Anti-Lipolysis ⇒ FFA circulation ↓ ⇒ VLDL ↓
   • Cholesterol ↓; HDL ↑; Lipoprotein(a) ↓
   • ☠: GIT Sx, glucose intolerance, vasodilation
3. **Triglyceride-effect only**
   Orlistat GIT lipase inhibition
   Ω-3 marine triglycerides

Porphyria

Def 1. Hereditary or acquired defects along various steps of haem biosynthetic pathway.
2. Causes one or combination of 3 clinical pictures, depending on step involved

Clinical	Biochemical abnormality	Organ
Neurological	Porphyrin precursor (ALA and PBG) ↑↑	Hepatic
Cutaneous	Photosensitive porphyrins (tetrapyrrolle ring) ↑↑	Hepatic / erythropoietic
Microcytic anaemia	Failure of haem synthesis	Erythropoietic

Hepatic porphyrias are commoner than erythropoietic porphyrias, even though 85% of body haem is synthesized in RBC, because in the liver, haem production is controlled by negative feeback, and so a failure to produce haem increases the rate of porphyrin production.

Haem synthetic pathway

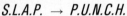

$S.L.A.P. \rightarrow P.U.N.C.H.$

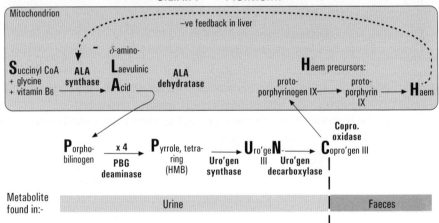

Types

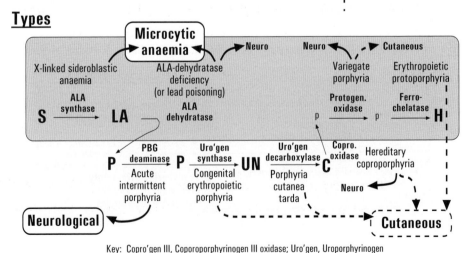

Key: Copro'gen III, Coporoporphyrinogen III oxidase; Uro'gen, Uroporphyrinogen

Acute intermittent porphyria

Epi   **I**nc: Commonest neurological porphyria. Autosomal dominant.
        Prev: 1 / 10,000 - PBG deaminase mutation; 1 / 100,000 - clinically affected (requires trigger)
   Age: Onset in teens - 30s
   Sex: F:M = 5:1, due to likely precipitants (premenstrual, pregnancy, 'pill', anorexia)
   Pre: *A.I.P. is Asymptomatic until Induced by Precipitants* (esp. enzyme-inducers)

> **A**lcohol, **A**nticonvulsants, **A**ntibiotics (sulphonamides, tetracyclines)
> **I**ntake ↓ (fasting), **I**nfection, **I**nhalation anaesthesia (halothane)
> **P**ill (estrogen), **P**ain-killers - opioids

PC   *A.I.P.*

> **A**cute abdomen - constipation or diarrhoea; fever, N + V; dysuria; arthralgia
> **I**ctus – fits, due to **I**CP rise and **I**nappropriate ADH secretion (Na ↓)
> **P**eripheral and autonomic neuropathy
> • PNS: acute bulbar, limb and respiratory weakness (like Guillain-Barré syndrome)
> • ANS: disproportionate tachycardia, hypertension; sweating, pallor; urinary retention
> **P**sychiatric: psychosis, mania, confusion, depression

Ix   **B**loods - WCC ↑, Na ↓, Urea ↑, LFT ↑
   Urine - Protein ↑, ALA and PBG (latter turns brown on standing, or pink with Ehrlich's aldehyde)
   Special - fibroblast culture for enzyme assay

Rx   1. High-glucose drink or 20% dextrose iv - inhibits ALA synthase
   2. Haematin (haem arginate iv) - inhibits ALA synthase
   3. Symptomatic: opioids; propranolol; diazepam or clonazepam ; fluid restrict (if SIADH); phenothiazine
   4. Prophylactic: avoid precipitants; screen relatives

Porphyria cutanea tarda

Epi   **I**nc: Commonest cutaneous porphyria. Acquired in majority, or Autosomal dominant.
   Pre: Chronic liver disease, esp. alcohol, autoimmune hepatitis, haemochromatosis, estrogen

PC   *P.C.T.*

> **P**hotosensitivity (erythema, bullae, pigmentation); **P**itting oedema
> **C**alcification of skin; **C**icatrix (scars); **C**irrhosis (cause)
> **T**richosis: hypertrichosis or hirsutism

Ix   **B**loods - LFTs deranged, Fe and Ferritin ↑ (always raised), Glucose ↑
   Urine - Uroporphyrinogen ↑ (ALA and PBG not raised due to compensatory PBG deaminase activity)

Rx   Chloroquine - complexes porphyrins; Venesection – for Fe overload; avoid sun, alcohol, estrogens

Renal Medicine

Acute Renal Failure

Causes

Pre-renal

Shock

S.H.O.C.K.

Sepsis

Haemorrhage
esp. peripartum
Path: Acute cortical necrosis

O: hyp**O**volaemia due to
D+V; pancreatitis; burns;
inadequate intake, esp. post-op.

Cardiogenic: heart failure

K: anaphyla**X**is /
blood transfusion reaction

Renovascular

S.T.E.N.T.A.B.L.E.

Stenosis, renal artery

Thrombosis:
atherosclerosis
hyperviscosity, sickle cell disease

Embolus

NSAIDs

Toxins, other:
e.g. ACE inhibitors, radiotherapy

Autoimmune:
scleroderma
vasculitis, inc. Takayasu's,
PAN, Wegener's

Blood pressure ↑:
malignant hypertension

Blood constituents:
DIC, TTP, HUS

Liver failure:
hepato-renal syndrome

Eclampsia, pre-

Electrolyte: hypercalcaemia

NB: Renovascular causes behave
biochemically like
'Renal'-type ARF

Renal

Glomerulonephritis

P.A.I.N.T.

Primary
proliferative,
membranoproliferative

Autoimmune
SLE, vasculitis,
anti-GBM,
IgA nephropathy

Infection
Post-streptococcal,
SBE, staphylococcus, syphilis,
HIV, HBV, HCV, malaria

Neoplasia: myeloma, lymphoma

Toxins: penicillamine, heroin

Tubulo-Interstitial Nephritis

T.I.N.

Toxins:
• Allergic: antibiotics, ACEI, NSAID
• Tubular: sulphonamides, aciclovir

Infection: Legionnaire's, leptospirosis,
brucellosis, CMV, Hanta virus,
Candida

Neoplasia: lymphoma; leukaemia

Acute Tubular Necrosis

A.T.N.

ABP ↓: patchy necrosis of tubules

Toxins: aminoglycosides,
cephalosporins, NSAID, cyclosporin,
contrast, paracetamol overdose,
paraquat,
ethylene glycol (oxalate crystals)

Necrosis:
• Rhabdomyolysis (myoglobin)
• Intravascular haemolysis (Hb)

Neoplasia:
• Tumour lysis (uric acid)
• Myeloma (BJP)

Nephritis, pyelo-

Post-renal

Ureteric Obstruction

Ureter or renal pelvis obstruction
may cause ARF if bilateral
involvement or unilateral with
only one functioning kidney

S.N.I.P.P.I.N.G.

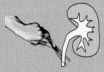

Stone

Neoplasia:
• Intrinsic: transitional cell ca.
• Extraluminal
• Colorectal / gynaecological cancer
• Lymphoma

Infection: TB, Schistosoma

Papillary necrosis

Pregnancy or other gynae.

Inflammation:
stricture / retroperitoneal fibrosis

Neurological

Genetic / congenital:
PUJ or VUJ stenosis, ureterocoele

Urinary retention

S.N.I.P.P.I.N.G.

Stone

Neoplasia: prostate, gynaecological

Infection: UTI

Papillary necrosis

Prostate: hyperplasia

Inflammation: stricture

Neurological:
• Neuropathy, cord lesion
• Toxins, post-operative atony
• Psychological

Genetic / congenital: valves

PC General 1. Anuria (or polyuria with TIN)
2. Fluid overload / hypertension
3. Electrolytes: K^+ – arrhythmia
Specific 1. Fever, arthralgia, rash – allergic TIN, autoimmune
2. Large tender kidneys – pyelonephritis, Hantavirus

Ix **B**loods: 1. Biochem:
- Urea / creatinine > 80 suggests pre-renal; 60–80 suggests renal
- K^+ ↑ (low in TIN), Mg^{2+} ↑, Ca^{2+} ↓, PO_4 ↑, ABGs show metabolic acidosis
- Underlying causes: Ca^{2+} ↑, uric acid ↑
2. Haem:
- FBC (normocytic anaemia suggests chronic renal failure or CRF)
- Eosinophils (TIN, vasculitis, cholesterol emboli), ESR, blood film
3. Immun:
- ANA, dsDNA, ENA, ANCA, anti-GBM, Ig, cryoglobulinaemia, serum electrophoresis
- C3 ↓ only   = post-streptococcal or membranoproliferative-II glomerulonephritis
- C3 and C4 ↓ = membranoproliferative-I glomerulonephritis, esp. SLE, HCV, MECG

Urine: 1. Dipstick:
- Blood – nephritis or may be myoglobin (false +ve); proteinuria; glycosuria – TIN
2. Cytology:
- RBC casts: GN; WBC casts: GN, pyelonephritis; eosinophiliuria: allergic TIN
- Epithelial casts, coarse granular casts – ATN
- Epithelial cells, hyaline casts, mildly granular casts – normal
3. Biochem:
- Urine Na: < 20 mmol/l   = pre-renal ARF
- Urine urea > 10 x plasma urea   = pre-renal ARF
  osmolal. > 1.5 x plasma osmolality   = pre-renal ARF
- Urine creatinine: to calculate Na filtration fraction:

$$\frac{Na_U \times Cr_P}{Cr_U \times Na_P} < 1 \quad – \text{pre-renal ARF}$$

- Urine protein: 30–300mg / day, or albumin:creatinine ratio > 3 = microalbuminuria
  > 3g / day   = nephrosis
- Urine protein electrophoresis: BJP, selectivity (use early morning urine or EMU)

Micro: 1. MSU; EMU x 3 (concentrated): AFB staining + ZN culture
2. Serology: ASO, antiDNAse B; HBV, HCV (ELISA or PCR); parasite film; serology
3. Blood cultures x 3

Monitor: 1. Fluid in and out; 2. Daily weights (insensible losses); 3. Temperature

ECG

Radio: 1. USS: large – obstruction; small – chronic renal failure; also stones, renal artery or vein duplex
2. CXR: pulmonary oedema; bones may show signs of renal osteodystrophy if CRF
3. PAXR / IVU (Functional) – stones, or other obstruction

Surgery: 1. Biopsy:
- Linear Ig deposits: SLE, anti-GBM disease ('ribbons'), diabetes
- Subepithelial granular IgG: post-Streptococcal GN
- Subepithelial spikes: membranous GN
- Subendothelial IgG: membranoproliferative GN
2. Cystoscopy

Rx **Underlying cause:**
- Pre-renal – fluid challenge
- Renal – steroids, antibiotics, etc.
- Post-renal – removal or bypass of obstruction

Fluid management: CVP monitoring, haemodialysis

Electrolytes: esp. K^+; Ca gluconate, insulin infusion; haemodialysis

Chronic Renal Failure – Causes

<u>Def</u> Permanent ↓ in GFR to < 50 ml/min (End-Stage Renal Failure: < 10 ml/min)

<u>Causes</u>

Renovascular

Renovascular
S.T.E.N.T.A.B.L.E.

Stenosis, renal artery
Thrombosis:
  atherosclerosis,
  sickle cell disease
Embolus
NSAIDs
Toxins, other:
  ACE inhibitors,
  radiotherapy
Autoimmune:
  scleroderma,
  vasculitis, inc. Takayasu's,
  PAN, Wegener's
Blood pressure ↑, which is...
Long-standing:
  hypertensive nephrosclerosis
  – **common**
Electrolyte: hypercalcaemia
  (also causes tubular disease)

Renal

Glomerulonephritis
P.A.I.N.T.S.

Primary:
  proliferative,
  minimal-change / membranous
  membranoproliferative
Autoimmune:
  SLE, vasculitis,
  anti-GBM, IgA nephropathy
Infection:
  post-streptococcal, HBV, HCV, HIV
Neoplasia: amyloid, myeloma
Toxins: penicillamine, heroin
Sclerosis (FSGS):
  1. Diabetes mellitus
  2. Sickle cell anaemia
  3. Renal ablation – see 'Structural'

Tubulo-Interstitial Nephritis
T.U.B.U.L.A.R. P.H.

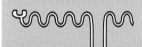

Toxins:
  NSAIDs, analgesics, lithium,
  cyclosporin, cisplatin
Ureteric reflux:
  VUR, chronic pyelonephritis
  chronic obstruction, e.g. TB
Blood pressure ↑
Uric acid (gout) / calcium ↑
Leukaemia, Lymphoma
Autoimmune: Sjögren's
Radiation / Renal transport

Polycystic kidneys – see 'Structural'

Hereditary:
  1. Alport's syndrome (X-linked)
  2. Fabry's syndrome (X-linked)

Structural

Developmental agenesis

Polycystic Kidneys
- Adult (APKD)
- Infant (IPKD)
- Medullary cystic disease

NB: Cystic kidneys may occur
  as a **consequence** of
  long-standing
  end-stage renal failure and
  dialysis

Neoplasia
- Renal cell carcinoma

Chronic Renal Failure - PC and O/E

S.C.A.R.R.I.N.G. T.U.B.E.S.

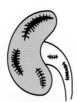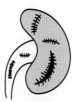

Skin
- Uraemia: pruritus (scratch marks), brown nails, hyperpigmented 'frost' or sallow, injected sclera
- Underlying cause: vasculitis, scleroderma, amyloid, partial lipodystrophy, angiokeratoma
- Complications: pallor (anaemia), subcutaneous or scleral calcification ($\downarrow Ca^{2+}$), tophi (gout)

Cardiac
- Fluid overload: pulmonary and peripheral oedema, JVP ↑ (or ↓ if salt-wasting)
- Pericarditis; tamponade (Kussmaul's sign – paradoxical JVP ↑ on inspiration), chest pain
- Ischaemic heart disease, dilated cardiomyopathy: multifactorial, inc. hypertriglyceridaemia, hyperhomocystinaemia, low HDL, insulin resistance, vascular calcification

ABP
- ↑: fluid overload (less commonly; ↓: salt-wasting with tubular disease)

Respiratory
- Pulmonary oedema (SOB), pleurisy (chest pain), pleural effusion, pulmonary fibrosis

Respiratory pattern
- Hiccups, uraemic fetor, Kussmaul's breathing (deep) due to metabolic acidosis

Immunocompromise, e.g. pneumonia

Neurological
- Encephalopathy: early – myoclonus, asterixis (hand flap), late – dementia, dysarthria, seizures
- Peripheral neuropathy, restless legs syndrome
- Myopathy: due to uraemia and osteomalacia

GIT
- Gastric ulcers due to gastrin ↑
- Haemorrhage, due to angiodysplasia and coagulopathy, impaired platelet function

Thrombocytopenia
- Purpura, GIT haemorrhage (also due to impaired platelet function and coagulopathy)

Urine
- Frequency or nocturia may occur with tubular disease
- Haematuria: IgA nephropathy, vasculitis or reflecting coagulopathy
- Loin pain, or renal mass – suggests renal cystic disease

Bones
- Osteomalacia (Vit D deficiency), osteoporosis

Endocrine
- Amenorrhoea, impotence, growth retardation (in children)

Systemic
- Anaemia (depression, fatigue)
- Anorexia, weight loss, cachexia; hypothermia

Chronic Renal Failure – Ix

Bloods

Biochemistry: *R.E.A.L.M.S.*

Renal

Urea ↑: endogenous and exogenous metabolite produced variably from amino-acid degradation
Creatinine ↑ • Metabolite produced at constant rate from phosphocreatine in muscle
• Inversely proportional to GFR: plot inverse-creatinine over time and extrapolate

Creatinine clearance = estimate of GFR:

$$\text{Clearance} = \frac{U_{Cr}.\ V}{P_{Cr}}$$

where P_{Cr} and U_{Cr} = plasma and urine concentration of creatinine
and V = volume of urine over 24 hrs

Adjust for surface-area (standard = 1.73 m^2); age; sex; diet and drugs
Clearance < 10 ml / min = End-Stage Renal Failure

Urea : creatinine ratio:

> 80: Urea generation ↑: meat, upper GI bleed, chronic sepsis, tetracycline
Urea resorption ↑: pre-renal or post-renal uraemia
Creat. generation ↓: wasting, amputation; steroid myopathy
60–80: Intrinsic renal failure
< 60: Urea generation ↓: low-protein intake (e.g. vegetarian), liver failure
Creatinine generation ↑: race (Blacks), rhabdomyolysis
Creatinine resorption ↑: trimethoprim, cimetidine; dialysis (urea lost more easily)

Electrolytes:

Na$^+$ ↓, K$^+$ ↑
Ca^{2+} ↓, PO$_4$ ↑, Mg^{2+} ↑, Vit D ↓, PTH ↑ due to –
tubular Ca resorption ↓, PO$_4$ excretion ↓, 1α-hydroxylation of cholecalciferol ↓

ABGs: Metabolic acidosis and respiratory compensation
LFTs: Alk. Phos. ↑ – osteomalacia; albumin ↓ – due to nephrosis, protein restriction, CAPD
Metabolic:

Glucose: ↑ due to insulin resistance and decreased insulin release
↓ (in diabetes) due to ↓ insulin catabolism and ↓ gluconeogenesis
Triglycerides, fasting ↑

Special: uric acid ↑; T4 ↑, T3 slightly ↓;
serum and urine electrophoresis (myeloma, amyloid – cause of CRF)

Haematology:

Hb: Normochromic, normocytic anaemia (bone marrow suppression, EPO production ↓); Film: Burr cells
WCC, platelets, clotting: impaired function for all and thrombocytopenia

Immunology: ANA, Rheumatoid factor, ANCA, cryoglobulins

Urine

1. Microscopy (early morning): haematuria; RBC or WBC casts
2. Protein (24-hour): glomerulonephritis
3. Amino acids, PO$_4$, glucose: tubular disease

Micro

1. MSU (UTI due to obstruction); *Schistosoma* urine microscopy
2. Hep B, C, HIV serology; malaria film

Monitor

1. ABP, fluid balance, weights: [oral + IV] vs [urine + faeces + vomit + insensible losses (weight)]
2. Glucose – insulin resistance

ECG

1. Sx. of K$^+$ ↓
2. LVH 2° to hypertension

Radiology

1. CXR: pulmonary oedema; CCF; AXR: calcification
2. USS: • Small kidneys suggests chronic renal failure (except early diabetes, obstruction, amyloid)
• Renal tract obstruction (reversible!); cysts, tumour
3. Functional: IVU / DMSA – Scarring due to VUR; DTPA or MAG3 + captopril – renovascular disease

Special

Renal biopsy – if cause unclear and renal size normal (i.e. potentially reversible!)

Chronic Renal Failure – Rx

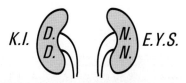

K.I. N.N. E.Y.S.

K$^+$ correct
- Particular concern during acute exacerbations
- Consider treating acidosis, but NaHCO₃ problematic due to high Na$^+$ content

Intake – salt / fluid
- Fluid-overload: ↓ salt and fluid intake, until normal CVP or JVP obtained
- Fluid-depleted: e.g. post-ATN, post-obstruction, chronic TIN – ↑ salt and fluid intake, until UO > 2l / day

Diuretics
- High-dose furosemide ± metolazone
- ACE inhibitors: renoprotective in diabetes; contraindicated in renal artery stenosis

Dialysis
- Haemodialysis:
    Method: 4 hrs / session; 3 sessions / week; 250 ml / min blood dialysed via forearm AV fistula
    Advantage: can vary dialysate composition; flow rate or pressure (∴ diffusion gradient)
    Disadvantage: low creatinine clearance: 6 ml/min; loss of amino acids, vitamins; no Vit D; EPO
    ☠: Arterial injury: haemorrhage, thrombosis, ischaemia ('steal'), **ABP**: postural hypotension
        Amyloid: β_2-microglobulin: carpal tunnel syndrome
        Aluminium toxicity: brain (dementia); bone marrow (anaemia); bone (osteomalacia)
- Chronic ambulatory peritoneal dialysis (CAPD):
    Method: introduce 2 l dialysate into peritoneum and replace 3–4 x /day
    Advantage: slightly better creatinine clearance: 7 ml/min, but still loses amino acids and vitamins
    ☠: Infection of catheter, peritonitis; blockage, leakage
        Intake fluid – mechanical back pain, genital oedema, hernia, haemorrhoids, hydrothorax
        Insulin resistance due to glucose loading from dialysate, obesity

Nutrition
- Low protein (0.5 g/kg/day - ↓es uraemic toxins and acidosis); high carbohydrate; low fat
- Haematinics (Fe, folate, Vit B12) and Vit C (as lost on dialysis)

NSAIDs – avoid; also avoid aminoglycosides

EPO (human recombinant erythropoeitin, slow-IV or subcut)
    ☠: ABP ↑; thrombocytosis; flu-like syndrome
    – may also require occasional blood transfusion with diuretic cover

Y: h**Y**perlipidaemia – simvastatin

h**Y**perglycaemia – avoid metformin, chlorpropamide; caution with insulins (due to risk of 'hypos')

h**Y**perPO4aemia – **Rx first** to avoid ectopic calcification: PO₄ restriction; oral PO₄ binders: MgCO₃ or CaCO₃

h**Y**poCalcaemia – 1α-hydroxylated cholecalciferol; calcitriol; CaCO₃, high-dose: ↓es PTH and ↓es PO₄

Symptomatic
- Hiccups or pruritus: chlorpromazine
- Peptic ulcers: omeprazole

Surgical – renal transplant
    ☠ : • Rejection (immunologic, ureteric anastomosis failure); immunosuppression (infections, neoplasia)
        • Vascular: polycythaemia, atherosclerosis, hypertension

Secondary renal failure: treat underlying cause – diabetes, hypertension, SLE, etc.

Haematuria – Causes

Pre-renal

Haematological

Bleeding diathesis:
- Coagulopathy
- Thrombocytopenia
- Platelet dysfunction

Haemoglobinuria, due to intravascular haemolysis:
- Hereditary:
  a) Sickle cell disease
  b) G6PD deficiency
- Acquired:
  a) Autoimmune haemolytic anaemia
  b) Paroxysmal cold haemoglobinuria
  c) RBC fragmentation, e.g. burns, trauma
  d) PNH, malaria

Ix: Urine microscopy

Renovascular

S.T.E.N.T.A.B.L.E.

Stenosis, renal artery
Thrombosis:
   atherosclerosis,
   sickle cell disease
Embolus
NSAIDs
Toxins, other:
   ACE inhibitors, radiotherapy
Autoimmune:
   scleroderma, vasculitis
   (Takayasu's, PAN, Wegener's)
Blood pressure ↑, which is ...
Long-standing
   hypertensive nephrosclerosis
   – **common**
Electrolyte: hypercalcaemia

Renal

Glomerulonephritis

P.A.I.N.T.S.

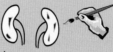

Primary:
   proliferative / RPGN,
   membranoproliferative
Autoimmune:
   SLE, scleroderma, vasculitis,
   anti-GBM, IgA nephropathy
Infection:
   endocarditis, visceral abscess,
   post-streptococcal,
   HBV, HCV, HIV
Neoplasia: lymphoma, leukaemia
Toxins: heroin
Syndromes, hereditary:
   1. Thin basement membrane disease
   2. Alport's disease

Tubulo-Interstitial Nephritis

T.I.N.

Toxins: 'allergic' – antibiotics, NSAIDs
Infection: Legionnaire's, leptospirosis
Neoplasia: lymphoma, leukaemia

Acute Tubular Necrosis

A.T.N.

ABP ↓ : severe haemorrhage
Toxins: aminoglycosides etc.
Necrosis: rhabdomyolysis (myoglobin)
Neoplasia: tumour lysis (uric acid)
Nephritis, pyelo-

Papillary Necrosis

1. Diabetes mellitus
2. Hypertension
3. Vasculitis
4. Sickle cell anaemia

Post-renal

Urinary Tract Obstruction

S.N.I.P.P.I.N.G.

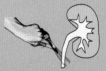

Stone / hypercalciuria
Neoplasia:
- Intrinsic: pelvis / ureters / bladder
- Extraluminal: e.g. colorectal / gynae

Infection: TB, schistosomiasis
Papillary necrosis
Pregnancy or other gynae
Inflammation:
   stricture / retroperitoneal fibrosis
Neurological (via UTIs)
Genetic / congenital:
   PUJ or VUJ stenosis, ureterocoele

Infection

<u>UTI</u>
<u>STD</u>
- Prostatitis (pyuria on PR massage)
- Vaginitis / urethritis

Structural

Kidneys
- Polycystic kidneys
  – Adult (APKD)
  – Infant (IPKD)
  – Medullary cystic disease
- Renal cell carcinoma

Prostate
Benign prostatic hyperplasia

---

1. **Non-urinary tract source,** e.g. PR, PV, enterocutanous fistula
2. **Pigmented urine:** dye ingestion (beetroot; rifampicin, L-DOPA); porphyria

IgA Nephropathy

<u>**Epi**</u> **I**nc: Commonest glomerulonephropathy, and commonest causes of hypertension in young men
      Age: 20–40s
      Sex: Men (commonest cause of hypertension in this group)
      Geo: Mediterranean, Asia; Blacks
      Aet: Autoimmune (assoc. HLA-B35 in French)

<u>**PC**</u> Renal-limited (or Berger's disease):
        1. Haematuria – recurrent, macroscopic: 1/3
        2. Proteinuria, inc. nephrosis: 1/3 (poor prognosis)
        3. Hypertension; CRF: 1/3

    Systemic: *G.R.O.S.S. Blood*

> **G**IT: • Coeliac, Crohn's, adenocarcinoma
>   • Biliary disease, chronic liver disease
> **R**espiratory: pneumonitis, obliterative bronchiolitis, adenocarcinoma
> **O**phthalmic: anterior uveitis; episcleritis
> **S**kin: vasculitis (Henoch–Schönlein purpura); dermatitis herpetiformis
> **S**pondylitis; Sjögren's syndrome
> **Blood**: monoclonal gammopathy of uncertain significance (IgA)

<u>**Ix**</u>   1. Serum IgA ↑ in 50%
     2. Complement: normal or ↑
     3. Biopsy: Light microscopy: • Mesangiocapillary glomerulonephritis
                             • Crescents; FSGS; tubulo-interstitial nephritis
         Immunofluoresence: mesangial IgA and C3 deposits

<u>**Rx**</u> 1. Fish oils ?
     2. Steroids: for nephrosis; active inflammation on biopsy

Thin Basement Membrane Disease
('Benign Haematuria')

<u>**Epi**</u> **I**nc: Commonest cause of asymptomatic haematuria
      Aet: Sporadic or hereditary (autosomal dominant: collagen Type IV, α4 chain mutation)

<u>**PC**</u> 1. Haematuria post-URTI
     2. Hypertension / proteinura – rare

<u>**Ix**</u> Light microscopy + IF: Normal
    Electron microscopy: Thin basement membrane (normal = 300–350 nm)

<u>**Rx**</u> Follow-up only

Proteinuria – Causes

Pre-renal

Overflow

- Acute-phase response:
  burns, fever, MI
- Myeloma:
  Bence-Jones proteinuria =
  Ig light-chain excess
  (**urine dipstick –ve!**, but
  salicylsulphonic acid test + ve)

Venous hypertension

- Physiological
  – Orthostatic:
    liver presses on IVC
  – Pregnancy
  – Strenuous exercise
- Congestive cardiac failure

Renovascular

S.T.E.N.T.A.B.L.E.

Stenosis, renal artery
Thrombosis: esp. renal **vein**
  due to venous hypertension
Embolus
NSAIDs
Toxins, other/radiotherapy
Autoimmune:
  • Scleroderma
  • Vasculitis, inc. PAN, Wegener's
Blood pressure ↑:
  hypertensive nephrosclerosis
Blood:
  • DIC, HUS, TTP
  • Hyperviscosity, e.g. CML
Liver: hepatorenal syndrome
Electrolyte: hypercalcaemia

Renal

Glomerulonephritis

P.A.I.N.T.S.

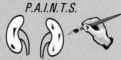

Primary:
membranous, minimal change,
FSGS, membranoproliferative
Autoimmune:
SLE, Sjögren's, sarcoid, PBC
IgA nephropathy
Infection: endocarditis,
visceral abscess, HCV, HIV,
malaria, schistosomiasis
Neoplasia:
amyloid, myeloma, solid tumours
Toxins: penicillamine, heroin, NSAIDs
Sclerosis, glomerulo-:
  1. **Diabetes mellitus**
  2. Sickle cell anaemia
  3. Glomerular capillary hypertension
  4. Alport's / Fabry's disease
Syndrome:
  'benign fixed proteinuria'
  Epi: young adult; normal ABP
  Ix: Glomerular pattern protein

Tubulo-Interstitial Nephritis

Acute: *T.I.N.*

Toxins: 'allergic' – antibiotics, NSAIDs
Infection: Legionnaire's, leptospirosis
Neoplasia: lymphoma, leukaemia

Chronic: *T.U.B.U.L.A.R.*

Toxins: NSAIDs, Li, cyclosporin
Ureteric reflux: **VUR**
Blood pressure ↑:
  hypertensive nephrosclerosis
Uric acid (gout); nephrocalcinosis
Lymphoma, leukaemia, myeloma
Autoimmune: - Sjögren's syn.
Radiation / transplant

Post-renal

Urinary tract obstruction

S.N.I.P.P.I.N.G.

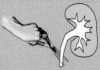

Stone / hypercalciuria
Neoplasia:
  • Intrinsic: pelvis / ureters / bladder
  • Extraluminal: e.g. colorectal / gynae
Infection: TB, schistosomiasis
Papillary necrosis / blood clot
Pregnancy
Inflammation:
  • Stricture
  • Retroperitoneal fibrosis
Neurological, via UTIs
Genetic / congenital:
  PUJ or VUJ stenosis, ureterocoele

Infection

<u>**UTI**</u>
<u>**STD**</u>

- Prostatitis (pyuria on PR massage)
- Vaginitis / urethritis

Structural

<u>**Kidneys**</u>

- Renal cell carcinoma

<u>**Bladder**</u>

- Polyp or carcinoma

---

1. **Urinary tract haemorrhage**
2. **False +ve urine dip-stick:** antibiotics; X-ray contrast media; alkalinuria

<u>Nephrotic Syndrome</u>

<u>PC</u>

N.E.P.H.R.O.T.I.C.

Nephritis: nephrotic syndrome may occur alone or as part of a general nephritis
- Alone: minimal-change, membranous, FSGS inc. diabetes mellitus, amyloidosis
- Nephritis: membranoproliferative renal artery or vein thrombosis
  malignant hypertension inc. eclampsia

Edema: • Generalized, esp. peri-orbital
- Pleural effusion; ascites
- GIT oedema: nausea, malabsorption, weight loss

Proteinuria: frothy urine

Hypoalbuminaemia:
- Hypovolaemia (postural hypotension; pre-renal ARF; $2°$ hyperaldosteronism: $K^+ \downarrow$)
- Growth retardation
- Poor wound healing

Raised lipids: LDL $\uparrow$, HDL $\downarrow$, triacylglycerides $\uparrow$
- PC: Atherosclerosis; xanthoma; pseudohyponatraemia
- Due to renal loss of apolipoprotein B

Osteomalacia: due to renal-loss of Vit D-binding globulin, which results in $Ca^{2+} \downarrow$

Thrombosis:
- DVT; CVA; renal vein thrombosis; pulmonary embolism
  – due to renal-loss of anti-thrombin-III; hypovolaemia; atherosclerosis

Infection, esp. pneumococcal peritonitis: loss of Igs + C3, C4

Chronic anaemia (hypochromic, but Fe-resistant): renal loss of transferrin

<u>Ix</u>

1. 24-hour Urine Protein

a) 150 - 500 mg / day: mild proteinuria (e.g. orthostatic; post-renal)
b) 500mg - 3 g / day: moderate proteinuria (e.g. glomerulonephritides, hypertension, UTI)
c) > 3g / day: heavy proteinuria, inc. nephrotic syndrome

2. Urine Electrophoresis: establishes 'selectivity' of glomerular disease

a) Selectivity: high (mid molecular weight – e.g. albumin): minimal-change glomerulonephritis
low (mid & high molecular wt. – e.g. IgG): membranous glomerulonephritis
b) Low-molecular weight (e.g. β_2- microglobulin): venous hypertension; proximal tubular disease
c) Bence-Jones protein: myeloma

<u>Rx</u>

Underlying cause: minimal change – steroids: treats proteinuria in 90%
– cyclosporin or cyclophosphamide if relapses
Diet: protein (caution if incipient renal failure); calories (overcome GIT oedema)
Fluid balance: salt and water intake; spironolactone or furosemide and amiloride; salt-free albumin 20%
Complications:
- Hypercholesterolaemia: simvastatin
- Infection: pneumococcal vaccine; IV benzylpenicillin
- DVT: LMW Heparin; antithrombin III supplements

Renovascular Disease

<u>**Causes**</u> *S.T.E.N.T.A.B.L.E.*

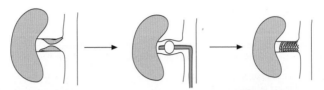

Stenosis, renal artery

Thrombosis, renal artery or vein

Embolus, renal artery
   1. Cardiogenic: AF, endocarditis, paradoxical (DVT via patent foramen ovale)
   2. Cholesterol emboli: from aortic atheroma, esp. post-aortic surgery; arteriography – Ix: eosinophilia

NSAIDs: vasodilate afferent and efferent arterioles, causing ↓ GFR

Toxins, other:
   1. Drugs - **A**CE inhibitors (and vasodilators); **A**mphotericin; **A**drenaline; cyclosporin **A**
   2. Radiotherapy

Autoimmune
   1. Scleroderma
   2. Vasculitides: Takayasu's, PAN, Wegener's granulomatosis
      Path: Intimal proliferation, medial thinning, fibrinoid necrosis of small arteries
      PC: • Microscopic haematuria, pyuria, cellular casts, mild proteinuria
             • Crisis: ARF, severe hypertension, microscopic angiopathic haemolytic anaemia (MAHA)

Blood pressure ↑
   1. Benign hypertensive nephrosclerosis
      Path: Intimal hyaline arteriosclerosis, necrotizing arteriolitis
      PC: Chronic renal failure
   2. Malignant hypertension
      Path: Fibrinoid necrosis, 'onion-skinning', 'flea-bitten kidney'
      PC: ARF, haematuria, nephrosis, microscopic angiopathic haemolytic anaemia (MAHA)

Blood constitutents
   1. Disseminated intravascular coagulation (DIC)
   2. Haemolytic uraemic syndrome (HUS)
      Epi: Commonest cause of ARF in children
      Cause: • Children: gastroenteritis, esp. verocytotoxicogenetic *E. coli* (VTEC), serotype 0157, H7
             • Adults: idiopathic, HIV, adenocarcinoma, SLE, post-partum, pre-eclampsia, genetic
      PC   • ARF: 'flea-bitten kidney' = cortical haemorrhagic microinfarcts
             • MAHA (fragmented RBCs)
             • Platelets ↓
   3. Thrombotic thrombocytopenic purpura (TTP) – as for HUS, plus:
             • Fever; WCC ↑
             • Infarcts: renal (ARF), brain-retina (focal neuro. Sx), bowel (mesenteric ischaemia)

Liver failure: hepatorenal syndrome
      Hepatic toxins and prostaglandins induce vasoconstriction

Eclampsia, pre-

Electrolyte: hypercalcaemia: • Vasoconstrictor
                                         • Also causes CRF via tubular and ureteric calcification

Stenosis, renal artery

Causes

1. Atherosclerosis
   Epi: Elderly; hypertension; ACE inhibitors (dilate efferent arteriole and so oppose physiological response)
   Site: Proximal; bilateral in 50%
2. Fibromuscular dysplasia
   Epi: Young women (30-40s; F:M = 4:1); smoking
   Site: **D**istal (**d**ysplasia); right-sided or bilateral

PC

1. Hypertension ± renal failure
2. Bruit: High-pitched

Ix

Bloods: • Creatinine ↑, K⁺ ↓, metabolic alkalosis
Radio: • Digital subtraction angiogram, duplex or MRA:
     fibromuscular dysplasia = 'string of beads'; smooth narrowing; local aneurysms; AVM; fistulae
    • Radionuclide scan (^{99m}Tc-DTPA or MAG3 scan ± captopril):
     captopril dilates efferent arteriole ⇒ dramatic ↓ in GFR and ↓ uptake of tracer (DTPA)
Special: • Captopril-induced hypotension: causes exaggerated ↑ in plasma renin activity
    • Renal vein renin ratio of > 1.5:1 between kidneys provides indication for surgery

Rx

1. Aspirin
2. Angioplasty
3. Surgery – better outcome

Thrombosis, renal artery or renal vein

Causes

1. Renal artery thrombus: *A.D.V.I.S.E. or H.E.P.A.R.I.N.I.S.E.*
   Vessel wall disease: **A**therosclerosis, **D**issection, **V**asculitis, **I**njury (inc. radiation), **S**tenosis
   Hypercoagulability: **H**ereditary - sickle cell disease, **E**strogens, **P**olycythaemia, inc. CML
2. Renal vein thrombus: *H.E.P.A.R.I.N.I.S.E.*
   Hereditary, **E**strogens, **P**olycythaemia, **A**utoimmune (antiphospholipid syn.)
   Renal (membranous glomerulonephritis, nephrotic syn), **I**njury, **N**eoplasia (renal cell carcinoma, adenocarcinoma)

PC

1. Pain in loin or flank: infarction (fever) or rupture (haemorrhagic shock)
2. Renal failure: • Acute: 'flash' pulmonary oedema; oliguria; hypertension
    • Chronic: remaining kidney develops focal segmental sclerosis
3. Pulmonary embolism: renal vein thrombosis

Ix

Bloods: creatinine ↑, LFT: AST ↑, ALP ↑, LDH ↑ (infarction)
Urine: • Renal artery thrombosis – mild proteinuria; micro. haematuria; pyuria
    • Renal vein thrombosis – heavy haematuria + proteinuria
Radio: angiogram (digital subtraction), duplex or MRA; MRV / selective renal venography

Rx

1. Heparin, warfarin, streptokinase
2. Thrombectomy
3. Nephrectomy in children with renal vein thrombosis

Glomerulonephritis

<u>**Def**</u> Glomerular inflammation

<u>**PC**</u> Causes classified according to predominant clinical syndrome:

Nephritic syndrome
Path: **Capillary proliferation**
PC: 1. Oliguria
      2. Hypertension
      3. Haematuria and pyuria
(presentation mimicked by renovascular disease, or acute tubulo-interstitial nephritis)

RPGN (Rapidly Progressive Glomerulonephritis)
Path: **Glomerular 'crescents'**
      = extreme form of capillary proliferation
PC: 1. Anuria (glomerular effacement)
      2. As for nephritic syndrome

Nephrotic syndrome
Path: **Membrane disease**
PC: 1. Proteinuria
      2. Oedema
      3. Hypercholesterolaemia

<u>Histology</u>

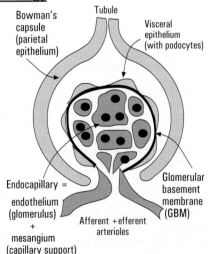

Bowman's capsule (parietal epithelium)
Tubule
Visceral epithelium (with podocytes)
Endocapillary = endothelium (glomerulus) + mesangium (capillary support)
Afferent + efferent arterioles
Glomerular basement membrane (GBM)

Segmental vs Global: glomerulus-level ascription
Focal vs Diffuse: kidney-level ascription

<u>NephrItic Syn. RPGN</u>

P.A.I.nts

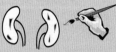

Primary: proliferative glomerulonephritis
- **Immune-complex:**
  Proliferation of endocapillaries
  Proliferative = sube**P**ithelial granular deposits ('starry sky')
  Ix: Low C3, C_H50
- **Pauci-immune:**
  Proliferation of endocapillary and parietal cell epithelium ('crescents')
  Focal necrosis
  Ix: normal C3, 4, C_H50 but p-ANCA +ve, and ESR, CRP ↑ as associated with vasculitis

Autoimmune
- **SLE, myositis:** as for immune-complex GN
- **Vasculitides**
  (e.g. PAN, Wegener's granulomatosis):
  As for pauci-immune glomerulonephritis
  Angiogram: aneurysms, infarcts
- **Anti-GBM disease**
  linear immune-complex deposits on GBM and tubules ('ribbon-like')
  Epi: smoking; hydrocarbons; flu; HLA DR-2, -4
  PC: Haematuria; haemoptysis ('Goodpasture's syndrome')
  Ix: – Anti-GBM in 50% of Goodpasture's = Ab against non-collagenous domain of collagen IV, $\alpha3$-chain
  C3, 4 normal, ANCA +ve in 20%, respiratory function (KCO), bronchoscopy

Infection
- *Streptococcus pyogenes:*
  Epi: 10-20 days post-pharyngitis / impetigo
  PC: smoky red urine (may persist for > 6 years), headache, N + V (ABP ↑), flank pain, acute renal failure that usually recovers within 1 month
  Ix: Serology:
      Anti-DNAseB, ASO, Anti-NADase (throat), antihyaluronidase (skin)
      C3, C_H50 ↓, Polyclonal IgG ↑
- **Chronic bacterial:**
  Bacterial endocarditis: C3, 4 ↓
  Visceral abscess: C3, C4 normal or ↑

NephrOtic Syndrome

P.A.I.N.T.S.

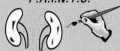

Primary
- **Membranous glomerulonephritis**
  Diffuse thickening of GBM
  Subepithelial immune-complex deposits
  ('silver spikes')
  Epi: 40% adult; < 5% child nephrotic syndrome
  70% membranous GN are idiopathic
  Ix: C3, 4 normal
- **Minimal-change disease:**
  No change / mild mesangial hypercellularity
  on light microscopy
  Diffuse effacement of podocyte foot processes
  on electron microscopy
  Epi: 20% adult; 80% child nephrotic syndrome
- **Focal segmental glomerulosclerosis:**
  Hyalinosis in parts of > 50% glomerulus

Autoimmune
- SLE, Sjögren's, Hashimoto's, Graves', PBC
  all cause membranous glomerulonephritis
- Atopy - associated with minimal-change GN

Infection
- Hep B or C, malaria, enterococcal SBE, syphilis
  all cause membranous glomerulonephritis
- HIV, immunization; URTI
  associated with minimal-change GN / FSGS

Neoplasia
- Amyloid (1° and 2° : Congo Red +ve); myeloma
- Lymphoma, renal-cell carcinoma – minimal-change
- Carcinoma, melanoma – membranous

Toxins
- Captopril, penicillamine, NSAIDs – membranous
- Ampicillin, rifampicin – minimal-change
- Opioids – FSGS

Sclerosis (other FSGS causes)
- Diabetes mellitus
  - also causes membranous; minimal-change GN
- Sickle cell anaemia
- Glomerular capillary hypertension:
  renal ablation, e.g. contralaleral renal agenesis
  or nephrectomy, renal artery thrombosis
  diffuse renal disease, e.g. reflux nephropathy

Sarcoidosis

Nephritic & Nephrotic Syn.

P.A.I.N.T.S.

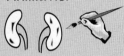

Primary
- **Membranoproliferative GN:**
  Mesangial proliferation ('mesangiocapillary GN')
  Diffuse thickening of GBM
  Types:
  1. Sube**N**dothelial and mesangial immune-complex
     deposits (mesa**N**gio)
     Ix: C3 + C4↓
     Course: Benign
  2. Linear, intramembranous dense C3 deposits due to
     'C3 nephritic factor', i.e. an IgG that stabilizes C3
     convertase of the alternative complement pathway
     Ix: C3↓ only
     Course: End-stage renal failure in 5–10 yrs
- **Focal segmental proliferative**
  causes are same as for proliferative GN

Autoimmune
- **SLE, Sjögren's, autoimmune hepatitis**
  all cause membranoproliferative GN
- **IgA nephropathy**
  Epi: **commonest glomerulonephritis** and cause
  of hypertension in young men
  PC: Haematuria 3 days post-URTI
  Types:
  1. Renal-limited (Berger's): 50% get CRF
  2. Cutaneous vasculitis (Henoch–Schönlein
     Purpura)
  3. Systemic disease-associated

Infection
- HBV, HCV (cryoglobulinaemia), HIV
- Staphylococcus – SBE, abscess, CSF 'shunt nephritis'
- Haemolytic uraemic syndrome
  all of these cause membranoproliferative GN

Neoplasia: Lymphoma, leukaemia

Toxins: Heroin

Syndromes
- Thin-basement membrane disease:
  Epi: Commonest cause of asymptomatic
  haematuria
  Aet: Autosomal dominant or sporadic;
  collagen type IV, α4-chain mutation
- Alport's disease
  Epi: Commonest hereditary nephritis (X-linked)
  Aet: Collagen type IV, α5-chain mutation
- Other: Nail-patella syn., partial lipodystrophy

Renal Tubular Disease

The effects of tubular disease depend on whether proximal or distal convoluted tubules are affected:

Proximal Tubular Disease

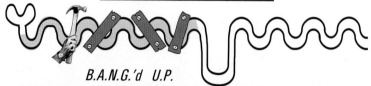

Types   *B.A.N.G.'d U.P.*

Bicarbonaturia **(Renal Tubular Acidosis – Type 2)**
  Causes: Hereditary (autosomal recessive or autosomal dominant), or acetazolamide
  PC: 1. Weakness; failure to thrive (mild acidosis, hypokalaemia)
        2. Rickets or osteomalacia (but **no** renal stones due to ↓ citrate resorption)
        3. Polyuria, polydipsia (due to increased $NaHCO_3$ in distal tubule, and hypokalemia)
  Ix: 1. 'Normal anion gap' metabolic acidosis:
         • Plasma HCO_3^-↓, Cl^-↑, K^+↓ ; urine HCO_3^-↑
         • Aciduria: minimum pH < 5.5 (due to ↓HCO_3^- filtration, ↑distal H^+ excretion)
        2. Plasma PO_4↓, Vit D↓; urine Ca^{2+}↑
  Rx: Bicarbonate

Amino aciduria (and low-molecular-weight proteinuria)
  Causes: 1. Overflow: phenylketonuria, maple syrup urine, homocystinuria; acquired liver failure
          2. PCT resorption ↓:
             a) Cystinuria: ↓ resorption of dibasic acids; PC: Renal stones
             b) Hartnup's disease: ↓ resorption of neutral AAs; PC: Pellagra (tryptophan deficiency)

Na$^+$ and K$^+$ wasting
  PC: Na^+ loss: hypovolaemia; K^+ loss: weakness

Glycosuria
  Causes: Overflow (diabetes, stress) or PCT resorption↓ (hereditary, pregnancy)
  PC: Polyuria, polydipsia

Uric aciduria

Phosphaturia
  Causes: 1. Overflow (paracetamol overdose)
           2. PCT resorption ↓ (X-linked dominant hypophosphataemic rickets)

'Fanconi's Syndrome'

  Def: generalized proximal tubule dysfunction of all or some of above defects
  Causes: *F.A.N.C.O.N.I.*

Familial: autosomal dominant, autosomal recessive, X-linked
Autoimmune: Sjögren's, autoimmune liver disease
Neoplasia: myeloma, amyloid
Calcium ↑/↓: primary or secondary hyperparathyroidism / chronic hypokalaemia
Other: outdated tetracycline, lead, mercury, cadmium, cisplatin, aspirin, neomycin
Necrosis, acute tubular
Inherited: Wilson's disease, cystinosis, Lowe's oculocerebrorenal disease, tyrosinaemia

PC: As above + chronic renal failure + Vit D deficiency + pyelonephritis
Rx: High fluid intake (sodium and water), $KHCO_3$, PO_4, α_1-calcidol

Distal Tubular Disease

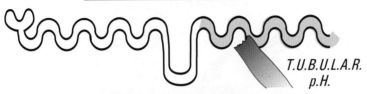

T.U.B.U.L.A.R.
p.H.

H⁺ Excretion Impairment (Renal Tubular Acidosis – Type 1)

Causes: *T.U.B.U.L.A.R. p.H.*

> **T**oxins: NSAIDs, lithium, amphotericin
> **U**reteric – vesico-, reflux: chronic pyelonephritis, urinary obstruction
> **B**lood pressure: hypertension
> **U**ric acid (gout) / Ca^{2+} ↑ (hyperPTHism, Vit D toxicity) / K^+ ↓
> **L**ymphoma, leukaemia, myeloma, amyloid
> **A**utoimmune: Sjögren's, SLE, autoimmune hepatitis
> **R**adiation nephritis, renal transplant
> **P**apillary necrosis: diabetes mellitus, sickle cell anaemia
> **H**ereditary: RTA-type 1 (autosomal dominant), medullary-sponge kidney

PC: 1. Weakness; failure to thrive (acidosis, hypokalaemia)
    2. Rickets or osteomalacia, **and** renal stones
    3. Polyuria, polydipsia

Ix: 1. 'Normal anion gap' metabolic acidosis: plasma HCO_3^-↓, Cl^-↑, K^+↓
       • Alkaluria: minimum pH > 5.5, and urine HCO_3^-↓ – cf. RTA type 2
       • Low urine NH_4^+ (as estimated by urine cation gap) – cf. GIT cause of acidosis
    2. Ca^{2+}↓, Vit D↓, PTH↑ ; urine Ca^{2+}↑
    3. Acid load test: loading with NH_4Cl fails to acidify urine (urine pH > 6.5)

Rx: KCl, followed by bicarbonate

Aldosterone Impairment (Renal Tubular Acidosis – Type 4)

Causes:
    1. Hyporeninism: diabetes mellitus, hypertensive nephrosclerosis
    2. Hypoaldosteronism: Addison's, adrenalectomy
    3. Aldosterone resistance: obstructive nephropathy, spironolactone

Ix: 1. Plasma: HCO_3^-↓, Cl^-↑, K^+↑ – cf. RTA types 1 and 2
    2. Urine: as for RTA type 1: alkaluria and urine HCO_3^-↓ (although minimum pH may be < 5.5)

Rx: 9α – Fludrocortisone (high-dose if resistance)

Diabetes Insipidus

Causes:
    1. Cranial: *D.I.V.I.N.I.T.Y.* – e.g. hereditary, sarcoid, pituitary adenoma
    2. Tubular: *T.U.B.U.L.A.R.* p.H. – e.g. toxins, ureteric reflux, blood pressure, uric acid ↑, Ca^{2+}↑

Ix: 1. Plasma osmolality > 300 mosm / kg
    2. Urine osmolality < 300 mosm / kg

Urinary Obstruction

Causes   The following cause obstruction in the renal pelvis, ureters, bladder or urethra:

S.N.I.P.P.I.N.G.

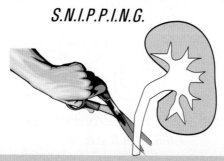

Stones

Neoplasia
1. Intrinsic: polyp / carcinoma – transitional cell (ureter / bladder) or squamous cell (urethra)
2. Extrinsic: colorectal, gynaecological or prostate carcinoma / lymphoma

Infection
1. TB: intrinsic fibrosis, or para-aortic lymph nodes
2. *Schistosoma haematobium* (Africa, Mediterranean)

Papillary necrosis
1. Diabetes mellitus / hypertension
2. Sickle cell anaemia / vasculitis
3. Acute tubular necrosis

Pregnancy (or other gynaecological) / **P**rostate
1. Pregnancy: due to direct compression, estrogen (smooth muscle relaxant)
   Other: fibroids, ovarian cyst, haematocolpos, haematometria (occurs at menses)
2. Prostate: benign prostatic hyperplasia, carcinoma, prostatitis (all cause bladder-neck obstruction)

Inflammation – fibrosis
1. Stricture: post-trauma, laparotomy (e.g. caesarian section – ureters), catheterization (urethra)
2. Retroperitoneal fibrosis, due to:
   - Primary: multifocal fibrosclerosis (66%); ESR ↑
   - Autoimmune: PAN
   - Infection: TB
   - Neoplasia: metastases, lymphoma, carcinoid
   - Toxins: methysergide
   - Surrounding inflammation: aortic aneurysm, pancreatitis, Crohn's, diverticulitis

Neurological – failure of peristalsis, e.g. anticholinergics

Genetic / congenital – urinary tract anomalies
1. Stenosis: PUJ (pelvic-ureteric junction) or VUJ (vesico-ureteric junction)
2. Ureter: ureterocoele; retrocaval ureter
3. Urethra: valves (commonest cause of bilateral hydronephrosis in boys), phimosis

PC   1. **Pain in flanks, suprapubically** – esp. stones, but also neoplasia, fibrosis
2. **Renal failure** – if obstruction of both ureters; one ureter if renal agenesis; bladder neck or urethra
3. **Urinary retention** – if obstruction of bladder neck or urethra

<u>Urinary Retention</u>

<u>Causes</u> The following cause obstruction in the bladder neck or urethra:

S.N.I.P.P.I.N.G.

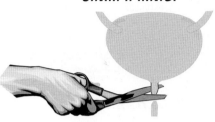

Stones

Neoplasia: carcinoma – bladder, prostate, colorectal, gynaecological

Infection: UTI, STD, abscess (e.g. bartholinitis, caruncle); PC: 'Holding on', strangury

Papillary necrosis

Pregnancy (or other gynaecological) / **P**rostate
    1. Pregnancy: retroverted uterus / other – fibroids; ovarian cyst, haematocolpos, haematometria
    2. Prostate: benign prostatic hyperplasia, carcinoma, prostatitis

Inflammation (fibrosis): stricture post-trauma, catheterization (urethra)

Neurological:
    1. LMN: diabetic neuropathy, cauda equina; UMN: multiple sclerosis, cord compression
    2. Atony: overdistension, e.g. diuretics, postoperative, binge-drinking
    3. Toxins, e.g. anticholinergics
    4. Psychological, inc. urethral myotonia (young women)

Genetic / congenital: urethral valves; phimosis

GIT: constipation (bladder neck obstruction)

<u>Types</u>

	Symptoms	Catheter residual volume	Renal function
Acute	Painful	< 1 litre	Normal
Chronic	Painless	> 1 litre	Renal failure
Acute-on-chronic	Painful	> 1 litre	Renal failure
(e.g. overfilling; UTI)		(normal < 600 ml)	

<u>Complications</u>
    1. Stones: form in diverticulae that develop between hypertrophied trabeculations
    2. Infection
    3. Renal failure

<u>Rx</u>
    1. Catheterize: measure residual volume, and leave for 1–2 days
    2. TWOC (trial without catheter): perform at midnight to allow daytime observation
    3. Indwelling catheterization, if TWOC failure, chronic retention, or prostatism, prostate carcinoma

Renal Stones

<u>**Epi**</u>   **I**nc: Lifetime risk = 1%
Age: 20–40s
Sex: M:F = 4:1 (opposite of gallstones)

<u>**Causes**</u>   Crystal formation depends on:

> **Chemical** factors: Ca^{2+} ↑, oxalate ↑, alkali ↑, citrate ↓
> **Crystallization** factors: stasis facilitates crystal nucleation

C.R.U.S.H.I.N.G.

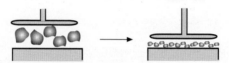

Calcium – hypercalciuria due to
   Path: Ca oxalate or phosphate stones (hydroxyapatite or brushite) occur in 80% all cases
   Causes: • Hypercalcaemia, esp. hyperparathyroidism
   • Normocalcaemia: hereditary hypercalciuria:
      PTH ↑ variant: intestinal absorption ↑ and bone resorption ↑
      PTH ↓ variant: renal PO_4 wasting and 2° intestinal absorption
   • Hypocitraturia: idiopathic, or due to hypokalaemia, e.g. from chronic diarrhoea
Renal tubular acidosis, type 1
   Path: Encourages stones due to alkaline urine; hypercalciuria; hypocitraturia
Uric acid
   Path: Uric acid or sodium monourate occurs in 5% cases
   Causes: • Hyperuricaemia (although only half of cases have gout)
   • Idiopathic, myeloproliferative states, chemotherapy, acidosis
Stasis
   • Renal cysts, bladder diverticulae, partial obstruction
Hereditary
   • Hyperoxaluria, due to hepatic oxalate synthesis ↑
   • Cystinosis: cystine stones form due to failure of proximal tubule resorption
   • Hypouricaemia: uric acid stones due to failure of proximal tubule resorption
Infection
   • *Proteus mirabilis* secretes urease that promotes alkaluria ⇒ struvite ($MgNH_4PO_4$ or $CaPO_4$)
   • Causes large, 'staghorn' calculi – makes up 10% cases
   • Assoc. women, chronic catheterization, chronic UTI
Nutrition: toxins
   1. Nutrition:
      • Hypercalciuria – high-salt diet
      • Oxalic acid – rhubarb or strawberries, tea or coffee, nuts or spinach, Vit C
      • Hyperuricaemia – purine-rich food, e.g. offal
      • Hyperlipidaemia – high-fat diet
   2. Toxins: sulphonamide, aciclovir, indinavir, Mg trisilicate (antacid), loop diuretics
GIT – fat malabsorption
   Causes: Crohn's, coeliac, chronic pancreatitis, bacterial overgrowth
   Path: Ca^{2+} binds to intraluminal fatty acids, releasing oxalate that gets absorbed

PC
1. Colic: loin → flank → iliac fossa pain
2. Strangury (urethral spasm), dysuria, passage of stone or gravel
3. Hematuria: micro- or macroscopic – essential!

Ix **B**lood   Renal: urea ↑ – volume depletion; creatinine ↑ – if only 1 functioning kidney / bilat. stones
                      Electrolytes: Ca^{2+}, PO_4 , PTH, uric acid, acidosis
                      FBC: WCC ↑ , ESR ↑

     Urine: Dipstick: RBC (essential); WBC, nitrite (infection); pH; protein + glucose
                   24-hr collection: calcium, oxalate, citrate, uric acid
                   Sediment microscopy; birefringence (+ve = Ca^{2+} oxalate); chemical analysis

Calcium		Struvite	Uric acid	Cystine
Dumb-bell	Bipyramidal	Staghorn	Small, amorphous	Yellow hexagons

     Micro: MSU – *Proteus mirabilis* (cause) or other UTI due to urinary stasis
     Radio: PAXR: opaque stones – 90%; lucent stones – 10% (*opposite of gallstones*)
                             calcium, struvite – radio-opaque; cystine – slightly opaque; uric acid – radiolucent
                             papillary nephrocalcinosis – medullary sponge kidney
                IVU, USS
     Special: • RTA type 1: NH_4Cl loading test
                  • Cystinuria: Na nitroprusside Test – urine turns cherry-red

Rx **General**
1. Fluid intake: aim for > 2 l / day urine; look for stone passage
2. Analgesia: morphine, indomethacin, propantheline
3. Stone removal:
    • Lithotripsy - extracorporeal, percutaneous ultrasound, or ureteric laser
    • Surgery: nephro - / ureterolithotomy; cystoscopy with ureteric flexible-basket ensnarement

Type-specific

Calcium:
    • Hypercalcaemia: treat accordingly
    • Normocalcaemic:
        – Thiazides; low-salt, high-potassium diet (↑ es tubular resorption of Ca^{2+})
        – Na-cellulose PO_4 (↓ es GIT absorption); oral PO_4 (urine PPi ↑ + Ca^{2+} ↓)

Renal tubular acidosis, type 1: KCl, bicarbonate

Uric acid: low-purine diet; allopurinol; K citrate – alkalize urine

Stasis: treat underlying cause

Hereditary
    • Hyperoxaluria: oral PO_4, pyridoxine, K citrate; liver + renal transplant
    • Cystinosis: penicillamine (cystine chelator); K citrate: alkalize urine

Infection: • Antibiotics
              • Acidify urine – methananime mandelate; urease inhibitor – acetohydroxamic acid

Nutrition: low-salt, high-potassium diet; low oxalic acid; low purines; low-fat diet

GIT: • correct fat malabsorption-lipase supplements
      • oxalate-binding resin-cholestyramine
      • oxalate precipitate-calcium lactate

Renal Enlargement

P.H.O.N.E. - shaped

 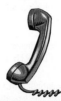

Polycystic kidneys / simple cysts:
   hereditary (APKD, IPKD, neurocutaneous)
Hypertrophy 2° to contralateral renal agenesis
Obstruction (hydronephrosis) /
Occlusion (renal vein thrombosis)
Neoplasia:
   • Renal cell carcinoma
   • Myeloma, lymphoma, amyloid
Endocrine: early diabetes mellitus

Renal Cysts

Large Kidneys

Adult polycystic kidney disease
Infant polycystic kidney disease
Neurocutaneous syndromes
   Epi: Autosomal dominant
   PC: Similar to adult polycystic kidneys +
      • Tuberous sclerosis: hyperplastic nodules, angiomyolipomas
      • Von Hippel-Lindau syndrome: renal cell carcinoma

Normal size

Medullary-sponge kidneys
   Epi: Majority are sporadic and congenital; few are autosomal dominant
   PC: 1. Incidental finding on AXR: papillary nephrocalcinosis
       2. Stones, haematuria, infection

Small Kidneys

Hereditary – nephronophthisis / medullary-cystic disease
   Epi: Nephronophthisis – autosomal recessive, children
        Medullary-cystic disease – autosomal dominant; adult-onset
   PC: 1. Renal failure, inc. polyuria
       2. Hepatic fibrosis, cerebellar ataxia (nephronophthisis)
Acquired – End-stage renal disease, dialysis
   PC: 1. Stones, infection, haematuria
       2. Polycythaemia (EPO secretion)
       3. Renal cell carcinoma

Adult Polycystic Kidney Disease

Epi   **AD**ults: renal failure > 20 yrs; usually 40–60 years
Autosomal **D**ominant
PKD1 gene, polycystin-1 (80%): cell–cell and cell–matrix membrane receptor
PKD2 gene, polycystin-2: Ca^{2+} channel that interacts with polycystin-1

PC   *M.I.S.H.A.P.E.N.*

Cysts originate from
all parts of nephron
and become detached from
parent nephron

Mass-effect: abdominal mass; flank pain
Infection
Stones, esp. uric acid
Haematuria or haemorrhage into cyst (acute pain)
ABP ↑: hypertension
Polyuria, nocturia: • Impaired tubular concentration
 • Renal failure
Extra-renal cysts: liver, pancreas, lungs, ovaries
Extra: colonic diverticulae, inguinal herniae
Neuro: cerebral berry aneurysms / subarachnoid haemorrhage
 + mitral valve prolapse; aortic aneurysm

Infant Polycystic Kidney Disease

Epi   Autosomal recessive
PKHD1 gene, fibrocystin

PC

Cysts originate from distal
tubule and collecting tubule,
and remain with nephron

Kidney • Abdominal masses in infant
 • Hypertension / renal failure in childhood
Systemic • Pulmonary hypoplasia
 • Liver failure due to hepatic fibrosis

Renal Cell Carcinoma

Def

Transformation of epithelial cells, predominantly from **proximal convoluted tubule:**

1. Clear cell   80%
   - von Hippel–Lindau tumour suppressor gene inactivation (chromosome 3p)
2. Chromophobic   10%
3. Oncocytic   5%
4. Collecting duct – medullary: 2%
   - Assoc: young people, sickle cell anaemia
   - Poor prognosis

Epi

Inc: Increasing incidence – currently 5% of all cancers
Age: 50–70 years
Sex: M:F = 3:1

Causes

V.I.C.T.O.R.Y.

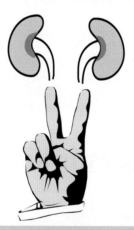

Von Hippel–Lindau (*VHL*) gene:
- Autosomal dominant

Inherited syndrome:
- Neurofibromatosis; tuberous sclerosis

Cystic disease:
- Adult polycystic kidney disease

Toxins:
- Smoking, cadmium, dry-cleaning; trichloroethylene

Obesity

Renal failure, end-stage:
- Esp. on chronic dial**Y**sis, due to acquired renal cysts

PC

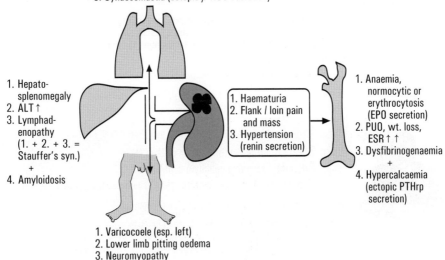

1. Pulmonary embolism 2° to renal vein thrombosis
2. Pulmonary metastases
3. Gynaecomastia (ectopic β-HCG secretion)

1. Hepato-
   splenomegaly
2. ALT ↑
3. Lymphad-
   enopathy
   (1. + 2. + 3. =
   Stauffer's syn.)
   +
4. Amyloidosis

1. Haematuria
2. Flank / loin pain
   and mass
3. Hypertension
   (renin secretion)

1. Anaemia,
   normocytic or
   erythrocytosis
   (EPO secretion)
2. PUO, wt. loss,
   ESR ↑ ↑
3. Dysfibrinogenaemia
   +
4. Hypercalcaemia
   (ectopic PTHrp
   secretion)

1. Varicocoele (esp. left)
2. Lower limb pitting oedema
3. Neuromyopathy

Ix rine: • Cytology
• Proteinuria – if heavy, may suggest renal vein thrombosis

Radio: • USS / IVU: renal mass
– Differential diagnosis = cyst, abscess, benign neoplasm (adenoma; angiomyolipoma)
• CT abdomen-pelvis-chest staging
• MRV: inferior vena cava and renal vein thrombosis

Rx

Local disease: radical nephrectomy
• En bloc removal of Gerota's fascia with adrenals, lymph nodes ± renal vein
Metastatic disease:
• Cytotoxics
• Hormonal therapy: progestagens
• Immunotherapy: interferon-α, interleukin-2
(☠ : capillary leakage syndrome, fever, shock)
• Surgery: palliation of local signs

Prog Poor, although some cases stabilize or even develop spontaneous regression

	5-year survival rate
Stage I (renal-confined)	70%
Stage III (renal vein thrombosis, lymphadenopathy)	40%
Stage IV (metastases)	10%

Testicular Tumours

Germ-Cell Tumours

Risk factors

1. Cryptorchidism: • Risk is higher for abdominal than inguinal site
   • Both testes at risk, even if one is in scrotum
2. Dysgenesis: Klinefelter's syndrome, testicular feminization syndrome
3. Isochromosome 12p reduplication

Seminoma

Epi: **S**emi, i.e. **middle**-aged (30–40s); commonest testis tumour

Path: **S**heets of large, uniform, clear cells
Spermatic cord and epididymis infiltrated
Synctium in 10% that secretes β-HCG and causes gynaecomastia

Ix: **T**umour markers: placental alkaline phosphatase

Prog: **S**crotal involvement only (stage 1) in 70%:
• Stage I: 5 yr survival rate 100%; stage II: 95%
• Good prognosis: spermatocytic seminoma – doesn't metastasize (50s+)

Rx: 1. Orchidectomy + retroperitoneal lymph-node dissection (RPLND)
2. Radiotherapy to abdominal lymph nodes

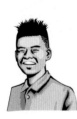

Teratoma

Epi: **T**wenties:
• Prognosis worsens with age, as tumours are less differentiated

Path: **T**otipotent tissue:
• Heterogeneous mix of differentiated cells
• Cartilage, bone, muscle, thyroid

Ix: **T**umour markers:
• AFP; β-HCG; hPL (human placental lactogen); LDH
N.B.: β-HCG and hPL may cause gynaecomastia

Prog: **T**errible prognosis (relative to seminoma):
• Rapid, disorderly growth: 60% present with lymph / vascular spread
PC: Back pain (retroperitoneal mets.) / dyspnoea (pulmonary mets.)
• Worst prognosis: undifferentiated 'embryonal carcinoma' or chorioca.
• Good prognosis: yolk-sac sumour (Ix: AFP), usually < 3 yrs old

Rx: 1. Orchidectomy + retroperitoneal lymph-node dissection (RPLND)
2. Chemotherapy – offers 80% remission

<u>Non-Germ-Cell Tumours</u>

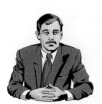

Sex cord–Stromal

Epi: **S**emi, i.e. **middle**-aged (30–40s)
Path: **S**teroid-producing, esp. Leydig-cell tumour
     PC: 1. Gynaecomastia (estrogen secretion)
         2. Precocious puberty (androgen or glucocorticoid secretion)
     Sertoli cell tumour / Androblastoma:
         – less hormone secretion.
     Spermatic cord and epididymis infiltrated

Prog: **S**crotal involvement only is usual: good prognosis

Lymphoma

Epi: **L**ater life (50s +)
Path: **L**arge-cell, diffuse, non-Hodgkin lymphoma
Prog: Poor

Ovarian Tumours

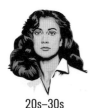

20s–30s

Germ-Cell Tumours

1. Teratoma
   - Epi: Twenties
   - Path: Totipotent tissue, due to unfertilized oocyte dividing and developing along 2 or 3 germ cell lines (endo-, meso-, or ectoderm): dermoid cyst (sebum, hair) + mamillary process (teeth, bone)
   - Ix: Tumour markers – only in variants with poor prognosis:
     AFP – yolk-sac tumour; β-HCG-choriocarcinoma
     Thyrotoxicosis ('struma ovarii')
   - Prog: *not Terrible – unlike testis teratomas*
     - Usually benign and cystic
     - Solid components may transform, e.g. skin – squamous cell carcinoma

2. Seminoma equivalent (= 'dysgerminoma')
   Unlike testis seminomas, ovarian dysgerminomas are usually *aggressive* due to early spread via blood

Functional Cysts (Non-Neoplastic)

1. Follicular: resolve spontaneously
2. Corpus luteum: unilateral pain; amenorrhoea
3. Theca-lutein: large bilateral mass
4. Endometriotic: pain; look like 'chocolate cysts' due to blood

---

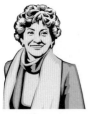

40s +

Adenoma or Adenocarcinoma (70%)

Aged (40s+); **A**bnormal ovarian function; **A**utosomal dominant – *See opposite*

Sex cord-Stromal Tumours

1. Granulosa-cell or theca-cell tumour:
   - PC: Secrete estrogen:
     - Amenorrhea (if premenopausal), menorrhagia, endometrial carcinoma
     - Breast enlargement; precocious puberty (if in children)
2. Sertoli-Leydig cell tumour or androblastoma:
   - PC: Secrete androgen:
     - Amenorrhea
     - Virilization, inc. cliteromegaly; breast atrophy
3. Fibroma:
   - PC: • Torsion upon pedicle
     - Ascites and pleural effusion (transudates) = 'Meig's syndrome'

Metastases

1. Gynaecological: endometrium, breast
2. GIT: gastric; colon, via transcoelomic or lymph spread ('Krukenberg tumour') mucus-secreting, signet-ring cells; bilateral

Ovarian Adenocarcinoma

Epi   Aged (40s +)

Aet   Abnormal ovarian function:
- Repeated ovulatory cycles induce epithelial trauma, repair and neoplasia:
  ∴ associated with nulliparity, early menarche, late menopause
- Persistent stimulation of ovaries by gonadotrophins:
  ∴ associated with clomiphene; protection offered by contraceptive pill

Autosomal dominant inheritance:
- *BRCA-1, -2*, hereditary non-polyposis colorectal carcinoma (Lynch syndrome)

Path   Derived from surface-epithelium (origins indicated)

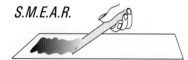

S.M.E.A.R.

Serous (Fallopian tube) – commonest adenocarcinoma:
Path: **S**ingle cavity with **S**urface exophytic papillary growths
Prog: **SER**ious: • Rapid transcoelomic spread and bilateral in 50%
　　　　　　　　 • Metastases common, but may regress after 1° removal

Mucinous-(endocervix):
Path: **M**ultilocular cyst – PC: large **M**ass
Prog: **M**ild – most are low-grade
　　　　　 Myxoma – 'pseudomyxoma peritonei': cyst may rupture with
　　　　　　　　　　 peritoneal seeding and mucin release

Endometrioid (endometrium):
Assoc: **E**ndometri**a**l carcinoma, **E**ndometri**o**sis

Author-named – **B**renner tumour:
Assoc: **B**leeding, postmenopausally, due to estrogen secretion

Renal-related = **C**lear-Cell tumour (like renal clear-cell carcinoma):
Assoc: **C**alcium elevation (PTH-related peptide secretion)
　　　　 Commonly recur

PC   Local: • Abdominal pain (chronic – mass effect; acute – bleed or torsion)
　　　　　 • Abdominal bloating (mass effect, ascites)
　　　　　 • Urinary frequency or constipation
　　　Extra-abdominal:
　　　　　 • Pleural effusions – DVT; paraneoplastic: limbic encephalitis

Ix   CA125 tumour marker

Rx   1. Surgery
　　　2. Carboplatin + paclitaxel

Prog
　　　　　　　　　　　　　　　　　　 5 yr survival rate
　　　Stage I – ovaries only　　　　　　　 80%
　　　　　　 II – pelvis extension　　　　　　 60%
　　　　　　 III – peritoneal, retroperitoneal spread　 30%
　　　　　　 IV – metastases in liver, pleura, etc.　 10%

Haematology

Anaemia

Def

Men:	Hb < 13.5 g/dl
Women:	Hb < 11.5 g/dl
Childern:	Hb < 11 g/dl
Newborn:	Hb < 15 g/dl

N.B. allowances should be made for changes in plasma volume, in the absence of changes in total red cell mass. This can be approximated by inspecting packed cell volume (PCV):

Normal PCV (haematocrit):
Men :   40–50%
Women: 35–50%

PC

Fatigue, SOB
Cardiac: palpitations; angina, CCF
Neuro: headaches, TIAs, retinal bleeds
Other: intermittent claudication

Presence of symptoms depend on:
- Severity < 10 g/dl = symptomatic
- Speed of onset: acute more symptomatic, as not compensated
- Age: reduced CVS compensation

O/E

Pale mucous membranes
Pruritus, koilonychia: Fe deficiency
Jaundice - haemolysis or megaloblastosis

Ix

1. **Blood:** FBC, film, reticulocytes: haematinics, transferrin saturation Haemolysis tests: e.g. Coombs' test
   Other: U+Es, LFTs, TFTs,
           ESR ($\uparrow$ with Hb $\downarrow$)
2. **Fine-needle aspirate and / or bone-marrow biopsy:** marrow cellularity, myeloid:erythroid ratio (range 3–12)
3. **Special:**
   Ferrokinetics (^{59}Fe):
   - Measures rate of Fe uptake from plasma = total erythropoiesis
   - Sacrum, liver, spleen uptake?
   RBC survival (^{51}Cr + RBC):
   - Measure radioactivity over liver and spleen over 3 weeks

Microcytic

MCV < 76 fl

1. Iron deficiency

Supply $\downarrow$:
- Diet, malabsorption

Demand $\uparrow$:
- Physiological (pregnancy, periods)
- Blood loss: GIT, urine, lung, haemolysis

Ix: Ferritin $\downarrow$, soluble transferrin receptor $\uparrow$

2. Haemolytic anaemias

Thalassaemia:
β: 1 gene on Chr 11 (100 mutations):-
β^0 = no globin; β^+ = $\downarrow$ globin

Major:	β^0/β^0 or β^+/β^+ or $\beta^+/$ E
Intermedia:	mild β^+/β^+ or $\beta^+/$ D
Minor or trait:	β/β^+ or β/β^0

α: 2 genes on Chr 16
α = globin; - = no globin

Hydrops fetalis:	Hb Barts (γ_4)	- - / - -
Intermedia:	Hb H disease (β_4)	- - /α -
Minor or trait:	α - /α - or - - /α α	
Carrier:	α - /α α	

Hereditary spherocytosis:
Commonest hereditary haemolytic anaemia in Whites, due to spectrin deficiency (auto dom)

3. Bone marrow hypoproduction

Chronic disease, anaemia of:
Cause: Infection, autoimmunity, neoplasia
Ix: Ferritin $\uparrow$, soluble transferrin receptor normal

Hereditary sideroblastic anaemia:
X-linked recessive; Rx: vitamin B6

Poisoning:
Lead:
PC: Abdominal pain, motor neuropathy, hypertension, renal tubular acidosis
O/E: Blue line along gums
Ix: 1. X-ray: epiphyseal sclerosis
     2. Film: basophilic stippling
     3. BM: ringed sideroblasts

Aluminium: e.g. renal dialysate

<u>Normocytic</u>
MCV 76–96 fl

1. Acute haemorrhage
Restoration of plasma volume (over hours) is quicker than RBC ↑ (over days)

2. Haemolytic anaemias
Hereditary:
- Haemoglobinopathy:
  Hb S (sickle cell);
  Unstable Hb or altered O_2 affinity
- Membrane defect:
  hereditary elliptocytosis
- Enzyme defect:
  G6PD or Pyruvate kinase deficiency

Acquired:
  Spleen enlargement
  PNH
  Liver disease
  Immune, e.g. SLE
  Toxin, e.g. MeDOPA
  Trauma to RBCs (MAHA)
  Infection, e.g. malaria
  Neoplasia, e.g. adenocarcinoma
  Graft, arterial

3. Bone marrow hypoproduction
Aplastic Anaemia: *A.P.L.A.S.T.I.C.*
  Acquired mutation, **P**NH, **L**eukaemia,
  Autoimmune, **S**niffing glue, **T**oxins,
  Infection, **C**ongenital
Bone marrow replacement:
- Myelofibrosis, myeloma, leukaemia
- Malignancy: osteoblastic metastases
- Infection: TB, *Brucella*, *Candida*
Chronic disease, anaemia of
  Path: Failure of iron recycling
  Cause: Infection, autoimmunity, malignancy
Diet: malnutrition, malabsorption (protein ↓)
Endocrine: Addison's, dysthyroidism

<u>Macrocytic</u>
MCV > 96 fl
M.A.R.M.A.L.A.D.E.

1. Megaloblastic
Vit B12 deficiency
  a) Intake ↓ : vegetarian, e.g. Hindus
  b) Absorption ↓ :
  - Stomach (IF and R protein synthesis):
      pernicious anaemia, gastrectomy
  - Duodenum, pancreas (R protein dissociation):
      coeliac, chronic pancreatitis
  - Small bowel (sequestration):
      bacterial overgrowth, e.g. blind-loop
  - Terminal ileum (absorption): Crohn's, TB
  c) Drugs: metformin, colchicine, N_2O anaesthesia

Folate deficiency
  a) Intake ↓ :   'tea + biscuits' diet – elderly
  b) Absorption ↓ : coeliac, Crohn's, AIDS
  c) Drugs:
      DHFR inhibitor: methotrexate, trimethoprim
      Dihydropteroate synthetase inhibitor:
          dapsone, sulphonamides, nitrofurantoin
      DNA antagonist: AZT, azathioprine, hydroxyurea
      + isoniazid, chloramphenicol
      + malabsorption: sulphasalazine, cholestyramine
      + inducers: phenytoin, phenobarbitone, OCP
  d) Demand ↑ :
  - Physiological: pregnancy, infancy
  - Neoplasia: myeloproliferative
  - Haemolysis, erythroderma, autoimmune

Other: orotic aciduria, transcobalamin-II deficiency

2. Alcoholic liver disease

3. Reticulocytosis
e.g. acute haemolysis or BM replacement

4. Myelodysplasia / Myeloma

5. Aplastic anaemia
chronic idiopathic, or Fanconi's

6. Leukaemia, acute: erythroleukaemia

7. Disordered iron ↑
haemochromatosis, or haemosiderosis

8. Endocrine: hypothyroidism

Bone Marrow Failure

The following cause either a peripheral blood pancytopenia or anaemia due to failure of haematopoeisis.

Normocytic anaemia

A.B.C.D.E.F.

Aplastic Anaemia
A.P.L.A.S.T.I.C. – **see opposite**
Ix: normocytic anaemia, but may be macrocytic in long-standing disease

Bone marrow replacement (myelophthisis)
- Malignancy: haematological – myelofibrosis, myeloma, leukaemia
- Malignancy: osteoblastic metastases
- Infection: TB, *Brucella, Coxiella, Legionella*
- Sarcoidosis

Chronic disease, anaemia of
Path: Failure of Fe recycling
Cause: Infection, autoimmunity, malignancy
Ix: Micro- or normocytic anaemia

Diet
- Malnutrition inc. anorexia nervosa
- Malabsorption (protein ↓)

Endocrine
- Addison's
- Dysthyroidism
- Hypogonadism

Failure
- Renal
- Liver

Megaloblastic anaemia

Folate or Vit B12 deficiency

Aplastic Anaemia

Def   Haematopoeitic stem-cell failure, in presence of bone marrow hypocellularity, leading to peripheral blood pancytopenia.

Causes

A.P.L.A.S.T.I.C.

Acquired mutation: telomerase reverse transcriptase (*TERT*)
- accounts for large proportion of 'idiopathic' cases

PNH (paroxysmal nocturnal haemoglobinuria) – recovery phase:
    Ix: Acid lysis test (Ham test); flow cytometry for GPI-linked proteins

Pregnancy

Leukaemia, acute; lymphoma or thymoma; myelodyplasia:
    Ix: Bone marrow shows abnormal cells; cytogenetic abnormalities

Autoimmune
- accounts for large proportion of 'idiopathic' cases
- SLE, eosinophilic fasciitis

Sniffing glue; ecstasy; pesticides (DDT)

Toxins:
    1. Dose-dependent: chemotherapy, methotrexate, chloramphenicol
    2. Idiosyncratic: chloramphenicol (1/50,000), tetracycline, sulphonamide
    3. Hypersensitivity: any drug after repeated exposure
    4. Radiation

Infection – viruses:
    1. Parvovirus B19 in hereditary haemolytic anaemia: causes pure red cell aplasia
    2. HAV, HBV, HCV (3 weeks - 8 months after)
    3. EBV, HIV

Congenital:
    1. Fanconi's anaemia (AR):
        Path: Chromosomal breaks and gaps due to failure of DNA repair mechanism
        PC: Skeletal hypoplasia; pigmented; heart or renal anomalies; AML
        Ix: Chromosome studies of peripheral blood cells
    2. Dyskeratosis congenita (AD):
        Path: Premature ageing due to *TERT* mutation (no chromosome breaks or gaps)
        PC: Dementia, ectodermal dysplasia (alopecia, nail dystrophy)
    3. Diamond–Blackfan syndrome – pure red-cell aplasia:
        PC: Short stature, sunken nasal bridge; hepatosplenomegaly and CCF (iron overload)

Rx

1. Supportive care:
    a) Packed cell transfusions using leucocyte-depleted products or HLA-matched platelets
    b) Antibiotics, antifungals
2. Medical:
    a) Androgens
    b) Anti-thymocyte globulin (☠: Serum–sickness) ± cyclosporin
3. Bone marrow transplantation – allogeneic

Haemolytic Anaemia – Causes

Hereditary

1. Haemoglobinopathy

Microcytic: thalassaemia: ineffective erythropoiesis and haemolysis
Normocytic: a) HbS (sickle cell), C, D, E, M
        b) Unstable Hb: Hb Koln, Hb Zurich
        c) Altered O_2 affinity: Hb Yakima ($\uparrow$), Hb Seattle ($\downarrow$)

2. Membrane Defect

Microcytic: Hereditary spherocytosis (autosomal dominant)
        commonest hereditary haemolytic anaemia in whites
        Path: Spectrin deficiency: spectrin is main structural unit of RBC membrane

Normocytic: a) Hereditary elliptocytosis (autosomal dominant):
        Path: Spectrin dimer or spectrin – ankyrin mutation $\Rightarrow$ RBCs are squashed in capillaries
        b) Hereditary stomatocytosis (autosomal dominant):
        Path: Na and K permeability $\uparrow$ $\Rightarrow$ swollen or dehydrated RBCs

3. Enzyme Defect

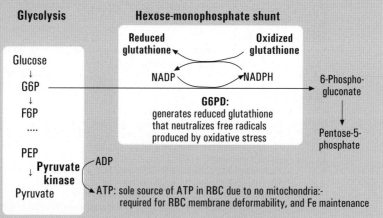

Normocytic:
   a) Glucose-6-phosphate dehydrogenase (G6PD) deficiency (X-linked)
      • Common in pts from Mediterranean (severe) and Africa
      • PC: Haemolytic crises and shock precipitated by oxidative stresses,
          viz. acute illness (e.g. infection, DKA); foods and drugs: *B.A.N. M.E.*
            Broad beans (fava); **A**spirin (high dose); **N**itrofurantoin, sulphonamides, ciprofloxacin;
          Malaria (chloroquine, primaquine); dapsone; **E**xtra: probenecid, soluble Vit K
   b) Pyruvate kinase deficiency (autosomal recessive)

N.B. HbS, elliptocytosis, G6PD heterozygotes provide malaria protection

<u>Acquired</u>

S.P.L.I.T.T.I.N.G.

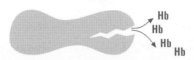

Spleen: hypersplenism – esp. due to to portal hypertension or infection

Paroxysmal nocturnal haemoglobinuria (PNH):
Path: clonal inactivatn of *pig-A* gene on X Chr ⇒ glycosyl phosphatidyl inositol (GPI) anchor deficiency
⇒ loss of RBC surface membrane complement inhibitors (e.g. decay accelerating factor)
⇒ haemolysis and platelet aggregation (arterial and venous thrombosis)

Liver:
a) Alcoholic cirrhosis: ↑RBC cholesterol: phospholipid ratio ⇒↓ membrane deformation (spur cells)
b) Wilson's disease: direct effect of copper

Immune, auto-: categorized according to optimal temperature at which Ig-RBC reaction
takes place:
a) Warm: *T.A.N.*:
Toxins: MeDOPA, L-DOPA (+apomorphine), high-dose penicillin, quinidine, sulphonamides
Autoimmune: SLE, Evans' syndrome (ITP + AIHA)
Neoplasia: Non-Hodgkin's lymphoma, CLL
b) Cold: *N.I.P.py*:
Neoplasia: benign monoclonal gammopathy, lymphoma
Infection: EBV, mycoplasma
Paroxysmal cold haemoglobinuria: primary autoimmune, measles, VZV, 3° syphilis
c) Other:
• Transfusion reaction (alloimmune)
• Rhesus disease of newborn (Rh –ve mother; Rh +ve neonate: isoimmune)
• Vasculitis, scleroderma: causes MAHA

Trauma to RBCs: micro-angiopathic haemolytic anaemia (MAHA) ⇒ RBC fragments
• Malignant hypertension, pre-eclampsia
• March haematuria (but no RBC fragments)

Thrombotic thrombocytopenic purpura (TTP):
MAHA: pregnancy, autoimmune, AIDS, *E. coli* (haemolytic uraemic syndrome)

Toxins:
• MAHA: benzene, arsenicals, chlorate, spider or animal bites
• Other: warm autoimmune haemolysis

Infection
• MAHA: menigococcaemia or pneumococcal septicaemia
• Other: i) Malaria (Blackwater fever); ii) *Bartonella* (Oroya fever);
iii) Leptospirosis (Weil's disease); iv) *Clostridium welchii*

Neoplasia: MAHA: mucinous adenocarcinoma

Glomerulonephritis or renal graft rejection: MAHA

Grafts: MAHA: prosthetic valves (esp. aortic) or arterial grafts

Haemolytic Anaemia – Clinical

<u>PC</u>   *A.B.C.D.*

1. **A**naemia
   due to haemolysis or associated aplastic crises (e.g. sickle cell disease, PNH)
2. **B**reakdown products:
   - Jaundice
   - Pigment stones
   - Haemoglobinuria
3. **C**ompensation:
   - Hepatosplenomegaly from erythropoietic hyperplasia
     (may also be *cause* of haemolysis if there is *hypersplenism*)
   - Medullary hyperplasia, e.g. bossed skull, prominent maxillae in children
   - Iron overload (p. 160) or *Yersinia* infections – due to many transfusions
4. **D**isease-specific:
   - Sickle cell: leg ulcers, dactylitis, chest crisis
   - PNH: venous or arterial thrombosis, pancytopenia due to myelofibrosis
   - Cold autoimmune: acrocyanosis; haemolysis on drinking cold liquids

<u>Ix - general</u>

1. Haematology
a) Reticulocytes > 5%
b) MCV:
   - Normocytic: most chronic haemolytic anaemias
   - Microcytic: thalassaemia, spherocytes, secondary iron loss with chronic haemolysis
   - Macrocytic: acute haemolysis due to reticulocytosis
c) Film
   - Polychromasia, due to immature cells
   - Specific red cell forms: spherocytes ($\downarrow$ surface area / volume); target cells ($\uparrow$ s.a. / vol.)
d) Bone marrow: erythroid hyperplasia

2. Chemistry:
a) LFTs:
   - Unconjugated BR $\uparrow$ ('acholuric' - i.e. absent in urine)
   - AST $\uparrow$ (but ALT normal)
   - LDH $\uparrow$ (esp. intravascular haemolysis)
b) α_2-haptoglobin $\downarrow$: binds to Hb and is cleared via reticuloendothelial system
c) Plasma haemoglobin (esp. intravascular haemolysis)

3. Urine:
a) Haemosiderin (intravascular haemolysis)
b) Haemoglobin (severe intravascular haemolysis)

Ix – specific

Hereditary

1. Haemoglobinopathy:

   Thalassaemia: MCV, HbA2, genetics
   Sickle cell: Film: drapanocytes, serum electrophoresis

2. Membrane defect:

   Hereditary spherocytosis: Film: microspherocytes (MCHC↑)
   osmotic fragility test; glucose incubation protects

3. Enzyme defect:

   G6PD deficiency: Film: blister, bite cells; Heinz bodies (oxidized Hb)
   enzyme assay (reticulocytes have normal activity)
   Pyruvate kinase deficiency: Film: poikilocytosis; prickle cells; enzyme assay

---

Acquired   *S.P.L.I.T*

Spleen: abdominal USS

Paroxysmal nocturnal haemoglobinuria (PNH):
   Complement-mediated lysis: acidify (Ham test) or add sucrose
   Flow cytometry for GPI-linked proteins, e.g. DAF, CD59

Liver: Film: spur cells

Immune, auto-:
   Warm AIHA:
      Direct Coombs' test: mix pt's RBCs + specific anti-IgG or anti-C3
         ⇒ agglutination with anti-IgG (penicillin, medopa), C3 (other drugs), or both (SLE)
      Indirect Coombs' test: pt's serum + normal RBCs + anti-IgG
   Cold AIHA:
      Direct Coombs' test:
         ⇒ agglutination with anti-C3 only, and at T < 30°C
      Cold agglutinin type:
         IgM anti-I (adult RBCs): monoclonal gammapathy, mycoplasma
         IgM anti-i (fetal RBCs): lymphoma, EBV
         IgG 'Donath–Landsteiner Ab': cold paroxysmal haemoglobinuria (do syphilis serology)

Trauma to RBCs: Film: schistocytes (RBC fragments)

Rx

PNH: 1. Steroids; 2. Androgens; anti-thymocyte globulin; 3. Bone marrow transplant
AIHA: 1. Immunosuppressants: steroids, azathioprine, cyclophosphamide, IVIg
      2. Splenectomy
      3. Blood transfusions, with prior adsorption of patient's 'panagglutinin antibodies',
         i.e. antibodies that cross-react with universal RBC antigens

Sickle Cell Anaemia

Def 1. Defective synthesis of β-globin chain due to point mutation: Glu $\longrightarrow$ hydrophobic Val
2. This results in less soluble HbS that tends to polymerize when deoxygenated

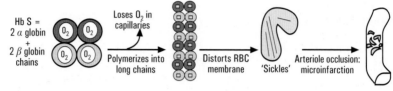

Hb S =
2 α globin
+
2 β globin chains

Loses O_2 in capillaries

Polymerizes into long chains

Distorts RBC membrane

'Sickles'

Arteriole occlusion: microinfarction

Epi Afro-Carribeans, Greeks

PC

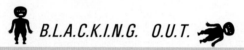 *B.L.A.C.K.I.N.G. O.U.T.*

Bone: 1. Pain : inc. dactylitis, finger shortening; Salmonella osteomyelitis
2. Avascular necrosis: femoral, humeral head, vertebral end-plates – growth retardation
3. Reshaping – frontal bossing in children due to widened diploe

Liver: pigmented gallstones

Anaemia: Hb 6–10 g/dl: not usually symptomatic

Crises: *S.H.A.R.P.* -
1. **S**equestration: spleen and liver venous occclusion – young children only
2. **H**aemolytic anaemia
3. **A**plastic anaemia: triggered by parvovirus or hepatitis infection
4. **R**espiratory ('chest crisis'): chest pain, SOB, fever, hypoxia:
due to pulmonary sickling leading to infarction, and pneumococcal infection
5. **P**ainful, vaso-occlusive: bones–joints–muscles, GIT, spleen – **commonest crisis**:
triggered by infection, dehydration, sympathetic activation

Kidney: 1. Medullary sickling: hyposthenuria (diabetes insipidus); renal tubular acidosis
2. Papillary necrosis: episodic haematuria, ureteric obstruction
3. Glomeruli: focal segmental glomerulosclerosis; membranous glomerulonephritis

Infection: due to hyposplenism following repeated splenic microinfarcts

Neuro: strokes: children – repeated infarcts; adults – haemorrhagic

Gonads: • Infertility; recurrent miscarriage; pre-eclampsia
• Priapism

Ophthalmological: proliferative retinopathy, vitreous haemorrhage, retinal detachment

Ulcers: leg, ankle – due to sluggish microcirculation

Thrombophilia: deep-vein thrombosis, pulmonary embolism, pulmonary hypertension,
coronary ischaemia (eventually cardiomyopathy)

Median age at death = 45 years, due to renal failure, pulmonary hypertension, cardiomyopathy

Ix

1. FBC: a) Hb 7–10 g/dl; MCV normal
      b) Reticulocytes ↑
      c) Neutrophils ↑

2. Film: a) Drapanocytes ('sickle cells')

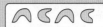

   b) Anisocytosis and poikilocytosis, inc. pencil cells

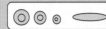

   c) Target cells

   d) Howell–Jolly bodies, due to hyposplenism

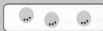

3. Electrophoresis
      a) Hb S/S (homozygote) or Hb S/A (trait)
      b) Hb F $(\alpha_2\gamma_2)$: ↑ 5–15%: higher levels correlate with less sickling and better prognosis

4. Sickling test:
      Reducing agent, e.g. Na metabisulphite, induces sickling by removing O_2

Rx

1. Prophylaxis
      a) Folic acid
      b) Penicillin V
      c) Vaccines: pneumococcal, *Haemophilus influenzae* b, meningitis A, C (in endemic areas)

2. Disease-modifying
      a) Hydroxyurea: ↑HbF levels, ↓neutrophils; ↓ no. of crises (☠: myelotoxic, carcinogenic)
      b) Exchange transfusions: given for pregnancy or frequent crises; recurrent CVA
      c) Allogeneic bone-marrow transplant

3. Sickle crisis
      a) O_2 and IV NaCl hydration – both decrease further sickling
      b) Opioids
      c) Antibiotics
      d) Exchange transfusion – reduces proportion of Hb S to < 30%

Variants

Sickle cell trait
Def: Heterozygotes i.e. HbSA = 40% HbS, 60% HbA (co-dominant expression)
PC: a) Normal Hb level; development; life expectancy
   b) Kidney: papillary sloughing – episodic painless haematuria, or ureteric obstruction (esp. boys)
   c) Crises: rare, but may be precipitated by high altitude; anaesthesia or pregnancy

Hb SC
Def: Hb C : Lysine amino-acid substitution at same position in β-globin chain as defect in Hb S
PC: Anaemia less severe (Hb 10–14 g/dl) but vaso-occlusion more likely as more RBCs, e.g. sea-fan retinopathy
Ix: Film: target cells prominent

Thalassaemia

<u>Def</u>   Heterogeneous group of genetic disorders of Hb synthesis that result in:
1. Ineffective erythropoeisis, due to decreased rate of globin synthesis
2. Haemolytic anaemia, due to production of abnormal RBCs (nucleated; abnormal globin)

HbA (96% adult Hb)	HbA2 (3% adult Hb)	HbF (fetal: 10 weeks + or 1% adult Hb)
2 α-globin chains	2 α-globin chains	2 α-globin chains

Haem molecule within each chain

| 2 β-globin chains | 2 δ-globin chains | 2 γ-globin chains |

<u>Epi</u>   Mediterranean Basin – N + W Africa; Middle East; SE Asia; also occurs sporadically

Classification schemes

1. Globin chain mutation:
     α : 2 genes on chromosome 16 (i.e. 4 genes per individual)
     β : 1 gene on chromosome 11 (i.e. 2 genes per individual)
2. Clinical severity:

Major:	Hb < 7 g/dl:	requires regular transfusion
Intermedia:	Hb 7–10 g/dl:	no regular transfusion; splenomegaly
Minor ('Trait'):	Hb 10–14 g/dl	
Carrier:	anaemia only occurs at high-altitudes or with general anaesthesia	

Types

α -Thalassaemia

No. of mutated genes		Name	Clinical
4	$- -\,/\,- -$	Hb Barts γ_4	'Hydrops fetalis': death in utero
3	$\alpha\,-\,/\,- -$	Hb H β_4	Thalassaemia Intermedia
2	$\alpha\,-\,/\,\alpha\,-$	Thalassaemia minor	Mild anaemia or asymptomatic
	$\alpha\alpha\,/\,- -$		
1	$\alpha\alpha\,/\,\alpha\,-$	Carrier	Asymptomatic

Key: α = normal gene;   - = mutated gene; γ_4 or β_4 represent alternative Hb type produced

β -Thalassaemia

No. of mutated genes		Name	Clinical
2	$\beta^0\,/\,\beta^0$	Thalassaemia major	Regular transfusions
	$\beta^+\,/\,\beta^+$ (different mutations)		
2	$\beta^+\,/\,\beta^+$ (mild mutations)	Thalassaemia intermedia	No regular transfusions
1	$\beta^0\,/\,\beta$		
	$\delta\beta$ fusion gene (Hb Lepore)		
1	$\beta^0\,/\,\beta$	Thalassaemia minor	
	$\beta^+\,/\,\beta$		

Key: β^0 = no β globin; β^+ = ↓ β globin (over 100 mutations recognized)

PC

Haemolytic anaemia from 3–6 months old, when fetal Hb → adult Hb
1. Anaemia: fatigue, pallor; leg ulcers; congestive cardiac failure
2. Haemolysis: mild jaundice (unconjugated bilirubin ↑); gallstones

Compensation of anaemia

1. Bones – medullary hyperplasia:
    a) Facies: bossed skull (X-ray = 'hair on end') /
           enlarged maxilla ('chipmunk facies')
    b) Pathological fractures, growth retardation:
           due to cortical thinning

2. Extramedullary haemopoeisis:
    hepatosplenomegaly, gingival hyperplasia

Compensation   **Therapy**

Therapy complications

1. Fe overload (see p. 160):
    2° to repeated transfusions and ↑ GIT uptake
    (hence also present in thalassaemia intermedia):
    e.g. myocardial damage, diabetes, cirrhosis → death in 30s!!

2. Infections:
    a) *Yersinia enterocolitica*: due to Fe overload and chelation therapy
    b) Capsulated bacteria, due to splenectomy
    c) Blood transfusion-associated

Ix

1. FBC: a) Anaemia – microcytosis, hypochromia:
        Hb < 7: major (β-thal only) ; Hb 7–11: intermedia (α- or β-thal); Hb 11–14: minor (α or β-thal)
     b) Red cell count ↑
     c) Reticulocytes – normal, ↓ or ↑ ; normal in thalassaemia intermedia
2. Film: a) 'Heinz bodies' due to oxidized Hb;
        'golf ball cells' due to α_4 or β_4 precipitation in β- or α-thalassaemia respectively
     b) Nucleated RBCs: normoblasts, reflect increased marrow turnover;
       nuclear remnants – Howell–Jolly bodies; basophilic stippling
     c) Other: target cells (haemolysis); siderocytes (iron inclusions); poikilocytes (α-thalassaemia)
3. Electrophoresis:
     a) β-thal major: Hb F ↑↑ (30–60%); Hb A absent!, Hb A2 variable
     b) β-thal intermedia: Hb F ↑
     c) β-thal minor: Hb F low; Hb A present, Hb A2 > 3.5%
     d) α-thal intermedia: **Hb H H**urries along, i.e. fast-moving band
4. Globin-chain synthesis studies or PCR or restriction-enzyme analyses:
        for family screening / prenatal diagnosis via cord blood or amniocentesis

Rx

1. Blood transfusions plus desferrioxamine (Fe chelator)
2. Folic acid: due to high RBC turnover predisposing to deficiency;
   Vit C (ascorbic acid) decreases Fe absorption
3. Splenectomy: decreases haemolysis, but wait until > 6 years old to reduce risk of infection
4. Bone marrow transplant

Folate and Vitamin B12 Metabolism

Structure

Tetrahydro**folate** Polyglutamate

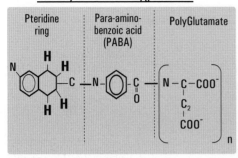

Pteridine ring | Para-amino-benzoic acid (PABA) | PolyGlutamate

Vitamin B12 (Cobalamin)

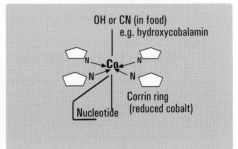

OH or CN (in food) e.g. hydroxycobalamin

Corrin ring (reduced cobalt)

Nucleotide

Absorption

Folic Acid

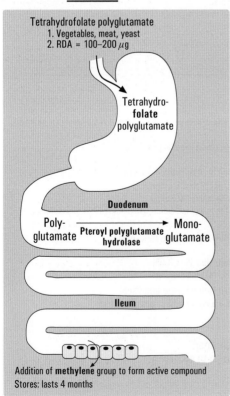

Tetrahydrofolate polyglutamate
1. Vegetables, meat, yeast
2. RDA = 100–200 μg

Tetrahydro-**folate** polyglutamate

Duodenum

Poly-glutamate → **Pteroyl polyglutamate hydrolase** → Mono-glutamate

Ileum

Addition of **methylene** group to form active compound
Stores: lasts 4 months

Vitamin B12

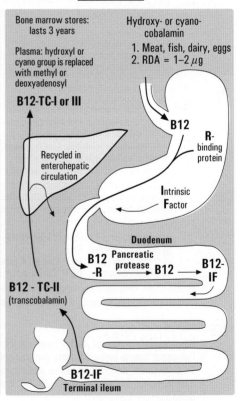

Bone marrow stores: lasts 3 years

Plasma: hydroxyl or cyano group is replaced with methyl or deoxyadenosyl

B12-TC-I or III

Hydroxy- or cyano-cobalamin
1. Meat, fish, dairy, eggs
2. RDA = 1–2 μg

B12

R-binding protein

Intrinsic **F**actor

Recycled in enterohepatic circulation

Duodenum

B12 -R → **Pancreatic protease** → B12 → B12-IF

B12 - TC-II (transcobalamin)

B12-IF
Terminal ileum

Metabolism

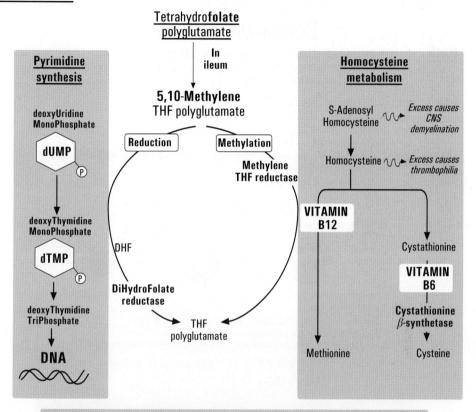

Other Metabolic Interactions

1. Folate: purine synthesis, amino-acid interconversions e.g. serine $\Rightarrow$ glycine
2. Vit B12 : methylmalonyl CoA $\Rightarrow$ SuccinylCoA

N.B. Deficiencies of DHF reductase, methylene THF reductase, or cystathionine β synthetase are responsible for homocystinuria

Ix

1. Deoxyuridine suppression test (folate or B12 deficiency):
    i) Administer ^{3}H-thymidine to dividing bone marrow precursors: $\longrightarrow$ measure DNA radioactivity
    ii) Remeasure DNA radioactivity after adding deoxyuridine (gets converted to dUMP)
    iii) Result: Normally, dUMP is converted to dTMP, and competes with ^{3}H-thymidine for incorporation into DNA

2. Urinary methylmalonyl CoA ↑ (B12 deficiency only)
3. Plasma homocysteine ↑ (folate or B12 deficiency)

Megaloblastic Anaemia

Def   1. Macrocytic anaemia
2. Erythroblasts have large, immature nuclei, reflecting diffuse, open chromatin structure
3. Due to defective DNA synthesis, esp. from Vit B12 or Folate deficiency (see p. 423)

Pernicious Anaemia

Path   1. Autoantibodies directed against parietal cells (95%) and intrinsic factor (70%)
2. Chronic atrophic gastritis (plasma cell infiltrate of gastric lamina propria) ⇒
    achlorhydria and gastric carcinoma

Epi   Inc: Most common cause of B12 deficiency in West
Age: Middle-aged or elderly
Sex: Females > males
Geo: North Europeans
Pre: 1. **A**utoimmunity, esp.vitiligo, thyroid or parathyroid disease, Addison's
       2. **A**gammaglobulinaemia
       3. **A**3 (HLA) or **A** blood group

PC

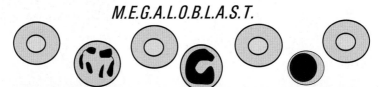

M.E.G.A.L.O.B.L.A.S.T.

Mucosal atrophy:
  1. Glossitis: beefy red, sore, smooth tongue, due to papillae loss
  2. Angular cheilitis – due to decreased epithelial turnover
  3. Impaired healing, including fractures – due to decreased osteoblast activity

Eyes – blue, **E**arly greying of hair, and wide-cheek bones (associations)

GIT: indigestion, episodic diarrhoea

Anorexia

Loss of weight

Organomegaly: splenomegaly

Bone marrow failure:
  1. Anaemia – pallor, cardiac failure
  2. Neutropenia – immunocompromise
  3. Thrombocytopenia – purpura

LFTs: jaundiced (lemon tinge), LDH ↑ due to haemolysis of abnormal RBCs

Autoimmune: vitiligo, infertility, Addison's, DM

Subacute combined degeneration of cord:
  Path: Posterior column degeneration (vibration / JPS ↓, Rombergism, Charcot joints)
  PC: Sensory disturbance in feet; gait ataxia; Charcot joints; extensor plantars, areflexia
     + dementia, optic atrophy, peripheral neuropathy

Tumour: gastric carcinoma in 4%

   N.B. Folate deficiency causes mucositis, anaemia, mild neuropathy

Ix **1. FBC**

RBCs	WBCs	Platelets
1. Film: • Oval, normochromic macrocytes • Megaloblasts (nucleated RBCs) • Polychromasia; basophilic stippling; Howell–Jolly bodies 2. Reticulocytes ↓ **N.B. neuropathy may occur even in presence of normal Hb and MCV**	1. Count: neutrophils ↓ 2. Film: hypersegmented neutrophils (≥ 6 lobes)	1. Count: ↓ 2. Film: abnormal appearance

2. Bone marrow

RBCs	WBCs	Platelets
Erythroid hyperplasia: large fine, stippled nuclei with normal haemoglobin	Giant metamyelocytes, band forms	Atypical megakaryocytes, hypersegmented nuclei

3. Chemistry

a) Haematinics:
- Serum Vit B12 ↓ (itself causes serum folate ↑ and red cell folate ↓)
- Red Cell Folate ↓ (reflects active THF polyglutamate form, cf. serum folate levels)
- Serum Fe and ferritin: ↑ or ↓ if co-existent malabsorption

b) Special tests to confirm Vit B12 deficiency
- Urinary methylmalonyl CoA ↑ (B12 deficiency only)
- Deoxyuridine suppression test on bone marrow cells

c) LFT: unconjugated BR ↑; LDH ↑

4. Identify underlying cause of Vit B12 or folate deficiency

a) Schilling test
- Part 1: Give oral radiolabelled B12 (^{58}Co), and measure urinary radioactivity
- Part 2: Give oral intrinsic factor while repeating part 1 (corrects pernicious anaemia)
- Part 3: Give tetracycline + metronidazole for week prior to part 1 (corrects blind-loop syndrome)

b) Autoantibodies:
- Pernicious anaemia: anti-parietal cell (95%); anti-intrinsic factor (70% +ve)
- Coeliac disease: anti-endomysium ot anti-tissue transglutaminase

c) Endoscopy:
- OGD: Pernicious anaemia, coeliac disease
- Colonoscopy: Crohn's or other causes of terminal ileal disease

d) Malabsorption studies, e.g. faecal fat, ^{14}C-labelled–glycholate bile salt breath test

Rx **1.Vit B12**

Method: IM hydroxycobalamin 1 mg od or alt. days for 1–3 weeks, then 1 mg every 3 months
Monitor: i) Reticulocytes ↑; ii) Hb ↑1g/dl per week; iii) Platelets + WCC normalize in 10 days

2. Folic acid

Method: 5 mg od for 4 months:
must correct B12 deficiency first to avoid neuropathy!

Lymphadenopathy

B.I.G. G.L.A.N.D.S.

Blood disorders

1. Lymphoproliferative:
   Localized: Hodgkin's; high-grade non-Hodgkin's lymphoma – localized
   Generalized: low-grade non-Hodgkin's lymphoma; CLL; acute leukaemia
2. Waldenström's macroglobulinaemia
3. Rare – Angioimmunoblastic lymphadenopathy
   – Sinus histiocytosis (massive lymphadenopathy)

Infection

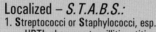

Localized – S.T.A.B.S.:
1. Streptococci or Staphylococci, esp.
   URTI: pharyngo-tonsillitis; otitis media; dental abscess
2. TB (scrofula) or
   Tropical: lymphogranuloma venereum (*Chlamydia trachomatis*), filariasis
3. Actinomyces
4. Bartonella henselae: cat-scratch fever
5. Syphilis, 1° (primary chancre)

Generalized:

1. Virus: EBV, CMV; hepatitis A–E; HIV; measles; rubella; pertussis
2. Bacterial: typhoid, septicaemia esp. with streptococci or staphylococci
3. Atypical bacteria: secondary syphilis, TB, atypical mycobacteria, *Brucella*
4. Toxoplasmosis
5. Tropical: schistosomiasis, *Echinoccocus*, leishmaniasis, trypanosomiasis

Granulomatous: sarcoidosis

Generalized: e.g. CLL, HIV, toxoplasmosis
Localized: e.g. Hodgkin's lymphoma, streptococci, TB, carcinoma
Autoimmune:

1. SLE, rheumatoid arthritis (Still's disease or Felty's syndrome)
2. Primary biliary cirrhosis
3. Graves' disease

Neoplasia:

1. Squamous cell carcinoma, e.g. head–neck, bronchial – localized
2. Adenocarcinoma, e.g. breast, gastric
3. Melanoma, malignant

Drugs: Phenytoin
Special:

1. Serum sickness, e.g. anti-lymphocyte globulin
2. Berylliosis (granulomatous)

<u>Splenomegaly</u>

B.I.G. S.P.A.A.N.

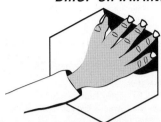

Blood disorders:
Neoplasia:
    1. Myeloproliferative: • Myelofibrosis, CML – massive
                               • PRV, ET   – medium
    2. Lymphoproliferative: • Prolymphocytic leukaemia ('hairy cell') – massive
                               • CLL, lymphoma, acute leukaemia
    3. Other: Waldenström's macroglobulinaemia (but not myeloma), histiocytosis X – (massive)

Functional hyperplasia – removal of defective RBCs, and extramedullary haematopoiesis:
    1. Inherited haemolytic anaemia: thalassaemia major or intermedia, hereditary spherocytosis
    2. Autoimmune: autoimmune haemolytic anaemia, ITP, pernicious anaemia, PNH
    3. Other: iron deficiency, aplastic anaemia

Infection:
    1. Virus: EBV, CMV; hepatitis A-E; HIV
    2. Bacterial: endocarditis, typhoid, septicaemia with splenic abscess
    3. Atypical bacteria: secondary syphilis, TB, atypical mycobacteria, *Brucella*
    4. Toxoplasmosis
    5. Tropical: chronic malaria (massive), schistosomiasis, *Echinoccocus*, leishmaniasis, trypanosomiasis

Granulomatous: sarcoid, primary biliary cirrhosis

Storage disease or other metabolic:
    1. Lipid storage disease: Gaucher's (massive splenomegaly), Niemann–Pick disease
    2. Hyperlipidaemia

Portal vein hypertension:
    1. Post-hepatic: Budd–Chiari syndrome, CCF
    2. Hepatic, esp. cirrhosis
    3. Pre-hepatic: splenic vein; portal vein thrombosis
    4. Pre-splenic: splenic artery aneurysm

Autoimmune:
    1. SLE, rheumatoid arthritis (Still's disease or Felty's syndrome)
    2. Graves' disease

Amyloid: AL or AA

Neoplasia:
    1. Renal cell carcinoma (Stauffer's syndrome)
    2. Metastases, esp. melanoma
    3. Cysts, inc. adult or infant polycystic kidney disease; hamartoma

Leucocytosis
I.N.N.A.T.E.

Neutrophilia

Infection:
1. Pyogenic
2. Atypical bacteria: Lyme, disseminated TB

Neoplasia:
1. Myeloproliferative:
   - CML, PRV, ET, myelofibrosis
   - AML, esp. M5 (Sweet's disease: acute febrile neutrophilic dermatosis)
2. Myelodysplasia: CMML
3. Solid tumours: carcinoma, melanoma, lymphoma

Necrosis:
1. Myocardial infarction (or even SVT)
2. Pulmonary, or bowel, infarction
3. Burns

Autoimmune:
1. Connective tissue disease, esp. myositis, rheumatoid arthritis (or acute gout)
2. Vasculitis, esp. PAN, PMR, Behçet's

Toxins:
1. Glucocorticoids (inhibits tissue margination); growth factors (G-CSF, GM-CSF)
2. Digoxin; adrenaline (including stress, excitement, vigorous exercise)
3. Poisoning: CO, mercury, lithium

Endocrine:
1. Diabetic ketoacidosis (or other acidotic states, e.g. uraemia)
2. Pregnancy

Extra:
1. Acute haemorrhage or haemolysis
2. Genetic: leucocyte adhesion deficiency
   = integrin β chain or selectin ligand deficiency
3. Hyposplenism, inc. splenectomy – also causes eosinophilia

Eosinophilia

Infection:
1. Helminths: nematodes, cestodes, trematodes (also scabies)
2. Bacteria: rebound post-sepsis; Lyme
3. Aspergillosis

Neoplasia:
1. Lymphoma: Hodgkin's or T-cell non-Hodgkin's (secretes IL-5)
2. AML – eosinophilic leukaemia
3. CML – hypereosinophilic syndrome

Nephrology:
1. Cholesterol emboli – acute renal failure
2. Allergic tubulointerstitial nephritis

Autoimmune:
1. Atopy: food or drug allergy, eczema, asthma
2. Vasculitis, esp. PAN; rheumatoid arthritis
3. Addison's

Toxins:
1. L-tryptophan
2. Poisoning: Spanish toxic oil, nickel – cause eosinophilic-myalgia syndrome

Eosinophilia - myofasciitis: PC: Pain, swelling in both arms; erythema; carpal tunnel syndrome

Extra:
1. Sarcoid
2. Splenectomy

Lymphocytosis

Infection:
1. Viruses: EBV, CMV, hepatitis A–E (all may cause atypical lymphocytes), influenza, mumps, rubella
2. Bacteria: post-sepsis, endocarditis, typhoid, pertussis
3. Atypical bacteria: TB, secondary syphilis, *Brucella*
4. Toxoplasmosis

Neoplasia:
1. Lymphoproliferative:
   - CLL, ALL
   - Non-Hodgkin's lymphoma
2. Myeloma
3. Carcinoma

Autoimmune: Organ-based: Graves' disease, myasthenia gravis, hypopituitarism

Monocytosis

Infection:
1. Viruses: EBV
2. Bacteria: septicaemia, endocarditis, typhoid, listeria
3. Atypical bacteria: TB, secondary syphilis, *Brucella*
4. Tropical: rickettsia, malaria, leishmaniasis, trypanosomiasis

Neoplasia:
1. Hodgkin's lymphoma
2. AML – monocytic variant
3. Myelodysplasia

<u>Acute Leukaemia - 1</u>

<u>Def</u>
1. Clonal proliferation of single abnormal progenitor, myeloid or lymphoid stem cell
2. Bone marrow infiltration > 30% with blast cells (usually > 50% at presentation)
3. Effects: a) Pancytopenia: normal haematopoiesis is 'crowded out' and actively inhibited
   b) Extreme leucocytosis: spill-over of long-living immature cells into blood

<u>Epi</u>
Inc: 5 / 100,000 p.a. : most common childhood malignancy; 5% adult malignancies
Age: Commoner in children and elderly

<u>Causes</u>   *T.R.I.G.G.ER.*

Toxins: alkylating agents, esp. with radiotherapy; smoking; benzene, esp. AML
Radiation: atom bomb survivors – AML peaked at 5–7 years; or in children of exposed fathers
Infection: HTLV-I virus – adult T-cell leukaemia/lymphoma (West Indies, Japan)
Genetic: • Chromosomal instability: Down's syn.(ALL or AML), ataxia telangiectasia, Fanconi's anaemia
         • Translocations: AML-M3 : t(15; 17) : PML–RARA (promyelocytic leukaemia – retinoic acid receptor)
Genetic: haematological transformation from: myeloproliferative disease, esp. CML, PRV,
         myelofibrosis; myelodysplasia
ER: electromagnetic radiation – pylons

<u>PC</u>

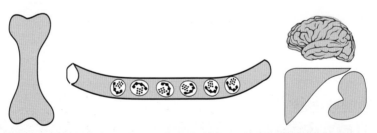

1. Bone pain: esp. children
2. Bone marrow failure:
a) Anaemia: fatigue, LOW
b) Infections:
   • Bacterial: PUO, mouth ulcers,
              Strep. pneumoniae
   • Viral: HSV, VZV, CMV, measles
   • Other: *Candida*, aspergillosis
c) Thrombocytopenia:
   purpura, excess bleeding time,
   cerebral or retinal bleeds
d) Clotting:
   DIC with AML-M3
   (procoagulant release
   from granules with chemoRx)

Hyperviscosity:
• Fatigue, confusion
• Seizures
• Stroke, blindness

Organ infiltration:

a) **Hepatosplenomegaly,**
   lymphadenopathy,
   sternal pain

b) **Meninges and eyes**
   (esp. ALL, AML-M4, M5):
   • Headaches, N+V
   • Papilloedema, CNPs
   • Fluid in anterior chamber

c) **Other:**
   • Spinal dura (AML-M2)
   • Gum hyperplasia, green skin,
     skin nodules (AML-M4, M5)
   • Renal failure, K+ ↑
     (AML-M5 due to lysozyme
     release from monocytes)

Ix

Blood: 1. FBC: a) Normochromic, normocytic anaemia
b) WBC: often 100–300 x 10⁹/l, esp.T-ALL and less differentiated AML,
but can be normal, or even low ('aleukaemic leukaemia')
c) Platelet: ↓ (esp. AML; M3 also causes DIC)

2. U+E: uric acid ↑; LDH ↑; calcium ↑

Radiology:
1. CXR: a) Infiltrates: due to leukaemia, infection or Rx, e.g. WBC transfusion, busulphan
b) Mediastinal lymph nodes, thymic enlargement
2. Bone: lytic lesions (childhood ALL)
3. Brain MRI: mass lesion: infiltrate or *Toxoplasma*; meningeal enhancement

Special: 1. Bone marrow aspirate and biopsy: blast cell proportion:
30% = acute leukaemia
5-30% = myelodysplasia
< 5% = remission (must also have normal FBC, no peripheral blasts or symptoms)
< 0.001% = minimal residual disease: only identifiable with immune or genetic markers
2. Lumbar puncture: ICP ↑ or blast cells

Typing

Progenitor stem cell — CD34

Myeloid stem cell

1. CD33
2. Persistent germ-line configuration
of VDJ genes: not involved in myeloid cells

Lymphoid stem cell

1. CD10
2. Terminal deoxynucleotidyl transferase
(TdT) +ve: adds extra bases to DJ genes

Acute Myeloid Leukaemia (AML)

M0: undifferentiated
M1,2: myeloblastic
M3: promyelocytic: t(15;17) translocation
M4,5: monocytic: commonest
extramedullary disease
M6: erythroleukaemia: elderly, MCV ↑
M7: megakaryocytic: bone marrow fibrosis

Myeloperoxidase +ve;   Auer rods   Budding
Sudan black +ve   (M7)
granules

Acute Lymphoblastic Leukaemia (ALL)

Pre B-ALL or T-ALL:
L1: small, uniform blasts,
large nucleus:cytoplasm ratios
L2: large, heterogeneous blasts,
small nucleus:cytoplasm ratios

B-ALL (leukaemic phase of lymphoma)
L3: blasts with vacuolated, basophilic
cytoplasm; t(8;14) translocation

Pre B-ALL and T-ALL can be differentiated by:
1. CD type:
B – CD19, 22; T – CD7
2. VDJ gene clonal rearrangement pattern:
B – Ig; T – T-cell receptor

Acute Leukaemia - 2

Rx

1. Bone marrow failure

RBCs	WBCs	Platelets
Packed RBC transfusions • If Hb < 9 g/dl • Use CMV –ve, if pt is seronegative • Use leucodepleted blood to avoid alloimmunization • ☠: Hyperviscosity (thrombi form in brain, lung, heart if WCC > 100 x10⁹); antibody formation with multiple transfusions	**Physical:** source isolate pasteurized food **Prophylaxis:** nystatin mouthwash, cotrimoxazole (PCP), VZV or measles Ig if exposed **Febrile neutropenic episode:** Broad-spectrum, e.g. piperacillin, tazobactam, gentamicin; fluconazole; aciclovir **Granulocyte transfusion or GM-CSF or G-CSF**	**Physical** avoid IM injections **Platelet concentrates** • If Plts < 20 x 10⁹/l • ☠: Antibody formation with multiple transfusions **Tranexamic acid** = anti-fibrinolytic **Leucopharesis:** if hyperviscosity

2. Chemotherapy ± radiotherapy

Induction:
  AML: *Ca.D.Et.*   (cytarabine, daunorubicin, etoposide)
  ALL: *D.O.P.A.*   (daunorubicin, vincristine (Oncovin), prednisolone, asparaginase)
• Consolidation therapy is essential for AML (repeat cycles of cytarabine), or
• Maintenance therapy required for ALL (out-patient Rx)

Sanctuary sites:
  a) CNS: Indications: ALL, M4, M5 during remission
        Rx: Systemic and intrathecal methotrexate + cranial irradiation (not children or elderly)
  b) Testes: irradiate

Alternative chemotherapy:
  a) All-*trans*-retinoic acid used in promyelocytic AML (M3):
        induces differentiation of promyelocyte clone, but resistance may develop
  b) Gemtuzumab (anti-CD33 monoclonal antibodies) used in relapsing AML
        Abs are linked to calicheamicin (cytotoxic), but resistance common
  c) Multi-drug resistance inhibitor, e.g. cyclosporin A: experimental

Supportive:
  a) Venous access: Hickman line insertion – tunnelled subcutaneously into SVC
  b) Nausea: metoclopramide, ondansetron, nabilone, steroids
  c) Gout: prophylactic allopurinol, hydration (tumour lysis syndrome)
  d) DIC: FFP and heparin used in M3 before chemotherapy

3. Bone marrow transplant

Indications: 1. Remission from AML with high-risk karyotype, or 1st relapse (in AML)
           2. Age < 60, and match present (for allogeneic)

Allogeneic grafting is associated with more adverse events (10% mortality rate, cf. 5% with autologous), due to graft-versus-host disease and graft rejection (inadequate chemoRx + irradiation), but is also more effective due to a graft-versus-leukaemia effect. Autologous transplants may also suffer from contamination with residual leukaemic cells. Both risk infection, esp. CMV.

Prognosis

Poor prognostic factors

General	Age: extremes: AML > 60 yrs ALL < 2 yrs or > 10 yrs (partly due to intolerance of chemotherapy) Sex: boys – testes becomes sanctuary site in ALL PMH: preceding myelodysplasia, CML, alkylating chemotherapy (AML)
PC	Extramedullary involvement, esp. CNS and hepatosplenomegaly
Ix	WCC > 50 x 10^9/l Morphology: Undifferentiated or hybrid leukaemia AML: M 0,5,6,7 (M3 best) ALL: L 3 (L1 best) Immunophenotype: ALL: B-ALL (surface Ig), or null-ALL (i.e. no B-cell markers) – worst T-ALL and c-ALL (common to B + T cells) have best prognosis Genetics: ALL: 1. Philadelphia chromosome +ve (cf. CML where it's good!) 2. Hypodiploidy (cf. hyperdiploidy – best prognosis) AML: multiple complex chromosome abnormalities
Rx	Time to acheive remission > 4 weeks

	AML	**ALL**
5-year disease-free survival	**40%** (20% in > 60 yrs; 70% with M3)	**80%** (for children with c-ALL)
1st remission	**80%** (40% in > 60 yrs)	**90%** (for children)

Chronic Myeloid Leukaemia

Def
1. Clonal proliferation of the pluripotent stem cell, with predominance of granulocyte lineage at all stages of maturity
2. Medullary and extramedullary proliferation

Epi
Inc: 1/100,000 p.a.
Age: Middle age (40–60); childhood variants (e.g. juvenile Ph –)
Sex: M slightly > F
Geo: 1. Factory workers – benzene; 2. Nuclear fallout – Hiroshima, Nagasaki, Chernobyl
Aet: 1. 95% exhibit the 'Philadelphia (Ph) chromosome' = t(9;22), found in all dividing progeny

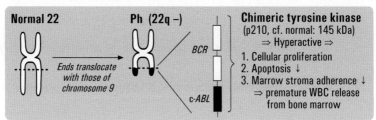

Normal 22	Ph (22q –)	Chimeric tyrosine kinase
		(p210, cf. normal: 145 kDa) ⇒ Hyperactive ⇒
	BCR	1. Cellular proliferation
Ends translocate with those of chromosome 9		2. Apoptosis ↓
		3. Marrow stroma adherence ↓
	c-ABL	⇒ premature WBC release from bone marrow

The Ph chromosome found in ALL has a short BCR component, resulting in a poorer prognosis

2. 5% are Ph– (worse prognosis)
    a) *BCR*–c-*ABL* rearrangement present, e.g. chronic monomyelocytic leukaemia
    b) *BCR*–c-*ABL* rearrangement not present, e.g. *RAS* gene mutation: poor prognosis

PC

Can be S.A.V.A.G.E.

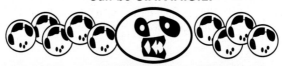

Splenomegaly, ± hepatomegaly:
    1. Left-upper quadrant pain or dragging sensation; dyspepsia; early satiety
    2. Pleuritic, L shoulder pain, pleural rub – splenic infarction

Anaemia / infections / purpura

Viscosity, hyper- (WCC > 500 x 10⁹/l):
    1. Neurological: headache, confusion, TIA–CVA, retinopathy (blurred vision)
    2. Other: Pulmonary infiltrates, skin nodules, priapism

Accelerated phase ⇒ **A**cute leukaemia
    1. Accelerated phase: pancytopenia, new cytogenetic abnormalities
        (cumulative transformation rate = 80%; annual rate = 20%)
    2. Acute leukaemia: > 30% blast cells in bone marrow
        80% develop AML (80% mortality); 20% develop ALL (50% mortality)
        (cumulative transformation rate = 70%; median occurence = 4 years)
    3. Myelofibrosis: alternative outcome following accelerated phase

Gout: give allopurinol with chemotherapy

Extra: 1. 'B symptoms': fever, night sweats, weight loss, anorexia; 2. Bone pain

Ix   **1. FBC**

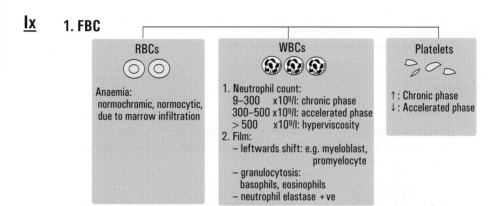

RBCs	WBCs	Platelets

Anaemia:
normochromic, normocytic,
due to marrow infiltration
	1. Neutrophil count:
	  9–300 x10⁹/l: chronic phase
	  300–500 x10⁹/l: accelerated phase
	  > 500 x10⁹/l: hyperviscosity
	2. Film:
	  – leftwards shift: e.g. myeloblast,
	                         promyelocyte
	  – granulocytosis:
	    basophils, eosinophils
	  – neutrophil elastase +ve
		↑: Chronic phase
		↓: Accelerated phase

2. Other bloods a) Neutrophil alkaline phosphatase ↓ (cf. myeloproliferative disease, infection)
                     b) Alkaline phosphatase ↑
                     c) Vit B12 levels and Vit B12 binding capacity ↑; uric acid ↑

3. Bone marrow biopsy: hypercellularity of all haematopoietic lineages, esp. granulocyte precursors

Rx   **1. Supportive**

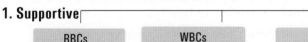

RBCs	WBCs	Platelets
RBC transfusion	Leucapharesis: – for hyperviscocity	Splenectomy or splenic irradiation: for spleen pain or pancytopenia

2. Medical:
  a) Imatinib (oral tyrosine kinase inhibitor):
      • Blocks ATP-binding site on p210 BCR–ABL fusion protein
      • ☠ : Fluid retention, nausea, cramps
  b) Interferon-α: direct anti-proliferative effect, RNase ↑, natural killer cells ↑; ☠ : lethargy, weight loss
  c) Cytotoxics: busulphan (☠ : pulmonary fibrosis), hydroxyurea (better at ↓ing platelets)
3. Allogeneic stem-cell transplant
      curative in 60%, providing < 65 yrs old, compatible donor, and early chronic phase

Prognosis   Median survival = 4 years; death due to acute leukaemia or bleeding

Poor prognostic factors

1. Ph –ve, e.g. elderly men, juvenile, CMML
2. Splenomegaly
3. FBC: Hb: persistent anaemia
       WBC: peripheral blasts; basophils; eosinophils
       Plt: thrombocytopenia or thrombocytosis

Polycythaemia

Def   Polycythaemia: increased number of RBCs, WBCs and platelets
Erythrocytosis: increased number of RBCs only

Causes

Relative

1. **Hypovolaemia:**   vomiting, burns; renal disease; diuretics, including alcohol
2. **Gaisbock's syndrome:**   assoc. obese, white, middle-aged men; hypertension; anxiety

True

1. **Tissue hypoxia**

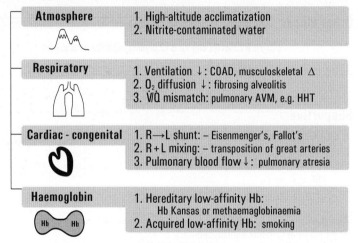

| **Atmosphere** | 1. High-altitude acclimatization |
| | 2. Nitrite-contaminated water |

Respiratory	1. Ventilation ↓ : COAD, musculoskeletal △
	2. O_2 diffusion ↓ : fibrosing alveolitis
	3. V̇/Q̇ mismatch: pulmonary AVM, e.g. HHT

Cardiac - congenital	1. R→L shunt: – Eisenmenger's, Fallot's
	2. R + L mixing: – transposition of great arteries
	3. Pulmonary blood flow ↓ : pulmonary atresia

Haemoglobin	1. Hereditary low-affinity Hb:
	Hb Kansas or methaemaglobinaemia
	2. Acquired low-affinity Hb: smoking

2. **Excess erythropoietin (EPO)**

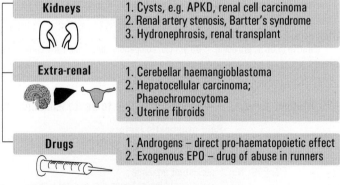

Kidneys	1. Cysts, e.g. APKD, renal cell carcinoma
	2. Renal artery stenosis, Bartter's syndrome
	3. Hydronephrosis, renal transplant

Extra-renal	1. Cerebellar haemangioblastoma
	2. Hepatocellular carcinoma;
	Phaeochromocytoma
	3. Uterine fibroids

| **Drugs** | 1. Androgens – direct pro-haematopoietic effect |
| | 2. Exogenous EPO – drug of abuse in runners |

3. **Polycythaemia rubra vera (PRV)**

Polycythaemia Rubra Vera (PRV)

Def
1. Red-cell count:
    a) Hb > 18 g/dl (may be masked by haemorrhge that is assoc. with disease)
    b) Haematocrit > 50%
    c) RBC mass – high (ascertained by dilution method using ^{51}Cr-labelled RBCs and ^{125}I -labelled plasma)
2. Secondary causes excluded, including normal EPO levels

PC   *P.R.V. G.O.*

Plethora: including conjunctival suffusion; acne rosacea

Pruritus: esp. after hot bath: due to histamine release from basophilia

Peptic ulcers: due to histamine release

Retinopathy and neurological deficits:
    1. Fundi: venule engorgement, haemorrhages, papilloedema
    2. Headaches ('fullness')
    3. Dizziness; fatigue; confusion

Vascular:
    1. Venous or arterial thrombosis – DVT, CVA
    2. Haemorrhage – e.g. cerebral: due to impaired platelet function
    3. Hypertension, CCF

Gout: due to hyperuricaemia

Organomegaly: hepatosplenomegaly (in 90%)

Ix
1. FBC (other than as in definition):
    a) WCC ↑;   neutrophil alkaline phosphatase (NAP) ↑, cf. CML, in which it is ↓
    b) Platelets ↑; but bleeding time ↑, due to abnormal platelet function
    c) ESR ↓
2. Chemistry:
    a) Vit B12 ↑ and transcobalamin-I ↑
    b) LDH ↓ , cf. myelofibrosis, in which it is ↑
3. Bone marrow biopsy:
    a) Erythropoiesis, granulopoiesis, megakaryocyte number and size – all increased
    b) Other: reticulin fibres (Ag stain) increased; Fe stores decreased; blast, colony-forming units
4. Special:
    a) Ferrokinetics (^{52}Fe): initially, ↑ increaesd uptake in axial skeleton → later, ↑ in liver, spleen
    b) Chromosomal studies: abnormal in 15%

Rx
1. Venesection: decrease haematocrit to < 46%, by venesecting 1 unit on alternate days
                       ☠ : DVT, and tolerated poorly in elderly

2. Myelosuppression: hydroxyurea, alkylating agents (e.g. chlorambucil, melphalan),
                         radioactive ^{32}P – ☠: malignant transformation

Prognosis

Median survival is 10 years if treated; but **transformation risk** to AML is 10%

Chronic Lymphocytic Leukaemia

Def
1. Slow, indolent, clonal proliferation of lymphocytes in mantle zone of 2° lymphoid follicles
2. B lymphocytes (CD19$^+$) with T-cell marker (CD5$^+$)
3. Immunodeficiency due to: a) Lymphocyte immaturity; lymphopenia; Ig $\downarrow$
   b) Neutropenia, due to marrow infiltration and hypersplenism

Epi
Inc: Commonest adult leukaemia: 3/100,000 p.a.
Age: Usually elderly (> 60). Middle-aged patients have aggressive variant
Sex: M : F = 2:1. Men have worse prognosis
Geo: 1. Factory workers (benzene, asbestos); farmers (soya bean production, herbicide)
   2. Whites > Blacks > Japanese, Chinese
Aet: 1. *bcl-2* proto-oncogene over-expression
   2. Chromosomal abnormalities, esp.
      • 13q deletion (75%) : good prognosis
      • 11 deletion (20%): poor prognosis; bulky lymphadenopathy

PC

B.L.O.B.B.I.E.S.

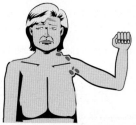

B symptoms (constitutional):
  • night sweats and weight loss
  • occur in late disease; or middle-aged aggressive variant, or Richter's syn. (*see opposite*)

Lymphadenopathy: painless, symmetric, diffuse, rubbery

Organomegaly: splenomegaly $\pm$ hepatomegaly
  esp. hairy cell or prolymphocytic variants

Bone marrow failure – anaemia (pallor)

Bone marrow failure – thrombocytopenia (purpura)

Immune dysfunction:
   1. Immunocompromised (cell-mediated immunity):
      herpes, esp. zoster (disseminated in 20%); pneumonia - bacterial, fungal
   2. Autoimmune:
      • Mikulicz's syn.: xerophthalmia, xerostomia, tonsil – salivary gland enlargement
      • Arthritis, effusions, vasculitis: esp. hairy cell, prolymphocytic or T-cell CLL
      • Hypersensitivity to insect bites or vaccinations ('vaccinia gangrenosum')

Excess
   1. Viscosity: esp. prolymphocytic CLL: WCC > 400 x 10^9/l (poor prognosis)
   2. Uric acid: gout, $\therefore$ give prophylactic allopurinol if chemoRx considered

Skin: nodules; vesicles; bullae; pruritus – 'L'homme rouge' (T-cell CLL)

Ix   **1. FBC**

RBCs	WBCs	Platelets

RBCs

Anaemia:
normochromic, normocytic,
due to:
1. Marrow infiltration
2. Autoimmune haemolysis:
  can be tested for with:
  • Direct Coombs Test
  • Warm agglutinins
  • Reticulocytes ↑

WBCs

1. Count:
  a) Lymphocytosis: 5–300 x 10^9/l
  b) Neutropenia   (T-CLL)
2. Immunophenotype:
  a) CD19⁺, CD 5⁺
  b) IgM, D surface expression ↓
  c) Light-chain restriction (κ or λ)
3. Film:
  a) Nucleus: cytoplasm ratio ↑
  b) Coarse, condensed chromatin

Platelets

Thrombocytopenia,
due to:
1. Marrow infiltration
2. ITP

Also:
'Smudge cells' –
artefactual WBC rupture

2. Other bloods: a) Bilirubin ↑ (nodes at porta hepatis), ALT ↑ (liver involvement), alk. phos. ↑, albumin ↓
b) IgG ↓ (paraproteinaemia in 5%); β_2-microglobulin ↑, LDH ↑ (poor prognosis)
c) Ca ↑, PO_4 ↓, uric acid ↑

3. Lymph node or bone marrow biopsy: lymphocytic replacement of > 30% (poor prognosis);
Richter's syndrome: rapid enlargement of lymph node by transformation into diffuse histiocytic lymphoma.

Rx   **1. Supportive**

RBCs	WBCs	Platelets

RBCs

1. RBC transfusion
2. Prednisolone:
  ↑ es all blood counts

WBCs

a) Pneumovax, flu vaccine
b) Prophylactic aciclovir; antifungals
  cotrimoxazole (PCP), isoniazid (TB)
c) IV immunogloblins

Platelets

Splenectomy or
splenic irradiation:
for spleen pain or
refractory ITP / AIHA

2. Medical:
  a) Cytotoxics - in high-stage disease:
    • Chlorambucil (alkylating agent) or fludarabine (purine analogues) ± cyclophosphamide
    • Combination CHOP chemoRx: for younger pts. to acheive ↑ er response rate
  b) Immunotherapy: anti-CD52 (alemtuzumab) or anti-CD20 (rituximab)
3. Radiotherapy: reduces lymph node and spleen size
4. Allogeneic therapies:
  a) Allogeneic stem-cell transplant + intensive chemoRx + TBI: if < 55 years old
  b) Allogeneic lymphocyte infusion + mild chemotherapy: enables graft vs. leukaemia reaction

Prognosis   Rai staging   Median survival

0:	WBC > 15 x 10^9/l (worse if > 5% prolymphocytes)	10 years
1:	Lymph nodes (worse if > 2 sites)	8 years
2:	Splenomegaly	6 years
3:	Hb < 10 g/dl	5 years
4:	Platelets < 100 x 10^9/l	2 years

Hodgkin's Lymphoma

<u>**Def**</u>
1. Tumour of main lymph node complex → orderly extension into contiguous sites
2. Reed–Sternberg (RS) cells = B cells with multinucleate, mirror-image, 'owl-eye' nuclei
3. Reactive inflammatory infiltrate: plasma cells, lymphocytes, histiocytes, eosinophils

<u>**Epi**</u>
Inc: 3/100,000 p.a.
Age: Bimodal: 20–30s (nodular sclerosis type), and > 60s (lymphocyte-depleted type)
Sex: M : F = 2:1. Women tend to have more favourable nodular sclerosis type
Geo: Low socioeconomic status; whites > blacks
Aet: 1. Inherited: HLA-DPB-1: monozygotic twins have 100 x risk
2. Infection: EBV (genome present in RS cells in 40%) or HIV: mixed cellularity type
3. Toxins: benzene, nitrous oxide, wood dust

<u>**PC**</u>

B.L.O.B.B.I.E.S.

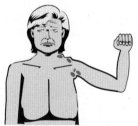

B symptoms (constitutional):
　1. Weight loss > 10% in 6 months
　2. Fever / night sweats: continuous or cyclical, high + swinging ('Pel–Ebstein'), or sepsis

Lymphadenopathy:
　1. Superficial: esp. cervical and axillary; discrete, continuous, matted mass;
　　　　　　firm, rubbery, painless (but pain with alcohol)
　2. Deep: • Mediastinal (superior vena cava obstruction), esp. nodular sclerosis type
　　　　　• Retroperitoneal (lower body oedema), esp. mixed cellularity type

Organomegaly: splenomegaly ± hepatomegaly

Bone marrow failure – pancytopenia

Bone pain - with alcohol

Immune dysfunction:
　1. Immunocompromised (cell-mediated immunity)
　　　　herpes, esp. zoster, CMV; TB; *Candida*; *Cryptococcus*
　2. Autoimmune
　　　　autoimmune haemolytic anaemia, ITP, paraneoplastic cerebellar degeneration

Extra: nephrotic syndrome

Skin: pruritus; erythema nodosum; icthyosis

Ix   **1. FBC**

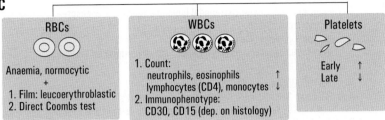

RBCs	WBCs	Platelets

Anaemia, normocytic
+
1. Film: leucoerythroblastic
2. Direct Coombs test
	1. Count:
	   neutrophils, eosinophils ↑
	   lymphocytes (CD4), monocytes ↓
	2. Immunophenotype:
	   CD30, CD15 (dep. on histology)
		Early ↑
		Late ↓

2. Other bloods   a) Bilirubin ↑ (nodes at porta hepatis), ALT ↑ (liver involvement), alk. phos. ↑, albumin ↓
b) IgG normal ; β_2-microglobulin ↑ and LDH ↑ (both suggest poor prognosis)
c) Ca ↑, PO$_4$↓, uric acid ↑

3. Lymph node ± bone-marrow biopsy

Nodular sclerosis	(50%)	fibrosis; lacunar variant of RS cell; eosinophilia; young women
Lymphocyte-predominant	(10%)	RS cells ↓; monoclonal B cells ↑; young men; good prognosis as ↑ inflammatory response
Mixed cellularity	(30%)	intermediate between lymphocyte predominant and depleted
Lymphocyte-depleted	(10%)	RS cells ↑; elderly men; poor prognosis

4. Staging CT, PET

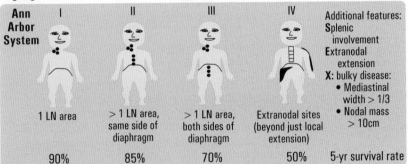

Ann Arbor System	I	II	III	IV	Additional features:
					Splenic
					   involvement
					Extranodal
					   extension
					X: bulky disease:
					   • Mediastinal
					     width > 1/3
					   • Nodal mass
					     > 10cm

	1 LN area	> 1 LN area, same side of diaphragm	> 1 LN area, both sides of diaphragm	Extranodal sites (beyond just local extension)	
	90%	85%	70%	50%	5-yr survival rate

Rx   1. **Supportive:** blood products, prophylactic aciclovir, cotrimoxazole, vaccinate, sperm–oocyte bank
2. **Medical – cytotoxics:**
   • MOPP (mustine, vincristine (Oncovin), procarbazine, prednisolone): ☠ infertility; AML, solid tumour
   • ABVD (doxorubicin (Adriamycin), bleomycin, vinblastine, dacarbazine): ☠ cardiomyopathy; pulmo. fibrosis
3. **Radiotherapy:** local; upper mantle (supra-diaphragmatic); inverted-Y (infra-diaphragmatic)
4. **Autologous stem-cell transplant** (+intensive chemotherapy +total-body irradiation):
   reserved for patients after 1st relapse → 25% long-term disease-free survival

Prognosis   Poor prognosis suggested by:

1. **Epi:** Elderly, male
2. **FBC:** Hb < 10 g/dl; WCC > 15 x 10^9/l; lymphocytes < 0.6 x 10^9/l
3. **Other:** ESR ↑, albumin ↓, β_2-microglobulin, LDH ↑

Non-Hodgkin's Lymphoma

Def
1. Tumour of nodal and/or extranodal lymphoid tissue → widespread dissemination via blood
2. Heterogeneous group:
   a) B or T lymphocyte
   b) Immature (central, high-grade) or mature (peripheral, low-grade)

Epi
Inc: 10/100,000 p.a.
Age: Bimodal: 1. Children – lymphoblastic or Burkitt's   – high-grade (like ALL)
                2. Adult   – small cell lymphocytic or follicular – low-grade (like CLL)
Sex: M slightly > F
Geo: Japan, Carribean (HTLV-I); Africa (EBV, malaria, HIV–Burkitt's)
Aet: 1. Infection: EBV + immunodeficiency state, e.g. HIV, malaria, HTLV-I, *H. pylori*
     2. Immunosuppression: post-transplant, chemoRx, radioRx (e.g. Hodgkin's lymphoma Rx)
     3. Immunodeficiency – hereditary: ataxia telangiectasia, Wiskott–Aldrich syndrome
     4. Autoimmune: coeliac, Crohn's, rheumatoid arthritis

PC

B.L.O.B.B.I.E.S.

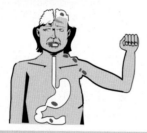

B symptoms (constitutional)
   As for Hodgkin's – but not prominent until advanced disease

Lymphadenopathy:
   1. Superficial: multiple, widespread, non-contiguous – suggests advanced disease
   2. Deep: mediastinal; retroperitoneal – esp. lymphoblastic
   3. Mucosa-associated (MALTomas):
       • Oral: pharynx ('Waldeyer's ring'): pharyngitis, dysphagia, stridor;
               mandible (Burkitt's lymphoma); salivary glands: xerostomia, xerophthalmia
       • Gastric: associated with *H. pylori*
       • Bowel ('Peyer's patches'): colic, D&V, clubbing, wasting –
               associated with T-cell lymphoma; coeliac; α heavy chain disease
       • Respiratory tract: cough, stridor
   4. CNS: associated with HIV, HTLV-I, lymphoblastic

Organomegaly: splenomegaly ± hepatomegaly

Bone marrow failure – pancytopenia

Bone pain – with alcohol

Immune dysfunction: autoimmune haemolytic anaemia, ITP

Endocrine: thyroid or testes infiltration

Skin: T-cell lymphoma (mycosis fungoides); icthyosis

<u>Ix</u> **1. FBC**

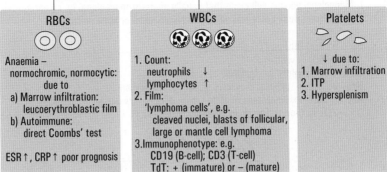

RBCs	WBCs	Platelets
Anaemia – normochromic, normocytic: due to	1. Count: neutrophils ↓ lymphocytes ↑	↓ due to: 1. Marrow infiltration 2. ITP 3. Hypersplenism
a) Marrow infiltration: leucoerythroblastic film	2. Film: 'lymphoma cells', e.g. cleaved nuclei, blasts of follicular, large or mantle cell lymphoma	
b) Autoimmune: direct Coombs' test	3. Immunophenotype: e.g. CD19 (B-cell); CD3 (T-cell) TdT: + (immature) or – (mature)	
ESR ↑, CRP ↑ poor prognosis		

2. Other bloods a) Bilirubin ↑ (nodes at porta hepatis), ALT ↑ (liver involvement), alk. phos. ↑, albumin ↓
b) IgG - total ↓, but paraproteinaemia in 15% (esp. indolent lymphomas)
c) Ca ↑ (esp. adult T-cell leukaemia-lymphoma), PO_4 ↓, uric acid ↑

3. Lymph node biopsy (or GIT, bronchial, brain, bone-marrow biopsy)

Grading: REAL classification (Revised European American Lymphoma)				
(5-year survival rates)	**B-cell**		**T-cell**	
Low-grade	MALToma	(75%)	Mycosis fungoides	(90%)
	Follicular	(70%)		
Intermediate-grade	Diffuse large cell	(50%)	Anaplastic	(75%)
	Mantle cell	(30%)	Peripheral	(25%)
High-grade	Burkitt's	(50%)	Adult-T-cell leukaemia–	
	Lymphoblastic	(50%)	lymphoma	(20%)

4. Staging: Whole-body CT, PET; CT Brain and CSF; OGD; colonoscopy; ENT exam
Ann Arbor System (see p. 453) – although staging less relevant to prognosis

<u>Rx</u> 1. Supportive: as for Hogkin's lymphoma (p. 453)
2. **Medical:** a) cytotoxic: CHOP (cyclophosphamide, doxorubicin (hydroxydaunorubicin), vincristine (Oncovin), prednisolone)
b) immunotherapy: interferon-α; rituximab (anti-CD20), alemtuzimab (anti-CD52)
3. Radiotherapy: a) Local – can be curative in stage I disease; b) Brain – CNS lymphoma
4. Autologous stem-cell transplant: (+ chemotherapy + total-body irradiation): if pt relapses
5. Special: a) **Splenic lymphoma with villous lymphocytes** – splenectomy (curative)
b) **CNS lymphoma** – brain irradiation; intrathecal (low-dose) and IV (high-dose) methotrexate

<u>**Prognosis**</u>   Poor prognosis suggested by grade and **International Prognostic Index:**

Epi:	Age > 60 (also AIDS)
PC:	Functional disability (Karnofsky score)
Bloods:	LDH ↑ (also pancytopenia, ESR or CRP ↑, albumin ↓, β_2-microglobulin)
Staging:	Ann Arbor stage 3 or 4; > 1 extranodal site (also bulky disease of > 10 cm)

Multiple Myeloma

Def   1. Monoclonal plasma cell clone that usually secretes monoclonal Ig, i.e.paraprotein
        2. Arises from **post-germinal centre** of lymph node, or bone marrow

Epi   Inc: 5 / 100,000 pa (1% all cancers)
        Age: > 40: ↑ with age
        Sex: Males slightly > females
        Geo: Blacks > Whites; survivors of nuclear irradiation
        Aet: 1. Chromosomal translocation – esp. *Myc* or *Ras* oncogene mutation
             2. IL-6: growth factor secreted by osteoclasts

PC   *P.O.P.U.L.A.T.I.O.N.*

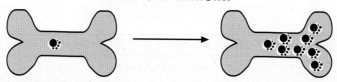

Plasma cells: in > 4% of bone marrow (usually > 30% in myeloma)

Osteolytic lesions:
     Path: Osteoclasts activated (via IL-1β, TNF-β); osteoblasts inhibited
     PC: 1. Bone pain, tenderness, worse with movement, during day, esp. back, shoulder, ribs
           2. Pathological fractures, e.g. wedge vertebral–cord compression; radicular pain
           3. Boney mass: skull, sternum, clavicle

Paraproteinaemia: > 30 g/l or rising
     Def: **Plasma:** monoclonal Ig &/or **Urine:** Bence-Jones protein (κ or λ light-chain restriction)
     Frequency: Plasma alone 20%; BJP alone 20%; both 58%; none 2% (esp. plasmacytomas)
     PC: 1. Hyperviscosity: esp. Ig M, A,D, IgG3, cryoglobulins ⇒ headache, visual blurring, Raynaud's
          2. Coagulopathy and impaired platelet function

U + Es:
     1. Urine: nephrotic syndrome; chronic renal failure (30%), due to:
                 a) Deposition of Bence-Jones protein; amyloid; infiltration of tumour
                 b) Other: calcium ↑, uric acid ↑; pyelonephritis (immunodeficient); NSAIDs
     2. Electrolytes: Ca ↑: due to osteolysis: ⇒ abdominal pain, N + V, polyuria, polydipsia
                Uric acid ↑: due to cell turnover ⇒ gout

Light chain amyloid (AL or primary) ⇒ nephrosis, neuropathy, cardiac failure

Anaemia: due to IL-1 myelosuppression

Thrombocytopenia

Immunodeficiency:
     Path: Due to polyclonal Ig ↓; cell-mediated immunity ↓; neutropenia; complement ↓
     PC: Bacterial respiratory and urinary tract infections - streptococci, staphylococci, Klebsiella

Organomegaly: hepatosplenomegaly

Neurological: peripheral neuropathy, papilloedema, P.O.E.M.S. syndrome =
     Peripheral neuropathy; **O**steosclerosis; **E**ndocrine (e.g. DM); **M**-band; **S**kin (e.g. hyperpigmentation)

1st three features are essential for diagnosis

<u>**Ix**</u> **1. FBC**

RBCs	WBCs	Platelets
1. Anaemia - normo- or macrocytic	1. Count: neutrophils ↓ (advanced disease)	1. Usually ↓ POEMS syn. ↑
2. Film: • Leucoerythroblastic • Rouleaux formation or ↑ background staining (due to ↑↑Ig)	2. Film: • Plasma cells (15%) • Mott cells: big cytoplasmic vacuoles • Flaming of cell rim	2. Platelet function: impaired
3. ESR ↑, CRP ↑	3. Immunophenotype e.g. surface expression of clonal Ig	3. Clotting times ↑ both 2 and 3 due to hyperviscosity

2. Chemistry

a) Electrophoresis: serum and urine

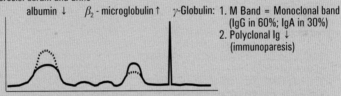

albumin ↓ β_2 - microglobulin ↑ γ-Globulin: 1. M Band = Monoclonal band (IgG in 60%; IgA in 30%) 2. Polyclonal Ig ↓ (immunoparesis)

b) U + E: urea ↑, creatinine ↑; Ca ↑, uric acid ↑
   Na ↓ (real and pseudohyponatraemia due to Ig ↑), Cl ↑ (∴ anion gap ↓)
c) LFT: LDH ↑; albumin ↓; alkaline phosphatase - normal as osteoblasts inactive

d) Urine: • Proteinuria – suggests renal disease (Bence-Jones protein is not detected by dipstick)
   • Glycosuria and aminoaciduria (Fanconi's syndrome, due to tubular damage)

3. Radiology

a) X-ray of limbs, spine, skull:
   • Focal or generalized osteoporosis, e.g. 'punched-out' holes in skull
   • Wedge fractures of spine
b) Tc bone scan: silent due to osteoblastic inhibition (may be + ve if sclerotic reaction occurs)

4. Bone-marrow biopsy

<u>**Rx**</u> 1. Supportive:
   • **Bone marrow suppression**: blood products; antibiotics; IVIg. **Bone lesions**: radiotherapy, surgery
   • **Hyperviscosity**: plasmapharesis. **Hypercalcaemia** - hydration, prednisolone, bisphosphonates
2. Medical - cytotoxics:
   • Elderly: single agent (melphalan or cyclophosphamide)
   • Young: VAD (vincristine, doxorubicin (Adriamycin), dexamethasone) ± IFN-α
3. Stem-cell transplant:
   • Autologous + high-dose melphalan: increases survival time; decreases remission rate
   • Allogeneic: 50% curative or long-term remission, although 30% mortality rate from procedure

<u>**Prognosis**</u>   5-year survival rate = 20%, i.e. *B.A.D.* = poor prognostic markers:

β_2-microglobulin ↑ (albumin ↓ M-band ↑); **B**ony lesions if extensive + symptomatic
Anaemia (ESR, CRP ↑↑); **D**ehydration (urea > 14; Ca ↑↑); L**D**H ↑

Paraproteinaemia

Malignant Paraproteinaemia

Criteria:

P.O.P.ulation

Plasma cells in bone marrow of > 4%
Osteolytic lesions on skeletal survey
Paraproteinaemia of > 20 g/l
  + immunoparesis – i.e. polyclonal IgG ↓

No Lymphadenopathy

Plasma cell neoplasm
1. Multiple myeloma
2. Localized myeloma = plasmacytoma
    a) Solitary Bone – osteolytic lesion
    b) Extramedullary – esp. MALToma of ENT,
              sinus, GIT, CNS, skin
      good prognosis, but bone type may transform
      into multiple myeloma
3. Plasma cell leukaemia = advanced myeloma
    hepatosplenomegaly, but less marrow
    involvement; poor prognosis

Lymphadenopathy

Immature B-cell neoplasm
1. CLL (5% produce paraproteinaemia)
2. B-cell lymphoma
3. Waldenström's macroglobulinaemia
    Epi: Men > 50 yrs
    Def: Lymphoplasmacytoid cell
        (early plasma cell) ⟶ IgM
    Path: Diffuse or localized tumour mass
    PC: • Hyperviscosity
        • B symptoms: fever, loss of weight
        • Lymphadenopathy, hepatosplenomegaly
    Ix: • Anaemia: 2° to aplasia, dilution, haemolysis
        • Cryoglobulins (Igs that precipitate in cold)
    N.B. a) X-rays = normal (cf. IgM Myeloma)
        b) U + E's = normal (IgM not excreted)
        c) Bence-Jones proteinuria in 20% (esp. κ)

Antibody fragment excess
1. Light-chain: AL amyloidosis
2. Heavy chain disease:
    α – Epi: • Arabs (Mediterranean / N. Africa)
              • Intestinal parasite infestation
        PC: • Villous atrophy, ileal malabsorption
              • GI lymphoma
    γ – PC: Lymphoma-like in elderly men
    μ – PC: CLL-like with lymphoplasmacytoid cells
        in bone marrow; hepatosplenomegaly

Benign Paraproteinaemia

Criteria:

P.O.P.ulation

Plasma cells in bone marrow of < 4%
Osteolytic lesions – absent
Paraproteinaemia of < 20 g/l

No Constitutional Symptoms

Monoclonal gammopathy of uncertain significance (MGUS)
Epi: 3% of > 70 yrs
Rx: Monitor for 3 years
Prognosis:
1. Transforms into:
    • Myeloma or lymphoma: 20% over next 10 yrs
    • Amyloid - 10%
2. Transient M-protein

Constitutional Symptoms

Systemic disease

1. Infection – esp. AIDS, parasites,
              chronic bacterial
2. Neoplasia – esp. carcinoma
3. Autoimmune

All may cause chronic cold haemagglutinins

<u>Hyperviscosity</u>

<u>Causes</u>

Cells
1. Polycythaemia: 1° (PRV) – commonest cause; 2° if severe
2. Chronic myeloid leukaemia
3. Acute leukaemia – if severe

Paraprotein
1. Waldenström's macroglobulinaemia: IgM
2. Multiple myeloma: IgM or IgA
3. Plasmacytoma

Iatrogenic
1. Packed cell products
2. Cryoprecipitate (given to haemophiliacs with circulating inhibitors): causes hyperfibrinogenaemia
3. IVIg therapy

<u>**PC**</u>

P.R.V. G.O.

Plethora, **P**ruritus, **P**eptic ulcers – all with PRV only

Purpura, **P**igmentation - reticulate, Raynaud's phenomenon, necrosis – esp. with cryoglobulinaemia, due to paraproteinaemia

Retinopathy / neurological deficits:
  1. 'Slow-flow retinopathy':
    PC: Visual disturbance: 'looking through a watery windscreen'
    Fundi: • Venule engorgement, constrictions: 'linked sausages'
        • Flame haemorrhages, exudates, papilloedema
  2. CNS: Headaches ('fullness'); dizziness;
      encephalopathy – fatigue, confusion, seizures
  3. PNS: peripheral neuropathy (demyelinating), due to anti-MAG Ab

Vascular:
  1. Venous or arterial thrombosis - DVT, CVA
  2. Haemorrhage – e.g. epistaxis, haematuria, cerebral:
      due to impaired platelet function and coagulopathy
  3. Hypertension, CCF

Gout: due to hyperuricaemia, but only with **cell** proliferation cause

Organomegaly: • Hepatosplenomegaly: PRV, CML, myeloma, lymphoma
             • Lymphadenopathy: Waldenström's macroglobulinaemia

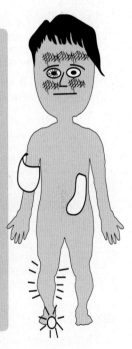

<u>**Ix**</u>
1. Bloods: FBC ↑: myeloproliferative; ↓: myeloma, Waldenström's
       ESR ↓: myeloproliferative; ↑: myeloma, Waldenström's
       Serum electrophoresis
2. Urine electrophoresis
3. Biopsy: • Bone marrow: myeloproliferative, myeloma
         • Lymph node: Waldenström's (lymphoplasmacytoid infiltrate)

<u>**Rx**</u>
Waldenström's: 1. Supportive: packed RBC transfusions; antibiotics
          2. Plasmapharesis: most effective for IgM as intravascularly confined
          3. Chemotherapy: cyclophosphamide + prednisolone: if symptomatic or cytopenic

<u>Amyloidosis</u>

<u>**Def**</u>   Accumulation of any fibrillar protein that folds abnormally into β-pleated-sheets:-

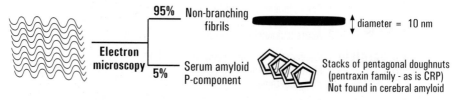

95% Non-branching fibrils — diameter = 10 nm

Electron microscopy

5% Serum amyloid P-component — Stacks of pentagonal doughnuts (pentraxin family - as is CRP) Not found in cerebral amyloid

<u>**Types**</u>   Distinguished by type of protein that forms in excess:

Systemic

1. **AL (1°)**   **L**ight chain - due to any cause of paraproteinaemia
   a) Light-chain secretion only: esp. λVI, or N-terminus of V_L – commonest
   b) B-cell neoplasm: e.g. multiple myeloma, plasmacytoma, lymphoma
   c) Benign monoclonal gammopathy

2. **AA (2°)**   **A**cute phase protein, protein A (breakdown product of serum amyloid A)
   a) Chronic inflammation (> 2 yrs): IL-1, IL-6 cytokines $\Rightarrow$ hepatocyte SAA secretion ↑es
      • Autoimmunity: rheumatoid arthritis (esp. Still's), ankolysing spondylitis, ulcerative colitis
      • Infection: bronchiectasis (staphylococci, TB), osteomyelitis, cellulitis
      • Neoplasm: Hodgkin's, renal cell carcinoma
   b) Hereditary periodic fever:
      • Familial Mediterranean fever (autosomal recessive): assoc: Sephardi Jews, Arabs
         type 1: recurrent serositis (pleurisy, peritonitis, synovitis) ; type 2: renal amyloid
      • Muckle–Wells syndrome

3. Autosomal dominant amyloidopathy:
   a) Transthyretin (carrier of thyroxine + retinol-binding protein; made in liver + choroid plexus)
         PC: lower limb and autonomic neuropathy, scalloped pupils, cardiac amyloid
   b) Gelsolin (actin modulator): assoc: Finnish
         PC: cranial and autonomic neuropathy, corneal and vitreous dystrophy
   c) Other: apolipoprotein AI, lysozyme, fibrinogen-α:
         PC: renal, cardiac, GIT amyloid (not neuropathy)

Organ-based

1. Cerebral:
      a) Amyloid β_2: dementia; cerebral lobar haemorrhage
      b) α-synuclein: Lewy body dementia, Parkinson's disease
      c) Prion protein (PrP): Creutzfeld–Jakob disease

2. Cardiac: transthyretin plus atrial natriuretic peptide – causes LVF and IHD in elderly

3. Endocrine
      a) Amylin (homology to calcitonin gene-related peptide): type 2 DM / Insulinoma
      b) Pro-calcitonin: medullary carcinoma of thyroid + other APUDomas

4. Soft tissue: e.g. β_2-microglobulin via haemodialysis: arthritis, carpal tunnel syndrome

<u>**PC**</u>   *O.R.G.A.N.I.S.E.D.*

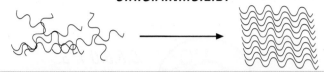

Organomegaly:
    1. Hepatosplenomegaly
    2. Lymphadenopathy: in AA amyloid and lymphoma

Renal:
    1. Proteinuria: nephrotic syndrome, renal vein thrombosis
    2. Chronic renal failure: glomerular + tubulo-interstitial + vascular disease
    3. Renal enlargement

GIT: 1. Macroglossia – dysphagia
    2. Bowel: malabsorption, diarrhoea, obstruction
    3. Liver: intrahepatic cholestasis; portal hypertension

Arthritis: rheumatoid-pattern, or large-joint monoarthritis; shoulder-pad sign

Neurological:
    1. Neuropathy: painful, sensory, autonomic, enlarged nerves
    2. Carpal tunnel syndrome
    3. 'Pseudomyopathy'

Skin: 1. Waxy plaques and papules
    2. Purpura: 'raccoon eyes' (factor X / fibrinogen deficiency)

Endocrine: goitre; adrenal, pituitary, pancreas enlargement (rarely deficiency)

Death due to:
    1. Cardiac: arrhythmias, heart block, digoxin hypersensitivity, restrictive cardiomyopathy,
       constrictive pericarditis, endocardial – valve disease
    2. Airway: larynx or bronchial thickening – stridor, dysphonia

N.B. Involvement of organs A.N.S.E.D. and macroglossia are usually only seen with 1° amyloid

<u>**Ix**</u> 1. Myeloma Ix:
      a) FBC, film, BM biopsy; b) Serum, urine electrophoresis, Ca, β_2-microglobulin; c) X-ray screen
    2. Biopsy: rectal; gingival; renal; abdominal fat pad aspirate
       Stain: H&E: **H**yaline, **E**osinophilic, **A**morphous, **P**roteinaceous material; Congo red + ve; birefringent
    3. SAP-scan: radiolabelled serum amyloid P scintigram (^{99}Tc)

<u>**Rx**</u> Treatment of underlying cause leads to regression of amyloid deposits, but prognosis poor for 1°

    1. AL: a) Chemotherapy: as for myeloma
          b) Serum amyloid P binding inhibitor: R-1-pyrrolidine carboxylic acid

    2. AA: a) Immunosuppressants, e.g. chlorambucil in Still's; or antibiotics for sepsis
          b) Colchicine for familial Mediterranean fever

    3. Transthyretin: liver transplant

    4. β_2-microglobulin: renal transplant (i.e. stopping haemodialysis)

Hyposplenism

Causes

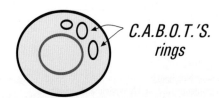

C.A.B.O.T.'S. rings

Congenital
1. Agenesis:
   associated immunodeficiency, e.g. Fanconi's anaemia
2. Congenital cyanotic heart disease

Autoimmune
1. SLE, rheumatoid arthritis (associated big spleen)
2. GIT: coeliac, inflammatory bowel disease,
   chronic active hepatitis (associated small spleen)
3. Graves' disease, Hashimoto's thyroiditis,
   hypopituitarism or growth hormone deficiency,
   glomerulonephritis
   (associated small spleen for all)

Blood disorder
1. Sickle cell: big spleen in infancy, but numerous microinfarcts
   cause gradual fibrosis and contraction
2. Thalassaemia; hereditary spherocytosis:
   often treated with elective splenectomy
3. Lymphoma •Sézary syndrome (T-cell)
   •Radiotherapy or graft-versus-host disease
4. Amyloid

Occlusion
   Splenic artery or vein thrombosis

Trauma / splenectomy

   Indications for elective splenectomy:
1. Autoimmune ITP or autoimmune haemolytic anaemia:
   both when steroid-resistant and chronic
2. Leukaemia or lymphoma:
   a) CML or myelofibrosis:
      ↓ symptoms of massive splenomegaly
      ↓ need for tranfusions
   b) CLL or lymphoma:
      ↓ thrombocytopenia
3. Thalassaemia major or intermedia; hereditary spherocytosis

Sarcoid

PC

1. **Infection**: due to decreased phagocytosis, chemotaxis, Ab production
2. **Thrombocytosis**: ischaemic heart disease; CVA; peripheral vascular disease
3. **Hypersplenism**: from accessory spleen enlargement at hilum, mesentery, or pancreas tail
4. **Autoimmunity**: due to impaired T cell suppression

Ix FBC and blood film: all cell counts ↑ due to less natural destruction

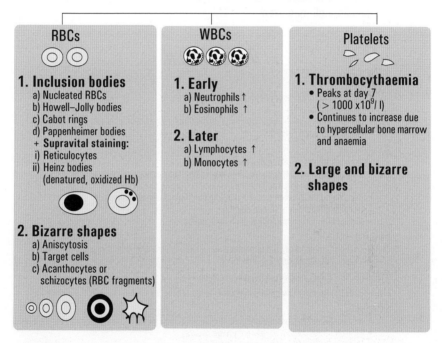

RBCs

1. Inclusion bodies
 a) Nucleated RBCs
 b) Howell–Jolly bodies
 c) Cabot rings
 d) Pappenheimer bodies
 + **Supravital staining**:
 i) Reticulocytes
 ii) Heinz bodies
 (denatured, oxidized Hb)

2. Bizarre shapes
 a) Aniscytosis
 b) Target cells
 c) Acanthocytes or
 schizocytes (RBC fragments)

WBCs

1. Early
 a) Neutrophils ↑
 b) Eosinophils ↑

2. Later
 a) Lymphocytes ↑
 b) Monocytes ↑

Platelets

1. Thrombocythaemia
 • Peaks at day 7
 (> 1000 x10^9/ l)
 • Continues to increase due
 to hypercellular bone marrow
 and anaemia

**2. Large and bizarre
 shapes**

Prophylaxis

1. Plan best time for splenectomy:
 delay splenectomy, as < 6 years-old are most susceptible to infection
2. Vaccines:
 a) PneumoVax (from 1 month before operation)
 b) Hib (*Haemophilus influenzae* b)
 c) MeningoVax A + C (esp. if travelling abroad)
3. Antibiotics:
 a) Penicillin V / erythromycin
 b) Anti-malarials (esp. if latent infection due to risk of reactivation or cerebral malaria)
 c) Salmonella infection
4. Anti-platelets: aspirin

Immunodeficiency – General

Causes

Causes can be categorized according to the part of the immune system affected:

Innate:

Mucosal defences: • Neuromuscular weakness; recumbency; smoking
• Iatrogenic: lines; cannulas; catheters; tracheostomy

Complement deficiency
Phagocytosis failure: respiratory viruses

B-cells: humoral
T-cells: cell-mediated

I.N.F.E.C.T.I.O.N.

Infection:
- HSV, influenza (*phagocytosis failure*)
- EBV (*B-cell defect*)
- HIV, malaria, lepromatous leprosy (*T-cell defect; HIV also affects phagocytosis*)
- Measles (*B- and T-cell defects*)

Neoplasia:
Leukaemia (*B- and T-cell defects*), esp.
- AML, CMML: acquired myeloperoxidase deficiency (*phagocytosis failure*)
     and IgA deficiency
- CLL, myeloma, thymoma: hypogammaglobulinaemia (*B-cell defect*)
- Hodgkin's lymphoma (*T-cell defect*)
- Metastatic carcinoma (*phagocytosis failure*)

Failure, organ:
- Cirrhosis, renal failure (*phagocytosis and B-cell defects, due to hypoproteinaemia*)
- Elderly (*T-cell defect*)

Endocrine: diabetes mellitus (*B- and T-cell defects*)

Congenital: primary immunodeficiencies (see p. 466)

Toxins:
- Alcohol (*phagocytosis failure*)
- Smoking (*cilia inhibition, phagocytosis failure*)
- Colchicine, NSAIDs (*phagocytosis failure*)
- Gold, penicillamine, steroids (*phagocytosis failure; B-cell defect*)
- Chemotherapy, radiotherapy, steroids (*global immune effects*)

Immune:
- SLE, rheumatoid arthritis
  (*phagocytosis and complement deficiency – classical pathway*)
- Sarcoidosis (*T-cell defect*)

Organomegaly - hypersplenism (*due to neutropenia*)

Nutritional:
- Malnutrition, malabsorption (*global immune effects*)
- Protein deficiency, esp. burns, protein-losing enteropathy, nephrosis (*B-cell defect*)
- Zinc deficiency (acrodermatitis enteropathica) (*B- and T-cell defects*)
- Fe deficiency (*T-cell defect*)

PC

Innate

Infection:

1. Pyogenic
   a) Boils, bronchiectasis – staphylococci:
      catalase +ve, and so can overcome peroxide-based defences
      when superoxide production is impaired in CGD
   b) Sinusitis, meningitis – streptococcus, *Haemophilus*
2. Fungi

B-cell

Infection:

1. Pyogenic – esp. encapsulated bacteria:
   Streptococcus pneumoniae, Haemophilus,
   Meningococcus, Salmonella
2. Viruses:
   a) VZV, recurrent
   b) HBV, chronic
   c) Enterovirus meningoencephalitis
   d) Live vaccines may cause disease
3. Fungi – *Pneumocystis pneumoniae* (hyperIgM)
4. Protozoa:
   a) Giardia (Bruton's agammaglobulinaemia)
   b) Malaria (splenectomy)

Autoimmunity:

1. Myositis (Bruton's agammaglobulinaemia)
2. SLE, rheumatoid arthritis, coeliac (IgA deficiency)
3. Atopy (IgA deficiency, hyperIgM)

Neoplasia: lymphoma (common variable immunodeficiency)

T-cell

Infection:

1. Pyogenic, inc. TB
2. Viruses – herpes: HSV, VZV, EBV, HHV-8
3. Fungi: Candida, PCP, Cryptococcus
4. Protozoa: cryptosporidia, toxoplasmosis

Autoimmunity: Sjögren's-like sicca syndrome

Neoplasia: Non-Hodgkin's lymphoma

Immunodeficiency – Primary

Causes

Innate

Mucosal Defences
Muscular dystophy, cystic fibrosis, Kartagener's

Complement
1. Classical pathway:
   C2, 1, 4 deficiency: causes SLE-like syndrome
2. Common pathway:
   - Membrane-attack complex – *Neisseria meningitis*
   - C3 deficiency – severe pyogenic infections
3. C1 esterase deficiency: angioedema
4. GPI cell anchor (protects against complement):
   paroxysmal nocturnal haemoglobinuria

Phagocytosis

Respiratory burst ↓
1. **CGD: chronic granulomatous disease:**
   Epi: X-linked – 60%; auto. recessive - 40%
   Path: NADPH oxidase deficiency ⇒ ↓ superoxide
   PC: a) Staphylococcal sepsis (being catalase +ve,
          it can overcome peroxide-based defences)
       b) Fungal sepsis
   Ix: Nitrazolium blue test
2. **Myeloperoxidase deficiency:**
   Epi: Autosomal recessive, 1/2000
   PC: a) Mild, unless concomitant diabetes mellitus
       b) Systemic candidiasis
3. **G6P dehydrogenase deficiency:**
   Immunodeficiency if < 5% G6PD activity

Chemotaxis ↓
1. **Leucocyte adhesion deficiency:**
   Path: Deficiency of integrin = C3b receptor
   PC: a) Recurrent gingivitis, skin, GU abscesses
       b) Delayed separation of umbilical stump
   Ix: Peripheral neutrophilia
2. **Lazy leucocyte syndrome**
3. **Job's syndrome**
   PC: a) Recurrent staphylococci, *Candida*
       b) Eczema; hyperIgE; eosinophilia
       c) Coarse facies; kyphoscoliosis

Granulocyte size ↑
Chediak–Higashi syndrome:
   Path: Deficient cathepsin G and elastase →
          inhibits fusion of phagolysosomes
   Ix: Blood film: large granules

Granulocyte number ↓
Kostmann syndrome: G-CSF receptor defect

B-Cell

Non-Selective Ig Deficiency
1. **Bruton's agammaglobulinaemia**
   Epi: 1/100,000; X-linked
   Path: a) Bruton's tyrosine kinase mutation
         b) B-cell count ↓; lymphoid hyperplasia
   PC: Presents in 1st year:
   ### A.G.A.M.M.A.G.LOB
   Autoimmune: dermatomyositis
   Gastroenteritis (giardia, enterovirus)
   Arthritis: mycoplasma (rheumatoid-pattern)
   Malabsorption; lactose intolerance
   Meningo-encephalitis (enterovirus)
   Anaemia, pernicious
   Growth hormone deficiency (X linkage)
   LOBar pneumonia; bronchiectasis; sinusitis
   Ix: Ig < 2 g/l

2. **Common variable immunodeficiency**
   Epi: 1/2000
   Path: a) Abnormalities in B- or Th-cell maturation
         b) Germinal centre hyperplasia
   PC: Presents in adulthood as for Bruton's, plus
       a) Fever
       b) Lymphadenopathy, hepatosplenomegaly,
          lymphoma, lymphocytosis, Hb ↓ platelets ↓
   Ix: Bone marrow: pre-B cells (no surface Ig)
   Rx: IVIg (for CVID and Bruton's)

Selective Ig Deficiency
1. **IgA deficiency**
   Epi: 1/600 Caucasians
   Path: 1°, congenital infection, penicillamine, phenytoin
   PC: **A**symptomatic, or immunodeficient (if ↓ IgG2, 4)
       Allergies: asthma, allergy to milk;
                blood transfusions (due to anti-IgA)
       Autoimmune: coeliac, CAH, SLE, RA
       Assoc: **A**taxia telangiectasia
       Absent vaccine response
   Ix: B cells bear IgM
   Rx: Use blood from IgA-deficient donor
2. **IgG subclass or functional IgG deficiency**
   PC: Asymptomatic ↔ pneumococcal infection

Hypergammaglobulinaemia
1. **Hyper IgM Immunodeficiency (XL)**
   Path: Neutrophils, IgG, A ↓; IgM, D ↑
   PC: a) Infections: bacterial, PCP, cryptosporidiosis
       b) Autoimmune liver disease
       c) Neoplasia
2. **Hyper IgE: Job syndrome**

T-Cell

Hypoparathyroidism-Associated

1. DiGeorge syndrome:
Path: Developmental defects of pharyngeal pouches 3 + 4

PC: *C.A.T.C.H. 22*

Cardiac anomalies
Artery △
Thymus aplasia: immunodeficiency
Craniofacial anomalies
Hypocalcaemia
22 = chromosome affected

Nezelof syn: thymus aplasia only (sporadic)

2. Chronic mucocutaneous candidiasis:
Path: deficient migratory inhibitory factor
PC: superficial *Candida* only
Assoc:
a) Polyglandular autoimmune syndrome –1
b) Fe deficiency

T-cell Defects

1. Ataxia telangiectasia:
Epi: Autosomal recessive
Path: Deficient DNA repair
PC: Presents in early childhood with:

Ataxia T.E.L.A.N.G.

Ataxia; apraxia of oculomotor system
Telangiectasia on sclera, elbows, ears
Endocrine: DM, hypogonadism
Liver: fatty liver / AFP ↑ ↑
Autoimmunity
Neoplasia: ALL, CLL, lymphoma; CEA ↑ :
  • In early 20s
  • 10% heterozygotes affected
  • Radiosensitive: risk of mammograms
Globulins: IgA deficiency

2. Wiskott–Aldrich syndrome:
Epi: X-linked
Path: Non-specific T-cell receptor (CD43)
PC: a) Recurrent Infections
b) Autoimmunity: ITP, AIHA / Eczema / JCA
c) Lymphoma in 20s
Ix: IgM ↓
IgA ↑

B- and T-Cell

SCID: Severe Combined Immunodeficiency

Epi: X-linked, autosomal recessive, Swiss-type
Path: Numerous mutations, inc.:
1. RAG 1 + 2: V(D)J recombination
2. DNA-dependent tyrosine kinase
3. Adenosine deaminase; ProteoNucleoProtein
4. IL-receptor γ chain (XL)
   ↓ T cells, ↓ NK cells, functionally defective B cells

Primary T-Cell Defects

(with 2ndary B-cell dysfunction)
1. MHC-II deficiency
2. TCR deficieny
3. ZAP70 tyrosine kinase deficiency
4. JAK3 protein kinase deficiency
   (similar to XL SCID)

Chromosomal defects

1. Aneuploidy: Down's, Turner's syndromes
2. Instability:
   a) Fanconi's anaemia
   b) Xeroderma pigmentosa
   c) Bloom's syndrome

Other

Transcobalamin deficiency
PC: Megaloblastic anaemia

Haemostasis

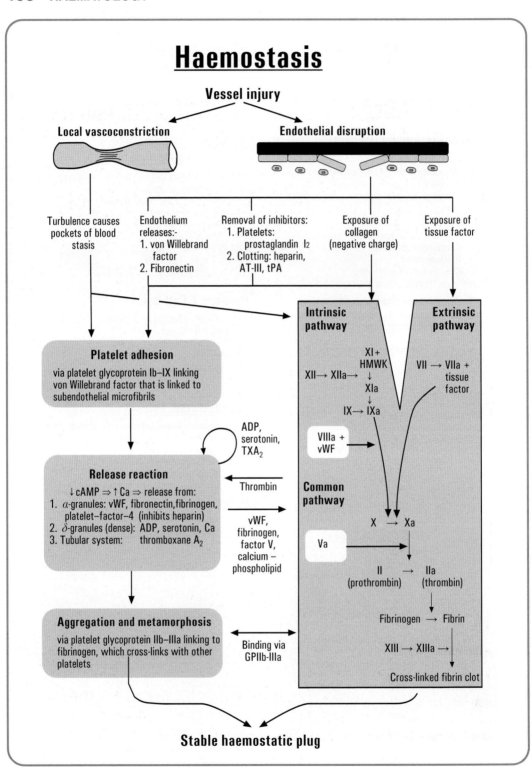

Vessel injury

Local vascoconstriction

Endothelial disruption

Turbulence causes pockets of blood stasis

Endothelium releases:-
1. von Willebrand factor
2. Fibronectin

Removal of inhibitors:
1. Platelets: prostaglandin I2
2. Clotting: heparin, AT-III, tPA

Exposure of collagen (negative charge)

Exposure of tissue factor

Intrinsic pathway

Extrinsic pathway

Platelet adhesion

via platelet glycoprotein Ib–IX linking von Willebrand factor that is linked to subendothelial microfibrils

XII→ XIIa→

XI + HMWK
↓
XIa
↓
IX→ IXa

VII → VIIa + tissue factor

ADP, serotonin, TXA₂

VIIIa + vWF

Release reaction

↓cAMP ⇒ ↑Ca ⇒ release from:
1. α-granules: vWF, fibronectin, fibrinogen, platelet–factor–4 (inhibits heparin)
2. δ-granules (dense): ADP, serotonin, Ca
3. Tubular system: thromboxane A₂

Thrombin

vWF, fibrinogen, factor V, calcium – phospholipid

Common pathway

X → Xa

Va

II → IIa
(prothrombin) (thrombin)

Aggregation and metamorphosis

via platelet glycoprotein IIb–IIIa linking to fibrinogen, which cross-links with other platelets

Binding via GPIIb-IIIa

Fibrinogen → Fibrin

XIII → XIIIa →

Cross-linked fibrin clot

Stable haemostatic plug

Haemostasis Control

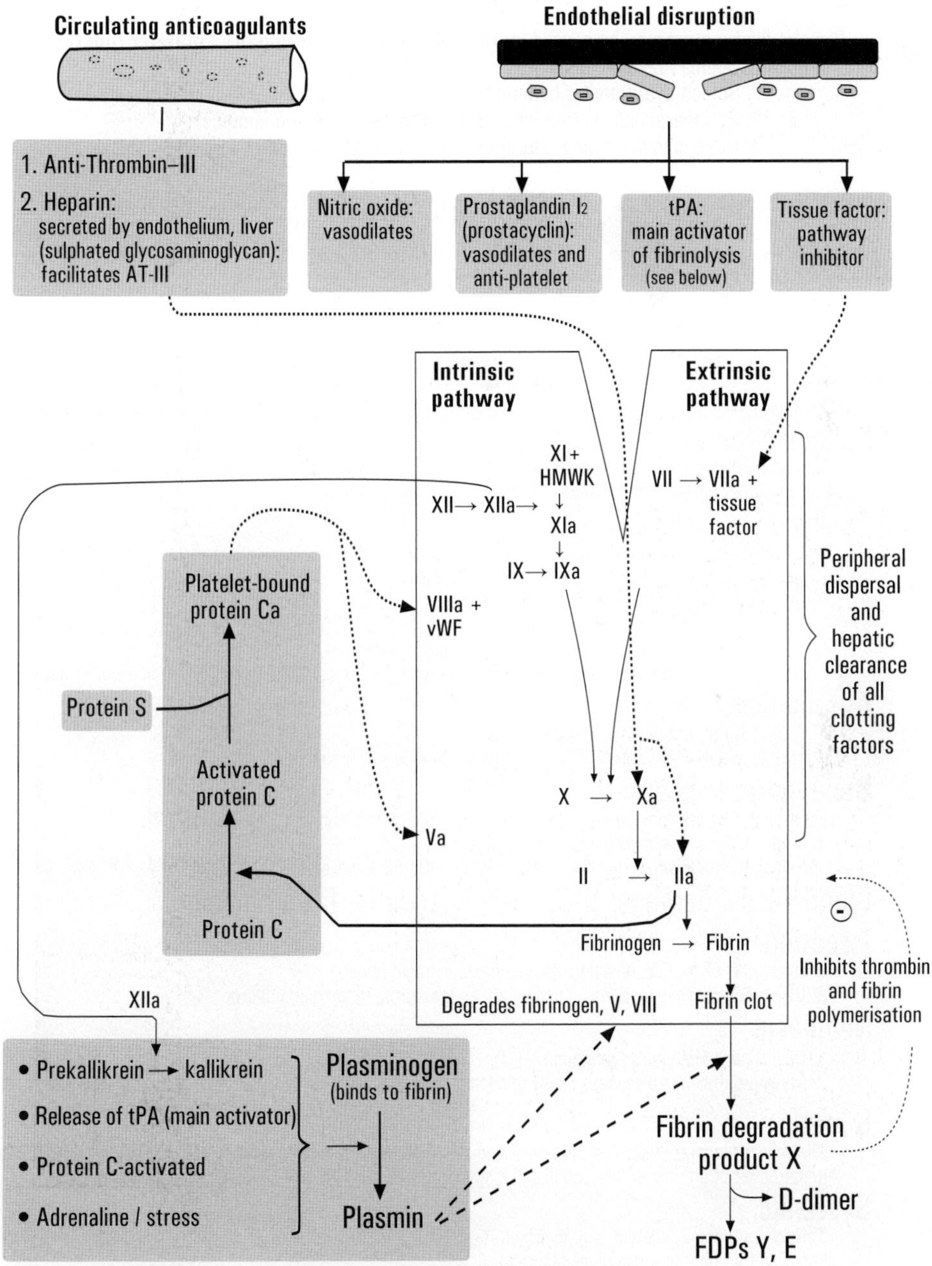

Circulating anticoagulants

Endothelial disruption

1. Anti-Thrombin–III
2. Heparin:
   secreted by endothelium, liver
   (sulphated glycosaminoglycan):
   facilitates AT-III

Nitric oxide:
vasodilates

Prostaglandin I₂
(prostacyclin):
vasodilates and
anti-platelet

tPA:
main activator
of fibrinolysis
(see below)

Tissue factor:
pathway
inhibitor

Intrinsic pathway

Extrinsic pathway

XI +
HMWK
↓
XIa
↓
IXa

XII → XIIa →

IX → IXa

VII → VIIa +
tissue
factor

Platelet-bound
protein Ca

VIIIa +
vWF

Peripheral
dispersal
and
hepatic
clearance
of all
clotting
factors

Protein S

Activated
protein C

Va

X → Xa

Protein C

II → IIa

XIIa

Fibrinogen → Fibrin

Degrades fibrinogen, V, VIII

Fibrin clot

⊖

Inhibits thrombin
and fibrin
polymerisation

• Prekallikrein → kallikrein

• Release of tPA (main activator)

• Protein C-activated

• Adrenaline / stress

Plasminogen
(binds to fibrin)

↓

Plasmin

Fibrin degradation
product X

↘ D-dimer

FDPs Y, E

All dotted lines represent inhibition; dashed lines represent proteolysis

Platelet Disorders

Causes

Platelet dysfunction may be caused by **thrombocytopenia** or **impaired platelet function**.
Thrombocytopenia may be caused by:

      1. Spleen overactivity: hypersplenism
      2. Peripheral destruction (immune) or consumption (non-immune)
      3. Bone marrow hypoproduction: megakaryocyte failure

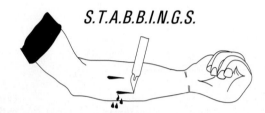

S.T.A.B.B.I.N.G.S.

Spleen: hypersplenism
Path: Phagocytes remove platelets, and large spleen sequesters 60–90% platelets (normal = 30%)
Causes: CML, portal hypertension, CCF (all cause pancytopenia)

Toxins
Path: Most are immune-mediated, but chemotherapy and alcohol have bone marrow suppressant effects.
Causes: *V.A.N.Q.U.I.S.H.E.D.*
      Valproate; **A**lcohol; **N**euro – benzodiazepines, cocaine; **QU**inine;
      Inflammatory – indomethacin, gold, penicillamine (NSAIDs inhibit platelet function);
      Sulphonylureas, sulphonamides (+penicillins); **H**eparin;
      Extra – blood transfusions (anti-HPA-1a in multiparous women); **D**igoxin, **D**iuretics – thiazides

Autoimmune
    1° : Immune thrombocytopenic purpura (ITP)
    2° : SLE, Evan's syndrome (ITP + autoimmune haemolytic anaemia)

Bone marrow failure
    1. Normocytic anaemia: aplastic anaemia, bone marrow replacement, diet (starvation)
    2. Megaloblastic anaemia: folate or B12 deficiency
    3. Selective megakaryocyte failure: e.g. Wiskott–Aldrich syndrome, HIV, alcohol

Blood vessel damage: DIC, TTP, vasculitis, fat embolism

Infection:
    1. Virus: HIV, EBV, VZV, measles; dengue haemorrhagic fever
    2. Other: septicaemia (esp. meningococcal), endocarditis, rickettsia, malaria

Neoplasia
    1. CLL (B-cell), Hodgkin's lymphoma – ITP
    2. Myeloproliferative disease; paraproteinaemia, esp. Waldenström's – causes impaired platelet function

Genetic
Thrombocytopenia: Wiskott–Aldrich or Chediak–Higashi syndromes: impaired megakaryocyte production
Impaired function: von Willebrand disease; glycoprotein, platelet granule or thromboxane deficiency

Systemic
Thrombocytopenia: dilution, e.g. overhydration
Impaired function: uraemia, liver failure
Artefactual: clotted blood or anti-platelet antibodies (dependent on EDTA, ∴ retake in citrated tube!)

<u>**PC**</u>

General: 1. Superficial: skin purpura or petechiae
2. Mucous membranes: epistaxis, gums, GIT, menorrhagia, haematuria
3. Deep: intracerebral haemorrhage

ITP: 1. Childhood: acute, mild, self-limiting
2. Adult: chronic, severe, relapsing–remitting

<u>**Ix**</u>

Bloods:
1. FBC, film, platelet size:
 a) Large platelets : ITP, myeloproliferative disease, grey platelet syn. (α-granule deficiency)
 b) Small platelets : CRF
2. Auto-antibodies:
 a) Anti-glycoprotein IIb–IIIa (IgG, M): ITP; anti-P1^{A1} : post-transfusion purpura
 b) ANA
 c) Direct Coombs' test (Evans' syndrome)
3. DIC tests: film showing schistocytes, clotting, FDPs, D-dimers, circulating fibrin monomer

Micro: HIV, EBV serology

Radio: abdominal USS – splenomegaly

Special:
1. Bone marrow – fine-needle aspirate and biopsy:
 • Megakaryocyte number ↓ : bone marrow failure
 • Megakaryocyte number ↑ : peripheral destruction
2. Aggregation times impaired with:
 • Adrenalin, ADP: δ-granule or COX–deficiency (genetic or aspirin), ET
 • Ristocetin: von Willebrand's disease
3. Other platelet studies:
 • Granule contents (↓ed in storage pool diseases, myeloproliferative disease)
 • Glycoprotein quantification, arachidonic acid metabolism, Ca flux studies
4. Ivy template bleeding time

Method: 2x incisions on volar forearm: 1 cm long, 1 mm deep
Result: +ve = bleeding time > 8 min
Interpretation: platelet count < 75 x 10^9/l, or impaired platelet function

<u>**Rx**</u>

ITP

Supportive: platelet transfusion: (half-life = hours)
Severe: prednisolone or IVIg
Chronic:
1. Immunosuppression: steroids, azathioprine, cyclophosphamide, rituximab
2. Other drugs: danazol, colchicine, IFN-α, high-dose Vit C
3. Splenectomy: if platelet count < 30 x 10^9/l, or intolerant of steroids, or young

Purpura

Def
1. Purpura = pink–red macules < 1 cm;
   Petechiae = very fine macules
2. Non-blanching – due to intradermal
   bleeding

PC The type of tissues in which bleeding
occurs suggests the underlying cause:-

Vascular:
Petechiae, purpura, bruises
Platelets:
1. Petechiae, purpura, bruises
2. Mucous membrane bleeds:
   epistaxis, gums, GIT, menorrhagia, urine
3. Deep: intracerebral
Clotting:
1. Petechiae, purpura, bruises
2. Mucous membrane bleeds
3. Deep: intracerebral, haemarthroses,
   subcutaneous (nerve palsies),
   teeth, tongue, trauma, bowel

Ix
Vascular:
1. FBC, film and clotting times are normal
2. Tourniquet Hess test:
   Blood pressure cuff inflated for 5 min:
   count petechiae within 2.5 cm diameter
   circle measured 4 cm below cubital fossa
   If > 20 petechiae = capillary fragility ↑
Platelets:
1. FBC: platelets ↓ or normal:
   • Platelet count ↓:
     film, bone marrow,
     autoAbs, FDPs
   • Platelet count normal:
     platelet function times, inc.
     Ivy template bleeding time:
     forearm incisions 1 cm long, 1 mm
     deep:
     if bleeding time > 8 mins ⇒ abnormal
     platelet function
Clotting:
1. Clotting times ↑
2. Dilution studies:
   Does normal serum correct?
3. Clotting factor, vWF assays
N.B. bleeding time normal

Causes
Vascular Defect

V.I.G.I.L.A.N.T.

Vitamin C deficiency – scurvy:
Path: Vit C is required for collagen cross-linking
O/E: 1. Perifollicular petechiae
     2. Gum bleeding

Infection: due to immune complexes:
1. Meningococcaemia
2. Rickettsia
3. Viruses: measles, dengue haemorrhagic fever
   (all also associated with low platelet count)

Genetic:
1. Collagen disease: ED-IV, OI, Marfan's
2. Pseudoxanthoma elasticum (AD / AR)
3. Hereditary haemorrhagic telangiectasia (AD):
   endoglin mutation

Injury:
1. Mechanical
2. Thrombotic thrombocytopenic purpura

Leg purpura:
chronic venous stasis or venous hypertension:
1. DVT
2. Excessive standing
3. Right-sided heart failure
4. Excessive coughing or vomiting

Limiting, self:
1. Senile purpura
2. Painful bruising syndrome:
   Epi: Women of child-bearing age
   PC: Prodromal tingling under skin;
       Bruising of limbs, trunk

Autoimmune:
1. Vasculitis: Henoch–Schönlein purpura,
                polyarteritis nodosa (men)
2. SLE, rheumatoid arthritis
3. Cryoglobulinaemia

Neoplasia:
Amyloid – esp. facial purpura from AL amyloid
(Ix: Serum and urine electrophoresis)

Toxins:
1. Steroid
2. Gold, penicillamine

Coagulopathy

V.I.G.I.L.A.N.T.

Vitamin K deficiency:
Path: Vit K epoxide Reductase causes γ-carboxylation
of glutamate residue on clotting factors
II, VII, IX, X $\Rightarrow$ enables Ca binding $\Rightarrow$
adsorption onto phospholipid surfaces
1. Malnutrition
2. Malabsorption – coeliac, chronic pancreatitis
3. Antibiotics
4. Haemorrhagic disease of newborn

Infection, due to DIC

Genetic
1. Haemophilias: VIII C (A), IX (B), XI, VII – mild;
XIII – severe
2. von Willebrand disease, type 3

Injury: due to DIC

Liver: obstructive jaundice:
due to ↓ Vit K absorption

Liver: hepatocellular dysfunction:
due to ↓ clotting factor synthesis,
↓ tPA detoxification, and DIC

Acute pancreatitis:
pancreatic proteases degrade clotting factors
PC: Bruising in flanks and umbilicus (Cullen's sign)

Autoimmune: circulating VIII inhibitors:
complication of haemophilia

Neoplasia:
1. Paraproteinaemia; amyloid:
due to factor X and fibrinogen deficiency
2. Acute myeloid leukaemia M3
3. Metastatic carcinoma – hyperplasminaemia

Toxins:
1. Anticoagulants: heparin, warfarin
2. Other: asparaginase, isoniazid (blocks XIII activity)

Transfusion, massive: dilutional effect

Thrombolysis:
1. tPA
2. Hyperplasminaemia: primary or secondary to
congenital cyanotic heart disease

Platelet Defect (p. 470)

S.T.A.B.B.I.N.G.S.

All cause **thrombocytopenia**, except where indicated
as causing **impaired platelet function**

Spleen: hypersplenism:
CML, portal hypertension, CCF

Toxins:

V.A.N.Q.U.I.S.H.E.D.
Valproate;
Alcohol;
Neuro – benzodiazepines, cocaine;
QUinine; **I**nflammatory – indomethacin, gold;
Sulphonylureas, sulphonamides (+ penicillins);
Heparin; **E**xtra – blood transfusions (anti-P1^{A1});
Digoxin, **D**iuretics – thiazides
+ impaired function (NSAIDs)

Autoimmune:
1. 1°: Immune thrombocytopenic purpura (ITP)
2. 2°: SLE, Evans' syndrome (ITP + haemolysis)

Bone marrow failure:
1. Normocytic anaemia:
• Aplastic anaemia
• Bone marrow replacement
• Diet (starvation)
2. Megaloblastic anaemia: folate or B12 deficiency
3. Selective megakaryocyte failure:
e.g. HIV, alcohol

Blood vessel damage:
DIC, TTP, vasculitis, fat embolism

Infection:
1. Viruses: HIV; EBV, VZV
2. Other: septicaemia, endocarditis; malaria

Neoplasia:
1. CLL (B-cell), Hodgkin's lymphoma: ITP
2. Myeloproliferative disease
3. Impaired function: paraproteinaemia,
esp. Waldenström's (hyperviscosity syndrome)

Genetic:
1. Thrombocytopenia: Wiskott–Aldrich or
Chediak–Higashi syndromes
2. Impaired function: von Willebrand disease;
glycoprotein, granule, TXA2 deficiency

Systemic:
1. Thrombocytopenia: dilution, e.g. overhydration
2. Impaired function: uraemia, liver failure
3. Artefactual: • Clotted blood
• Anti-platelet antibodies

Thrombosis

Prothrombotic states are summarized by Virchow's triad of pathological processes:
1. Endothelial injury: arterial thrombosis
2. Stasis: venous or cardiac thrombosis
3. Hypercoagulability: venous > arterial thrombosis

Each pathology tends to be associated with thrombosis in particular parts of the circulation, as shown. However, all 3 processes are probably involved at each instance of thrombosis, e.g. an atherosclerotic plaque may rupture causing endothelial injury; exposure of procoagulants, and turbulence with pockets of stasis.

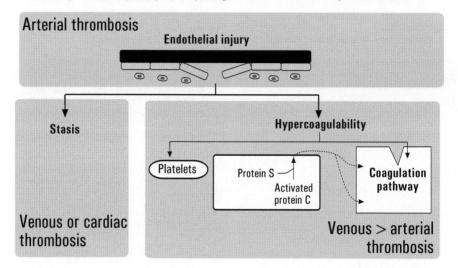

Causes   *A.D.V.I.S.E. O.R. H.E.P.A.R.I.N.I.S.E.*

Endothelial injury

Atherosclerosis: hypertension, DM, cholesterol, smoking
Arteriosclerosis: hypertension, DM

Dissection: hypertension, connective tissue mutation – Ehlers–Danlos, Marfan's
Dysplasia: fibromuscular

Vasculitis: • Autoimmune (e.g. polyarteritis nodosa, giant-cell arteritis, SLE)
              • Infection (e.g. TB, syphilis, Pneumococcus, Chlamydia)
Valvulitis: endocarditis, aortic stenosis

Injury: trauma, catheterization (angioplasty), indwelling central line
Injury: radiation

Spasm: migraine, variant angina
Sarcoidosis

External compression: e.g. tumour, cervical rib
Embolism: should be considered as a mechanism in any case of arterial ischaemia

Stasis

Obesity
Operation: esp. hip or other orthopaedic, or for cancer
Recumbency: e.g. long-haul flight, peripartum, debilitated
Right-sided heart failure: or other venous hypertension, inc. varicose veins

Hypercoagulability

Hereditary:
    1. Prothrombin mutation
    2. Factor V Leiden mutation (activated protein C resistance);
        protein S or C deficiency; anti-thrombin-III deficiency
    3. Fibrinolysis defect: fibrinogen or plasminogen mutation; tPA ↓; tPA inhibitor ↑
    4. Homocystinuria

Endocrine:
    1. Estrogens: • Pregnancy: phlegmasia alba dolens (3rd trimester / Puerperium)
                 • OCP: ↑ Vit K-dependent CFs, VIII; ↓ AT-III, tPA
                 • HRT: Although ↓ LDL / HDL and hence ↓ IHD
    2. Androgens: anabolic steroids, danazol (anti-estrogen), 'Dianette' (anti-androgen)
    3. Diabetes mellitus: esp. due to HONK

Polycythaemia; **P**araproteinaemia; **PNH** (paroxysmal nocturnal haemoglobinuria):
    1. Polycythaemia, including myeloproliferative disease (hyperviscosity)
    2. Paraproteinaemia (hyperviscosity)
    3. Other haematological: PNH, sickle cell disease, Fe deficiency, DIC, TTP

Autoimmune:
    1. Antiphospholipid syndrome (primary or associated with SLE)
    2. Vasculitis: Behçet's syndrome, PAN, Wegener's, Sjögren's syndrome
    3. Ulcerative colitis
    + Sarcoidosis

Renal:
    1. Nephrosis: due to glomerular loss of AT-III
    2. Dehydration

Injury; **I**nfarction: due to increased sympathetic response and CRP elevation

Neoplasia:
    1. Adenocarcinoma (mucin / protease-secreting), e.g. pancreas, bronchus, breast, bowel
        PC: 'Trousseau's phenomenon' = migratory thrombophlebitis
    2. Acute leukaemia (AML or ALL)
    3. Local: • Portal vein thrombosis, secondary to carcinoma of pancreas, liver, adrenal
              • Cerebral vein thrombosis, secondary to head–neck squamous cell carcinoma

Infection
    1. Systemic: endotoxinaemia (lipopolysaccharide), TB, Chlamydia
    2. Local: cellulitis (DVT); otitis media, sinusitis (cerebral vein thrombosis)

Smoking; **S**enility (increasing age)

Exogenous: chemotherapy (L-asparaginase, methotrexate); steroids; COX-2 inhibitors

<u>Disseminated Intravascular Coagulation</u>

<u>**Def**</u>   Disseminated Intravascular Coagulation (DIC) =
1. Run-away control of haemostasis
2. Triggered by: a) Extensive endothelial disruption, e.g. infection, trauma, AVM
                   b) Procoagulant release, e.g. neoplasia, placental disruption
3. Results in consumption, and consequently depletion, of platelets and clotting factors

<u>Causes</u>   *Make sure you N.O.T.I.C.E. it !!*

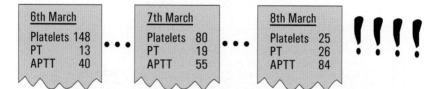

6th March		7th March		8th March
Platelets 148	● ● ●	Platelets 80	● ● ●	Platelets 25
PT 13		PT 19		PT 26
APTT 40		APTT 55		APTT 84

Neoplasia
1. Mucin-secreting adenocarcinoma: pancreas, gastric, breast, bronchus
2. AML: acute promyelocytic leukaemia – M3

Obstetric
1. Abortion: septic, missed, retained products of conception
2. Peri-partum: eclampsia; placental abruption; amniotic fluid embolism

Trauma
1. Crush injury, surgery, burns
2. Hyperthermia or hypothermia
3. Hypoxia (acute)

Infection
1. Bacterial: meningococcaemia, coliforms (endotoxin),
              Clostridium perfringens, leptospirosis
2. Viral: purpura fulminans, esp. CMV, VZV, hepatitis
3. Malaria – *Plasmodium falciparum*: large procoagulant release

Congenital
AVM, e.g. Kasabach–Merritt syndrome: giant haemangioma in infants

Extra
1. Acute anaphylaxis
2. Blood transfusion reaction
3. Liver failure

<u>**Prognosis**</u>   1. Large spectrum of severity, including asymptomatic cases
             2. 50% mortality rate (because of associated condition)

<u>Path</u>

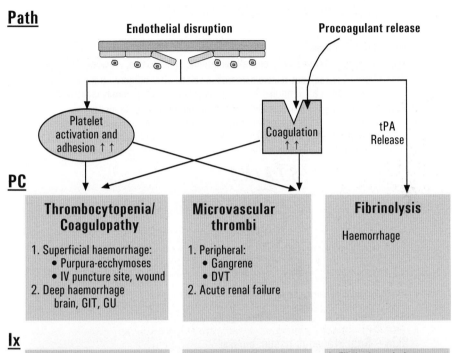

<u>PC</u>

Thrombocytopenia/ Coagulopathy	**Microvascular thrombi**	**Fibrinolysis**
		Haemorrhage
1. Superficial haemorrhage: • Purpura-ecchymoses • IV puncture site, wound 2. Deep haemorrhage brain, GIT, GU	1. Peripheral: • Gangrene • DVT 2. Acute renal failure	

<u>Ix</u>

1. Platelets ↓ 2. Clotting APTT↑, PT↑, TT↑, Fibrinogen ↓ N.B. Clotting times may be normal in DIC, due to presence of activated clotting factors!	1. Film - schistocytes, due to microangiopathic haemolytic anaemia (MAHA) 2. AT-III ↓	1. Fibrin degradation products X + Y ↑ 2. D-dimer ↑ 3. Euglobin clot lysis time ↓ 4. Circulating fibrin monomer: ethanol–gelatin test

<u>Rx</u> Underlying condition +

1. Platelet concentrates • Fresh frozen plasma • Cryoprecipitate (fibrinogen) 2. Fresh whole blood	Heparin: for dangerous thrombosis, e.g. DVT, PE, PVD	Anti-fibrinolytics: 1. ε-aminocaproic acid 2. Aprotinin ☠: Acute renal failure, so need to give adjunctive low-dose heparin

Haemophilias

Haemophilia A (Factor VIII Deficiency)

Epi   **I**nc: 1/10,000 males

Age: Presents in 1st year, e.g. cephalhaematoma, circumcision, crawling (bruising)

Sex: Males (X-linked), but female carriers may bleed after surgery / trauma due to 'lyonization', i.e.– if normal X-chromosome is disproportionately inactivated

Aet: 1. Hereditary – 75%: X-linked disease: numerous mutations on Xq
Sporadic – 25%, i.e. new mutation or latent carriership for several generations
2. ↓ Synthesis of VIII from liver, spleen, kidney + lymphoid tissue
3. Anti-VIII:C antibodies in 20%

PC   *S.T.A.I.N.S.*

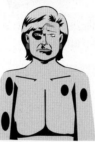

Skin – **S**ubcutaneous tissue: bruising

Teeth (dental extraction) / **T**ongue (haematoma → stridor)

Arthritis:
   i) Acute haemarthroses: esp. hip, knee, ankle
   ii) Osteoarthritis: due to recurrent haemarthroses → ankylosis + muscle atrophy
   iii) Bony pseudotumours / cysts: due to subperiosteal bleeding → pathological fractures

Intestine–urinary haemorrhage:
   i) GIT haemorrhage: due to coagulopathy / NSAIDs for arthritis / hepatitis C
   ii) GU haemorrhage / ureteric colic, papillary necrosis due to antifibrinolytic use

Neurological:
   i) CVA (Bleed): Commonest cause of death
   ii) Femoral nerve compression – 2° to retroperitoneal–psoas sheath haematoma
   iii) Compartment syndrome due to muscle / fascial haemorrhage

Nose: epistaxis

Side-effects of Rx:
   1: AIDS, hepatitis A–G from transfusions pre-1990s (HIV), pre-2000 (HCV)
   2: Factor VIII inhibitor in 20% of pts
   3: Thrombosis, due to antifibrinolytics, DDAVP, prothrombin complex

Severity depends on % VIII activity: 20–5%: mild bleeding post-op. or trauma
                                         5–1%: infrequent spontaneous bleeding
                                         < 1%: frequent, severe spontaneous bleeds

Ix

1. Clotting times
APTT: ↑
1. 50:50 mix with normal plasma: normalizes APTT
2. 50:50 VIII-deficient plasma: - APTT still ↑:
   allows quantification or determination of carrier status (< 75% VIII activity)
3. Immune assay of individual factors: VIII, IX, vWF
PT: Normal
TT: Normal

2. Genetic screening
Methods: RFLP; DNA hybridization; PCR
Used to amplify chorionic villus sampled blood (10–12 weeks) or umbilical vein (18–20 weeks)

Rx

Conservative
1. Avoidance: contact sports, unnecessary dental Rx; NSAIDs; IM injections
2. Vaccines: Hep B; regular LFTs
3. Haemarthrosis: rest, splint, elevate; physiotherapy: prevents joint fibrosis

Factor VIII concentrate
1. Source: FFP, cryoprecipitate; lyophilized (virus-inactivated);
   immunoaffinity (adsorbed + eluted onto monoclonal Abs); recombinant DNA
2. Indications: Used to raise VIII activity to > 30% activity in acute haemorrhage, or as
   prophylaxis, e.g. before sports or dental procedures
3. ☹: a) Inhibitors i.e. Anti VIII IgG
   Rx: • High-dose VIII; only if low Ig titre; porcine VIII
   • Prothrombin complex concentrates = trace quantities of activated clotting factors
   • Immunosuppression; immunodepletion
   b) Autoimmune haemolytic anaemia – due to anti-A and -B in intermediate-purity concentrates
   c) Allergy

DDAVP (Desmopressin = ADH) – IVI or nasal snuff:
1. Releases VIII + vWF from endothelium; stabilizes VIII in plasma
2. Indications: acute haemorrhage in mild disease, as endothelium contains only limited stores
3. ☹: Thrombosis esp. in elderly; hyponatraemia

Antifibrinolytics tranexamic acid or ε-aminocaproic acid (IV, PO, mouth wash):
1. Inhibits plasmin formation by tPA (which is also released from endothelium by DDAVP!)
2. Indications: acute haemorrhage or prophylaxis; as an adjunct to DDAVP.

Haemophilia B (Factor IX Deficiency) or 'Xmas Disease'

Epi: 1/3 rd as common as haemophilia A, but also X- linked
PC: As for haemophilia A
Ix: Immune assay reveals IX deficiency; otherwise as for haemophilia A
Rx: Factor IX concentrate – longer half-life than VIII (less frequent infusions); **DDAVP is ineffective!**

Factor XI Deficiency

Mild bleeding disorder, tends to occur in Ashkenazi Jews, and is autosomal recessive

Factor XIII Deficiency

Severe bleeding disorder with infertility and abortions. Rare and autosomal recessive
Ix: Urea-dissolution test (XIII assay)

Blood Transfusion Complications

Incidence   Any reaction = 2%; death = 2/100,000

Early

Haemolytic Reaction – Immediate   (1/12,000 transfusions)
Causes:
    1. Blood-group mismatch:
      ABO – intravascular haemolysis: IgG, IgM, classical complement pathway
      RhD, Kell – extravascular haemolysis: IgG, C3b, mononuclear phagocytic system
    2. Mechanical: faulty blood warmer; pumps, tubes
PC: 1. General: fever, shock, acute renal failure
    2. GIT symptoms: N+V, diarrhoea, abdominal–back pain
    3. Chest symptoms: chest pain, SOB, wheeze
    4. Skin symptoms: pruritus, jaundiced (haemolysis)
Ix: 1. Sample donor and recipient blood: serology, cross-match, direct Coombs' test, blood culture
    2. Haemolysis tests: unconjugated BR, AST, LDH; reticulocytes, α2-haptoglobin
      Intravascular haemolysis: haemoglobinuria, haemosiderinuria
    3. Complications:- screen for DIC (FDPs and D-dimers) and MAHA (film: schistocytes)
Rx: 1. Fluids, blood, FFP; 2. Hydrocortisone, chlorpheniramine; 3. 'Renal' dopamine, adrenaline, haemodialysis

Immune Reactions – Non-haemolytic

Non-haemolytic febrile transfusion reaction (N.H.F.T.R.)   (1/50 transfusions)
Path: Anamnestic response to HLA-I and -II on WBCs, and platelets (HLA-I only),
      due to previous transfusion or pregnancies
PC: fever at 30 min – 2 hr; flushing; tachycardia
Prophylaxis: WBC-depleted products ('buffy-coat depleted'); in-line filters

Allergy – types -   (1/50 transfusions)
1. Atopy: plasma proteins of donor, e.g. Igs, react in atopic pt $\Rightarrow$ mild urticaria (continue transfusion)
2. IgA deficiency: reaction against donor IgA $\Rightarrow$ anaphylactic shock
3. Inadvertent donor antigen: e.g. C4-albumin, penicillin, ethylene oxide

Pulmonary leucagglutinin reaction   (1/5000 transfusions)
Path: Donor or recipient has high anti-granulocyte Ab titre due to past transfusion or multiparity
PC: 1. Non-cardiogenic pulmonary oedema due to agglutination and leucostasis in lungs
    2. Neutropenia (cytotoxicity); 3. Shock (complement-driven vasodilation)

Infection

Endotoxin (Rx: anti-endotoxin IgM)
Bacteria, e.g. coliforms, Pseudomonas, Yersinia (Rx: piperacillin + gentamicin)

Overload – fluid: Presents as features of congestive cardiac failure

   + delivery problems: thrombophlebitis; air embolism
   + massive transfusion complications:
        1. Hypothermia
        2. Ion toxicity (transfused citrate $\Rightarrow$ Ca$\downarrow$; K$\uparrow$; acid–base disturbance)
        3. Clotting factor and platelet depletion / DIC (give platelets and FFPs after 4 units)

<u>Late</u>

Haemolytic Reaction – Delayed   (1/1000 transfusions)

Cause   • Due to delayed, $2°$ immune response to RBC alloantigen other than those routinely screened for
         • It is not detected pre-transfusion by cross-matching because of low recipient antibody levels
         • Risk increased by previous transfusions or in multiparous women
         • Extravascular haemolysis

PC: 1. Occurs 1 day–2 weeks after transfusion
        2. Hb fails to rise; jaundice (but may be life-threatening)

Ix: 1. Direct Coombs' test
        2. Indirect Coombs' test: Ab screen against wide RBC Ag assay; quantify by no. of units lysed
        3. Type donor blood given

Immune Reactions – Non-haemolytic

Alloantigen sensitization = Abs generated to RBC or HLA antigens, without reaction:
  predisposes to future transfusion reactions, including haemolytic disease of the newborn

Post-transfusion purpura
        Cause: • Where recipient lacks platelet antigen HPA-1a (GPIIIa receptor), transfusion
                 leads to development of anti-platelet antibodies to both donor and self platelets
               • 2% population lack HPA-1A; Abs more likely in multiparous women
        PC: Thrombocytopenia at 7–10 days post-transfusion

GVHD or immunosuppression
  • Immunocompromised patients may develop GVHD by donor T-cell activity
  • Lymphopenia may occur in post-surgery transfusion

Infection

Bacteria: syphilis, *Salmonella*, *Brucella*
Viruses: hepatitis B,C,E,G; HTLV-I; HIV; CMV (significant if recipient immunocompromised)
Parasites: malaria, toxoplasmosis, microfilariasis
Other: prion

Overload – Iron

At-risk groups = recurrent transfusions:
    1. Congenital: thalassaemia major or intermedia; pure red-cell aplasia (Diamond–Blackfan syndrome)
    2. Acquired: aplastic anaemia; myelodysplasia, myelofibrosis

Complications (as for $1°$ haemochromatosis – see p. 160

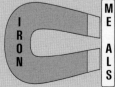

M yocardial deposition: dysrhythmias
E ndocrine: Pituitary (growth failure; hypogonadism)
                   Pancreas (DM); Parathyroid (Ca ↓) / thyroid (T4 ↓)
A rthritis
L iver: cirrhosis
S kin: pigmentation due to haemosiderin and melanin

Glossary

1,25-DHCC	1,25-dihydroxycholecalciferol
17-KS	17-ketosteroids
2,3-DPG	2,3-diphosphoglycerate
25-HCC	25-hydroxycholecalciferol
2-D	two-dimensional
3-D	three-dimensional
3TC	lamivudine
5-HIAA	5-hydroxyindoleacetic acid
5-HT	serotonin (5-hydroxytryptamine)
5-HT$_3$	type 3 serotonin receptor
5-HTP	5-hydroxytryptophan
11BHSD	11β-hydroxysteroid dehydrogenase
AA	amino acid(s)
AAA	abdominal aortic aneurysm
AAFB	alcohol- and acid-fast bacilli
Ab	antibody
ABG	arterial bypass graft, arterial blood gases
ABP	arterial blood pressure
ABPA	allergic bronchopulmonary aspergillosis
ABVD	doxorubicin, bleomycin, vinblastine and dacarbazine
AcAc	acetoacetate
AcCoA	acetyl coenzyme A
ACE	angiotensin-converting enzyme
ACEI	ACE inhibitor
Ach	acetylcholine
AchR	acetylcholine receptor
ACTH	adrenocorticotrophic hormone
AD	autosomal dominant
ADEM	acute disseminated encephalomyelitis
ADH	antidiuretic hormone (=AVP)
ADHD	attention deficit hyperactivity disorder
ADP	adenosine diphosphate
AE	air entry or adverse effects
AED	anti-epileptic drug
AF	atrial fibrillation
AFB	acid-fast bacilli
AFP	α-fetoprotein
Ag	antigen
AICA	anterior inferior cerebellar artery
AIDP	acute inflammatory demyelinating polyneuropathy
AIDS	acquired immunodeficiency syndrome
AIHA	autoimmune haemolytic anaemia
A-II	angiotensin-II receptor
AION	anterior ischaemic optic neuropathy
Al(OH)$_3$	aluminium hydroxide
ALA	aminolaevulinic acid
Alb	albumin
Alk. Phos.	alkaline phosphatase
ALL	acute lymphoblastic leukaemia
ALP	alkaline phosphatase
α$_1$-AT	α$_1$-antitrypsin
ALS	amyotrophic lateral sclerosis
ALT	alanine aminotransferase (transaminase)
AMA	antimitochondrial antibody
AM(S)AN	acute motor (and sensory) axonal neuropathy
AML	acute myeloid leukaemia
AMML	acute myelomonocytic leukaemia
ANA	antinuclear antibodies
ANCA	antineutrophil cytoplasmic antibodies
Ank. Spond.	ankylosing spondylitis
ANP	atrial natriuretic peptide
Anti-LKM	antibodies to liver-kidney microsomes
AP	anteroposterior, abdominoperineal
APB	apex beat
APC	adenomatous polyposis coli
APKD	adult polycystic kidney disease
APSAC	anisoylated plasminogen streptokinase activator complex
APTT	activated partial thromboplastin time
APUD	amine precursor uptake and decarboxylation
AR	aortic regurgitation, autosomal recessive
ARAS	ascending reticular activating system
ARC	AIDS-related complex
ARDS	adult respiratory distress syndrome
ARF	acute renal failure
AS	aortic stenosis
ASD	atrial septal defect
ASH	asymmetric septal hypertrophy
ASIS	anterior superior iliac spine
ASO	anti-streptolysin O
AST	aspartate aminotransferase (transaminase)
AT	antitrypsin
AT-III	anti-thrombin III
ATN	acute tubular necrosis
ATP	adenosine triphosphate
AV	aortic valve, arteriovenous, atrioventricular
A-V	atrioventricular
AVM	arteriovenous malformation
AVN	atrioventricular node
AVNRE	atrioventricular nodal re-entry (tachycardia)
AVP	arginine vasopressin (=ADH)
AVRE	atrioventricular re-entry (tachycardia)
AVRT	atrioventricular re-entry tachycardia
AXR	abdominal X-ray
Aza/AZA	azathioprine

AZT	azidothymidine (zidovudine)	CIDP	chronic inflammatory demyelinating polyneuropathy
Ba	barium	CJD	Creutzfeldt-Jakob disease
BAL	bronchoalveolar lavage	CK	creatine kinase
BCG	bacille Calmette-Guérin	Cl^-	chloride
β-B	beta blockers	CLL	chronic lymphocytic leukaemia
β-HCG	β human chorionic gonadotrophin	CMC	carpometacarpal
BHB	β-hydroxybutyrate	CMI	cell-mediated immunity
BHC	benzene hexachloride	CML	chronic myeloid leukaemia
BHL	bihilar lymphadenopathy	CMML	chronic myelomonocytic leukaemia
BJP	Bence Jones protein	CMT	Charcot-Marie-Tooth (disease)
blk	block	CMV	cytomegalovirus
BM	bone marrow or name of manufacturer of 'BM stick'	CMZ	carbamazepine
		CNS	central nervous system
BMPR	bone morphogenetic protein receptor	CO	cardiac output, carbon monoxide
BNH	bilateral nodular hyperplasia	CO_2	carbon dioxide
BO	bowel opening	CO_3	carbonate
BP	blood pressure	CoA	coenzyme A
bpm	beats per minute	COAD	chronic obstructive airways disease
BPPV	benign paroxysmal positional vertigo	COMT	catechol-*O*-methyltransferase
BR	bilirubin	COX	cyclooxygenase
BSE	bovine spongiform encephalopathy	CPAP	continuous positive airway pressure
Bx	biopsy	CPH	chronic persistent hepatitis
BXO	balanitis xerotica obliterans	CPR	cardiopulmonary resuscitation
ca./Ca.	carcinoma	CPT	carnitine palmitoyltransferase
Ca/Ca^{2+}	calcium	Cr	chromium, or creatinine
CABG	coronary artery bypass graft	CRAG	cryptococcal antigen
$CaCO_3$	calcium carbonate	CREST	calcinosis, Raynaud's, oesophageal and gut dysmotility, sclerodactyly, and telangiectasia
CADASIL	cerebral autosomal dominant arteriopathy with subcortical infarcts and leucoencephalopathy		
		CRF	chronic renal failure
CAG	cytosine-adenine-guanine	CRH	corticotrophin-releasing hormone
CAH	congenital adrenal hyperplasia, chronic autoimmune hepatitis	CRION	chronic relapsing inflammatory optic neuropathy
cAMP	cyclic adenosine monophosphate	CRP	C-reactive protein
c-ANCA	cytoplasmic anti-neutrophil cytoplasmic antibodies	CS	Churg-Strauss (syndrome)
		CSF	cerebrospinal fluid
CAPD	chronic ambulatory peritoneal dialysis	CSM	carotid sinus massage
CBD	corticobasal degeneration	CSU	catheter-specimen urine
CCF	congestive cardiac failure	CT	computed tomography
CCHD	cyanotic congenital heart disease	CTZ	chemoreceptor trigger zone
CCK	cholecystokinin	Cu	copper
CCl_4	carbon tetrachloride	CVA	cerebrovascular accident
CCU	coronary care unit	CVID	common variable immunodeficiency
CD	cluster differentiation antigen	CVP	central venous pressure
CEA	carcinoembryonic antigen	CVS	cardiovascular system
Cef	cefuroxime	CXR	chest X-ray
CF	cystic fibrosis, clotting factor	Cyt	cytochrome
CFA	cryptogenic fibrosing alveolitis	Δ	disorder, difference
CFTR	cystic fibrosis transmembrane regulator	D+V	diarrhoea and vomiting
CGD	chronic granulomatous disease	DA_2	type 2 dopamine receptor
cGMP	cyclic guanosine monophosphate	DAF	decay accelerating factor (CD55)
C_H50	complement functional assay	DAG	diacylglyceride
CHOP	cyclophosphamide, doxorubicin, vincristine and prednisolone	DBP	diastolic blood pressure
		DC	direct current
Chr	chromosome	*DCC*	deleted in colon cancer gene
CI	contraindication		

DDAVP®	desmopressin (1-deamino-8-D-arginine vasopressin)
ddC	zalcitabine (dideoxycytidine)
DDD	dual-chamber pacemaker
ddI	didanosine (dideoxyinosine)
DEET	diethyltoluamide
def.	deficiency
DEXA	dual-energy X-ray absorptiometry
DH	drug history
DHEA	dehydroepiandrostenedione
DHF	dihydrofolate
DHFR	dihydrofolate reductase
DI	diabetes insipidus
DIC	disseminated intravascular coagulation
DIDMOAD	diabetes insipidus, diabetes mellitus, optic atrophy, deafness + bladder atony
DIP	distal interphalangeal
DKA	diabetic ketoacidosis
DM	diabetes mellitus, dermatomyositis
DMARD	disease-modifying anti-rheumatoid drug
DMD	Duchenne muscular dystrophy
DMSA	dimercaptosuccinic acid
DMT-1	divalent metal transporter
DNA	deoxyribonucleic acid
DNase	deoxyribonuclease
DOC	11-deoxycorticosterone
DOTS	directly observed therapy
DRPLA	dentatorubral-pallidoluysian atrophy
dsDNA	double-stranded DNA
dTMP	deoxythymidine monophosphate
DTPA	diethylenetriamine pentaacetic acid
dUMP	deoxyuridine monophosphate
DVT	deep vein thrombosis
DXM	dexamethasone
DZ	dizygotic
E2	oestradiol
EBV	Epstein-Barr virus
ECC	ecchondroma
ECG	electrocardiography
ECHO	echocardiography, echovirus
ED	Ehlers-Danlos (syndrome)
EDTA	ethylenediamine tetraacetic acid
EEG	electroencephalography
ELISA	enzyme-linked immunosorbant assay
EMD	electromechanical dissociation, also termed pulseless electrical activity (PEA)
EMG	electromyography
EMU	early-morning urine
ENA	extractable nuclear antigen
ENC	enchondroma
ENT	ear, nose and throat
EPO	erythroporetin
ER	endoplasmic reticulum

ERCP	endoscopic retrograde cholangiopancreatography
ESM	ejection systolic murmur
ESR	erythrocyte sedimentation rate
ET	endotracheal
ET	essential thrombocythaemia
ethinylE2	ethinyloestradiol
F6P	fructose-6-phosphate
FAP	familial amyloid polyneuropathies
FB	foreign body
FBC	full blood count
FBPase	fructose-1,2-biphosphatase
FDP	fibrin degradation products
Fe	iron
FEV_1	forced expiratory volume in 1 second
FFA	free fatty acids
FFP	fresh frozen plasma
FH	family history, familial hyperlipidaemia
FiO_2	fractional concentration of oxygen in inspired air
FNA	fine-needle aspiration
FO	faeco-oral
FSGS	focal segmental glomerulosclerosis
FSH	facioscapulohumeral (dystrophy), follicle-stimulating hormone
fT3	free triiodothyronine
fT4	free thyroxine
FTA	fluorescent treponemal assay
FVC	forced vital capacity
G&S	Group and Save
G6Pase	glucose 6-phosphatase
G6PD	G6P dehydrogenase
GBM	glomerular basement membrane
GBS	Guillain-Barré syndrome
GCA	giant-cell arteritis
GCS	Glasgow Coma Scale
G-CSF	granulocyte colony-stimulating factor
GFR	glomerular filtration rate
GGP	glucose-6-phosphate
GGT	γ-glutamyl transpeptidase
GH	growth hormone
GHRH	growth hormone-releasing hormone
GI	gastrointestinal
GIT	gastrointestinal tract
Glu	glucose, glutamate
GLUT	glucose transporter
Gly	glycine
GM-CSF	granulocyte-macrophage colony-stimulating factor
GN	glomerulonephritis
GnRH	gonadotrophin-releasing hormone
G-O	gastro-oesophageal
GOR	gastro-oesophageal reflux
GP	glycoprotein
GPI	glycosylphosphatidylinositol
GRA	glucocorticoid-remediable aldosteronism

GTN	glyceryl trinitrate
GTP	guanosine triphosphate
GU	genitourinary
GVHD	graft-versus-host disease
H^+	hydrogen ion (proton)
H_1	type 1 histamine receptor
H_2	hydrogen, type 2 histamine receptor
H_2O_2	hydrogen peroxide
H_2S	hydrogen sulphide
HAART	highly active antiretroviral therapy
HACEK	*Haemophilus* spp., *Actinobacillus actinomycetemcomitans, Cardiobacterium hominis, Eikenella corrodens* and *Kingella kingae*
HAV	hepatitis A virus
HB	heart block
Hb	haemoglobin
HBV	hepatitis B virus
HCC	hepatocellular carcinoma
HCl	hydrochloric acid
HCO_3^-	bicarbonate
HCV	hepatitis C virus
HDL	high-density lipoprotein
HDV	hepatitis D virus
Hep	hepatitis
HGPRT	hypoxanthine-guanine phosphoribosyl transferase
HHT	hereditary haemorrhagic telangiectasia
HHV	human herpesvirus
HIV	human immunodeficiency virus
HLA	human leucocyte antigen
HMG CoA	3-hydroxy-3-methylglutaryl coenzyme A
HMMA	4-hydroxy-3-methoxymandelic acid (=VMA)
HMWK	high-molecular-weight kininogen
HNPCC	hereditary non-polyposis colon cancer
HOCM	hypertrophic obstructive cardiomyopathy
HONK	hyperosmolar non-ketoacidosis
HPA	human platelet antigen
hPL	human placental lactogen
HPOA	hypertrophic pulmonary osteoarthropathy
HPV	human papillomavirus
HR	heart rate
HRT	hormone-replacement therapy
HS	heart sounds
HSAN	hereditary sensory and autonomic neuropathy
HSP	Henoch-Schönlein purpura
HSV	herpes simplex virus
HT	hypertension
HTLV	human T-cell lymphotrophic virus
HUS	haemolytic-uraemic syndrome
I/I^-	iodine/iodide
IBD	inflammatory bowel disease
IBM	inclusion body myositis
ICP	intracranial pressure

ICS	intercostal space
IDDM	insulin-dependent diabetes mellitus
IDL	intermediate-density lipoprotein
IF	immunofluorescence
IFN	interferon
Ig	immunoglobulin
IGF	insulin-like growth factor
IHD	ischaemic heart disease
IL-1 (etc.)	interleukin-1 (etc.)
IL-1R (etc.)	interleukin-1 receptor (etc.)
IM/im	intramuscular
IND	indication
INR	International Normalized Ratio
IP	interphalangeal (joint)
IPKD	infant polycystic kidney disease
IPPV	intermittent positive-pressure ventilator
IQ	intelligence quotient
IRMA	intraretinal microvascular abnormalities
ISMN	isosorbide mononitrate
ITP	idiopathic thrombocytopenic purpura
ITU	intensive therapy unit
IUCD	intrauterine contraceptive device
IUD	intrauterine (contraceptive) device
IV/iv	intravenous
IVC	inferior vena cava
IVDU	intravenous drug user
IVI	intravenous infusion
IVIg	intravenous immunoglobulin
IVU	intravenous urography
JCA	juvenile chronic arthritis
JPS	joint position sense
JVP	jugular venous pressure
K/K^+	potassium ion
KCl	potassium chloride
$KClO_4$	potassium perchlorate
KCO	gas transfer coefficient (diffusion rate) across alveoli
KI	potassium iodide
KOH	potassium hydroxide
L	left
LBBB	left bundle branch block
LA	left atrium
LAD	left atrial dilatation, left axis deviation
LADP	left atrial diastolic pressure
LAP	left atrial pressure
LATS	long-acting thyroid stimulator (anti-TSH-R stimulating antibodies)
LCAT	lecithin:cholesterol acyltransferase
LDH	lactate dehydrogenase
LDL	low-density lipoprotein
LE	lupus erythematosus
LEMS	Lambert-Eaton myasthemic syndrome
LFT	liver function tests
LH	luteinizing hormone
LHOA	Leber's hereditary optic atrophy
LHRH	luteinizing hormone-releasing hormone

LHS	left hand side		MIBG	*m*-iodobenzylguanidine
LIF	left iliac fossa		MIP	maximum inspiratory pressure
LKM	(antibodies to) liver kidney microsomes		MMN	multifocal motor neuropathy with conduction block
LL	lepromatous leprosy		MMR	measles, mumps and rubella
LMN	lower motor neurone		MND	motor neurone disease
LMW	low-molecular-weight		Mø	macrophage
LN	lymph node		MODY	maturity-onset diabetes of young
LOC	loss of consciousness		MOPP	mustine, vincristine, procarbazine and prednisolone
LOS	lower oesophageal sphincter			
LOW	loss of weight		MPO	myeloperoxidase
LP	lumbar puncture		MPTP	1-methyl-4-phenyl-1,2,5,6-tetrahydropyridine
LPL	lipoprotein lipase			
LSE	left sternal edge		MR	mitral regurgitation, mortality rate
LSH	left side of heart		MRA	magnetic resonance angiography
LTB4	leukotriene B4		MRI	magnetic resonance venography
LV	left ventricle		mRNA	messenger RNA
LVEDP	left ventricular end-diastolic pressure		MRSA	methicillin-resistant *Staphylococcus aureus*
LVEDV	left ventricular end-diastolic volume			
LVF	left ventricular failure		MS	mitral stenosis, multiple sclerosis
LVH	left ventricular hypertrophy		MSA	multiple systems atrophy
LVP	left ventricular pressure		MSU	midstream urine
Ly	lymphocyte		MTP	metatarsophalangeal
mAchR	muscarinic acetylcholine receptor		MTX	methotrexate
MAD	mandibular advancement device		MuSK	muscle-specific kinase
MADSAM	multifocal acquired demyelinating sensory and motor (neuropathy)		MV	mitral valve
			MVP	mitral valve prolapse
MAG	myelin-associated glycoprotein		MVR	mitral valve replacement
MAG3	mercaptoacetyl triglycine (technetium scan)		MZ	monozygotic
			N	nerve
MAHA	microangiopathic haemolytic anaemia		N. Saline	normal saline
MAI	*Mycobacterium avium intracellulare*		N+V (+D)	nausea and vomiting (and diarrhoea)
MALT	mucosa-associated lymphoid tissue		N_2	nitrogen
MAO	monoamine oxidase		N_2O	nitrous oxide
MAOI	MAO inhibitor		Na	sodium
MAT	microscopic agglutination test		NABQI	*N*-acetyl-*p*-benzoquinoneimine
Mb	myoglobin		nAchR	nicotinic acetylcholine receptor
MCHC	mean corpuscular haemoglobin concentration		NaCl	sodium chloride
			NADH/NAD+	nicotinamide adenine dinucleotide (reduced/oxidized forms)
MCP	metacarpophalangeal			
MCTD	mixed connective tissue disease		NADPH	nicotinamide adenine dinucleotide phosphate
MCV	mean cell volume			
MDI	metered-dose inhaler		NAG	*N*-acetylglucosamine
MDR	multi-drug resistant		$NaHCO_3$	sodium bicarbonate
MECG	mixed essential cryoglobulinaemia		NAM	*N*-acetylmuramic acid
MELAS	mitochondrial encephalomyopathy, lactic acidosis and stroke-like episodes		NAP	neutrophil alkaline phosphatase
			NARTI	nucleoside analogue reverse transcriptase inhibitor
MEN	multiple endocrine neoplasia			
met	metastasis		NBM	nil by mouth
Mg/Mg^{2+}	magnesium		N.chromic	normochromic
$MgSiO_3$	magnesium silicate		N.cytic	normocytic
$MgSO_4$	magnesium sulphate		Neutroø	neutrophil
MGUS	monoclonal gammopathy of uncertain significance		NG	nasogastric
			NGT	nasogastric tube
MHC-I	major histocompatability complex class I molecule		NH_4^+	ammonium
			NIDDM	non-insulin-dependent diabetes mellitus
MI	myocardial infarction			

NK	neurokinin
NMJ	neuromuscular junction
NNARTI	non-nucleoside-analogue reverse transcriptase inhibitor
NO_2	nitrogen dioxide
NREM	non rapid eye movement
NSAID	non-steroidal anti-inflammatory drug
NSTEMI	non-ST-elevation myocardial infarction
O_2	oxygen
OA	osteoarthritis
OCP	oral contraceptive pill
OGD	oesophagogastroduedenoscopy
OGTT	oral glucose tolerance test
OI	osteogenesis imperfecta
OM	osteomalacia
OSA	obstructive sleep apnoea
OT	occupational therapy
P	phosphorus
P:S	pulmonary-to-systemic
P:SVR	ration of pulmonary to systemic vascular resistance
PABA	*p*-aminobenzoic acid
$PaCO_2$	partial pressure of carbon dioxide in arterial blood
PAF	platelet activating factor
PAN	polyarteritis nodosa
p-ANCA	perinuclear anti-neutrophil cytoplasmic antibodies
PaO_2	partial pressure of oxygen in arterial blood
PAO_2	alveolar partial pressure of oxygen
PAS	periodic acid-Schiff (stain)
PAWP	pulmonary arterial wedge pressure
PAXR	plain abdominal X-ray
PBC	primary biliary cirrhosis
PBG	porphobilinogen
PC	presenting complaint (used in a loose sense to include signs and abnormal tests)
PCOS	polycystic ovarian syndrome
PCP	*Pneumocystis carinii* pneumonia
PCR	polymerase chain reaction
PCT	proximal convoluted tubule
PCV	packed cell volume
PD	Parkinson's disease
PDA	patent ductus arteriosus
PDH	pyruvate dehydrogenase
PE	pulmonary embolism
PEEP	positive end-expiratory pressure
PEFR	peak expiratory flow rate
PEG	percutaneous endoscopic gastrostomy
PEP	phosphoenolpyruvate
PET	position-emission tomography
PET	pancreatic endocrine tumours
PFK	phosphofructokinase
PGAS	polyglandular autoimmune syndrome

PGE_1	prostaglandin E_1
PGL	persistent generalized lymphadenopathy
PH	personal history (e.g. smoking, alcohol, drugs)
Ph	Philadelphia chromosome
Phaeo.	phaeochromocytoma
PHT	pulmonary hypertension
PI	protease inhibitor
PICA	posterior inferior cerebellar artery
PID	pelvic inflammatory disease
PION	posterior ischaemic optic neuropathy
PIP	proximal interphalangeal
PIP	phosphatidylinositol phosphate
PKA	protein kinase A
PKU	phenylketonuria
Plts	platelets
PM	polymyositis
PMF	progressive massive fibrosis
PMH	past medical history
PML	progressive multifocal leucoencephalopathy
PML	promyelocytic leukaemia
PMP22	peripheral myelin protein 22 gene
PMR	polymyalgia rheumatica
PNET	primitive neuroectodermal tumour
PNH	paroxysmal nocturnal haemoglobinuria
PNS	peripheral nervous system
PO	*per os* (by mouth)
pO_2	partial pressure of oxygen
PO_4^{3-}	phosphate
POEMS	polyneuropathy, organomegaly, endocrinopathy, monoclonal gammopathy and skin changes
POTS	postural orthostatic tachycardia syndrome
PP	pancreatic polypeptide
PPD	purified protein derivative
PPI	proton-pump inhibitor
PPi	free (inorganic) pyrophosphate
PPM	permanent pacemaker
PPr	peroxisome proliferator-activated (receptor)
PR	*per rectum* (by/from rectum) and pulmonary regurgitation
PRL	prolactin
Prox.	prophylaxis
PrP	prion protein
PRPP	phosphoribosyl pyrophosphate
PRV	polycythaemia rubra vera
PS	pulmonary stenosis
PSC	primary sclerosing cholangitis
PSM	pansystolic murmur
PSM	progressive supranuclear palsy
pt	patient
PT	prothrombin time
PTH	parathyroid hormone

PTH-rp	parathyroid hormone-related peptide		SARS	severe acute respiratory syndrome
PTT	partial thromboplastin time		SBE	subacute bacterial endocarditis
PTU	propylthiouracil		SBP	systolic blood pressure
PU	peptic ulcer		SC/sc	subcutaneous
PUJ	pelvic-ureteric junction		SCA	spinocerebellar ataxia
PUO	pyrexia of unknown origin		SCID	severe combined immunodeficiency
PV	*per vaginam* (by/from vagina)		SE	side effects
PVD	pulmonary venous dilatation		SEP	serum electrophoresis
PXE	pseudoxanthoma elasticum		SER	smooth endoplasmic reticulum
R	right		SERM	selective oestrogen receptor modulator
RBBB	right bundle branch block		SH	social history
RA	right atrium, rheumatoid arthritis		SHBG	sex hormone-binding globulin
RAAS	renin-angiotensin-aldosterone system		SI	sacro-iliac
RAD	right axis deviation		SIADH	syndrome of inappropriate antidiuretic
RARA	retinoic acid receptor ·			hormone secretion
RAST	radio-allergosorbent test		SK	streptokinase
RBC	red blood cells		SLA	(antibodies to) soluble liver antigen
RCA	right coronary artery		SLE	systemic lupus erythematosus
REM	rapid eye movement		SMA	spinal muscular atrophy
RF	radiofemoral		SNRI	serotonin and noradrenaline reuptake
RFLP	restriction fragment length polymorphism			inhibitor
Rh	rhesus		SO_2	sulphur dioxide
RhF	rheumatoid factor		SOB	shortness of breath
RHS	right hand side		SOBOE	shortness of breath on exercise
RIF	right iliac fossa		SOD	superoxide dismutase
RIPE	rifampicin, isoniazid, pyrazinamide and		SR	survival rate
	ethambutol		SRP	signal recognition particle
RNA	ribonucleic acid		SS-A	Sjögren's syndrome antibodies A
RNase	ribonuclease		SS-B	Sjögren's syndrome antibodies B
RNP	ribonucleoprotein		ssDNA	single-stranded DNA
RPGN	rapidly progressive glomerulonephritis		SSPE	subacute sclerosing panencephalitis
RPLND	retroperitoneal lymph-node dissection		SSRI	selective serotonin reuptake inhibitor
RPR	rapid plasma reagin		SST	short Synacthen test
RR	respiratory rate		STD	sexually transmitted disease
RS	Reed-Sternberg (cell)		STEMI	ST-elevation myocardial infarction
RSE	right sternal edge		SUFE	slipped upper femoral epiphysis
RSH	right-sided heart		SUNCT	short-lasting unilateral neuralgia with
RSV	respiratory syncytial virus			conjunctival injection and tearing
rT3	reverse triiodothyronine		SV	supraventricular
RTA	renal tubular acidosis		SVC	superior vena cava
RTI	respiratory tract infection		SVCO	superior vena cava obstruction
rtPA	recombinant tissue-type plasminogen		SVT	supraventricular tachycardia
	activator		SX	symptoms, signs
RUQ	right upper quadrant		syn.	syndrome
RV	right ventricle, residual volume		T4	thyroxine
RVEDP	right ventricular end-diastolic pressure		TAC	trigeminal-autonomic cephalgia
RVF	right ventricular failure		TAG	triacylglyceride
RVH	right ventricular hypertrophy		TAPVD	total anomalous pulmonary venous
RVOTO	right ventricular outflow tract obstruction			drainage
SAA	serum amyloid A		TB	tuberculosis
SAH	subarachnoid haemorrhage		TBB	transbronchial biopsy
SALT	speech and language therapy		TBG	thyroxine-binding globulin
SAM	systolic anterior motion		Tc	technetium-99m
SAN	sino-atrial node		TCA	tricyclic antidepressant
SAP	radiolabelled serum amyloid P scintigram		TCR	T-cell receptor
	(^{99}Tc)		TdT	terminal deoxynucleotidyltransferase

TED	transverse elastic graduated		UC	ulcerative colitis
temp	temporary		UDP	uridine diphosphate
TENS	transcutaneous electrical nerve stimulation		UIP	usual interstitial pneumonitis
			ULN	upper limit of normal
TERT	telomerase reverse transcriptase		UMN	upper motor neurone
TFTs	thyroid function tests		UO	urine output
TG	thyroglobulin		URT	upper respiratory tract
TG	triglycerides		URTI	upper respiratory tract infection
TGA	transposition of the great arteries		USS	ultrasound scan
TGF	transforming growth factor		UTI	urinary tract infection
T_H	helper T (cell)		UVA	ultraviolet A
THF	tetrahydrofolate		V/Q	ventilation/perfusion
TIA	transient ischaemic attack		VAD	vincristine, doxorubicin and dexamethasone
TIBC	total iron-binding capacity			
TIN	tubulo-intestinal nephritis		Val	valine
TIPSS	transjugular intrahepatic porto-systemic shunt		VDRL	Venereal Diseases Research Laboratory (syphilis serological test)
TLC	total lung capacity		VE	ventricular extrasystole
TLCO	total lung diffusion coefficient		VF	ventricular fibrillation
TMJ	temporomandibular joint		VG	voltage-gated
TNF	tumour necrosis factor		VHL	von Hippel-Lindau (disease)
TnI	troponin I		ViM	ventral intermediate
TOE	transoesophageal echocardiography		VIP	vasoactive intestinal peptide
top	topical		Vit	vitamin
TORCH	toxoplasmosis, other (e.g. syphilis), rubella, cytomegalovirus, herpes (and hepatitis)		VLDL	very low-density lipoprotein
			VMA	vanillylmandelic acid (=HMMA)
			VMN	ventromedial nucleus (of thalamus)
tPA	tissue-type plasminogen activator		VPB	ventricular premature beat
TPHA	*Treponema pallidum* haemagglutination assay		VRE	vancomycin-resistant enterococci
			VSD	ventricular septal defect
TPI	*Treponema pallidum* immobilization		VT	ventricular tachycardia
TPN	total parenteral nutrition		VTEC	verocytotoxicogenetic *Escherichia coli*
TPR	temperature, pulse and respiration		VUJ	vesico-ureteric junction
TR	tricuspid regurgitation		VUR	vesico-ureteric reflux
TRH	thyrotrophin-releasing hormone		vWF	von Willebrand factor
tRNA	transfer RNA		VZV	varicella-zoster virus
TSH	thyroid-stimulating hormone		WBC	white blood cell
TSH-R	TSH receptor		WCC	white cell count
TT	tuberculoid leprosy		WG	Wegener's granulomatosis
TTP	thrombotic thrombocytopenic purpura		WPW	Wolff-Parkinson-White (syndrome)
TURP	transurethural resection of the prostate		X-match	cross-match blood type
TV	tricuspid valve		XL	X-linked
TVF	tactile vocal fremitus		xsome	chromosome
TWOC	trial without catheter		xteristics or	
TXA_2	thromboxane A_2		xters	characteristics
U&E/U+E	urea and electrolytes		Zn	zinc
UA	unstable angina		ZN	Ziehl-Neelsen (stain)

Index

A

abdominal examination 114
abdominal masses 115
abdominal pain 102–3
abscess
  amoebic 186
  Brodie's 256
  liver 186
  lung 83
absences 281
achondroplasia 252
acid–base balance 366–7
acidosis 366–7
acromegaly 332
actinomycoses 172
acute confusional state 264–5
acute coronary syndromes 24–5
acute leukaemia 442–5, 475
acute lymphoid leukaemia 443–5
acute myeloid leukaemia 443–5
acute pancreatitis 136–7
acute promyelocytic leukaemia 476
acute renal failure 392–3
acute tubular necrosis 392–3
acute visual loss 298–9
acute weakness 284
Addison's disease 344–5
adenocarcinoma
  lung 93
  mucin-secreting 475–6
  ovarian 418–19
adenoviruses 176, 181
adrenal gland
  phaeochromocytoma 358
  steroid synthesis 349
adrenal insufficiency 344
adult polycystic kidney disease 394, 413
adult respiratory distress syndrome 91
agammaglobulinaemia 220, 465–6
  Bruton's 465–6
Albright hereditary osteodystrophy 376
aldosterone 348, 375
aldosterone impairment 407
alkalosis 366–7
allergic alveolitis 79
allergy, blood transfusion-related 480
alloantigen sensitization 481
Alport's disease 252
alveolitis, extrinsic allergic 79
Alzheimer's disease 269
amegakaryocytic thrombocytopenia 470
amenorrhoea 350–3
  causes 350

investigations 352
treatment 353
ε-aminocaproic acid 479
amoebae 169, 186
amoebic abscess 186
amoeboma 186
amyloidosis 460–1
amyotrophic lateral sclerosis 290–1
ANA (anti-nuclear Abs) 237, 239
anaemia 422–37, 470
  aplastic anaemia 423, 425, 470
  autoimmune acquired haemolytic anaemia 427
  Fanconi's anaemia 425
  haemolytic anaemia 422–3
  iron deficiency anaemia 422
  macrocytic anaemia 423–4
  megaloblastic anaemia 423–4, 436–7, 470
  microcytic anaemia 388, 422
  normocytic anaemia 423–4, 426, 470
  pernicious anaemia 436–7
  sickle cell anaemia 430–1
analgesia 223
anamnestic reaction, HLA-1 480
anaphylaxis 476
ANCA (anti-neutrophil cytoplasmic Abs) 237
aneurysmal cysts 256
angina 37
ankylosing spondylitis 230, 255
anterior horn diseases 290
antibiotics 174–6
  sites of action 175
anticoagulants 469
antifibrinolytics 479
antinuclear antibodies 237, 239
antiphospholipid syndrome 475
antiretroviral drugs (HAART) 199
aortic regurgitation 6, 9
aortic stenosis 6, 8
aplastic anaemia 423, 425, 470
aprotinin 477
APTT 479
APUDomas 358
arachnids 168
arrhythmias 9
arterial thrombosis 474–5
arteritis
  giant-cell 263
  polyarteritis 246–7
  Takayasu's arteritis 246–7
  see also vasculitides
arthrodesis 223
arthropathies, seronegative 228–35
arthroplasty 223

arthropods 168
asbestosis 78
Ascaris lumbricoides 214
ascites 150–1
asthma
  acute severe 72–3
  chronic 66–7
  drugs 69–71
  general management 68–9
ataxia–telangiectasia 467
atlanto–axial dislocation 225
atrial fibrillation 18–19
atrial septal defect 50
atrioventricular conduction defect 22–3
auto-antibodies 237–9, 243, 471
  pernicious anaemia 437
autoimmune acquired haemolytic anaemia 427
autoimmune diseases 236–46
  polyglandular autoimmune syndromes 363
  vasculitis 475

B

B-cell immunodeficiency syndromes 465–7
babesiosis 169
bacillary dysentery 185
Bacillus anthracis infection 172
Bacillus cereus infection 172
back pain 254–5
bacteria 172–3
  cell wall 175
  Gram-positive/negative 173, 174
bacterial gastroenteritis 184
bacterial infections 172–85
  Helicobacter pylori 172–85
Bacteroides spp. 173
balanitis 191
balantidiasis 187
Balantidium coli infection 187
basement membrane disease 399
Behçet's syndrome 475
Bell's palsy 305
β_2-agonists 70, 71
bile salts 131
bilharzia 217
biliary cirrhosis 158
bilirubin disorders 140–1
bismuth poisoning 257
blackouts 27
blood groups, haemolytic reaction 480–1
blood pressure, raised see hypertension

blood transfusion 480–1
bone cysts 256
bone marrow
    failure 424, 444
    hypoproduction 422–3
    megaloblastic anaemia 437
    transplantation 444
Borrelia burgdorferi infection 170, 208
botulism 295
bowel obstruction 103
bradycardia 22–3
Brodie's abscess 256
bronchiectasis 82
bronchitis, COAD 74–5
bronchospasm 70, 71
Brugia malayi infection 215
Bruton's agammaglobulinaemia
    465–6
Budd–Chiari syndrome 153
Buerger's disease 246
bulbospinal muscular atrophy 290

C

caliciviruses 181
Calymmatobacterium granulomatis
    infection 190–1
Campylobacter jejuni infection 180
candidiasis 169, 467
capsular fibrosis 223
carcinoid syndrome 360
carcinoid tumours 360–1
cardiac examination 4–5
cardiac failure 34–5, 37
    fluid overload 480
cardiac tamponade 3
cardiac thrombosis 474–5
cardiology 1–51
    mnemonics
        ALAS I'M TRAPPED 26
        ATRIAL SWITCH 18
        CARNAGE 2, 33
        DIVISIONS 23
        I AM HURTIN 42
        I'M QVICK 21
        PASSES 38–9
        PREDICTION 32
        SHOCKING 30
        THE CHOP + MEAT 35
    treatments 36–7
cardiomyopathy 46–7
Carney complex 362
carpal tunnel syndrome 250–1
cellulitis 475
cerebellar disease 276–7
cerebral vein thrombosis 475
cestodes 168, 216
chancroid 191
Charcot–Marie–Tooth disease 220
Chediak–Higachi syndrome 466, 470
chemotherapy 444
chest examination 54
chest pain 2–3

acute coronary syndromes 24–5
chest X-ray 62–3
chickenpox 176, 193
Child–Pugh score 148
Chlamydia pneumoniae infection 170,
    178
Chlamydia trachomatis infection 170,
    178, 189, 190
cholera 183
cholesterol 386–7
chondrosarcoma 257
Christmas disease 479
chronic autoimmune hepatitis 157
chronic granulomatous disease 466
chronic lymphocytic leukaemia 450–1
chronic mucocutaneous candidiasis
    467
chronic myeloid leukaemia 446–7
chronic obstructive airways disease
    (COAD) 74–5
chronic renal failure 394–7
Churg–Strauss syndrome 246–7
ciliate protozoa 187
cirrhosis, primary biliary 158
CJD 171
clinical chemistry 366–89
    mnemonics
        AIP PCT 389
        CARDIAC 367, 374–5
        DIVINITY 372
        DRIED 371
        I AM 376
        INVITE IS FREE 366
        KILLER TRIGGER 367
        OX CHOPS 387
        PEARLS 386
        PENSIONERS 382
        PINTS 369
        PV BONES 385
        SICK BONE 381
        STONES 378
        TUBULAR pH 372
        VIBRATIN 376
Clostridium botulinum infection 172,
    180–1
Clostridium difficile infection 185
Clostridium perfringens infection 172,
    180–1, 476
clotting times 479
clubbing 56
coagulation 468–9
coagulopathies 473–7
    disseminated intravascular
        coagulation 476–7
    hypercoagulopathy 474–5
    procoagulant release 476–7
coal worker's pneumoconiosis 78
cobalamin (vit. B12) 423, 434–5, 437
coeliac disease 134–5
cold sore 194
colitis
    amoebic 186

ulcerative 126–9, 475
collagen diseases 252–3
colorectal carcinoma 130–1
coma 266–7
    myxoedematous 337
common variable immunodeficiency
    466
compartment syndrome 478
complement disorders 466
congenital heart disease
    cyanotic 48–9
    non-cyanotic 50–1
congestive cardiac failure, fluid
    overload 480
connective tissue diseases 252–3
constipation 105
cord compression 288
coronary syndromes, acute 24–5
cortical Lewy body disease 269
corticosteroids
    deficiency 374
    excess 348, 375
Corynebacterium diphtheriae
    infection 172
Coxiella burnetti (Q-fever) 170, 178,
    210
Creutzfeldt–Jakob disease 171
Crohn's disease 126–9
cryoglobulinaemia 249
cryptogenic fibrosing alveolitis 77
Cryptosporidium infection 169, 186
crystal deposition
    gout 234–5
    osteoarthritis 223
Cushing's syndrome 346–7
cutaneous larva migrans 215
cyanosis 57
cyanotic congenital heart disease
    48–9
cystic fibrosis 84–5
cytomegalovirus (CMV) infection 176

D

dactylitis 256
DDAVP (desmopressin) 479
deafness 303
dementia 268–9
dermatomyositis 244–5
dermatophytes 169
desmopressin 479
diabetes insipidus 372–3, 407
diabetes mellitus 310–23
    chronic complications 316–17
    conservative treatment 320
    diagnosis/monitoring 318–19
    hyperosmolar non-ketotic 314
    lactic acidosis 315
    oral hypoglycaemics 323
    treatment of complications 321
    types 1 & 2 310
diabetic ketoacidosis 312–14
Diamond–Blackfan syndrome 425

diarrhoea 104
  giardiasis 187
  travellers' 184
DiGeorge syndrome 467
dilated cardiomyopathy 46–7
Diphyllobothrium latum 216
disc prolapse 255
disseminated intravascular
    coagulation 476–7
dizziness 279
DMARDs (disease-modifying anti-
    rheumatoid drugs) 227
DNA viruses 171, 176–7
donovanosis 190–1
dorsal root ganglionopathy 293
Dracunculus medinensis 215
ductus arteriosus, patent 51
dysentery 185
dyskeratosis congenita 425
dysphagia 110–11
dystonia 273

E

ecchondroma 257
Echinococcus granulosus 216
eczema herpeticum 194
Ehlers–Danlos syndrome 252
Eisenmenger's syndrome 49, 98
elastic tissue diseases 252–3
elastin defects 253
electrocardiogram (ECG),
    interpretation 12–17
elephantiasis 215
emphysema 75
encephalitis 194
enchondroma 256, 257
endocrinology 310–63
  mnemonics
    ADDISONS'S 344
    CANNONICAL 316
    CAPITALS 358
    DELAYS 320
    DIVINE 356–7
    DIVINITY 326
    FASTING 325
    FIVE HT AMINE 360
    GAIN OF FUNCTION 338, 342
    GAMES 356
    GIANT CONK 333
    GIVES GAS 359
    GLARGINE 322
    GLUCOSE AMINO ACIDS 346
    HATRED 334, 342
    HONK 314
    IATROGENIC 324
    PAPA'S FAMILY 343
    PATENTS 354
    PECTORALIS 354
    PEPSI & COKE 310
    PGAS TOAD 363
    Sex GUITAR 327–9
    SHAPE 351

    SHOWING OFF 335, 339
    STRICT 340
    TAINT 357
    WASHED OUT 345
endothelial injury 474–7
endotoxinaemia 475
Entamoeba histolytica infection 169,
    186
enteric fever 182
Enterobius vermicularis 214
eosinophilia 440
epidermolysis bullosa 252
epilepsia partialis continua 274
epilepsy 280–1
epistaxis 112
Epstein–Barr virus (EBV) 195
erythema infectiosum (fifth disease)
    176, 193
erythema multiforme 194
erythropoietin, excess 448
Escherichia coli infection 184
Ewing's sarcoma 257
extrinsic allergic alveolitis 79

F

facial examination 4, 54, 114, 142
facial nerve palsy 304–5
factor IX deficiency 479
factor V Leiden mutation 475
factor VIII concentrate 479
factor VIII deficiency 478–9
factor XI deficiency 479
factor XIII deficiency 479
Fallot's tetralogy 48–9
Fanconi's anaemia 425
Fanconi's syndrome 406–7
Felty's syndrome 224
femoral nerve compression 478
fibrillin defects 253
fibrinolysis defects 475
fibrosing alveolitis 76–7
fibrosis, capsular 223
fifth disease 176, 193
filariasis 168, 215
finger clubbing 56
flagellate protozoa 169, 187
flatworms 168
fluid overload, congestive cardiac
    failure 480
flukes 217
fluorosis 257
folate
  deficiency 423–4, 437
  metabolism 434–5
  synthesis 175
food poisoning 180
foot ulcers, diabetes mellitus 317
frontotemporal dementia 268–9
fungal infections 169

G

G6PD deficiency 429

Gaisbock's syndrome 448
gait disturbance 287
galactosaemia 324
gallstones 164–5
gastric neoplasia 124–5
gastrinoma 359
gastroenteritis 181
  bacterial 184
  ileal-based 182–3
gastroenterology 101–65
  mnemonics
    AFFLICTS 164
    AN ABP 148
    BIG METS 162
    BIG SPAN 115
    BOSSES 105
    BULGIN 110
    BURNS 117
    CLANKING 161
    CRAGGY 132
    DINNERS 123
    DRIPPING TAPS 113
    GIN & TONICS 106
    GIT SCARS 120
    HIDDEN 130
    HOPING 121
    INTERNALS 108–9
    INVISIBLE 105
    IRRITANTS 116
    JAPANS SHAME 124
    MAIN 153
    MEALS 160
    MUCOSA 122
    OPEN IT WIDE 105
    PAT PINTS 150
    PHONE 115
    PINCHES 146
    POTENTIAL 102
    REALMS 143
    SCARED SLOUCHERS 127
    SNACKS 129
    SOILINGS 104
    TABOOS 152, 162
    VANISHING 103
    VERY SICK 181
    VINTAGE 112
genetic screening 479
genital discharge 188–9
genital ulceration 190–1
genu varum 223
germ-cell tumours 416, 418
giant-cell arteritis 263
giant-cell tumour 256
giardiasis 169, 187
gingivostomatitis 194
glandular fever 195
glaucoma 298
glomerulonephritis 404–5
glucagonoma 359
glucose tolerance test 318
glucose-6-phosphate deficiency 429
glycogen storage diseases 324

goitre 342
gonadal failure 355, 357
gonorrhoea 189
gout 234–5
graft-vs-host disease (GVHD) 481
granuloma inguinale 190–1
granulomatosis, Wegener's 246–7
granulomatous disease 466
Graves' ophthalmopathy 341
growth hormone 332–3
Guillain–Barré syndrome 285
guinea worm 168, 215
gynaecomastia 354

H

haem, synthesis 388
haemarthroses 478
haematemesis 112
haematology 421–81
  mnemonics
    ABCD 428
    ABCDEF 424
    ADVISE or HEPARINISE 474
    AGAMMAGLOB 466
    APLASTIC 423, 425
    ATELANG 467
    BIG GLANDS 438
    BIG SPAAN 439
    BLACKING OUT 430
    BLOBBIES 450, 452, 454
    CABOT'S 462
    CATCH22 467
    INFECTION 464
    INNATE 440
    MARMALADE 423
    MEGALOBLAST 436
    NOTICE 476
    ORGANISED 461
    POPULATION 456, 458
    PRV GO 449, 459
    SAVAGE 446
    SHARP 430
    SPLIT 429
    SPLITTING 427
    STABBINGS 470, 473
    STABS 438
    STAINS 478
    TRIGGER 442
    VANQUISHED 470
    VIGILANT 472–3
haematuria 398, 399
haemochromatosis 160
haemoglobinopathies 426
haemolytic anaemia 422–3
  causes 426–7
    acquired 427
    hereditary 426
  clinical 428–9
  thalassaemia 422, 432–3
haemolytic reactions 480–1
  post blood transfusion 480–1
haemolytic–uraemic syndrome 184

haemophilias 478–9
Haemophilus ducreyi infection 190–1
haemorrhage 478–9
  rectal bleeding 113
haemorrhagic colitis 184
haemorrhagic stroke 282
haemostasis 468–9, 476–7
hands
  examination 4, 54, 114, 142, 225
  wasting 286
headache, acute and chronic 260–3
heart
  cardiac examination 4–5
  cardiomyopathy 46–7
heart block 22
heart failure 34–5, 37
  fluid overload 480
Helicobacter pylori infection 120–2
Henoch–Schönlein disease 246–7
hepatitis
  chronic autoimmune 157
  infective 156–7
hepatomegaly 115
hereditary spherocytosis 429
herpesviruses 176
  herpes gladiatorum 194
  herpes labialis 194
  herpes simplex virus-2 191
  herpetic whitlow 194
hexose-monophosphate shunt 426
HIV infection 196–9
  clinical 198–9
  pathogenesis 196
HLA-1, anamnestic reaction 480
Hodgkin's lymphoma 452–3
homocystinuria 475
hormone replacement,
    hypopituitarism 329
hydrocephalus, obstructive 299
Hymenolepis nana 216
hyperaldosteronism 348, 375
hypercalcaemia 378–9
hypercholesterolaemia 386–7
hypercoagulopathy 474–5
hypergammaglobulinaemia 466
hyperkalaemia 374
hyperlipidaemia 386–7
hypermineralocorticoidism 348, 375
hypernatraemia 371
hyperosmolar non-ketotic diabetes
    mellitus 314
hyperparathyroidism
  primary 256, 378
  secondary 257
hyperprolactinaemia 330–1
hypertension 32–3, 36
  portal 146–7
  pulmonary 98–9
hyperthyroidism
  causes 338
  complications 341
  treatment 340

hypertriglyceridaemia 386–7
hypertrophic cardiomyopathy 46
hyperviscosity 459
hypoaldosteronism 348, 375
hypocalcaemia 376–7
hypoglycaemia 324–5
hypoglycaemics, oral 323
hypokalaemia 375
hyponatraemia 368–9
hypoparathyroidism, primary 376
hypoparathyroidism-associated
    immunodeficiency 467
hypopituitarism 326–9
  causes 326
  treatment 329
hypothalamic–pituitary failure 326–9,
    357
hypothyroidism 334–7
  causes 334
  complications 337
  treatment 336

I

idiopathic thrombocytopenic purpura
    470–1
IgA deficiency 466
IgA nephropathy 399
immune reaction, post blood
    transfusion 480
immunocompromised patients,
    pneumonia 179
immunodeficiency
  common variable 466
  general 464–5
  primary 466–7
  severe combined 467
immunosuppression, GVHD 481
impotence 354
inclusion bodies 463
inclusion body myositis 245
infant polycystic kidney disease 413
infectious diseases 167–217
  mnemonics
    ANGRY 199
    BLAND 172
    BOLT 170
    CHAINFREE 171, 177
    CIRCULAR 179
    CLOUDY AGAIN 206
    CRAPPERS 189
    FALCIPARUMS 212
    FRICTION 211
    GO SALMONELLA 182
    GO SOON 194
    GOA 189
    GOES SLOWLY 195
    GUCCIS VAGINA 188
    MAI needs CARE 204
    MEASLES MUMPS RUBELLA
        192
    MOURNS 209

OPERA 171
PITHY 184
PSEUDO 173
QUARTILES 170
RANSACKS 201
RIPPERS 203
SCARED SLOUCHERS 127
SHAGGIN SCARS 190
SHIGA 185
SNACK 208
SNAKE 214
SORE FACE 193
SPY SEEKS GBH PVC and L 173
TAX SLUM 170, 204
infective endocarditis 40–1
infective hepatitis 156–7
inflammatory bowel disease 126–9
insects 168
insulin 311, 322, 324
intestinal obstruction 103
iron deficiency anaemia 422
iron overload, blood transfusion 481
ischaemic ulcer 317

J

jaundice 140–1
Job syndrome 466
joint effusion 223
JVP 5

K

Kasabach–Merritt syndrome 476
Kawasaki's disease 246
Kennedy's disease 290
keratoconjunctivitis 194, 224
kidney disease
  adult polycystic 394, 413
  glomerulonephritis 404–5
  IgA nephropathy 399
  infant polycystic 413
  nephritic syndrome 404–5
  nephrosis 475
  nephrotic syndrome 401, 404–5
  tubulointerstitial nephritis 370, 392
  see also renal
Klebsiella infection 178
Klinefelter's syndrome 357
Kostmann syndrome 466

L

lactic acidosis 315
large cell carcinoma 93
lateral sclerosis 290–1
lead poisoning 257
Legionella pneumophila infection 178
leishmaniasis 169
leprosy 205
Leptospira interrogans infection 170, 209
leucagglutinin reaction 480
leucocyte adhesion deficiency 466

leucocytosis 440–1
leukaemia 442–51
  acute leukaemia 442–5, 475
  acute lymphoid leukaemia 443–5
  acute myeloid leukaemia 443–5
  acute promyelocytic leukaemia 476
  chronic lymphocytic leukaemia 450–1
  chronic myeloid leukaemia 446–7
leukoplakia 191
leukotriene receptor antagonists 70, 71
Lewy body disease 269
lice, pubic 191
lichen sclerosus et atrophicus 190–1
Listeria monocytogenes infection 172
liver (amoebic) abscess 186
liver failure 142–4
  acute 152–3
  chronic 154–5
liver flukes 217
liver transplant 145
liver tumours 162
Loa loa 215
lower motor neurone lesions 304
lower motor neurone syndrome 290
lumbar spinal stenosis 255
lung abscess 83
lung carcinoma 92–3
lung flukes 217
lupus erythematosus 238–9
Luschka, neurocentral joints 225
lymphadenopathy 438
  lymphoma 452–5
  paraproteinaemia 458
lymphocytosis 441
lymphogranuloma venereum 191
lymphoma 452–5
  testicular 417
lymphoproliferative disorders 439
lyonization, X chromosome 478

M

McCune–Albright syndrome 356
macrocytic anaemia 423–4
macroglobulinaemia, Waldenström's 439, 470
macular degeneration 298
malabsorption 132–3
malaria 212–13
Malassezia furfur infection 169
male infertility 355
male sexual problems 354
Marfan syndrome 253
mast-cell stabilizers 70, 71
measles 192
megakaryocytic failure 470
megaloblastic anaemia 423–4, 436–7, 470
meningitis 194
meningococcaemia 476
metabolic acidosis 366–7

metabolic alkalosis 366–7
metastases
  from bone 256
  to bone 257
metatarsal heads, volar subluxation 225
methylxanthines 70, 71
microcytic anaemia 388, 422
Microsporidium infection 186
middle ear infection 305
migraine 260–3
migratory thrombophlebitis 475
Mikulicz's syndrome 243, 450
mitral regurgitation 7, 11
mitral stenosis 6, 10, 98
monoclonal gammopathy of uncertain significance 458
monocytosis 441
mononeuropathy multiplex 293
motor neurone disease 291
  lower motor neurone syndrome 290
mucocutaneous candidiasis 467
multiple endocrine neoplasia 362
multiple myeloma 456–7
mumps 192
murmurs 6–7
muscarinic antagonists 70, 71
myasthenia gravis 294–5
mycobacteria 170, 202–4
Mycoplasma spp. 170, 178
myeloma 257
myelopathy 288–9
myeloperoxidase deficiency 466
myeloproliferative disorders 439, 470, 475
myocardial infarction 26–31
myocarditis 44
myoclonus 274
myopathy 296–7
myositis 244–5
myxoedematous coma 337
myxoma 45

N

Naegleria fowleri infection 169
nausea and vomiting 106–7
Necator americanus 214
Neisseria gonorrhoeae infection 189
nematodes 168, 214–15
nephritic syndrome 404–5
nephrosis 475
nephrotic syndrome 401, 404–5
neurocentral joints of Luschka 225
neurocutaneous diseases 307
neuroendocrine tumours 358–62
neurofibromatosis 306
neurogenic claudication 255
neurology 260–307
  mnemonics
    A SKINNY MAN 290
    ABSENCE 281

ACTION 294
ADVISE OR HEPARINIZE 282
APPLES 291
ATAXIC 293
BEATINGS 275
CAFE NOIR 306
CHOREA 272
CRASH 278–9
DANISH PASTRY 277
DIVINITY 268, 270, 276, 280,
   288–9, 301, 303
FAMILIAL 268
GBS = AIDP 285
HAEMATOMA 283
HEATING 293
HITTING ME 272–3
IMBALANCE 302
INVITE PASS IS FREE 264–6
IT'S THIN 292
LARGE 293
MATCHING SITES 262
OPTIC 299, 300
PAIN ENDINGS HURT 292
RAPID TAPS 274
STAND UP 278
THINNER 296
TRAPPED 271
VICIOUS 260
VISION 299, 301
WIDENING 303
neuromuscular junction disease
   294–5
neuropathic ulcer 317
neuropathies 286
   mononeuropathy multiplex 293
   peripheral 292–3
   small-fibre 293
neutropenia, leucagglutinin reaction
   480
neutrophilia 440
Nocardia infection 172
non-germ-cell tumours 417
non-Hodgkin's lymphoma 454–5
non-steroidal anti-inflammatory drugs
   227, 235
normocytic anaemia 423–4, 426, 470
NSTEMI 25
   management 28

O

obstruction
   intestinal 103
   ureteric 392–3
   urinary 408
obstructive hydrocephalus 299
obstructive sleep apnoea 94–5
occupational lung diseases 78–9
oesophageal carcinoma 118–19
oesophageal varices 148–9
oesophagitis 116
Ollier's syndrome 256
Onchocerca volvulus 215

ophthalmopathy, diabetic 317
opportunistic infection in AIDS 199
optic atrophy 300
oral glucose tolerance test 318
oral hypoglycaemics 323
oral ulceration 109
osteoarthritis 220–3
osteochondritis 221
osteochondroma 257
osteodystrophy, renal 257
osteogenesis imperfecta 220, 252
osteoma, osteoid 257
osteomalacia 380–1
osteomyelitis 221, 256
osteonecrosis 221
osteophytes 223
osteoporosis 223, 382–3
osteosarcoma 257
osteotomy, Keller's 223
ovarian failure 350, 353
ovarian tumours 418–19

P

Paget's disease 257, 384–5
pancreatic disease 132
   acute pancreatitis 136–7
   chronic pancreatitis 138–9
   endocrine tumours 163, 359
   exocrine tumours 163, 475
papillitis 300–1
papilloedema 301–2
papovaviruses 176
paraproteinaemia
   amyloidosis 460
   malignant and benign 456, 458,
      475
parathyroid hormone 378–9
paratyphoid fever 182
parkinsonism 270–1
paroxysmal nocturnal
   haemoglobinuria 425, 427,
   475
parvovirus infection 174, 176, 193
patent ductus arteriosus 51
pathological processes, Virchow's
   triad 474
peptic ulcers 120–3
pericardial disease 42–3
peripheral neuropathy 292–3
peritonitis 103
pernicious anaemia 436–7
Perthes' disease 221
phaeochromocytoma 358
phlegmasia alba dolens 475
phosphate, deficiency 376, 381
phosphorus poisoning 257
Phthirus pubis 191
Pick bodies 269
pinta 207
pituitary apoplexy 299
pituitary causes of amenorrhoea 353

placental disruption 476–7
Plasmodium falciparum infection 186,
   212–13
platelet disorders 470–3
   disseminated intravascular
      coagulation 476–7
pleural effusion 88–9
Plummer–Vinson syndrome 118
pneumoconioses 78
pneumonia 64–5
   community-acquired 178
   immunocompromised 179
   nosocomial 179
pneumothorax 86–7
POEMS syndrome 257
poisoning, lead, radium, bismuth,
   phosphorus 257
polyarteritis 246–7
polycystic kidney disease 394, 413
polycythaemia 448, 475
polycythaemia rubra vera 449
polydipsia 370
polyglandular autoimmune
   syndromes 363
polymyositis 245
polyuria 370
porphyria 388–9
portal hypertension 146–7
portal vein thrombosis 475
postural hypotension 278
poxviruses 176
precordium
   auscultation 5
   palpation 5
primary biliary cirrhosis 158
prions 171
progressive bulbar palsy 291
prolactin, hyperprolactinaemia 330–1
prolactinoma 353
proteins C and S 474–5
proteinuria 400
prothrombin, mutation 475
proton pump inhibitors 122
protozoans 169, 186–7
pruritus vulvae 191
pseudohermaphroditism 350
pseudohypoparathyroidism 376
pseudomembranous colitis 185
Pseudomonas aeruginosa infection
   173, 174
pseudotuberculosis 185
pseudotumours 478
pseudoxanthoma elasticum 253
psoriatic arthropathy 231
puberty
   delayed 357
   precocious 356
pubic lice 191
pulmonary embolism 96–7
pulmonary hypertension 98–9
pulmonary leucagglutinin reaction
   480

pulmonary oedema 90–1
pulse 5
purpura 472–3
    fulminans 476
    idiopathic thrombocytopenic (ITP)
        470–1
    immune thrombocytopenic (ITP)
        473
    post blood transfusion 481
pyruvate kinase deficiency 429

Q

Q-fever 170, 178, 210

R

radiculopathy 255
radium poisoning 257
Raynaud's phenomenon 248
rectal bleeding 113
Reed–Sternberg cells 452
Reiter's syndrome 231
relapsing fever 208
renal, *see also* kidney disease
renal artery stenosis 402–3
renal artery thrombosis 403
renal cell carcinoma 414–15
renal cysts 412
renal enlargement 115, 412
renal failure 392–3
renal medicine 392–419
    mnemonics
        ADVISE or HEPARINISE 403,
            474
        BANG UP 406
        CRUSHING 410
        FANCONI 406
        GROSS 399
        KIDDNNEYS 397
        MISHAPEN 413
        NEPHROTIC 401
        PAINT TIN ATN 392, 398
        PAINTS 394, 398, 400, 404–5
        PHONE 115, 412
        REALMS 396
        SCARRING TUBES 395
        SHOCK 392
        SMEAR 419
        SNIPPING 392, 398, 400, 408–9
        STENTABLE 392, 394, 398, 400,
            402
        TUBULAR pH 394, 400, 407
        VICTORY 414
    tubulointerstitial disease 370
renal osteodystrophy 257
renal stones 410–11
renal tubular disease 406–7
renal vein thrombosis 403
renovascular disease 392–4, 402–3
respiratory acidosis 366–7
respiratory alkalosis 366–7
respiratory medicine 53–99

examination 54
mnemonics
    ACUTE 137
    AGITATES ME 136
    anti-GLIADINS 134
    ASTHMA 66
    BLOBS 92
    BOMBERS 93
    CABBIE 60
    CHEST INSULATION 88
    COILED 90
    FINE, FANGS 62
    GRANULOMAS 80
    HARMFUL 64
    INTRAHEPATIC 140
    PANCREAS 137
    PENTAHOUSE 76
    RAMP 72
    REALMS 135
    SINS 163
    STINK 83
    STRIP 86
    TIGHT 91
    TOXIC 91
respiratory failure 58–9
respiratory function tests 60–1
restrictive cardiomyopathy 47
reticular cell sarcoma 257
retinal detachment 298
rheumatic fever 38–9
rheumatoid arthritis 224–7, 255
rheumatoid factor 237
rheumatology 220–57
    mnemonics
        ANNOYIN SCARS 224
        ATTACK 235
        BONE1M 255–6
        CRACKING 240, 244
        CREST 240
        ELASTIC 253
        FINALITY 221
        GOA 231
        GOUTY 234
        ITS ACHIN MEE 220
        LOAF SIDS 251
        MADDENING PAIN 254
        OWTCHA 221
        PAINT 246
        PENNIES 256–7
        POMEGRANATE 250–1
        RAPERS 228
        SAFE 256
        SAMPLING 227
        SAUNA PAIN 249
        SCARED SLOUCHERS 229–30
        SOS ANA SOS ANA 238
        SURROUNDINGS 242, 247
        WILLIAM 253
rickets 380–1
Rickettsiae 170
river blindness 215
RNA viruses 171, 176–7

rotaviruses 177, 181
roundworms 168, 214–15
rubella 192

S

Salmonella infection 180, 182
sarcoidosis 80–1, 475
Sarcoptes scabiei (scabies) 191
Schilling test 437
schistosomiasis 217
Schmidt's syndrome 363
scleroderma 240–1
sclerosis 257
scurvy, vitamin C deficiency 470
seizures 280–1
seminoma 416
septic arthritis 232–3
seronegative arthropathies 228–35
severe combined immunodeficiency
    467
sex-cord stromal tumours 417, 418
Shigella infections 181, 185
shock 30–1
SIADH 368–9
sickle cell anaemia 430–1
silicosis 78
sinus (junctional) rhythm 22–3
Sjögren's syndrome 242–3
slapped cheek syndrome 176, 193
small cell carcinoma 93
small-fibre neuropathy 293
sore throat 108–9
spherocytosis, hereditary 429
spinal cord
    cord compression 288
    intrinsic cord disease 289
    myelopathy 288–9
spinal muscular atrophy 290
spinal stenosis 255
spirochaetes 170
spirometry 60
spleen
    hypersplenism 470
    hyposplenism 462–3
    splenomegaly 115, 439
spondylosis 255
sporozoan prototozoa 169, 186
squamous cell carcinoma 93, 118
staphylococcal infection (*S. aureus*)
    172, 174, 180
stasis 475
STEMI 25
    management 29
steroids 70, 71
    osteoarthritis 223
    synthesis 349
streptococcal infection 172, 174, 178
stroke
    haemorrhagic 282
    ischaemic 282
Strongyloides stercoralis 214
Sturge–Weber syndrome 307

subchondral cysts 223
subchondral sclerosis 223
synovitis 223
syphilis 190, 206
syringomyelia 220
systemic lupus erythematosus 238–9
systemic sclerosis 240–1

T

T-cell defects, primary 467
T-cell immunodeficiency syndromes 465–7
tachycardia 16–17
  ventricular 20–1
Taenia solium 216
Takayasu's arteritis 246–7
tapeworms 168, 216
temporal arteritis 263
teratoma 416, 418
testicular failure 355, 357
testicular tumours 356, 416–17
thalassaemia 422, 432–3
thin basement membrane disease 399
Thomas' test 222
threadworms 214
thrombocythaemia 463
thrombocytopenia 470–1, 477
thrombophlebitis, migratory 475
thrombosis 474–5
  arterial 474–5
  cardiac 474–5
  cerebral vein 475
  portal vein 475
  renal artery 403
  venous 474–5
thyroid tumours 343
thyrotoxicosis, neonatal 341
thyroxine 336
tinea cruris 191
Toxocara canis 215
Toxoplasma gondii infection 169
tranexamic acid 479
trematodes 168, 217
tremor 274–5
Treponema pallidum infection (syphilis) 190, 206
treponemes, non-venereal 207

Trichinella spiralis 215
Trichomonas vaginalis infection 169
Trichophyton infection 169, 191
Trichuria trichuris 214
trigeminal–autonomic cephalgias 262–3
Trousseau's phenomenon 475
Trypanosoma spp. 169
tuberculosis 200–3
tuberous sclerosis 307
tubulointerstitial nephritis 370, 392
Turner's syndrome 357
typhoid fever 182
typhus 210, 211

U

ulcerative colitis 126–9, 475
ulcers
  diabetes mellitus 317
  genital 190–1
  ischaemic 317
  neuropathic 317
  oral 109
  peptic 120–3
urea dissolution test 479
Ureaplasma spp. 170
ureteric obstruction 392–3
urethral discharge 188–91
urinary obstruction 408
urinary retention 392–3, 409

V

vaccinia virus infection 176
vaginal discharge 188–91
varicella (chickenpox) 176, 193
varices 147–9
vascular defects, causing purpura 472–3
vascular dementia 268–9
vasculitides 236, 246–7, 472–3
  autoimmune 475
  see also arteritis
venous thrombosis 474–5
ventricular septal defect 51
ventricular tachycardia 20–1
vertigo 302
Vibrio cholerae infection 183
Vibrio parahaemolyticus infection 180

Vincent's angina 208
VIPomas 359
Virchow's triad (pathological processes) 474
viruses
  DNA and RNA 171, 176–7
  exanthema 192–3
visceral larva migrans 215
visual loss 298–9
vitamin B12
  deficiency 423, 437
  metabolism 434–5
vitamin C, deficiency 470
vitamin D
  deficiency 376, 381
  physiology 380
vitamin K, deficiency 473
vitreal haemorrhage 298
von Hippel–Lindau disease 307, 362
von Willebrand disease 470

W

Waldenström's macroglobulinaemia 439, 470
walking disturbance 287
water-deprivation test 373
weakness, acute 284
Wegener's granulomatosis 246–7
Werner–Morrison syndrome 359
Williams' syndrome 253, 378
Wilson's disease 161
Wiscott–Aldrich syndrome 467, 470
Wuchereria bancrofti 215

X

X chromosome, lyonization 478
xanthalesma 387

Y

yaws 207
yeasts 169
Yersinia enterocolitica infection 185

Z

Ziehl–Neelsen staining 186
Zollinger–Ellison syndrome 359